D0524586

# *M*ASTERING
# HEALTHCARE TERMINOLOGY

# Contents

# *M*ASTERING
# HEALTHCARE TERMINOLOGY

**4TH** EDITION

BETSY J. SHILAND

MS, RHIA, CCS, CPC, CPHQ, CTR
AHIMA Approved ICD-10-CM/PCS Trainer

Assistant Professor
Allied Health Department
Community College of Philadelphia
Philadelphia, Pennsylvania

ELSEVIER

*With 500 illustrations*

## ELSEVIER
MOSBY

3251 Riverport Lane
St. Louis, Missouri 63043

MASTERING HEALTHCARE TERMINOLOGY

ISBN: 978-0-3230-8032-3

**Copyright © 2013, 2010, 2006, 2003 by Mosby, Inc., an affiliate of Elsevier Inc.**

No part of this publication may be reproduced or transmitted in any form or by any means, electronic or mechanical, including photocopying, recording, or any information storage and retrieval system, without permission in writing from the publisher. Details on how to seek permission, further information about the Publisher's permissions policies and our arrangements with organizations such as the Copyright Clearance Center and the Copyright Licensing Agency, can be found at our website: www.elsevier.com/permissions.

This book and the individual contributions contained in it are protected under copyright by the Publisher (other than as may be noted herein).

---

### Notices

Knowledge and best practice in this field are constantly changing. As new research and experience broaden our understanding, changes in research methods, professional practices, or medical treatment may become necessary.

Practitioners and researchers must always rely on their own experience and knowledge in evaluating and using any information, methods, compounds, or experiments described herein. In using such information or methods they should be mindful of their own safety and the safety of others, including parties for whom they have a professional responsibility.

With respect to any drug or pharmaceutical products identified, readers are advised to check the most current information provided (i) on procedures featured or (ii) by the manufacturer of each product to be administered, to verify the recommended dose or formula, the method and duration of administration, and contraindications. It is the responsibility of practitioners, relying on their own experience and knowledge of their patients, to make diagnoses, to determine dosages and the best treatment for each individual patient, and to take all appropriate safety precautions.

To the fullest extent of the law, neither the Publisher nor the authors, contributors, or editors, assume any liability for any injury and/or damage to persons or property as a matter of products liability, negligence or otherwise, or from any use or operation of any methods, products, instructions, or ideas contained in the material herein.

---

**Library of Congress Cataloging-in-Publication Data**

Shiland, Betsy J.
    Mastering healthcare terminology / Betsy J. Shiland.—4th ed.
        p. ; cm.
    Includes bibliographical references and index.
    ISBN 978-0-323-08032-3 (pbk.)
    I. Title.
    [DNLM: 1. Terminology as Topic—Problems and Exercises. W 15]
    610.1'4—dc23
                                                    2011035524

*Publisher:* Jeanne Olsen
*Managing Editor:* Linda Woodard
*Publishing Services Manager:* Julie Eddy
*Senior Project Manager:* Celeste Clingan
*Designer:* Jessica Williams

Printed in the United States of America

Last digit is the print number:   9   8   7   6   5   4   3   2   1

Working together to grow
libraries in developing countries

www.elsevier.com | www.bookaid.org | www.sabre.org

ELSEVIER    BOOK AID International    Sabre Foundation

# Contributor

*Erinn Kao, Pharm.D, R.Ph.*
Pharmacist
GE Healthcare
St. Louis, Missouri

# Reviewers

*Randal Beard, MEd, RMA*
Instructor
Medical Careers Institute
Virginia Beach, Virginia

*Elaine H. Blankenship, MA, HS-BCP*
HST Clinical Coordinator
Darton College
Albany, Georgia

*Sandra Hertkorn, LVN*
Certified Coder Reimbursement Specialist
Instructor, Health Information Management
Bryan College, Sacramento
Sacramento, California

*Bridgette Hudson, RN, MSN, NREMT-P*
Assistant Professor
Tarrant County College
Hurst, Texas

*Cherlynda Livingston, BA, MDS Certified*
Director of Education
MedTech Institute
Tucker, Georgia

*Alice M. Noblin, PhD, RHIA, CCS, LHRM*
Health Informatics and Information Management
    Program Director and Instructor
University of Central Florida
Orlando, Florida

*Teresa M. Pirone, CNA, LMT*
Danbury, Connecticut

*Barbara A. Root, R.T. (R) (M) CMAA*
CMAA Instructor
ALG Computer Training Center
Solon, Ohio

*Paulette L. Washington, RHIT, MS*
Medical Transcriptionist
Nuance
Burlington, Massachusetts

*Barbareta A. Welch McGill, RN, BSN, MSN, DRS*
Assistant Professor/Interim Assistant Chair,
    Department of Nursing
North Carolina Central University
Durham, North Carolina

*Ruby Wertz, MSHA, BSN, RN*
Assistant Dean
Nevada State College
Henderson, Nevada

*Carole Stemple Zeglin, MSEd, BS MT, RMA*
Assistant Professor and Director, Medical Assisting
    and Phlebotomy Programs
Westmoreland County Community College
Youngwood, Pennsylvania

Beginning a healthcare career is like visiting a foreign country. If you want to converse with the inhabitants, you need to speak their language. If you are interested in a career in healthcare, fluency in its terminology is required. The goal of **Mastering Healthcare Terminology** is to help you learn the large number of terms that describe very specific healthcare conditions or procedures in the easiest, most effective manner possible.

We don't often think about what makes up our language, perhaps because we are so familiar with it. Prefixes, suffixes, and word roots make up both the English language and healthcare language. A student of terminology can develop a sizable vocabulary by learning these decodable word parts and the rules necessary to join them together. Memorizing eponyms, abbreviations, symbols, and nondecodable terms completes a healthcare professional's vocabulary.

## ORGANIZATION OF THE BOOK

**Mastering Healthcare Terminology** has been designed for your success. Each feature has been chosen to help you learn this new language quickly and effectively.

To get you started, Chapters 1 and 2 orient you to the basic concepts necessary to learn healthcare terminology. Chapter 1 is focused on word parts and basic building and decoding skills. Chapter 2 explains the organization of the body, as well as positional and directional terms. You will use the material in both of these chapters throughout the remainder of the text.

Chapters 3 through 15 are body system chapters, each organized in the same way. The function of each system is introduced first, followed by the anatomy and physiology. A summary table of common anatomy and physiology word parts for the system functions as an excellent study tool. Once the terms for normal function are covered, pathologic terms, diagnostic techniques, therapeutic interventions, pharmacologic terms, and common abbreviations are presented. Chapter 16 covers cancer terminology for all the body systems.

The internal structure of each chapter consists of small learning segments or "chunks." Concepts, terms, and abbreviations for a topic are covered and then immediately followed by exercises that reinforce and assess your understanding and retention of the material. Pathology and procedure terms are organized into tables that include phonetic pronunciations followed by the terms' component word parts and their meanings. Special boxes alert you to terminology pitfalls. Electronic healthcare records and engaging end-of-chapter exercises provide you the opportunity to practice the terminology you've learned.

## FEATURES

We've loaded **Mastering Healthcare Terminology** with special features to help you quickly and correctly learn the medical terminology you need to effectively communicate in the clinical setting.

- **Word parts next to their text mentions** in the anatomy and physiology section demonstrate the origins of terms.

Word parts and meanings next to their text mentions in the anatomy and physiology sections demonstrate the origin of terms.

| | |
|---|---|
| **small intestine** = enter/o | |
| **duodenum** = duoden/o | |
| **lumen** = lumin/o | |
| **jejunum** = jejun/o | |
| **ileum** = ile/o | |
| **fold, plica** = plic/o | |
| **villus** = vill/o | |
| **lipid, fat** = lipid/o, lip/o | |
| **large intestine, colon** = col/o, colon/o | |

**⊗ Be Careful!**

*The combining form* **gastr/o** *refers only to the stomach. The combining forms* **abdomin/o,** **lapar/o,** *and* **celi/o** *refer to the abdomen.*

**ileocecal**
    ile/o = ileum
    cec/o = cecum
    -al = pertaining to

**cecum** = cec/o

**appendix** = appendic/o, append/o

**feces** = fec/a

**sigmoid colon** = sigmoid/o

**rectum, straight** = rect/o

**anus** = an/o

**rectum and anus** = proct/o

**⊗ Be Careful!**

*Don't confuse the term* **ilium,** *meaning part of the hip bone, with* **ileum,** *meaning part of the small intestine.*

## Small Intestine

Once the chyme has been formed in the stomach, the pyloric sphincter relaxes a bit at a time to release portions of it into the first part of the **small intestine,** called the **duodenum** (doo AH deh num). The small intestine gets its name, not because of its length (it is about 20 feet long), but because of the diameter of its **lumen** (LOO mun) (a tubular cavity within the body). The second section of the small intestine is the **jejunum** (jeh JOO num) and the distal part of the small intestine is the **ileum** (ILL ee um).

Multiple circular folds in the small intestines, called **plicae** (PLY see), contain thousands of tiny projections called **villi** (VILL eye) (*sing.* villus), which contain blood capillaries that absorb the products of carbohydrate and protein digestion. The villi also contain lymphatic vessels, known as **lacteals** (LACK tee uls), that absorb **lipid** (LIH pid) substances from the chyme. A lipid is a fatty substance.

The suffix *-ase* is used to form the name of an enzyme. It is added to the name of the substance upon which the enzyme acts: for example, **lipase,** which acts on lipids, or amylase, which acts on starches. *-ose* is a chemical suffix indicating that a substance is a carbohydrate, such as *glucose.*

## Large Intestine

In contrast to the small intestine, the **large intestine** or **colon** (Fig. 5-4) is only about 5 feet long, but it is much wider in diameter. The primary function of the large intestine is the elimination of waste products from the body. Some synthesis of vitamins occurs in the large intestine, but unlike the small intestine, the large intestine has no villi and is not well suited for absorption of nutrients. The **ileocecal** (ILL ee oh SEE kul) valve is the exit from the small intestine and the entrance to the colon. The first part of the large intestine, the **cecum** (SEE kum), has a wormlike appendage, called the **vermiform appendix** (VUR mih form ah PEN dicks) (*pl.* appendices), dangling from it. Although this organ does not seem to have any direct function related to the digestive system, it is thought to have a possible immunologic defense mechanism.

No longer called chyme, whatever has not been absorbed by the small intestines is now called **feces** (FEE sees). The feces pass from the cecum to the **ascending colon** (KOH lin), through the **transverse colon,** the **descending colon,** the **sigmoid colon** (the S-shaped part of the large intestine), and on to the **rectum** (the last straight part of the colon), where they are held until released from the body completely through the **anus** (the final sphincter in the GI tract.) The process of releasing feces from the body is called **defecation,** or a bowel movement (BM).

**⊗ Be Careful!**

*Do not confuse* **-cele,** *the suffix meaning herniation, with* **celi/o,** *a combining form for abdomen.*

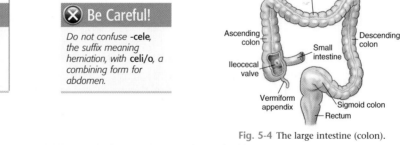

Fig. 5-4 The large intestine (colon).

**⊗ Be Careful!**

*Do not confuse* **an/o,** *the combining form for anus;* **ana-,** *the prefix meaning up or apart; and* **an-,** *the prefix meaning no, not, or without.*

**Be Careful! Boxes remind students of potentially confusing look-alike or sound-alike word parts and terms.**

170      Chapter 5

## Exercise 4: Stomach and Intestines

*Label the drawing with correct anatomic terms and combining forms where appropriate.*

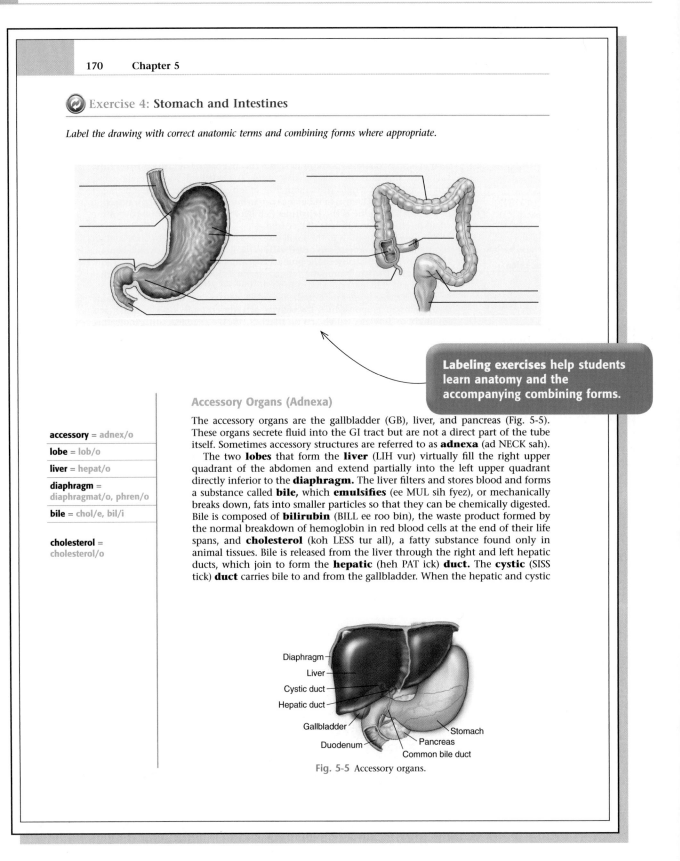

> **Labeling exercises help students learn anatomy and the accompanying combining forms.**

### Accessory Organs (Adnexa)

The accessory organs are the gallbladder (GB), liver, and pancreas (Fig. 5-5). These organs secrete fluid into the GI tract but are not a direct part of the tube itself. Sometimes accessory structures are referred to as **adnexa** (ad NECK sah).

The two **lobes** that form the **liver** (LIH vur) virtually fill the right upper quadrant of the abdomen and extend partially into the left upper quadrant directly inferior to the **diaphragm.** The liver filters and stores blood and forms a substance called **bile,** which **emulsifies** (ee MUL sih fyez), or mechanically breaks down, fats into smaller particles so that they can be chemically digested. Bile is composed of **bilirubin** (BILL ee roo bin), the waste product formed by the normal breakdown of hemoglobin in red blood cells at the end of their life spans, and **cholesterol** (koh LESS tur all), a fatty substance found only in animal tissues. Bile is released from the liver through the right and left hepatic ducts, which join to form the **hepatic** (heh PAT ick) **duct.** The **cystic** (SISS tick) **duct** carries bile to and from the gallbladder. When the hepatic and cystic

**accessory** = adnex/o

**lobe** = lob/o

**liver** = hepat/o

**diaphragm** = diaphragmat/o, phren/o

**bile** = chol/e, bil/i

**cholesterol** = cholesterol/o

Diaphragm
Liver
Cystic duct
Hepatic duct
Gallbladder
Duodenum
Stomach
Pancreas
Common bile duct

**Fig. 5-5** Accessory organs.

> Age Matters boxes highlight important concepts and terminology for both pediatric and geriatric patients.

## Age Matters

### Pediatrics

GI congential disorders are cleft palate, esophageal atresia, Hirschsprung disease, and pyloric stenosis. Although none of these are common, they do require medical intervention. Gastroenteritis and appendicitis—with their possible complications, respectively, of dehydration and peritonitis—are the most common reasons for hospital admissions of children.

### Geriatrics

An aging digestive system is more likely to develop new dysfunctional cell growths (both benign and malignant), so statistics for polyps and colorectal cancer are high for the senior age group. Other diagnoses that appear more often are GERD and dysphagia, hemorrhoids, and type 2 diabetes mellitus.

To practice spelling the pathology terms that you have learned in this chapter. click on **Hear It, Spell It.** To see how well you pronounce the pathology terms in this chapter, click on **Hear It, Say It.** To review the pathology terms in this chapter, play **Medical Millionaire.**

## DIAGNOSTIC PROCEDURES

### Terms Related to Imaging

Visualizing the internal workings of the digestive system can be achieved through a wide variety of techniques but is usually accomplished through either radiographic imaging or endoscopy, or a combination of the two. Most of the procedures below are a form of radiography, or "taking x-rays." However, because the tissues of the digestive system are soft (as opposed to bone), a radiopaque contrast medium may be necessary to outline the digestive tract. This substance may be introduced into the body through the oral or anal opening, or it may be injected. Fluoroscopy provides instant visual access to deep tissue structures.

| Term | Word Origin | Definition |
|---|---|---|
| **barium enema (BE)**<br>BAIR ee um<br>EN nuh mah | | Introduction of a barium sulfate suspension through the rectum for imaging of the lower digestive tract to detect obstructions, tumors, and other abnormalities. |
| **barium swallow (BaS)** | | Radiographic imaging done after oral ingestion of a barium sulfate suspension; used to detect abnormalities of the esophagus and stomach (Fig. 5-21). |

*Continued*

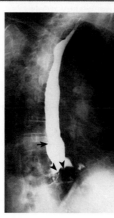

Fig. 5-21 Barium swallow.

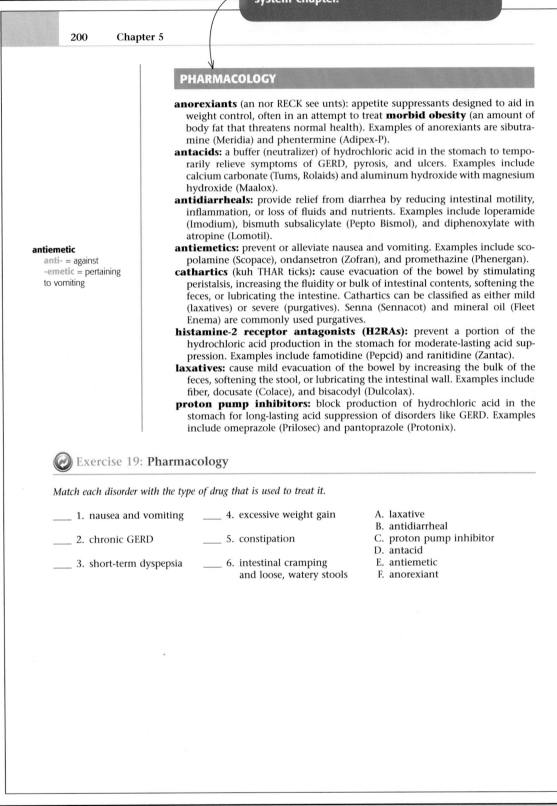

Pharmacology is included in each body system chapter.

200    Chapter 5

## PHARMACOLOGY

**anorexiants** (an nor RECK see unts): appetite suppressants designed to aid in weight control, often in an attempt to treat **morbid obesity** (an amount of body fat that threatens normal health). Examples of anorexiants are sibutramine (Meridia) and phentermine (Adipex-P).

**antacids:** a buffer (neutralizer) of hydrochloric acid in the stomach to temporarily relieve symptoms of GERD, pyrosis, and ulcers. Examples include calcium carbonate (Tums, Rolaids) and aluminum hydroxide with magnesium hydroxide (Maalox).

**antidiarrheals:** provide relief from diarrhea by reducing intestinal motility, inflammation, or loss of fluids and nutrients. Examples include loperamide (Imodium), bismuth subsalicylate (Pepto Bismol), and diphenoxylate with atropine (Lomotil).

**antiemetics:** prevent or alleviate nausea and vomiting. Examples include scopolamine (Scopace), ondansetron (Zofran), and promethazine (Phenergan).

**cathartics** (kuh THAR ticks): cause evacuation of the bowel by stimulating peristalsis, increasing the fluidity or bulk of intestinal contents, softening the feces, or lubricating the intestine. Cathartics can be classified as either mild (laxatives) or severe (purgatives). Senna (Sennacot) and mineral oil (Fleet Enema) are commonly used purgatives.

**histamine-2 receptor antagonists (H2RAs):** prevent a portion of the hydrochloric acid production in the stomach for moderate-lasting acid suppression. Examples include famotidine (Pepcid) and ranitidine (Zantac).

**laxatives:** cause mild evacuation of the bowel by increasing the bulk of the feces, softening the stool, or lubricating the intestinal wall. Examples include fiber, docusate (Colace), and bisacodyl (Dulcolax).

**proton pump inhibitors:** block production of hydrochloric acid in the stomach for long-lasting acid suppression of disorders like GERD. Examples include omeprazole (Prilosec) and pantoprazole (Protonix).

**antiemetic**
anti- = against
-emetic = pertaining to vomiting

Exercise 19: **Pharmacology**

*Match each disorder with the type of drug that is used to treat it.*

_____ 1. nausea and vomiting    _____ 4. excessive weight gain

_____ 2. chronic GERD    _____ 5. constipation

_____ 3. short-term dyspepsia    _____ 6. intestinal cramping and loose, watery stools

A. laxative
B. antidiarrheal
C. proton pump inhibitor
D. antacid
E. antiemetic
F. anorexiant

Electronic medical records present a variety of actual medical reports in an EHR format.
Case studies to accompany each medical record increase the human connection between patients, providers, and healthcare documentation.

Gastrointestinal System    173

## Case Study    Peter Jacobs

JACOBS, PETER E - 613446 Opened by  JEROME, ALAN MD    _ ☐ ✕

Task   Edit   View   Time Scale   Options   Help

As Of 06:15

**JACOBS, PETER E**

Age: 62          Sex: Male        Loc: WHC-SMMC
DOB: 08/20/1950  MRN: 613446      FIN: 3506004

Reference Text Browser | Form Browser | Medication Profile

Orders | Last 48 Hours | ED | Lab | Radiology | Assessment | **Surgery** | Clinical Notes | Pt. Info | Pt. Schedule | Task List | I & O | MAR

Flowsheet: Surgery    …    Level: Operative Report        ⦿ Table  ○ Group  ○ List

Navigator    ✕
✓  Operative Report

PREOPERATIVE DIAGNOSIS:          Rule out GI pathology
POSTOPERATIVE DIAGNOSIS:         See "Impression" below
OPERATION:                       Upper GI endoscopy

Patient was brought into the endoscopy suite where continuous oximetry, blood pressure, and ECG monitoring was placed. He was given 50 mg of fentanyl before procedure. The GIF Olympus 150 video endoscope was introduced through the pharynx without difficulty. Proximal portion of the esophagus appeared normal. At approximately mid esophagus, there were noted streaks of erythema extending up into the esophagus. The squamocolumnar junction was at 33 cm where there was a smooth concentric narrowing of the esophagus. There was mild friability of this tissue and distally was a moderate hiatal hernia. The scope was advanced through this into the gastric fundus, which was visualized in both the forward and retroflexed manner. Mucosa appeared quite normal. Distally, there was marked erythema of the antrum, particularly surrounding the pylorus. Biopsy was taken for *H. pylori*. The duodenum was difficult to intubate but appeared normal. Scope was withdrawn again to the level of the lower esophageal sphincter at 36 cm. Biopsies were taken from that area and circumferentially up to approximately 32 cm. There was minimal bleeding. Patient tolerated the procedure well.

IMPRESSION:
1. Reflux esophagitis with stricture at 33 cm
2. Moderate hiatal hernia
3. Probably Barrett esophagus
4. Diffuse antral gastritis, biopsy pending

PROD | MAHAFC | 23 August 2012 | 06:15

## Exercise 7: Operative Report

*Using the operative report above, answer the following questions. Use a dictionary as needed for this exercise.*

1. What was the route of the endoscope? _____

2. The portion of the esophagus that appeared normal was (close to/far from) the mouth. Circle one.

3. The mucosa was normal in which part of the stomach? _____

4. What are synonyms for the "lower esophageal sphincter"? _____

Choose **Hear It, Spell It** to practice spelling the anatomy and physiology terms that you have learned in this chapter. To practice pronouncing anatomy and physiology terms choose **Hear It, Say It.**

Frequent reference to online games and activities alert students to opportunities for interactive learning.

Newly revised review exercises encourage word building and practical use of terminology.

## WORDSHOP

| Prefixes | Combining Forms | Suffixes |
|----------|-----------------|----------|
| a- | cheil/o | -al |
| an- | chol/e | -eal |
| dys- | cholecyst/o | -ectomy |
| peri- | choledoch/o | -ia |
| pre- | col/o | -iasis |
| syn- | esophag/o | -ic |
| trans- | gastr/o | -itis |
|  | hepat/o | -pepsia |
|  | lapar/o | -phagia |
|  | lith/o | -plasty |
|  | nas/o | -rrhea |
|  | odont/o | -stomy |
|  | py/o | -tomy |
|  | stomat/o | -tresia |

*Build the following terms by combining the word parts above. Some word parts may be used more than once. Some won't be used at all. The number in parentheses indicates the number of word parts needed to build the term.*

| Definition | Term |
|------------|------|
| 1. pertaining to the stomach and esophagus (3) | |
| 2. condition of no opening (2) | |
| 3. pertaining to surrounding the teeth (3) | |
| 4. pertaining to the nose and stomach (3) | |
| 5. new opening of the colon (2) | |
| 6. inflammation of the gallbladder (2) | |
| 7. new opening between the stomach and esophagus (3) | |
| 8. removal of the gallbladder (2) | |
| 9. discharge of pus (2) | |
| 10. condition of difficult/painful swallowing (2) | |
| 11. condition of bad digestion (2) | |
| 12. condition of gallstones (3) | |
| 13. condition of stones in the common bile duct (3) | |
| 14. incision of the abdomen (2) | |
| 15. surgical repair of the mouth (2) | |

## STUDENT RESOURCES

**Electronic assets for students** on Evolve include entertaining interactive games and activities that have been designed to test specific areas of knowledge as you prepare for quizzes and exams. Breeze through the challenges of learning health-care terminology, and quickly learn to speak the language of your future career! Included with *Mastering Healthcare Terminology, Fourth Edition,* are a variety of learning aids intended to make your study of healthcare terminology as efficient and enjoyable as possible.

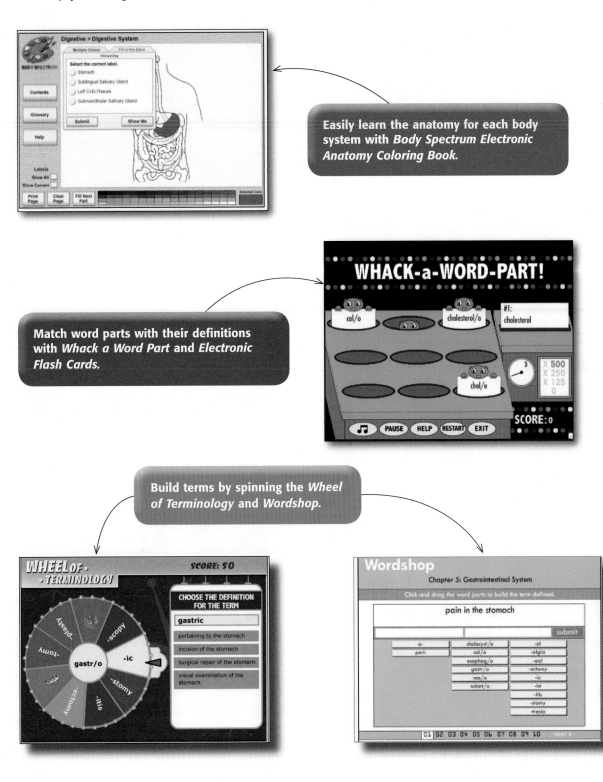

Easily learn the anatomy for each body system with *Body Spectrum Electronic Anatomy Coloring Book.*

Match word parts with their definitions with *Whack a Word Part* and *Electronic Flash Cards.*

Build terms by spinning the *Wheel of Terminology* and *Wordshop.*

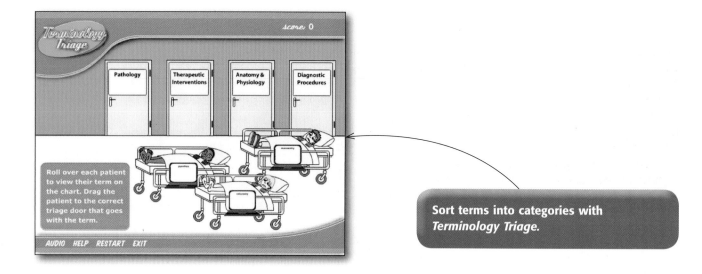

Learn medical terminology by playing *Medical Millionaire* and *Tournament of Terminology.*

Sort terms into categories with *Terminology Triage.*

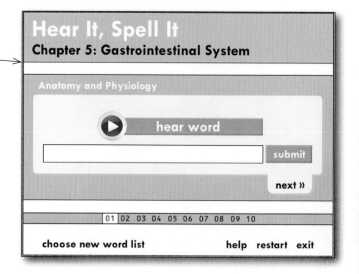

Practice pronouncing and spelling medical terms with *Hear It, Spell It* and *Hear It, Say It*. Download *iTerms* to listen to all the terms and definitions from the text.

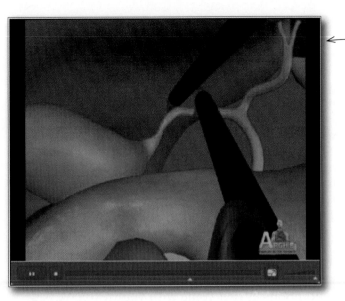

Watch *medical animations* to help you visualize pathologic and procedural terms.

## Mosby's Medical Terminology Online

*Mosby's Medical Terminology Online for Mastering Healthcare Terminology, Fourth Edition,* is a great resource to supplement your textbook. This web-delivered course supplement, available for separate purchase, provides a range of visual, auditory, and interactive elements to reinforce your learning and synthesize concepts presented in the text. Interactive lesson reviews at the end of each module provide you with testing tools that are actually fun. Clicking on a bolded term provides you with the pronunciation, definition, and Spanish translation. Related internet resources can be accessed by clicking on the hypertext links provided throughout the text.

This online course supplement is accessible only if you have purchased the access code packaged with your book. If you did not purchase the book/access package, ask your instructor for information or visit http://evolve.elsevier.com/Shiland to purchase.

# To the Instructor

You are the most important driving force behind your students' mastery of medical terminology. That's why we have provided you with all the resources you will need to teach this new language to your students:

- A **PowerPoint presentation** includes over 1000 slides to make teaching from Shiland a breeze. Slides are enhanced with additional images.
- **A test bank** consists of over 4500-questions. Multiple-choice, fill-in-the-blank, and true/false questions that can be sorted by subject, objective, and type of questions using Examview.
- **Handouts** can be used for classroom quizzes or homework.
- **Emailable, gradable quizzes** on the student site can be used for extra credit.
- **Image collection** in PPT and jpeg formats.
- **TEACH Lesson Plans** help you prepare for class and make full use of the rich array of ancillaries and resources that come with your textbook.
  TEACH is short for "Total Education and Curriculum Help," which accurately describes how these lesson plans and lecture materials have been providing creative and innovative instructional strategies to both new and experienced instructors to the benefit of their students.
  Each lesson plan contains:
- 50-minute lessons that correlates chapter objectives with content and teaching resources
- Convenient lists of key terms for each chapter
- Classroom activities and critical-thinking questions that engage and motivate students

Visit http://evolve.elsevier.com/Shiland/ for more information.

# From the Author

My greatest joy as a teacher has been to run into students long after they have finished one of my classes: students now practicing the career of their choice that they had begun so many years before. Students tell me how much they have used what they learned, how glad they are that they took the course, and, finally, how much fun it was. Certainly, healthcare terminology is a serious subject, but there is no reason not to have fun while you are learning. The Evolve website that accompanies this text will allow you to practice all aspects of terminology, while playing games that test your knowledge of all that serious stuff. Research shows that you need to be in contact with a new term at least six times to remember it. By attending class, reading the chapters, completing the exercises, and playing the games, you will have easily met that goal.

I am deeply grateful to all the people who have helped me in get this fourth edition to print. Thanks are due:

- To my past and present students: for your questions, your enthusiasm, and your drive to accomplish a career in healthcare.
- To **Erinn Kao** for updating the pharmacology information and to **Jeanne Robertson**, who expertly turned my thoughts into beautiful illustrations for the text.
- To my Elsevier cohorts: **Jeanne Olson**, for her calm leadership; **Linda Woodard**, for her relentless drive for quality in every aspect of the book; to **Celeste Clingan** for her production expertise, and to **Jessica Williams** for her beautiful design—thank you all for guiding me once again through the process.
- To the my family: brother and sister-in-law, **Thomas** and **Maureen Shiland**, both National Board Certified teachers, who have provided many discussions and resources that helped me solidify my thinking on the structure of the exercises and games. And most important of all: thanks to my son, **Thomas**, who continues to inspire, encourage, and support me.

**Betsy Shiland**
**bshiland@ccp.edu**

# Contents

# 1

*They do certainly give very strange, and newfangled, names to diseases.*
*—Plato*

## OBJECTIVES

- State the derivation of most healthcare terms.
- Use the rules given to build, spell, and pronounce healthcare terms.
- Use the rules given to change singular terms to their plural forms.
- Recognize and recall an introductory word bank of prefixes, suffixes, and combining forms and their respective meanings.

# Introduction to Healthcare Terminology

## CHAPTER AT A GLANCE

*Use this list of key word parts and terms to assess your knowledge. Check off the ones you have mastered.*

### KEY WORD PARTS

#### PREFIXES
- ☐ ante-
- ☐ anti-
- ☐ dys-
- ☐ endo-
- ☐ hyper-
- ☐ hypo-
- ☐ neo-
- ☐ per-
- ☐ peri-

#### SUFFIXES
- ☐ -al
- ☐ -algia
- ☐ -ectomy
- ☐ -graphy
- ☐ -itis
- ☐ -logy
- ☐ -plasty
- ☐ -scope
- ☐ -tomy

#### COMBINING FORMS
- ☐ arthr/o
- ☐ cardi/o
- ☐ col/o
- ☐ cyst/o
- ☐ enter/o
- ☐ gastr/o
- ☐ gloss/o
- ☐ hepat/o
- ☐ hyster/o
- ☐ mamm/o
- ☐ nat/o
- ☐ neur/o
- ☐ ophthalm/o
- ☐ oste/o
- ☐ path/o
- ☐ ped/o
- ☐ rhin/o
- ☐ therm/o

### KEY TERMS
- ☐ acronym
- ☐ acute
- ☐ chronic
- ☐ combining form
- ☐ decodable term
- ☐ diagnosis
- ☐ eponym
- ☐ nondecodable term
- ☐ prefix
- ☐ prognosis
- ☐ sign
- ☐ suffix
- ☐ symptom
- ☐ word root

## DERIVATION OF HEALTHCARE TERMS

Healthcare terminology is a specialized vocabulary derived from Greek and Latin word components. This terminology is used by professionals in the medical field to communicate with each other. By applying the process of "decoding," or recognizing the word components and their meanings and using these to define the terms, anyone will be able to interpret literally thousands of medical terms.

The English language and healthcare terminology share many common origins. This proves to be an additional bonus for those who put forth the effort to learn hundreds of seemingly new word parts. Two excellent and highly relevant examples are the **combining forms** (the "subjects" of most terms) gloss/o and lingu/o, which mean "tongue" in Greek and Latin, respectively. Because the tongue is instrumental in articulating spoken language, Greek and Latin equivalents appear, not surprisingly, in familiar English vocabulary. The table below illustrates the intersection of our everyday English language with the ancient languages of Greek and Latin and can help us to clearly see the connections. **Suffixes** (word parts that appear at the end of some terms) and **prefixes** (word parts that appear at the beginning of some terms) also are presented in this table. Special notice should be given to the pronunciation key that is provided directly under the examples: You will have to use your tongue to say them! *Please remember that terminology is spoken as well as written and read.* You must take advantage of the many resources that this text provides if you wish to fully communicate as a healthcare professional.

| Ancient Word Origins in Current English and Healthcare Terminology Usage | | |
| --- | --- | --- |
| Term | Word Origins | Definition |
| **gloss**ary (GLAH sur ee) | *gloss/o* tongue (Greek) *-ary* pertaining to | An English term meaning "an alphabetical list of terms with definitions." |
| **gloss**itis (glah SYE tiss) | *gloss/o* tongue (Greek) *-itis* inflammation | A healthcare term meaning "inflammation of the tongue." |
| bi**lingu**al (by LIN gwal) | *bi-* two *lingu/o* tongue (Latin) *-al* pertaining to | An English term meaning "pertaining to two languages." |
| sub**lingu**al (sub LIN gwal) | *sub-* under *lingu/o* tongue (Latin) *-al* pertaining to | A healthcare term meaning "pertaining to under the tongue." |

Did you notice that healthcare terms use the word origins literally, while English words are related to word origins but are not exactly the same? Fortunately, most healthcare terms may be assigned a simple definition through the use of their word parts.

## TYPES OF HEALTHCARE TERMS

### Decodable Terms

Decodable terms are those terms that can be broken into their Greek and Latin word parts and given a working definition based on the meanings of those word parts. Most medical terms are decodable, so learning word parts is important. The word parts are:

- **Combining form:** word root with its respective combining vowel
  - **Word root:** word origin
  - **Combining vowel:** a letter sometimes used to join word parts. Usually an "o" but occasionally an "a", "e", "i" or "u".
- **Suffix:** word part that appears at the end of a term. Suffixes are used to indicate whether the term is an anatomic, pathologic, diagnostic, or therapeutic intervention term.
- **Prefix:** word part that sometimes appears at the beginning of a term. Prefixes are used to further define the absence, location, number, quantity, or state of the term.

In our first examples, gloss/ and lingu/ are word roots with an "o" as their combining vowel. Gloss/o and lingu/o are therefore combining forms, -ary, -al and -itis are suffixes and bi- and sub- are prefixes. Figs 1-1 and 1-2 demonstrate the decoding of the terms **glossitis** and **sublingual**. Throughout the text, we will be using combining forms, so that you will learn the appropriate combining vowel for that particular term.

## Nondecodable Terms

Not all terms are composed of word parts that can be used to assemble a definition. These terms are referred to as **nondecodable terms,** that is, words used in medicine whose definitions must be memorized without the benefit of word parts. These terms will have a blank space in the word origin tables presented in the text or will include only a partial notation because the word origins either are not helpful or don't exist. Examples of nondecodable terms include the following:

- **Cataract:** From the Greek term meaning "waterfall." In healthcare language, this means progressive opacification of the lens.
- **Asthma:** From the Greek term meaning "panting." Although this word origin is understandable, the definition is a respiratory disorder characterized by recurring episodes of paroxysmal dyspnea (difficulty breathing).
- **Diagnosis:** The disease or condition that is named after a healthcare professional evaluates a patient's signs, symptoms, and history. Although the term is built from word parts (dia-, meaning "through," "complete"; and -gnosis, meaning "state of knowledge"), using these word parts to form the definition of diagnosis, which is "a state of complete knowledge," really isn't very helpful.
- **Prognosis:** Similar to *diagnosis,* the term *prognosis* can be broken down into its word parts (pro-, meaning "before" or "in front of"; and -gnosis, meaning "state of knowledge"), but this does not give the true definition of the term, which is "a prediction of the probable outcome of a disease or disorder."
- **Sequela** (suh KWELL ah): A condition that results from an injury or disease.
- **Acute:** A term that describes an abrupt, severe onset (acu- means "sharp") to a disease.
- **Chronic:** Developing slowly and lasting for a long time (chron/o means "time"). Diagnoses may be additionally described as being either acute or chronic.
- **Sign:** An objective finding of a disease state (e.g., fever, high blood pressure, rash)
- **Symptom:** A subjective report of a disease (pain, itching)

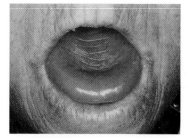

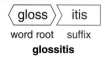
word root   suffix
**glossitis**

**Fig. 1-1** Decoding of the term **glossitis**.

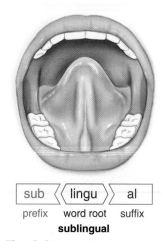

sub   lingu   al
prefix   word root   suffix
**sublingual**

**Fig. 1-2** Decoding of the term **sublingual**.

Other types of terms that are not built from word parts include the following:

- **Eponyms:** terms that are named after a person or place associated with the term.* Examples include:
  - **Alzheimer disease,** which is named after Alois Alzheimer, a German neurologist. The disease is a progressive mental deterioration.
  - **Achilles tendon,** a body part named after a figure in Greek mythology whose one weak spot was this area of his anatomy. Tendons are bands of tissue that attach muscles to bone. The Achilles tendon is the particular tendon that attaches the calf muscle to the heel bone (calcaneus). Unlike some eponyms, this one does have a medical equivalent, the calcaneal tendon.

## Abbreviations and Symbols

Abbreviations are terms that have been shortened to letters and/or numbers for the sake of convenience. Symbols are graphic representations of a term. Abbreviations and symbols are extremely common in written and spoken healthcare terminology but can pose problems for healthcare workers. The Joint Commission has published a "DO NOT USE" list of dangerously confusing abbreviations, symbols, and acronyms that should be avoided (see Appendix C). The Institute of Safe Medical Practice, Inc., has provided a more extensive list. Each healthcare organization should have an official list, which includes the single meaning allowed for each abbreviation or symbol. Examples of acceptable abbreviations and symbols include the following:

- **Simple abbreviations:** A combination of letters (often, but not always the first of significant word parts) and sometimes numbers
  - IM: abbreviation for "intramuscular" (pertaining to within the muscles)
  - C2: second cervical vertebra (second bone in neck)
- **Acronyms:** Abbreviations that are also pronounceable
  - CABG: coronary artery bypass graft (a detour around a blockage in an artery of the heart)
  - TURP: transurethral resection of the prostate (a surgical procedure that removes the prostate through the urethra)
- **Symbols:** Graphic representations of terms
  ♀ stands for female
  ♂ stands for male
  ↑ stands for increased
  ↓ stands for decreased
  + stands for present
  − stands for absent

## Exercise 1: Derivation of Healthcare Terms and Nondecodable Terms

*Match the following types of healthcare terms with their examples.*

____ 1. symbol                ____ 4. eponym                A. CABG
                                                             B. Alzheimer disease
____ 2. decodable term        ____ 5. nondecodable term     C. ♀
                                                             D. glossitis
____ 3. simple abbreviation   ____ 6. acronym               E. C2
                                                             F. asthma

*This text presents terms without the possessive 's. This practice is in accordance with the American Medical Association (AMA) and the American Association of Transcriptionists (AAMT).

Many students find that flash cards help them remember word parts. If this is a strategy that could work for you, now is a great place to start, whether the cards are purchased or handmade. One card will be needed for each word part, with the part on one side and the definition on the reverse. The Evolve website that accompanies this text provides electronic flash cards that can be sorted by chapter, by type of word part (prefix, suffix, combining form) and by abbreviation.

## DECODING TERMS

### Check, Assign, Reverse, Define (CARD Method)

Using Greek and Latin word components to decipher the meanings of healthcare terms requires a simple four step process. You need to:

- **Check** for the word parts in a term.
- **Assign** meanings to the word parts.
- **Reverse** the meaning of the suffix to the front of your definition.
- **Define** the term.

Using Figure 1-3, see how this process is applied to your first patient, Alex.

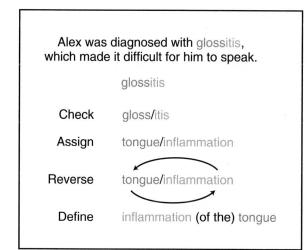

Fig. 1-3 How to decode a healthcare term using the **CARD** method.

Most of the terms presented in this text appear in standardized tables. The term and its pronunciation appear in the first column, the word origin in the second, and a definition in the third. A table that introduces five healthcare terms that include five different combining forms and suffixes is provided on p. 6. (The use of prefixes will be introduced later.) Success in decoding these terms depends on how well you remember the 12 word parts that are covered in the table below. Once you master these 12 word parts, you will be able to recognize and define many other medical terms that use these same word parts—a perfect illustration of how learning a few word parts helps you learn many healthcare terms. The "wheel of terminology" included on Fig. 1-4 demonstrates how the different suffixes in the table on p. 6. can be added to a combining form to make a variety of terms.

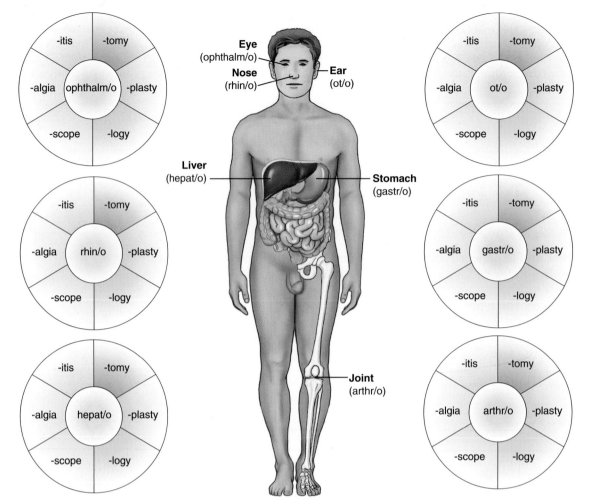

**Fig. 1-4** Body parts and their combining forms. Surrounding the figure are "terminology wheels" that show how different suffixes can be added to a combining form to make a variety of terms.

## Common Combining Forms and Suffixes

### Combining Forms

arthr/o = joint
gastr/o = stomach
ophthalm/o = eye
ot/o = ear
rhin/o = nose
hepat/o = liver

### Suffixes

-algia = pain
-tomy = incision
-scope = instrument to view
-logy = study of
-plasty = surgical repair
-itis = inflammation

The following table demonstrates how terms are presented in this book. Notice that the first column includes the term and its pronunciation. The second column breaks the term down into word parts and their meanings. The third column includes the definition of the term and any synonyms.

## Samples of Decodable Terms

| Term | Word Origins | Definition |
|------|-------------|------------|
| arthralgia<br>ar THRAL jah | *arthr/o* joint<br>*-algia* pain of | Pain of a joint. |
| gastrotomy<br>gass TROT uh mee | *gastr/o* stomach<br>*-tomy* incision | Incision of the stomach. |
| ophthalmoscope<br>off THAL muh skohp | *ophthalm/o* eye<br>*-scope* instrument to view | Instrument used to view the eye. |
| otology<br>oh TALL uh jee | *ot/o* ear<br>*-logy* study of | Study of the ear. |
| rhinoplasty<br>RYE noh plass tee | *rhin/o* nose<br>*-plasty* surgical repair | Surgical repair of the nose. |
| hepatitis<br>heh peh TYE tiss | *hepat/o* liver<br>*-itis* inflammation | Inflammation of the liver. |

## Exercise 2: Combining Forms

*Match the combining forms with their meanings.*

____ 1. ear      ____ 4. eye      A. rhin/o

                                      B. arthr/o

____ 2. stomach      ____ 5. joint      C. ot/o

                                      D. gastr/o

____ 3. nose                                            E. ophthalm/o

## Exercise 3: Suffixes

*Match the suffixes with their meanings.*

____ 1. pain      ____ 4. incision      A. -tomy

                                      B. -algia

____ 2. surgical repair      ____ 5. study of      C. -logy

                                      D. -plasty

____ 3. instrument to view                              E. -scope

## Exercise 4: Decoding the Terms Using Check, Assign, Reverse, and Define

*Using the method shown in Figure 1-3 and the 12 word parts you have just memorized, decode and define these five NEW terms.*

1. ophthalmology _____

2. otoplasty _____

3. gastralgia _____

4. arthroscope _____

5. rhinotomy _____

## BUILDING TERMS

Now that you've seen how terms are decoded, we will discuss how they are built. First, a few rules on how to spell healthcare terms correctly.

### Spelling Rules

With a few exceptions, decodable healthcare terms follow five simple rules.

1. If the suffix starts with a vowel, a combining vowel is *not* needed to join the parts. For example, it is simple to combine the combining form **arthr/o** and suffix **-itis** to build the term **arthritis**, which means "an inflammation of the joints." The combining vowel "**o**" is not needed because the suffix starts with the vowel "**i**."

2. If the suffix starts with a consonant, a combining vowel *is* needed to join the two word parts. For example, when building a term using **arthr/o** and **-plasty**, the combining vowel is retained and the resulting term is spelled **arthroplasty**, which refers to a surgical repair of a joint.

3. If a combining form ends with the same vowel that begins a suffix, one of the vowels is dropped. The term that means "inflammation of the inside of the heart" is built from the suffix **-itis** (inflammation), the prefix **endo-** (inside), and the combining form **cardi/o. Endo-** + **cardi/o** + **-itis** would result in *endocardiitis*. Instead, one of the "i"s is dropped, and the term is spelled **endocarditis**.

4. If two or more combining forms are used in a term, the combining vowel is retained between the two, regardless of whether the second combining form begins with a vowel or a consonant. For example, joining **gastr/o** and **enter/o** (small intestine) with the suffix **-itis**, results in the term **gastroenteritis**. Notice that the combining vowel is *kept* between the two combining forms (even though **enter/o** begins with the vowel "e"), and the combining vowel is *dropped* before the suffix **-itis**.

5. Sometimes when two or more combining forms are used to make a medical term, special notice must be paid to the order in which the combining forms are joined. For example, joining **esophag/o** (which means esophagus), **gastr/o** (which means stomach), and **duoden/o** (which means duodenum, [the first part of the small intestines]) with the suffix **-scopy** (process of viewing), produces the term esophagogastroduodenoscopy. An **esophagogastroduodenoscopy** is a visual examination of the esophagus, stomach, and duodenum. In this procedure, the examination takes place in a specific sequence, that is, esophagus first, stomach second, then the duodenum. Thus the term reflects the direction from which the scope travels through the body (Fig. 1-5).

### Suffixes

The body systems chapters in this text (Chapters 3 through 15) include many combining forms that are used to build terms specific to each system. These combining forms will not be seen elsewhere, except as a sign or symptom of a particular disorder. **Suffixes**, however, are used over and over again throughout the text. Suffixes usually can be grouped according to their purposes. The following tables cover the major categories.

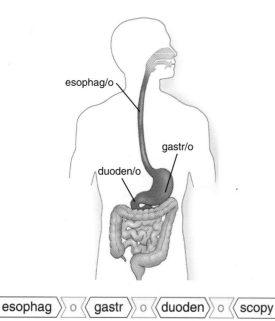

Fig. 1-5 The decoding of the term **esophagogastroduodenoscopy (EGD)**.

## Noun-Ending Suffixes

Noun endings are used most often to describe anatomic terms. Noun endings such as -icle, -ole, and -ule describe a diminutive structure.

| Noun-Ending Suffixes | | | | |
|---|---|---|---|---|
| Suffix | Meaning | Example | Word Origins | Definition |
| -icle | small, tiny | cuticle | *cut/o* skin<br>*-icle* small | Small skin (surrounding the nail). |
| -is | structure, thing | hypodermis | *hypo-* under<br>*derm/o* skin<br>*-is* structure | Structure under the skin. |
| -ole | small, tiny | arteriole | *arteri/o* artery<br>*-ole* small | Small artery. |
| -ule | small, tiny | venule | *ven/o* vein<br>*-ule* small | Small vein. |
| -um | structure, thing, membrane | endocardium | *endo-* within<br>*cardi/o* heart<br>*-um* structure | Structure within the heart. |
| -y | process of | atrophy | *a-* no, not, without<br>*troph/o* development<br>*-y* process of | Process of no development. |

## Adjective Suffixes

Adjective suffixes such as those listed below usually mean "pertaining to." For example, when the suffix **-ac** is added to the combining form **cardi/o**, the term *cardiac* is formed, which means "pertaining to the heart." Remember that when you see an adjective term, you need to see what it is describing. For example, cardiac pain is pain of the heart, and cardiac surgery is surgery done on the heart. An adjective tells only half of the story.

## Adjective Suffixes

| Suffix | Meaning | Example | Word Origins | Definition |
|--------|---------|---------|--------------|------------|
| -ac | pertaining to | cardiac | *cardi/o* heart<br>*-ac* pertaining to | Pertaining to the heart. |
| -al | pertaining to | cervical | *cervic/o* neck<br>*-al* pertaining to | Pertaining to the neck. |
| -ar | pertaining to | valvular | *valvul/o* valve<br>*-ar* pertaining to | Pertaining to a valve. |
| -ary | pertaining to | coronary | *coron/o\** heart, crown<br>*-ary* pertaining to | Pertaining to the heart. |
| -eal | pertaining to | esophageal | *esophag/o* esophagus<br>*-eal* pertaining to | Pertaining to the esophagus. |
| -ic | pertaining to | hypodermic | *hypo-* below<br>*derm/o* skin<br>*-ic* pertaining to | Pertaining to below the skin. |
| -ous | pertaining to | subcutaneous | *sub-* under<br>*cutane/o* skin<br>*-ous* pertaining to | Pertaining to under the skin. |

*Coron/o literally means "crown," but is used most frequently to describe the arteries that supply blood to the heart; so the meaning "heart" has been added.

### Pathology Suffixes

Pathology suffixes describe a disease process or a sign or symptom. The meanings vary according to the dysfunctions that they describe.

## Pathology Suffixes

| Suffix | Meaning | Example | Word Origins | Definition |
|--------|---------|---------|--------------|------------|
| -algia | pain | cephalalgia | *cephal/o* head<br>*-algia* pain | Pain in the head. |
| -cele | herniation | cystocele | *cyst/o* bladder, sac<br>*-cele* herniation, protrusion | Herniation of the bladder. |
| -dynia | pain | cardiodynia | *cardi/o* heart<br>*-dynia* pain | Pain in the heart. |
| -emia | blood condition | hyperlipidemia | *hyper-* excessive<br>*lipid/o* fats<br>*-emia* blood condition | Excessive fats in the blood. |
| -ia | condition | agastria | *a-* without<br>*gastr/o* stomach<br>*-ia* condition | Condition of having no stomach. |
| -itis | inflammation | gastroenteritis | *gastr/o* stomach<br>*enter/o* small intestine<br>*-itis* inflammation | Inflammation of the stomach and small intestine. |

## Pathology Suffixes—cont'd

| Suffix | Meaning | Example | Word Origins | Definition |
|---|---|---|---|---|
| -malacia | softening | chondromalacia | *chondr/o* cartilage<br>*-malacia* softening | Softening of the cartilage. |
| -megaly | enlargement | splenomegaly<br>(Fig. 1-6) | *splen/o* spleen<br>*-megaly* enlargement | Enlargement of the spleen. |
| -oma | tumor, mass | osteoma | *oste/o* bone<br>*-oma* tumor, mass | Tumor of a bone. |
| -osis | abnormal condition | psychosis | *psych/o* mind<br>*-osis* abnormal condition | Abnormal condition of the mind. |
| -pathy | disease process | gastropathy | *gastr/o* stomach<br>*-pathy* disease process | Disease process of the stomach. |
| -ptosis | prolapse, drooping, sagging | hysteroptosis | *hyster/o* uterus<br>*-ptosis* prolapse | Prolapse of the uterus. |
| -rrhage,<br>-rrhagia | bursting forth | hemorrhage | *hem/o* blood<br>*-rrhage* bursting forth | Bursting forth of blood. |
| -rrhea | discharge, flow | otorrhea | *ot/o* ear<br>*-rrhea* discharge, flow | Discharge from the ear. |
| -rrhexis | rupture | cystorrhexis | *cyst/o* bladder, sac<br>*-rrhexis* rupture | Rupture of the bladder. |
| -sclerosis | abnormal condition of hardening | arteriosclerosis | *arteri/o* artery<br>*-sclerosis* abnormal condition of hardening | Abnormal condition of hardening of an artery. |
| -stenosis | abnormal condition of narrowing | tracheostenosis | *trache/o* trachea, windpipe<br>*-stenosis* abnormal condition of narrowing | Abnormal condition of narrowing of the trachea or windpipe. |

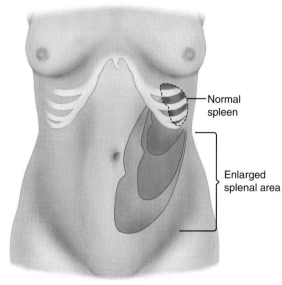

Normal spleen

Enlarged splenal area

Fig. 1-6 Splenomegaly.

### ⊗ Be Careful!

*Don't confuse* -**malacia,** *meaning softening with* -**megaly,** *meaning enlargement.*

### ⊗ Be Careful!

*Don't confuse* -**sclerosis,** *meaning hardening with* -**stenosis,** *meaning narrowing.*

### ⊗ Be Careful!

*Don't confuse* -**rrhage** *and* -**rrhagia,** *meaning bursting forth with* -**rrhea,** *meaning a discharge.*

## Exercise 5: Noun-Ending, Adjective, and Pathology Suffixes

*Match the suffixes with their meaning.*

_____ 1. -icle, -ole, -ule      _____ 6. -malacia       A. softening
                                                        B. abnormal condition of hardening
_____ 2. -megaly               _____ 7. -algia          C. pain
                                                        D. prolapse
_____ 3. -um                   _____ 8. -ptosis         E. small, tiny
                                                        F. blood condition
_____ 4. -ic, -al, -ous        _____ 9. -emia           G. enlargement
                                                        H. abnormal condition of herniation, protrusion
_____ 5. -cele                 _____ 10. -sclerosis     I. pertaining to
                                                        J. structure, thing, membrane

*Using the method shown in Figure 1-3 and the new word parts introduced in the tables above, decode and define these five NEW terms.*

11. cardiomegaly _____

12. osteomalacia _____

13. valvulitis _____

14. cephalic _____

15. gastroptosis _____

### Diagnostic Procedure Suffixes

Diagnostic procedure suffixes indicate a procedure that helps to determine the diagnosis. Although a few diagnostic procedures also can help to treat a disease, most are used to establish a particular disease or disorder.

| Diagnostic Procedure Suffixes | | | | |
|---|---|---|---|---|
| Suffix | Meaning | Example | Word Origins | Definition |
| -graphy | process of recording | mammography | *mamm/o* breast<br>*-graphy* process of recording | Process of recording the breast. |
| -metry | process of measuring | spirometry (Fig. 1-7) | *spir/o* breathing<br>*-metry* process of measuring | Process of measuring breathing. |
| -opsy | process of viewing | biopsy | *bi/o* living, life<br>*-opsy* process of viewing | Process of viewing living tissue. |
| -scopy | process of viewing | esophagogastroduodenoscopy | *esophag/o* esophagus<br>*gastr/o* stomach<br>*duoden/o* duodenum<br>*-scopy* process of viewing | Process of viewing the esophagus, stomach, and duodenum. |

## Therapeutic Intervention Suffixes

Therapeutic intervention suffixes indicate types of treatment. Treatments may be medical or surgical in nature.

### Therapeutic Intervention Suffixes*

| Suffix | Meaning | Example | Word Origins | Definition |
|--------|---------|---------|--------------|------------|
| -ectomy | removal, resection, excision | tonsillectomy | *tonsill/o* tonsil<br>*-ectomy* cut out | Removal of the tonsils. |
| -plasty | surgical repair | rhinoplasty | *rhin/o* nose<br>*-plasty* surgical repair | Surgical repair of the nose. |
| -rrhaphy | suture | splenorrhaphy | *splen/o* spleen<br>*-rrhaphy* suture | Suture of the spleen. |
| -stomy | new opening | colostomy | *col/o* colon, large intestine<br>*-stomy* new opening | New opening of the colon or large intestine (Fig. 1-8). |
| -tomy | incision, cutting | osteotomy | *oste/o* bone<br>*-tomy* incision | Incision into the bone. |
| -tripsy | crushing | lithotripsy | *lith/o* stone<br>*-tripsy* crushing | Crushing of stones. |

*In October 2013, the institution of ICD-10-CM will change how we define these suffixes. The current definitions of removal, resection and excision will each have distinctly different meanings. After 2013, using only one of these words in defining a medical term gives it a very specific and potentially misleading meaning.

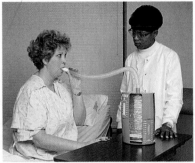

Fig. 1-7 Spirometry.

### ⊗ Be Careful!

*Don't confuse* **-ectomy,** *meaning a removal with* **-stomy,** *meaning a new opening or* **-tomy,** *meaning an incision.*

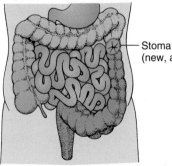

Stoma
(new, artificial opening)

Fig. 1-8 Colostomy.

## Instrument Suffixes

Instruments are indicated by yet another set of suffixes. Note the obvious similarities to their diagnostic and therapeutic "cousins." For example, electrocardiography is a diagnostic procedure that is done to measure the electrical activity in the heart; an electrocardiograph is the instrument that is used to perform electrocardiography.

## Instrument Suffixes

| Suffix | Meaning | Example | Word Origins | Definition |
|--------|---------|---------|--------------|------------|
| -graph | instrument to record | electrocardiograph | *electr/o* electricity<br>*cardi/o* heart<br>*-graph* instrument to record | Instrument to record the electricity of the heart. |
| -meter | instrument to measure | thermometer | *therm/o* temperature, heat<br>*-meter* instrument to measure | Instrument to measure temperature. |
| -scope | instrument to view | ophthalmoscope | *ophthalm/o* eye<br>*-scope* instrument to view | Instrument to view the eye. |
| -tome | instrument to cut | osteotome | *oste/o* bone<br>*-tome* instrument to cut | Instrument to cut bone (Fig. 1-9). |
| -tripter | machine to crush | lithotripter | *lith/o* stone<br>*-tripter* machine to crush | Machine to crush stone. |
| -trite | instrument to crush | lithotrite | *lith/o* stone<br>*-trite* instrument to crush | Instrument to crush stone (Fig. 1-10). |

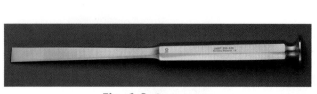

Fig. 1-9 Osteotome.

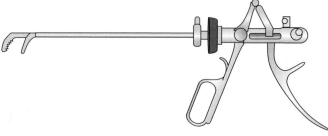

Fig. 1-10 Lithotrite.

### Specialty and Specialist Suffixes

Specialties and specialists require yet another category of suffixes. Someone who specializes in the study of the heart would be called a *cardiologist*. **Cardi/o** means "heart" and **-logist** means "one who specializes in the study of."

## Specialty and Specialist Suffixes

| Suffix | Meaning | Example | Word Origins | Definition |
|--------|---------|---------|--------------|------------|
| -er | one who | polysomnographer | *poly-* many, much, excessive, frequent<br>*somn/o* sleep<br>*graph/o* record<br>*-er* one who | One who records many (aspects of) sleep. |
| -iatrician | one who specializes in treatment | geriatrician | *ger/o* old age<br>*-iatrician* one who specializes in treatment | One who specializes in treatment of old age (patients). |

## Specialty and Specialist Suffixes—cont'd

| Suffix | Meaning | Example | Word Origins | Definition |
|---|---|---|---|---|
| -iatrics | treatment | pediatrics | *ped/o* children<br>*-iatrics* treatment | The treatment of children. |
| -iatrist | one who specializes in treatment | psychiatrist* | *psych/o* mind<br>*-iatrist* one who specializes in treatment | One who specializes in treatment of the mind. |
| -iatry | process of treatment | psychiatry | *psych/o* mind<br>*-iatry* process of treatment | Process of treatment of the mind. |
| -ist | one who specializes | dentist | *dent/i* teeth<br>*-ist* one who specializes | One who specializes in the teeth. |
| -logist | one who specializes in the study of | psychologist* | *psych/o* mind<br>*-logist* one who specializes in the study of | One who specializes in the study of the mind. |
| -logy | study of | neonatology | *neo-* new<br>*nat/o* born, birth<br>*-logy* study of | The study of the newborn (Fig. 1-11). |

*A psychologist usually has a master's or a doctoral degree; a psychiatrist holds a medical degree.

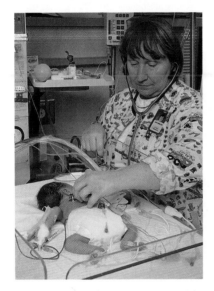

**Fig. 1-11** Neonatology.

## Exercise 6: Diagnosis, Therapy, Instrument, and Specialty/Specialist Suffixes

*Match the suffixes with their meanings.*

____ 1. -tome    ____ 6. -scope    A. removal, resection
B. new opening
____ 2. -logy    ____ 7. -scopy    C. instrument to view
D. process of viewing
____ 3. -graphy    ____ 8. -ectomy    E. instrument to cut
F. instrument to measure
____ 4. -meter    ____ 9. -tomy    G. incision, cutting
H. process of recording
____ 5. -logist    ____ 10. -stomy    I. study of
J. one who specializes in the study of

*Using the method shown in Figure 1-3 and the new word parts introduced in the preceding tables, decode and define these five NEW terms.*

11. osteologist _____

12. spirometer _____

13. hysteroscopy _____

14. cystoscope _____

15. splenectomy _____

## Prefixes

Prefixes modify a medical term by indicating a structure's or a condition's:

- Absence
- Location
- Number or quantity
- State

Sometimes, as with other word parts, a prefix can have one or more meanings. For example, the prefix **hypo-** can mean "below" or "deficient." To spell a term with the use of a prefix, simply add the prefix directly to the beginning of the term. No combining vowels are needed!

| Prefixes | | | | |
|---|---|---|---|---|
| Prefix | Meaning | Example | Word Origins | Definition |
| a- | no, not, without | apneic | *a-* without<br>*pne/o* breathing<br>*-ic* pertaining to | Pertaining to without breathing. |
| an- | no, not, without | anophthalmia | *an-* without<br>*ophthalm/o* eye<br>*-ia* condition | Conditon of without an eye. |
| ante- | forward, in front of, before | anteversion | *ante-* forward<br>*vers/o* turning<br>*-ion* process of | Process of turning forward. |
| anti- | against | antibacterial | *anti-* against<br>*bacteri/o* bacteria<br>*-al* pertaining to | Pertaining to against bacteria. |
| dys- | abnormal, difficult, bad, painful | dystrophy | *dys-* abnormal<br>*-trophy* process of nourishment | Process of abnormal nourishment. |
| endo-, end- | within | endoscopy | *endo-* within<br>*-scopy* process of viewing | Process of viewing within. |
| epi- | above, upon | epigastric | *epi-* above<br>*gastr/o* stomach<br>*-ic* pertaining to | Pertaining to above the stomach. |

## Prefixes—cont'd

| Prefix | Meaning | Example | Word Origins | Definition |
|---|---|---|---|---|
| hyper- | excessive, above | hyperglycemia | *hyper-* excessive, above<br>*glyc/o* sugar, glucose<br>*-emia* blood condition | Blood condition of excessive sugar. |
| hypo- | below, deficient | hypoglossal | *hypo-* below<br>*gloss/o* tongue<br>*-al* pertaining to | Pertaining to below the tongue. |
| inter- | between | intervertebral | *inter-* between<br>*vertebr/o* vertebra, backbone<br>*-al* pertaining to | Pertaining to between the backbones. |
| intra- | within | intramuscular | *intra-* within<br>*muscul/o* muscle<br>*-al* pertaining to | Pertaining to within the muscle. |
| neo- | new | neonatal | *neo-* new<br>*nat/o* birth, born<br>*-al* pertaining to | Pertaining to a newborn. |
| par- | near, beside | parotid | *par-* near<br>*ot/o* ear<br>*-id* pertaining to | Pertaining to near the ear. |
| para- | abnormal | paraphilia | *para-* abnormal<br>*phil/o* attraction<br>*-ia* condition | Condition of abnormal attraction. |
| per- | through | percutaneous | *per-* through<br>*cutane/o* skin<br>*-ous* pertaining to | Pertaining to through the skin (Fig. 1-12). |
| peri- | surrounding, around | pericardium | *peri-* surrounding<br>*cardi/o* heart<br>*-um* structure | Stucture surrounding the heart. |
| poly- | many, much, excessive, frequent | polyneuritis | *poly-* many, much, excessive, frequent<br>*neur/o* nerve<br>*-itis* inflammation | Inflammation of many nerves. |
| post- | after, behind | postnatal | *post-* after<br>*nat/o* birth, born<br>*-al* pertaining to | Pertaining to after birth. |
| pre- | before, in front of | prenatal | *pre-* before<br>*nat/o* birth, born<br>*-al* pertaining to | Pertaining to before birth. |
| sub- | under, below | subhepatic | *sub-* under<br>*hepat/o* liver<br>*-ic* pertaining to | Pertaining to under the liver. |
| trans- | through, across | transurethral | *trans-* through<br>*urethr/o* urethra<br>*-al* pertaining to | Pertaining to through the urethra. |

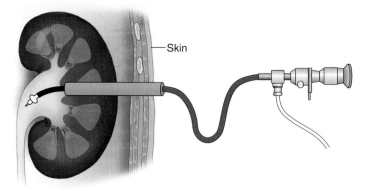

Fig. 1-12 Percutaneous endoscopic gastrotomy (PEG).

| ⊗ **Be Careful!** | ⊗ **Be Careful!** | ⊗ **Be Careful!** | ⊗ **Be Careful!** |
|---|---|---|---|
| *Don't confuse **inter-** meaning between with **intra-** meaning within.* | *Don't confuse **ante-** meaning forward with **anti-** meaning against.* | *Don't confuse **per-** meaning through with **peri-** meaning surrounding and **pre-** meaning before.* | *Don't confuse **hyper-** meaning excessive, above with **hypo-** meaning below, deficient.* |

## Exercise 7: Prefixes

*Match the prefixes with their meanings.*

____ 1. anti-     ____ 6. dys-     A. under, below
                                   B. above, excessive
____ 2. inter-    ____ 7. intra-   C. against
                                   D. bad, difficult, painful, abnormal
____ 3. poly-     ____ 8. peri-    E. within
                                   F. many
____ 4. ante-     ____ 9. sub-     G. through
                                   H. between
____ 5. hyper-    ____ 10. per-    I. forward
                                   J. around, surrounding

*Using the method shown in Figure 1-3 and the new word parts introduced in the preceding tables, decode and define these five terms.*

11. subhepatic _____

12. pericardium _____

13. dyspneic _____

14. percutaneous _____

15. hypoglycemia _____

## SINGULAR/PLURAL RULES

Because most healthcare terms end with Greek or Latin suffixes, making a healthcare term singular or plural is not always done the same way as it is in English. The following table gives the most common singular/plural endings and the rules for using them. Examples of unusual singular/plural endings and singular/plural exercises will be included throughout the text.

### Rules for Using Singular and Plural Endings

| If a Term Ends in: | Form the Plural by: | Singular Example | Plural Example | Plural Pronounced as: |
|---|---|---|---|---|
| -a | dropping the -a and adding -ae | vertebra (a bone in the spine) VUR tuh brah | vertebrae VUR tuh bray | Long a, e, or i, depending on the term |
| -is | dropping the -is and adding -es | arthrosis (an abnormal condition of a joint) ar THROH sis | arthroses ar THROH seez | seez |
| -ix or -ex | dropping the -ix or -ex and adding -ices | appendix ap PEN dicks | appendices ap PEN dih seez | seez |
| -itis | dropping the -itis and adding -itides | arthritis (inflammation of a joint) ar THRY tiss | arthritides ar THRIH tih deez | deez |
| -nx | dropping the -nx and adding -nges | phalanx (a bone in the fingers or toes) FAY lanks | phalanges fuh LAN jeez | ng (as in sing) and jeez |
| -um | dropping the -um and adding an -a | endocardium (the structure inside the heart) en doh KAR dee um | endocardia en doh KAR dee ah | ah |
| -us | dropping the -us and adding an -i | digitus (a finger or toe) DIJ ih tus | digiti DIJ ih tye | eye |
| -y | dropping the -y and adding -ies | therapy (a treatment) THAIR ah pee | therapies THAIR ah peez | eez |

### Exercise 8: Plurals

*Change the singular terms to plural using the rules given in the preceding table.*

1. esophag**us** (the tube joining the throat with the stomach) _____

2. lary**nx** (the voice box) _____

3. forn**ix** (an arched structure) _____

4. pleu**ra** (the sac surrounding the lungs) _____

5. diagno**sis** _____

6. myocardi**um** _____

7. cardiomyopath**y** _____

8. hepat**itis** _____

## Pronunciation of Unusual Letter Combinations

| Spelling | Pronunciation | Term | Meaning |
|---|---|---|---|
| eu | you | **eu**thyroid<br>yoo THIGH royd | Good, healthy thyroid function. |
| ph | f (fill) | **ph**alanx<br>FAY lanks | One of the bones of the fingers or toes. |
| pn | n (no) | **pn**eumonitis<br>noo moh NYE tis | Inflammation of the lungs. |
| ps | s (sort) | **ps**ychology<br>sye KALL uh jee | Study of the mind. |
| pt | t (top) | **pt**osis<br>TOH sis | Prolapse, drooping. |
| rh, rrh | r (row) | **rh**initis<br>rye NYE tis | Inflammation of the nose. |
| x | z (zoo) | **x**eroderma<br>zeer oh DUR mah | Condition of dry skin. |

## Exercise 9: Pronunciation of Unusual Letter Combinations

| If you hear a term starting with the sound and it's not under that letter in the dictionary: | Try looking for it under _____ in the dictionary. |
|---|---|
| z |  |
| f |  |
| n |  |
| u |  |
| t |  |
| s |  |

## Common Combining Forms

| Combining Form | Meaning | Combining Form | Meaning |
|---|---|---|---|
| arteri/o | artery | lith/o | stone |
| arthr/o | joint | mamm/o | breast |
| bacteri/o | bacteria | muscul/o | muscle |
| bi/o | living, life | my/o | muscle |
| cardi/o | heart | nat/o | birth, born |
| cephal/o | head | neur/o | nerve |
| cervic/o | neck, cervix | ophthalm/o | eye |
| chondr/o | cartilage | oste/o | bone |
| col/o | large intestine, colon | ot/o | ear |
| coron/o | crown, heart | path/o | disease |
| cut/o | skin | ped/o | child |
| cutane/o | skin | phil/o | attraction |
| cyst/o | bladder, sac | pne/o | breathing |
| dent/i | tooth | psych/o | mind |
| derm/o | skin | rhin/o | nose |
| duoden/o | duodenum | somn/o | sleep |
| electr/o | electricity | spir/o | breathing |
| enter/o | small intestine | splen/o | spleen |
| esophag/o | esophagus | therm/o | heat, temperature |
| gastr/o | stomach | tonsill/o | tonsil |
| gloss/o | tongue | trache/o | trachea, windpipe |
| glyc/o | glucose, sugar | troph/o | nourishment |
| hem/o | blood | urethr/o | urethra |
| hepat/o | liver | valvul/o | valve |
| hyster/o | uterus | ven/o | vein |
| lingu/o | tongue | vers/o | turning |
| lipid/o | lipid, fat | vertebr/o | backbone, vertebra |

# Chapter Review

*Match the word parts to their definitions.*

## WORD PART DEFINITIONS

| Prefixes | | Definition | |
|---|---|---|---|
| *a-* | 1. | _____ | between |
| *anti-* | 2. | _____ | through |
| *dys-* | 3. | _____ | near, beside |
| *inter-* | 4. | _____ | within |
| *intra-* | 5. | _____ | against |
| *par-* | 6. | _____ | no, not, without |
| *para-* | 7. | _____ | surrounding, around |
| *per-* | 8. | _____ | abnormal |
| *peri-* | 9. | _____ | before, in front of |
| *poly-* | 10. | _____ | many, much, excessive, frequent |
| *pre-* | 11. | _____ | under, below |
| *sub-* | 12. | _____ | abnormal, difficult, painful, bad |

| Suffixes | | Definition | |
|---|---|---|---|
| *-ar* | 13. | _____ | pain |
| *-dynia* | 14. | _____ | discharge, flow |
| *-ectomy* | 15. | _____ | narrowing |
| *-graphy* | 16. | _____ | tumor, mass |
| *-ia* | 17. | _____ | instrument to crush |
| *-itis* | 18. | _____ | inflammation |
| *-logy* | 19. | _____ | bursting forth |
| *-meter* | 20. | _____ | process of viewing |
| *-oma* | 21. | _____ | study of |
| *-osis* | 22. | _____ | incision, cutting |
| *-pathy* | 23. | _____ | surgical repair |
| *-plasty* | 24. | _____ | removal, resection, excision |
| *-rrhage* | 25. | _____ | process of recording |
| *-rrhaphy* | 26. | _____ | instrument to measure |
| *-rrhea* | 27. | _____ | suture |
| *-scopy* | 28. | _____ | new opening |
| *-stenosis* | 29. | _____ | abnormal condition |
| *-stomy* | 30. | _____ | disease process |
| *-tomy* | 31. | _____ | pertaining to |
| *-tripter* | 32. | _____ | condition |

## WORDSHOP

| Prefixes | Combining Forms | Suffixes |
|----------|-----------------|----------|
| an- | arteri/o | -al |
| endo- | cardi/o | -algia |
| epi- | cephal/o | -ectomy |
| hypo- | col/o | -graphy |
| neo- | enter/o | -ia |
| para- | gastr/o | -ic |
| per- | hepat/o | -id |
| peri- | hyster/o | -itis |
| poly- | nat/o | -logy |
| pre- | ophthalm/o | -megaly |
| sub- | ot/o | -scope |
| trans- | rhin/o | -scopy |
| | somn/o | -stomy |
| | splen/o | -um |

Build the following terms by combining the above word parts. Some word parts may be used more than once. Some may not be used at all. The number in parentheses indicates the number of word parts needed.

| Definition | Term |
|------------|------|
| 1. condition of without an eye (3) | |
| 2. pertaining to near the ear (3) | |
| 3. pertaining to under the liver (3) | |
| 4. inflammation of the stomach and small intestines (3) | |
| 5. instrument to view the ear (2) | |
| 6. structure surrounding the heart (3) | |
| 7. new opening of the colon (2) | |
| 8. process of recording an artery (2) | |
| 9. process of viewing within (2) | |
| 10. removal of the uterus (2) | |
| 11. the study of (many) sleep (3) | |
| 12. pertaining to before birth (3) | |
| 13. pain in the head (2) | |
| 14. pertaining to above the stomach (3) | |
| 15. enlargement of the spleen (2) | |

## *Case Study*  Studying Healthcare Terminology

Students taking a healthcare terminology class may be right out of high school, returning to college to explore a new career, or starting college after working in other fields. These students are ready to learn, to apply what they know, and to absorb the material as efficiently as possible. Maya has come straight from being senior class president in a Kansas high school, whereas Izaak is returning to college after a stint in the Peace Corps in central Africa during which he realized he wanted to become a nurse. Lukas worked for several years for the Chicago Transit Authority but now is interested in trying out a new career. Working together, these three students can bring new insights and learning strategies to a study group.

A regular time to study should be a priority for a student. For every hour of class, a student should budget 2 hours of study time outside of class. For example, Maya uses the time between her classes at school and after dinner to study. Lukas schedules his study time during part of his lunch break and after his children go to bed. Izaak studies while riding the bus to work and on weekends.

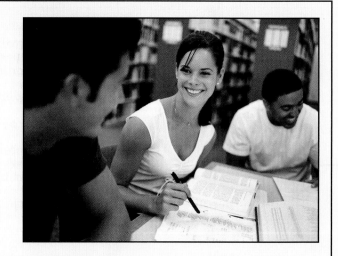

Lukas, Maya, and Izaak know that their terminology textbook is just an introduction to healthcare terminology. As professionals in the healthcare field, they will need to learn to use reference materials to enhance their understanding of terminology. For this reason, they team up and discuss the types of references and websites available to the public. Each photocopies or prints out a sample page for the others. As a result, when these are exchanged, each has a sample that illustrates that source. This familiarizes each of them with the references they may very well use some day—either in research or on the job.

You'll find fun interactive learning on the Shiland Evolve site at **http://evolve.elsevier.com/Shiland.**
Evolve Student Resources include:

- **Terminology Triage game**—sort terms into categories.
- **Wheel of Terminology game**—build terms by spinning the wheel.
- **Tournament of Terminology game**—answer questions in a multitude of med term categories.
- **Whack-a-Word Part game**—match word parts with definitions.
- **Medical Millionaire game**—earn a "million dollars" by answering questions about pathology terms.
- **Wordshop**—practice building terms.
- **Hear It, Spell It**—listen to a term, then spell it correctly.
- **Hear It, Say It**—listen to a term being pronounced, then record and listen to your own pronunciation.
- **Flash cards**—learn word parts and their definitions.
- **Body Spectrum Electronic Anatomy Coloring Book**—review anatomy.
- **iTerms audio**—listen to all terms and definitions from the text.

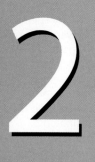

*What a piece of work is a man! How noble in reason! How infinite in faculties! In form and moving, how express and admirable! In action how like an angel! In apprehension, how like a god! the beauty of the world! the paragon of animals!*
**—William Shakespeare**

## CHAPTER OUTLINE

## OBJECTIVES

- Recognize and use terms associated with the organization of the body.
- Recognize and use terms associated with positional and directional vocabulary.
- Recognize and use terms associated with the body cavities.
- Recognize and use terms associated with the abdominopelvic regions and quadrants.
- Recognize and use terms associated with planes of the body.

# Body Structure and Directional Terminology

## CHAPTER AT A GLANCE

*Use this list of key word parts and terms to assess your knowledge. Check off the ones you have mastered.*

### KEY WORD PARTS

#### PREFIXES
- [ ] bi-
- [ ] contra-
- [ ] epi-
- [ ] ipsi-
- [ ] meta-
- [ ] mid-
- [ ] uni-

#### SUFFIXES
- [ ] -ad
- [ ] -um

#### COMBINING FORMS
- [ ] abdomin/o
- [ ] anter/o
- [ ] crani/o
- [ ] cyt/o
- [ ] dist/o
- [ ] dors/o
- [ ] hist/o
- [ ] infer/o
- [ ] later/o
- [ ] medi/o
- [ ] pelv/i
- [ ] poster/o
- [ ] proxim/o
- [ ] super/o
- [ ] thorac/o
- [ ] umbilic/o
- [ ] ventr/o
- [ ] viscer/o

### KEY TERMS

- [ ] abdominal
- [ ] anterior
- [ ] bilateral
- [ ] caudad
- [ ] cephalad
- [ ] contralateral
- [ ] cranial
- [ ] deep
- [ ] distal
- [ ] dorsal
- [ ] epigastric
- [ ] frontal plane
- [ ] hypochondriac
- [ ] hypogastric
- [ ] inferior
- [ ] inguinal
- [ ] ipsilateral
- [ ] lateral
- [ ] lumbar
- [ ] medial
- [ ] midsagittal plane
- [ ] pelvic
- [ ] posterior
- [ ] proximal
- [ ] spinal
- [ ] superficial
- [ ] superior
- [ ] thoracic
- [ ] transverse plane
- [ ] umbilical
- [ ] unilateral
- [ ] ventral
- [ ] visceral

## ORGANIZATION OF THE HUMAN BODY

The human body and its general state of health and disease may be understood by studying the various **body systems,** such as the digestive and respiratory systems. Each body system is composed of different **organs,** such as the stomach and lungs. These organs are made up of combinations of **tissues,** such as epithelial and muscular tissue, which in turn are composed of various **cells** that have very specialized functions.

All of these levels of organization are involved in a continual process of sensing and responding to conditions in the organism's environment. A negative change at one level of one system may cause a reaction throughout the entire body. **Homeostasis** (hoh mee oh STAY sis) is the normal dynamic process of balance needed to maintain a healthy body. When the body can no longer compensate for trauma or pathogens, disease, disorder, and dysfunction result.

### Cells

The smallest unit of the human body is the cell. Although there are a number of different types of cells, all of them share certain characteristics, one of them being **metabolism** (muh TAB boh lih zum). Metabolism is the act of converting energy by continually building up substances by **anabolism** (an NAB boh lih zum) and breaking down substances by **catabolism** (kuh TAB boh lih zum) for use by the body. Metabolism can be described as an equation:

$$\text{Metabolism} = \text{Anabolism} + \text{Catabolism}$$

See Fig. 2-1 for an illustration of a cell and the corresponding table below for a brief description of the pictured organelles and their functions.

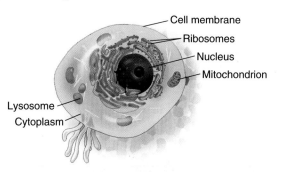

Fig. 2-1 The cell.

**homeostasis**
home/o = same
-stasis = controlling

**metabolism**
meta- = change, beyond
bol/o = throwing
-ism = state of

**anabolism**
ana- = up, apart
bol/o = throwing
-ism = state of

**catabolism**
cata- = down
bol/o = throwing
-ism = state of

## Cell Parts

| Cell Part | Word Origin | Function |
|---|---|---|
| **cytoplasm**<br>SYE toh plaz um | *cyt/o* cell<br>*-plasm* formation | Holds the organelles of the cell. |
| **lysosome**<br>LYE soh sohm | *lys/o* dissolving<br>*-some* body | Organelle that serves a digestive function for the cell. |
| **ribosome**<br>RYE boh sohm | *rib/o* ribose<br>*-some* body | Site of protein formation; contains RNA. |
| **mitochondrion** (*pl.* mitochondria)<br>mye toh KAHN dree un | *mitochondri/o* mitochondria<br>*-on* structure | Converts nutrients to energy in the presence of oxygen. |
| **nucleus** (*pl.* nuclei)<br>NOO klee us | *nucle/o* nucleus<br>*-us* structure | Control center of cell; contains DNA, which carries genetic information. |

You can review the cell structure by clicking on **Body Spectrum Electronic Anatomy Coloring Book → Cell Structure.**

## Tissues

There are four major categories of **tissue.** Within each type, the tissue either is supportive (**stromal** [STROH mull] tissue) or does the actual work (**parenchymal** [pair EN kuh mull] tissue) of the organ. For example, parenchymal nerve cells are the neurons that conduct the nervous impulse. Neuroglia are stromal nerve cells that enhance and support the functions of the nervous system. The four types of tissue include the following:

**Epithelial** (eh puh THEE lee ul): acts as an internal or external covering for organs, for example, the outer layer of the skin or the lining of the digestive tract. Note that the derivation of the term includes a combining form for the nipple (thel/e). Originally the term epithelium was used to describe the membrane covering the nipple. Later the usage was expanded to include all surface membranes whether on the skin or mucosal membrane surfaces that communicate with the outside of the body.

**Connective:** includes a variety of types, all of which have an internal structural network. Examples include bone, blood, and fat.

**Muscular:** includes three types, all of which share the unique property of being able to contract and relax. Examples include heart muscle, skeletal muscle, and visceral muscle.

**Nervous:** includes cells that provide transmission of information to regulate a variety of functions, for example, neurons (nerve cells).

## Organs

Organs, also referred to as **viscera** (VIH sur ah) (*sing.* viscus), are arrangements of various types of tissue that accomplish specific purposes. The heart, for example, is made up of muscle tissue, called **myocardium** (mye oh KAR dee um), and it is lined with epithelial tissue known as **endocardium** (en doh KAR dee um). Organs are grouped within body systems but do have specific terms to describe their parts.

### Parts of Organs

Organs can be divided into parts and have a set of terms that describe these various parts. See the table on p. 30.

---

**tissue** = hist/o

**stromal** = strom/o

**parenchymal**
  par- = near
  en- = in
  chym/o = juice
  -al = pertaining to

**epithelial**
  epi- = upon
  thel/e = nipple
  -al = pertaining to

**muscle** = my/o

**nervous** = neur/o

**organ** = viscer/o

**myocardium**
  my/o = muscle
  cardi/o = heart
  -um = structure

**endocardium**
  endo- = within
  cardi/o = heart
  -um = structure

## Parts of Organs

| | Term | Combining Form | Definition |
|---|---|---|---|
| | **apex**<br>A pecks | *apic/o* | The pointed extremity of a conical structure (*pl.* apices). |
| | **body** (corporis)<br>KOR por iss | *corpor/o*<br>*som/o*<br>*somat/o* | The largest or most important part of an organ. |
| | **fornix**<br>FOR nicks | *fornic/o* | Any vaultlike or arched structure (*pl.* fornices). |
| | **fundus**<br>FUN dis | *fund/o* | The base or deepest part of a hollow organ that is farthest from the mouth of the organ (*pl.* fundi). |
| | **hilum**<br>HYE lum | *hil/o* | Recess, exit, or entrance of a duct into a gland, or of a nerve and vessels into an organ (*pl.* hila). |
| | **lumen**<br>LOO min | *lumin/o* | The space within an artery, vein, intestine, or tube (*pl.* lumina). |
| | **sinus**<br>SYE nus | *sin/o, sinus/o* | A cavity or channel in bone, a dilated channel for blood, or a cavity that permits the escape of purulent (pus-filled) material (*pl.* sinuses). **Antrum** (*pl.* antra) and **sinus** are synonyms. |
| | **vestibule**<br>VES tih byool | *vestibul/o* | A small space or cavity at the beginning of a canal. |

## Exercise 1: Intracellular Functions

*Match each cell part with its function.*

____ 1. mitochondria  ____ 4. lysosomes     A. directs and replicates the cell

                                            B. watery solution within cell, holds organelles

____ 2. ribosomes     ____ 5. cytoplasm     C. contain enzymes to digest material

                                            D. responsible for energy production

____ 3. nucleus                             E. synthesize proteins

## Exercise 2: Types of Tissue

*Match the characteristics of the tissue with its type.*

____ 1. contracts tissue      ____ 3. has an internal structural network      A. nervous

____ 2. transmits information    ____ 4. is an internal/external body covering    B. epithelial
     C. muscular
     D. connective

## Exercise 3: Organ Parts

*Match the combining forms with their meanings.*

____ 1. fund/o      ____ 6. fornic/o      A. cavity/channel in bone/organ

____ 2. lumin/o     ____ 7. hil/o      B. pointed extremity of conical structure
     C. archlike structure

____ 3. sin/o      ____ 8. corpor/o      D. base or deepest part of a hollow organ
     E. entrance/exit/recess for ducts/vessels

____ 4. apic/o      F. space within an artery or tube
     G. largest, most important part of organ, body

____ 5. vestibul/o      H. small space at beginning of a canal

## Exercise 4: Pertaining to Organ Parts

*Fill in the blanks with the definitions of the following terms.*

1. intraluminal _____

2. hilar _____

3. periapical _____

4. antral _____

5. nuclear _____

6. cytoplasmic _____

7. extracorporeal _____

8. vestibular _____

9. fundal _____

*Fill in the blank with the correct organ part.*

10. Fatty deposits may form in the _____ (space within) of the arteries, resulting in atherosclerosis.

11. Hector had a stone that was obstructing urine flow at the level of the _____ (exit/entrance) of the right kidney.

12. The x-rays showed a blunted _____ (tip) of the left lung.

13. The _____ (largest part) of the stomach was described as inflamed.

14. The paranasal _____ (cavities in bone) were completely blocked.

## Body Systems

⊗ **Be Careful!**

*Do not confuse **my/o**, the combining form for muscle, and **myel/o**, the combining form for spinal cord or bone marrow.*

The organs of the body systems work together to perform certain defined functions. For example, movement is a function of the musculoskeletal system. Although each system has a number of functions, one must remember that the systems interact, and problems with one system can affect the function of other systems. For example, in the condition called *secondary hypertension*, disease in one body system (usually the lungs) causes a pathologic increase in blood pressure in the cardiovascular system. This hypertensive pressure is secondary to the primary cause (lung disease). Once the disorder of the initial system resolves, the hypertension disappears.

The following table lists each body system, its function, its related organs, and some of the combining forms used to describe conditions and disorders.

## Body Systems

| Body System | Functions |
|---|---|
| **musculoskeletal**<br>muss kyoo loh SKELL uh tul | Support, movement, protection |
| **integumentary**<br>in teg yoo MEN tuh ree | Cover and protection |
| **gastrointestinal**<br>gass troh in TESS tih nul | Nutrition |
| **urinary**<br>YOOR ih nair ee | Elimination of nitrogenous waste |
| **reproductive** | Reproduction |
| **blood/lymphatic/immune**<br>lim FAT tick | Transportation of nutrients/waste, protection |
| **cardiovascular**<br>kar dee oh VASS kyoo lur | Transportation of blood |
| **respiratory**<br>RESS pur ah tore ee | Delivers oxygen to cells and removes carbon dioxide |
| **nervous/behavioral**<br>NER vus | Receive/process information |
| **special senses** | Information gathering |
| **endocrine**<br>EN doh krin | Effects changes through chemical messengers |

## Exercise 5: Body Systems and Functions

____ 1. information gathering

____ 2. delivers oxygen to cells and removes carbon dioxide

____ 3. reproduction

____ 4. cover and protection

____ 5. transportation of nutrients/waste, protection

____ 6. effects changes through chemical messages

____ 7. receive/process information

____ 8. nutrition

____ 9. transportation of blood

____ 10. support, movement, protection

____ 11. elimination of nitrogenous waste

A. integumentary
B. gastrointestinal
C. male reproductive
D. musculoskeletal
E. endocrine
F. special senses
G. blood, lymphatic, and immune
H. respiratory
I. female reproductive
J. nervous
K. urinary
L. cardiovascular

## Combining Forms for Body Organization

| Meaning | Combining Form | Adjective Form |
|---|---|---|
| blood | hem/o, hemat/o | hematic |
| bone | oste/o, osse/o | osseous, osteal |
| breakdown, dissolve | lys/o | lytic |
| cell | cyt/o, cellul/o | cellular |
| epithelium | epitheli/o | epithelial |
| fat | adip/o | adipose |
| heart | cardi/o | cardiac |
| heart muscle | myocardi/o | myocardial |
| juice | chym/o | chymous |
| muscle | my/o, muscul/o | muscular |
| nerve | neur/o | neural |
| nipple | thel/e | thelial |
| nucleus | kary/o, nucle/o | nuclear |
| organ, viscera | organ/o, viscer/o | visceral |
| same | home/o | |
| stroma | strom/o | stromal |
| system | system/o | systemic |
| tissue | hist/o | |
| to throw, throwing | bol/o | |

## Prefixes for Body Organization

| Prefix | Meaning |
|---|---|
| ana- | up, apart, away |
| cata- | down |
| en- | in |
| endo- | within |
| epi- | above, upon |
| meta- | beyond, change |
| para- | near, beside, abnormal |
| supra- | upward, above |

## Suffixes for Body Organization

| Suffix | Meaning |
|---|---|
| -al, -ous | pertaining to |
| -ia, -ism | condition, state of |
| -on | structure |
| -plasm | formation |
| -some | body |
| -stasis | controlling, stopping |
| -um | structure, thing, membrane |
| -us | structure |

## Specialties/Specialists and General Terms

The levels of organization of the body are accompanied by a number of specialties and their associated specialists.

| Term | Word Origin | Definition |
|---|---|---|
| **cytology**<br>sigh TALL uh gee | *cyt/o* cell<br>*-logy* study of | The study of the cells. A **cytologist** specializes in the study of the cell. The suffix **-logist** means "one who specializes in the study of." |
| **histology**<br>his TALL uh gee | *hist/o* tissue<br>*-logy* study of | The study of tissues. A **histologist** specializes in the study of tissues. |
| **anatomy**<br>ah NAT uh mee | *ana-* up, apart, away<br>*-tomy* incision, cutting | To cut apart; the study of the structure of the body. An **anatomist** specializes in the structure of the body. |
| **physiology**<br>fiz ee ALL uh gee | *physi/o* growth<br>*-logy* study of | The study of growth; the study of the function of the body. A **physiologist** specializes in the study of the function of the body. |
| **pathology**<br>pah THOL uh gee | *path/o* disease<br>*-logy* study of | The study of disease. A **pathologist** specializes in the study of disease. |
| **biopsy**<br>BYE op see | *bi/o* life, living<br>*-opsy* process of viewing | Process of viewing living tissue that has been removed for the purpose of diagnosis and/or treatment. |
| **necropsy**<br>NEH krop see | *necr/o* death, dead<br>*-opsy* process of viewing | Process of viewing dead tissue. |
| **autopsy**<br>AH top see | *auto-* self<br>*-opsy* process of viewing | Process of viewing by self; term commonly used to describe the examination of a dead body to determine cause(s) of death. |

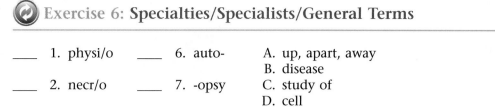

## Exercise 6: Specialties/Specialists/General Terms

____ 1. physi/o      ____ 6. auto-       A. up, apart, away
                                         B. disease
____ 2. necr/o       ____ 7. -opsy       C. study of
                                         D. cell
____ 3. ana-         ____ 8. path/o      E. self
                                         F. one who specializes in the study of
____ 4. bi/o         ____ 9. -logy       G. death, dead
                                         H. process of viewing
____ 5. cyt/o        ____ 10. -logist    I. life, living
                                         J. growth

## Exercise 7: Decoding Terms

*Write the meanings of the following terms.*

1. cytology _____

2. pathologist _____

3. necropsy _____

4. histologist _____

5. biopsy _____

## ANATOMIC POSITION AND SURFACE ANATOMY

Now that you understand the levels of organization of the body, you need the terms that describe locations, positions, and directions on the body. A standard frame of reference, the **anatomic position**, is the position in which the body stands erect with face forward, arms at the sides, palms forward, with toes pointed forward. This position is used to describe the surface anatomy of the body, both front (ventral) and back (dorsal). Figure 2-2 shows the anatomic position, both front and back, and is labeled with all the surface anatomy labels you will encounter throughout this text.

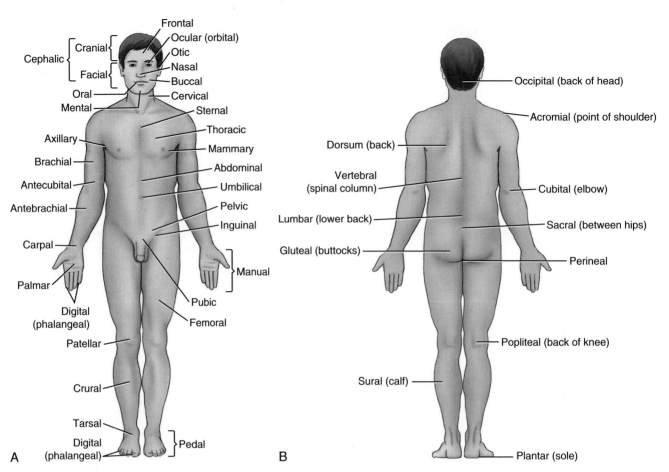

**Fig. 2-2 A,** Ventral surface anatomy. **B,** Dorsal surface anatomy.

## Ventral Surface Anatomy Terms (Head and Neck)

| Term | Word Origin | Definition |
|---|---|---|
| **buccal** <br> BUCK uhl | *bucc/o* cheek <br> *-al* pertaining to | Pertaining to the cheek. |
| **cephalic** <br> seh FAL ik | *cephal/o* head <br> *-ic* pertaining to | Pertaining to the head. |
| **cervical** <br> SUR vik uhl | *cervic/o* neck <br> *-al* pertaining to | Pertaining to the neck. **Collum** is a term that refers to the entire neck. |
| **cranial** <br> KRAY nee uhl | *crani/o* skull <br> *-al* pertaining to | Pertaining to the skull. |
| **facial** <br> FAY shuhl | *faci/o* face <br> *-al* pertaining to | Pertaining to the face. |
| **frontal** <br> FRUN tuhl | *front/o* front <br> *-al* pertaining to | Pertaining to the front, the forehead. |
| **mental** <br> MEN tuhl | *ment/o* chin <br> *-al* pertaining to | Pertaining to the chin. |

## Ventral Surface Anatomy Terms (Head and Neck)—cont'd

| Term | Word Origin | Definition |
|------|-------------|------------|
| **nasal**<br>NAY zuhl | *nas/o* nose<br>*-al* pertaining to | Pertaining to the nose. |
| **ocular**<br>AHK you lar | *ocul/o* eye<br>*-ar* pertaining to | Pertaining to the eye. |
| **oral**<br>OR uhl | *or/o* mouth<br>*-al* pertaining to | Pertaining to the mouth. |
| **otic**<br>OH tik | *ot/o* ear<br>*-ic* pertaining to | Pertaining to the ear. Also called **auricular**. |

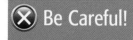 **Be Careful!** *The term **mental** means pertaining to the chin as well as pertaining to the mind.*

## Ventral Surface Anatomy (Trunk)

| Term | Word Origin | Definition |
|------|-------------|------------|
| **abdominal**<br>ab DOM ih nuhl | *abdomin/o* abdomen<br>*-al* pertaining to | Pertaining to the abdomen. |
| **axillary**<br>AKS ih lay ree | *axill/o* axilla (armpit)<br>*-ary* pertaining to | Pertaining to the armpit. |
| **coxal**<br>KOKS uhl | *cox/o* hip<br>*-al* pertaining to | Pertaining to the hip. |
| **deltoid**<br>DELL toyd | *delt/o* triangular<br>*-oid* resembling | Pertaining to the deltoid muscle covering the shoulder. The combining form **om/o** is often used for the shoulder. |
| **inguinal**<br>IN gwin uhl | *inguin/o* groin<br>*-al* pertaining to | Pertaining to the groin. |
| **mammary**<br>MAM ah ree | *mamm/o* breast<br>*-ary* pertaining to | Pertaining to the breast. |
| **pelvic**<br>PELL vik | *pelv/o, pelv/i* pelvis<br>*-ic* pertaining to | Pertaining to the pelvis. |
| **pubic**<br>PEW bik | *pub/o* pubis<br>*-ic* pertaining to | Pertaining to the pubis. |
| **sternal**<br>STIR nuhl | *stern/o* sternum (breastbone)<br>*-al* pertaining to | Pertaining to the breastbone. |
| **thoracic**<br>thor AS ik | *thorac/o* chest<br>*-ic* pertaining to | Pertaining to the chest. Also called **pectoral**. |
| **umbilical**<br>um BILL ih kuhl | *umbilic/o* umbilicus (navel)<br>*-al* pertaining to | Pertaining to the umbilicus. |

## Ventral Surface Anatomy (Arms and Legs)

| Term | Word Origin | Definition |
|------|-------------|------------|
| **antecubital**<br>an tee KYOO bit uhl | *ante-* forward, in front of, before<br>*cubit/o* elbow<br>*-al* pertaining to | Pertaining to the front of the elbow. |
| **brachial**<br>BRAY kee uhl | *brachi/o* arm<br>*-al* pertaining to | Pertaining to the arm. **Antebrachial** means pertaining to the forearm. |
| **carpal**<br>KAR puhl | *carp/o* wrist<br>*-al* pertaining to | Pertaining to the wrist. |
| **crural**<br>KRUR uhl | *crur/o* leg<br>*-al* pertaining to | Pertaining to the leg. |
| **digital**<br>DIJ ih tuhl | *digit/o* finger/toe<br>*-al* pertaining to | Pertaining to the finger/toe. **Phalangeal** means pertaining to the bones in the fingers/toes. |
| **femoral**<br>FEM or uhl | *femor/o* thigh<br>*-al* pertaining to | Pertaining to the thigh. |
| **manual**<br>MAN you uhl | *man/u* hand<br>*-al* pertaining to | Pertaining to the hand. |
| **palmar**<br>PALL mar | *palm/o* palm<br>*-ar* pertaining to | Pertaining to the palm. Also termed **volar**. |
| **patellar**<br>pah TELL ar | *patell/o, patell/a* kneecap<br>*-ar* pertaining to | Pertaining to the kneecap. |
| **pedal**<br>PED uhl | *ped/o* foot<br>*-al* pertaining to | Pertaining to the foot. |
| **plantar**<br>PLAN tur | *plant/o* sole<br>*-ar* pertaining to | Pertaining to the sole of the foot. |
| **tarsal**<br>TAR suhl | *tars/o* ankle<br>*-al* pertaining to | Pertaining to the ankle. |

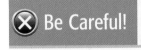 **Be Careful!** *Ped/o means foot in the term pedal, but it can mean child or children in terms such as pediatrics and pedodontics.*

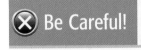 **Be Careful!** *Man/o means pressure or scanty but* **man/u** *and* **man/i** *mean hand.*

## Dorsal Surface Anatomy Terms

| Term | Word Origin | Definition |
|------|-------------|------------|
| **acromial**<br>ak ROH mee uhl | *acromi/o* acromion<br>*-al* pertaining to | Pertaining to the acromion (highest point of shoulder). |
| **dorsal**<br>DOR suhl | *dors/o* back<br>*-al* pertaining to | Pertaining to the back. |
| **gluteal**<br>GLOO tee uhl | *glute/o* buttocks<br>*-al* pertaining to | Pertaining to the buttocks. |

## Dorsal Surface Anatomy Terms—cont'd

| Term | Word Origin | Definition |
|------|-------------|------------|
| lumbar<br>LUM bar | *lumb/o* lower back, loin<br>*-ar* pertaining to | Pertaining to the lower back. |
| nuchal<br>NOO kull | *nuch/o* neck<br>*-al* pertaining to | Pertaining to the neck, especially the back of the neck. |
| olecranal<br>oh LEK rah nuhl | *olecran/o* elbow<br>*-al* pertaining to | Pertaining to the elbow. |
| perineal<br>pair ih NEE uhl | *perine/o* perineum<br>*-al* pertaining to | Pertaining to the perineum. The perineum is the space between the external genitalia and the anus. |
| popliteal<br>pop lih TEE uhl | *poplit/o* back of knee<br>*-eal* pertaining to | Pertaining to the back of the knee. |
| sacral<br>SAY kruhl | *sacr/o* sacrum<br>*-al* pertaining to | Pertaining to the sacrum. |
| scapular<br>SKAP yoo luhr | *scapul/o* scapula, shoulderblade<br>*-ar* pertaining to | Pertaining to the scapula. |
| sural<br>SOO ruhl | *sur/o* calf<br>*-al* pertaining to | Pertaining to the calf. |
| vertebral<br>ver TEE bruhl | *vertebr/o* vertebra, spine<br>*-al* pertaining to | Pertaining to the spine. |

## Exercise 8: Surface Anatomy Terms

*Match the word parts with their definitions.*

____ 1. cephal/o  ____ 11. glute/o

____ 2. cervic/o  ____ 12. vertebr/o

____ 3. brachi/o  ____ 13. ot/o

____ 4. sur/o  ____ 14. or/o

____ 5. ped/o  ____ 15. crani/o

____ 6. axill/o  ____ 16. man/u

____ 7. thorac/o  ____ 17. cubit/o

____ 8. mamm/o  ____ 18. plant/o

____ 9. digit/o  ____ 19. bucc/o

____ 10. carp/o  ____ 20. tars/o

A. armpit
B. wrist
C. mouth
D. breast
E. elbow
F. buttocks
G. head
H. cheek
I. backbones
J. arm
K. calf
L. ankle
M. neck
N. hand
O. sole
P. chest
Q. ear
R. foot
S. skull
T. fingers/toes

## Exercise 9: **Surface Anatomy**

*Label the regions with the appropriate surface anatomy terms.*

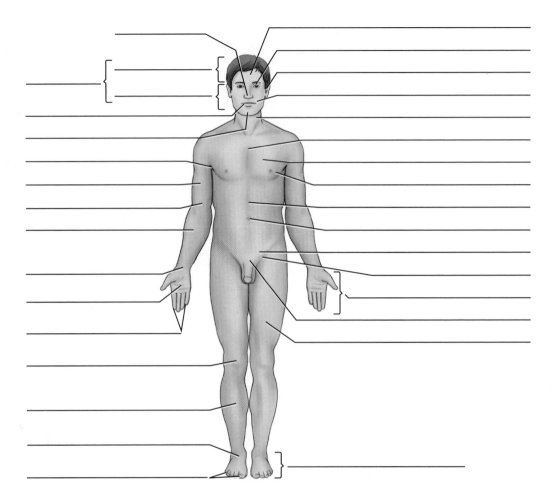

## POSITIONAL AND DIRECTIONAL TERMS

Positional and directional terms are used in healthcare terminology to describe up and down, middle and side, and front and back. Because people may be lying down, raising their arms, and so on, standard English terms cannot be used to describe direction. The following table lists directional and positional terms as opposite pairs, with their respective combining forms or prefixes and illustrations. For example, x-rays may be taken from the front of the body to the back—an anteroposterior (AP) view—or from the back to the front—a postero-anterior (PA) view (Figs. 2-3 and 2-4). The midline of the body is an imaginary line drawn from the crown of the head down between the eyes, through the chest, and separating the legs.

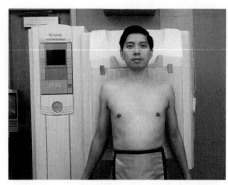

Fig. 2-3 Patient positioned for anteroposterior (AP) x-ray of the chest.

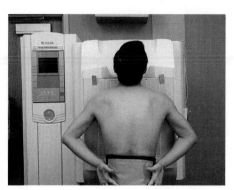

Fig. 2-4 Patient positioned for posteroanterior (PA) x-ray of the chest.

## Positional and Directional Terms

| | Term | Word Origin | Definition |
|---|---|---|---|
| | **anterior (ant)**<br>an TEER ee or<br>**ventral**<br>VEN truhl | *anter/o* front<br>*-ior* pertaining to<br>*ventr/o* belly<br>*-al* pertaining to | Pertaining to the front.<br><br>Pertaining to the belly side. |
| | **posterior (pos)**<br>poss TEER ee or<br>**dorsal**<br>DOR suhl | *poster/o* back<br>*-ior* pertaining to<br>*dors/o* back<br>*-al* pertaining to | Pertaining to the back.<br><br>Pertaining to the back of the body. |
| | **superior (sup)**<br>soo PEER ee or<br>**cephalad**<br>SEFF uhl add | *super/o* upward<br>*-ior* pertaining to<br>*cephal/o* head<br>*-ad* toward | Pertaining to upward.<br><br>Pertaining toward the head. |

*Continued*

## Positional and Directional Terms—cont'd

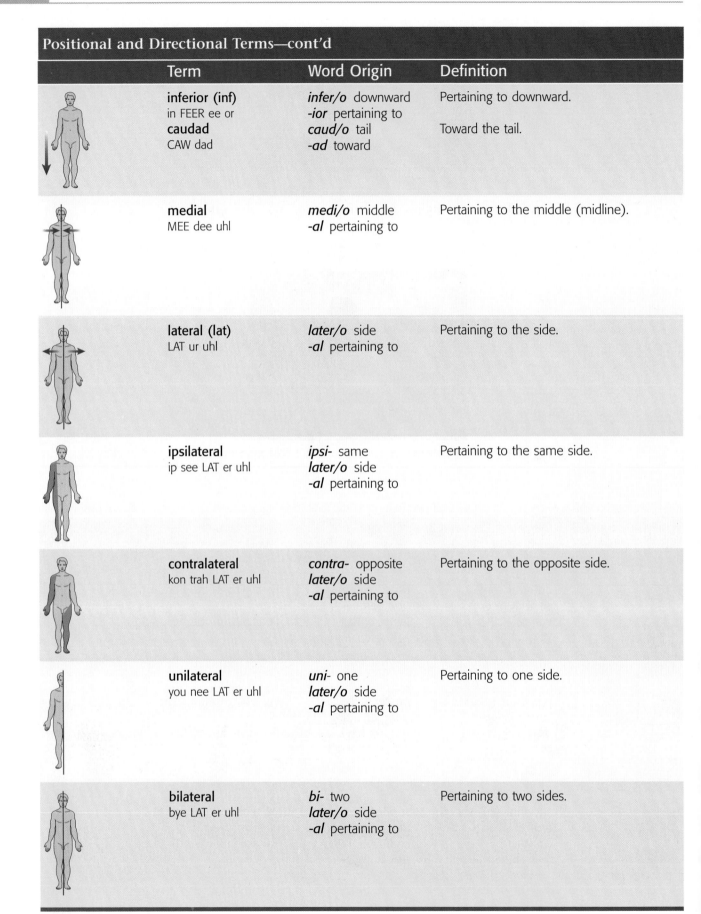

| | Term | Word Origin | Definition |
|---|---|---|---|
| | **inferior (inf)**<br>in FEER ee or<br>**caudad**<br>CAW dad | ***infer/o*** downward<br>***-ior*** pertaining to<br>***caud/o*** tail<br>***-ad*** toward | Pertaining to downward.<br><br>Toward the tail. |
| | **medial**<br>MEE dee uhl | ***medi/o*** middle<br>***-al*** pertaining to | Pertaining to the middle (midline). |
| | **lateral (lat)**<br>LAT ur uhl | ***later/o*** side<br>***-al*** pertaining to | Pertaining to the side. |
| | **ipsilateral**<br>ip see LAT er uhl | ***ipsi-*** same<br>***later/o*** side<br>***-al*** pertaining to | Pertaining to the same side. |
| | **contralateral**<br>kon trah LAT er uhl | ***contra-*** opposite<br>***later/o*** side<br>***-al*** pertaining to | Pertaining to the opposite side. |
| | **unilateral**<br>you nee LAT er uhl | ***uni-*** one<br>***later/o*** side<br>***-al*** pertaining to | Pertaining to one side. |
| | **bilateral**<br>bye LAT er uhl | ***bi-*** two<br>***later/o*** side<br>***-al*** pertaining to | Pertaining to two sides. |

## Positional and Directional Terms—cont'd

| | Term | Word Origin | Definition |
|---|---|---|---|
| | **superficial** (external)<br>soo per FISH uhl | | On the surface of the body. |
| | **deep** (internal) | | Away from the surface of the body. |
| | **proximal**<br>PROCK sih muhl | *proxim/o* near<br>*-al* pertaining to | Pertaining to near the origin. |
| | **distal**<br>DISS tuhl | *dist/o* far<br>*-al* pertaining to | Pertaining to far from the origin. |
| | **dextrad***<br>DEKS trad | *dextr/o* right<br>*-ad* toward | Toward the right. |
| | **sinistrad***<br>SIN is trad | *sinistr/o* left<br>*-ad* toward | Toward the left. |
| | **afferent**<br>AF fur ent | *af-* toward<br>*fer/o* to carry<br>*-ent* pertaining to | Pertaining to carrying toward a structure. |
| | **efferent**<br>EF fur ent | *ef-* away from<br>*fer/o* to carry<br>*-ent* pertaining to | Pertaining to carrying away from a structure. |
| | **supine**<br>SOO pine | | Lying on one's back. |
| | **prone**<br>PROHN | | Lying on one's belly. |

*This is the *patient's*, not the reader's, right and left.

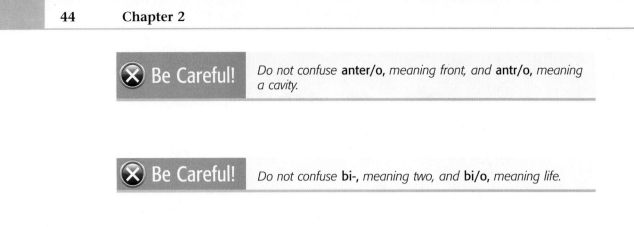

## Exercise 10: Word Parts for Positional and Directional Terms

*Match the word parts with their definitions.*

| | | | |
|---|---|---|---|
| ____ 1. bi- | ____ 10. contra- | A. same | |
| | | B. side | |
| ____ 2. infer/o | ____ 11. super/o | C. toward (suffix) | |
| | | D. upward | |
| ____ 3. anter/o | ____ 12. af- | E. right | |
| | | F. opposite | |
| ____ 4. ef- | ____ 13. sinistr/o | G. left | |
| | | H. pertaining to | |
| ____ 5. medi/o | ____ 14. ipsi- | I. two | |
| | | J. near | |
| ____ 6. proxim/o | ____ 15. dist/o | K. back | |
| | | L. away from, out | |
| ____ 7. uni- | ____ 16. dextr/o | M. middle | |
| | | N. front | |
| ____ 8. later/o | ____ 17. -ad | O. toward, in (prefix) | |
| | | P. downward | |
| ____ 9. poster/o | ____ 18. -ior | Q. far | |
| | | R. one | |

## Exercise 11: Positional and Directional Terms

*Match the definition with the correct term.*

| | | |
|---|---|---|
| ____ 1. medial | ____ 7. prone | A. pertaining to downward |
| | | B. pertaining to carrying away from a structure |
| ____ 2. inferior | ____ 8. deep | C. pertaining to the middle |
| | | D. pertaining to the opposite side |
| ____ 3. distal | ____ 9. contralateral | E. away from the surface of the body |
| | | F. pertaining to far from the origin |
| ____ 4. anterior | ____ 10. ipsilateral | G. pertaining to carrying toward a structure |
| | | H. pertaining to the same side |
| ____ 5. dorsal | ____ 11. afferent | I. pertaining to the back of the body |
| | | J. lying on one's back |
| ____ 6. supine | ____ 12. efferent | K. pertaining to the front |
| | | L. lying on one's belly |

# *Case Study* John Greco

John Greco has been suffering for years from heartburn and the sensation of food getting stuck partway down his throat. He has been taking 30 mg of Prevacid daily for the past 5 years and has been careful about what he eats, staying away from spicy foods and carbonated beverages. Lately, however, his heartburn has become worse, and his physician refers him to a gastroenterologist. Dr. Perez performs an endoscopy, which reveals a narrowing close to the cardiac sphincter. She also performs a biopsy, which is positive for the bacterium *Helicobacter. pylori*. John's stricture (narrowing) is dilated, and he is given an antibiotic to treat the *H. pylori*.

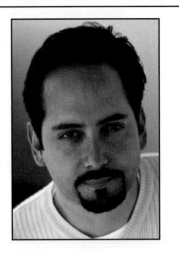

---

Greco, John J - 759990 Opened by Perez, Raechel, MD

Task   Edit   View   Time Scale   Options   Help

| Greco, John J | Age: 33 years | Sex: Male | Loc: CMH-STL |
|---|---|---|---|
| | DOB: 01/27/1979 | MRN: 759990 | FIN: 5411777 |

Reference Text Browser | Form Browser | Medication Profile

Orders | Last 48 Hours | ED | Lab | Radiology | Assessments | **Surgery** | Clinical Notes | Pt. Info | Pt. Schedule | Task List | I & O | MAR

Flowsheet: Surgery   Level: Operative Report   ● Table ○ Group ○ List

**Navigator**
✓ Operative Report

Preoperative diagnosis:     Esophagitis with stricture
Postoperative diagnosis:    Same, along with gastritis
Surgical procedure:          Upper GI endoscopy with biopsy

33-year-old male with a long history of gastroesophageal reflux, history of strictures, recommended for GI endoscopy. The patient was taken to the endoscopy suite, and under topical anesthetic, the endoscope was inserted without difficulty. The **proximal** and midesophagus were normal. The **distal** esophagus showed signs of reflux with circumferential structure. Upon entering the stomach, it was filled with bile. No **proximal** lesions. A biopsy was performed on the antrum for *Helicobacter*. Pyloric channel and duodenum were clean. J-maneuver revealed no fundic abnormalities. The endoscope was withdrawn, and the patient then was dilated with a #42 French with Hurst dilators. The patient tolerated the procedure well and returned to the recovery room in stable condition.

PROD | MAHAFC | 26 March 2012 | 12:11

## Exercise 12: Operative Report

*Using the operative report on p. 45, answer the following questions.*

1. Which organ was described as inflamed before the operation? _____

2. After the operation, which organ/organs were described as inflamed? _____

3. Translate "The proximal and midesophagus were normal." _____

4. Which end of the esophagus was farthest from the point of origin? Circle one. *(proximal esophagus, midesophagus, distal esophagus)*

## BODY CAVITIES

**dorsal = dors/o**

**ventral = ventr/o**

The body is divided into five cavities (Fig. 2-5). Two of these five cavities are in the back of the body and are called the **dorsal** (DOOR sul) **cavities.** The other three cavities are in the front of the body and are called the **ventral** (VEN trul) **cavities.** Most of the body's organs are in one of these five body cavities.

### Dorsal Cavities

**cranial = crani/o**

**spinal = spin/o**

The **cranial** (KRAY nee ul) **cavity** contains the brain and is surrounded and protected by the cranium, or skull. The **spinal** (SPY nul) **cavity** contains the spinal cord and is surrounded and protected by the bones of the spine, or vertebrae.

### Ventral Cavities

**thoracic = thorac/o**

**sternum = stern/o**

**vertebrae = vertebr/o**

**pleural = pleur/o**

**mediastinum = mediastin/o**

The **thoracic** (thoh RASS ick) cavity contains the heart, lungs, esophagus, and trachea (windpipe) and is protected by the ribs, the **sternum** (breastbone), and the **vertebrae** (backbones). This chest cavity is further divided into the two **pleural** (PLOOR ul) **cavities** that contain the lungs; the **mediastinum** (mee dee uh STY num), the space between the lungs; and the **pericardial** (pair ih KAR dee ul) **cavity** that holds the heart.

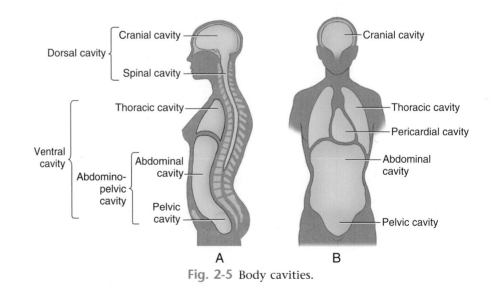

**Fig. 2-5** Body cavities.

The pleura is a double-folded serous (watery) membrane that serves to provide a small amount of lubrication that allows the lungs to contract and expand with minimal friction. The side of the membrane that is closest to the lung is called the **visceral pleura,** while the side that is closest to the body wall is the **parietal pleura.**

The pericardial cavity shares a similar structure to the pleural cavity, again having a double-folded serous membrane designed to avoid friction on the organ that it encloses. In this case the inner membrane is termed the **visceral pericardium,** while the outer membrane is the **parietal pericardium.**

The **abdominopelvic** (ab DOM ih noh PELL vick) **cavity** is composed of two cavities (abdominal and pelvic) that are not separated by any physical structure. Because nothing physically separates the abdominal and pelvic cavities, they are often collectively referred to as the abdominopelvic cavity.

The abdominal cavity contains the stomach, liver, gallbladder, pancreas, spleen, and intestines, while the pelvic cavity contains the bladder and reproductive organs. The only anterior protection for the abdominal cavity are the skin and muscles covering it, and in the back, just the vertebrae. It is separated from the thoracic cavity by a broad dome-shaped muscle called the **diaphragm** (DYE uh fram).

The **pelvic** (PELL vick) **cavity** contains the bladder and reproductive organs. These organs are cradled on the sides and in the back by the pelvic bones.

The entire abdominopelvic cavity is lined with yet another serous membrane called the **peritoneum** (pair ih tih NEE urn). The **parietal** (puh RYE uh tul) layer of the peritoneum lines the abdominopelvic cavity, while the **visceral** (VISS er ul) layer surrounds its organs. The term parietal is derived from a Latin term for wall, hence this layer is always the one closest to the body wall. The visceral layer of the peritoneum (or pericardium) is the one that is closest to the organ or organs that it encloses. The greater and lesser **omenta** (oh MEN tah) are extensions of the visceral peritoneum that hold and support the cavity's organs. The fold of the peritoneum that joins the parietal and visceral layers and attaches it to the posterior wall of the abdominal cavity is called the **mesentery** (MEZ eh tair ee).

---

**abdomen** = abdomin/o, celi/o, lapar/o

**diaphragm** = diaphragmat/o, diaphragm/o, phren/o

**pelvis** = pelv/o, pelv/i

**peritoneum** = peritone/o

**organ** = viscer/o

**wall** = pariet/o

❌ **Be Careful!**

The term **abdomen** refers to a region, whereas the **stomach** is an organ.

---

🔄 Exercise 13: **Body Cavities**

*Match the organ with the appropriate body cavity.*

| | | |
|---|---|---|
| ____ 1. cranial | ____ 4. spinal | A. spinal cord |
| | | B. bladder |
| ____ 2. abdominal | ____ 5. thoracic | C. stomach |
| | | D. brain |
| ____ 3. pelvic | | E. heart |

## ABDOMINOPELVIC REGIONS

The **abdominopelvic regions** are the nine regions that lie over the abdominopelvic cavity (Fig. 2-6). The area in the center of the abdominopelvic region is called the **umbilical** (um BILL ih kul) area. Laterally, to the left and right of this area, are the **lumbar** (LUM bar) regions. They are called the lumbar regions because they are bound by the lumbar vertebrae. Superior to the lumbar regions, and below the ribs, are the **hypochondriac** (hye poh KON dree ack) regions. Medial to the hypochondriac regions, and superior to the umbilical region, is

---

**abdominopelvic**
  abdomin/o = abdomen
  pelv/o = pelvis
  -ic = pertaining to

**umbilical** = umbilic/o, omphal/o

**lumbar** = lumb/o

**hypochondriac**
  hypo- = under
  chondr/o = cartilage
  -iac = pertaining to

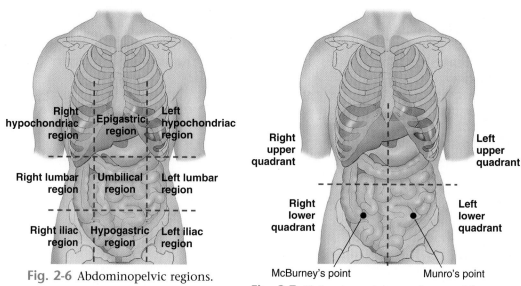

Fig. 2-6 Abdominopelvic regions.

Fig. 2-7 Abdominopelvic quadrants with Munro's and McBurney's points.

**epigastric**
　epi- = upon, above
　gastr/o = stomach
　-ic = pertaining to

**hypogastric**
　hypo- = under
　gastr/o = stomach
　-ic = pertaining to

**iliac** = ili/o

**inguinal** = inguin/o

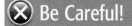 **Be Careful!**

*Do not confuse **hypo-**, meaning under or deficient, and **hyper-**, meaning above or excess.*

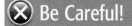 **Be Careful!**

*Do not confuse **ile/o**, meaning ileum (part of the intestine), and **ili/o**, meaning ilium (part of the hip).*

**sagittal** = sagitt/o

**mid-** = middle

**frontal** = front/o

the **epigastric** (eh pee GASS trick) region. Inferior to the umbilical region is the **hypogastric** (hye poh GASS trick) region, and lateral to the sides of the hypogastric region are, respectively, the right and left **iliac** (ILL ee ack) regions, sometimes referred to as the **inguinal** (ING gwih nul) regions.

## ABDOMINOPELVIC QUADRANTS

A simpler method of naming a location in the abdominopelvic area is to divide the area into quadrants, using the navel as the intersection. These quadrants are referred to as either right or left, upper or lower (Fig. 2-7). In the right upper quadrant (RUQ) lies the liver. In the left upper quadrant (LUQ) lie the stomach and the spleen. The appendix is in the right lower quadrant (RLQ). If a patient complains of pain in the area of **McBurney's point,** the area that is approximately two thirds of the distance between the navel and the hip bone in the RLQ, appendicitis is suspected. Except for the appendix, the left lower quadrant (LLQ) contains organs similar to the lower right. In the LLQ, halfway between the navel and the hip bone, is **Munro's point.** This is a standard site of entrance for surgeons who perform laparoscopic surgery.

## PLANES OF THE BODY

Another way of describing the body is by dividing it into planes, or flat surfaces, that are imaginary cuts or sections through the body. The use of plane terminology is common when imaging of internal body parts by computed tomography (CT) scans, magnetic resonance imaging (MRI), positron emission tomography (PET) scans, or other imaging techniques. Figs. 2-8 to 2-10 show the three body planes and corresponding views of the brain.

**Sagittal** (SAJ ih tul) **planes** are vertical planes that separate the sides from each other (see Fig. 2-8). A **midsagittal plane,** also termed the **median plane,** separates the body into equal right and left halves. The **frontal** (or **coronal** [koh ROH nul]) **plane** divides the body into front and back portions (see Fig. 2-9). The **transverse plane** (also called **cross-sectional**) divides the body horizontally into an upper part and a lower part (see Fig. 2-10). And finally, the **oblique plane,** not as commonly used as the first three, divides the body at a slanted angle.

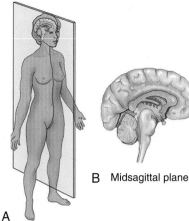
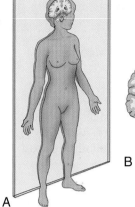

**Fig. 2-8 A,** Midsagittal plane.
**B,** Midsagittal section of the brain.

**Fig. 2-9 A,** Frontal plane. **B,** Frontal section of the brain.

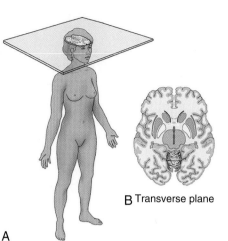

**Fig. 2-10 A,** Transverse plane.
**B,** Transverse section of the brain.

## Combining and Adjective Forms for Body Cavities, Abdominopelvic Quadrants and Regions, and Planes

| Meaning | Combining Form | Adjective Form |
|---|---|---|
| abdomen | abdomin/o, celi/o, lapar/o | abdominal, celiac |
| back | dors/o | dorsal |
| cartilage | chondr/o | chondral |
| cranium (skull) | crani/o | cranial |
| diaphragm | diaphragmat/o, diaphragm/o, phren/o | diaphragmatic, phrenic |
| front, bellyside | front/o, ventr/o | frontal, ventral |
| groin | inguin/o | inguinal |
| ileum | ile/o | ileal |
| ilium | ili/o | iliac |
| lower back, loin | lumb/o | lumbar |
| mediastinum | mediastin/o | mediastinal |
| organ | viscer/o, organ/o | visceral |
| pelvis | pelv/i, pelv/o | pelvic |
| peritoneum | peritone/o | peritoneal |
| pleura | pleur/o | pleural |
| spine | spin/o | spinal, spinous |
| sternum | stern/o | sternal |
| stomach | gastr/o | gastric |
| thorax (chest) | thorac/o | thoracic |
| umbilicus (navel) | umbilic/o, omphal/o | umbilical, omphalic |
| vertebra | vertebr/o | vertebral |
| wall | pariet/o | parietal |

## Prefixes for Body Cavities, Abdominopelvic Quadrants and Regions, and Planes

| Prefix | Meaning |
|--------|---------|
| epi- | above, upon |
| hyper- | excessive, above |
| hypo- | deficient, below, under |
| mid- | middle |
| trans- | through, across |

## Suffixes for Body Cavities, Abdominopelvic Quadrants and Regions, and Planes

| Suffix | Meaning |
|--------|---------|
| -ant, -iac, -ic | pertaining to |
| -verse | to turn |

Click on **Hear It, Spell It** to practice spelling the body structure and directional terms that you have learned in this chapter. To practice pronouncing body structure and directional terms, click on **Hear It, Say It.**

## Exercise 14: Abdominopelvic Regions

*Using your knowledge of directional terms and the nine abdominopelvic regions, answer the following questions.*

1. Superior to the umbilical region is the _____ region.

2. Lateral to the umbilical region are the left and right _____ regions.

3. Medial to the left and right inguinal regions is the _____ region.

4. Inferior to the lumbar regions are the left and right _____ regions.

5. Lateral to the epigastric region are the right and left _____ regions.

## Exercise 15: Abdominopelvic Regions

*Label the abdominopelvic regions.*

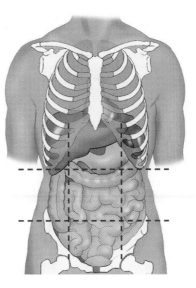

## Exercise 16: Planes of the Body

1. Which plane divides the body into superior and inferior portions? _____

2. Which plane divides the body into equal left and right sections? _____

3. Which plane divides the body into anterior and posterior sections? _____

## *Case Study*  *Elise Duncan*

Elise Duncan is a star forward on her high school's basketball team. During a game, she jumps up to grab a rebound, and as she comes down, she steps on another player's foot. Her ankle twists severely, and she falls. She is unable to stand or walk on the affected foot because of the severe pain and rapid swelling. The trainer applies ice and wraps the ankle, and Elise is taken to the ER by her parents. X-rays reveal that her ankle is broken, and that surgery is necessary to repair it. Elise is unhappy that her season has been ended prematurely, but she knows that the surgery is necessary. She undergoes surgery the next day, and it is successful.

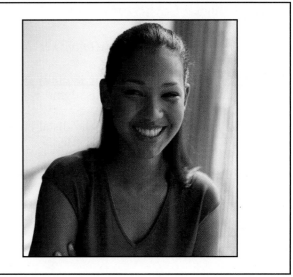

## Case Study  Elise Duncan

Duncan, Elise M - 554427 Opened by Andersen, Michelle J        _ 🗗 ✕

Task   Edit   View   Time Scale   Options   Help

As Of 07:32

| Duncan, Elise M | Age: 17 years | Sex: Female | Loc: CMH-STL |
|---|---|---|---|
| | DOB: 12/21/1995 | MRN: 554427 | FIN: 5411777 |

Reference Text Browser   Form Browser   Medication Profile

Orders | Last 48 Hours | ED | Lab | Radiology | Assessments | **Surgery** | Clinical Notes | Pt. Info | Pt. Schedule | Task List | I & O | MAR

Flowsheet: Surgery ▼ ...   Level: Operative Report ▼        ⦿ Table  ○ Group  ○ List

Navigator                      ✕

✔   Operative Report

The patient was brought to the operating room, given a spinal anesthetic, and placed in the supine position. The right ankle then was prepped and draped in the usual sterile manner. The operation was performed under tourniquet control.

(1) An incision was made laterally over the distal fibula. Initial incision went through skin and subcutaneous tissue. Bleeders throughout the procedure were treated, clamped, and electrocoagulated. The fascia then was incised, and the fracture was identified. The fracture ends were cleared and clamped in anatomic position. A 6-hole, one-third semitubular plate was placed posterolater-ally and transfixed with the screws. Anatomic position was achieved.

We then proceeded medially, (2) where a short incision was made over the medial malleolus. Initial incision went through skin and subcutaneous tissue. Bleeders throughout the procedure were treated, clamped, and electrocoagulated. The fascia was incised, and a large medial malleolar fracture fragment was identified. The fracture was freshened and then clamped. Three 3-M staples then were used to transfix the fracture. (3 and 4) Intraoperative x-rays then were taken, AP and lateral, which showed anatomic position of all fractures with the ankle joint in anatomic position.

The wound was thoroughly irrigated. Both sides were closed with 3-0 Dexon, subcutaneous tissue with 2-0 Dexon, and the skin with skin clips. A compressive dressing was applied, followed by the application of a short leg cast.

PROD | MAHAFC | 8 June 2012 | 07:32

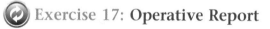

## Exercise 17: Operative Report

*Refer to the operative report above to answer the following questions. Underline the correct answer.*

1. "The incision (that) was made laterally over the distal fibula." If you know that the fibula is one of the lower lateral leg bones, the distal end is *(closer to the hip/closer to the toes)*.

2. The malleoli are processes at the distal ends of the fibula and tibia. The medial malleolus is on the *(inner surface/outer surface)* of the leg.

3. The "intraoperative x-rays" were taken *(before/during/after)* the operation.

4. The AP view of the ankle joint fracture was taken from *(back to front/front to back)*.

## Abbreviations

| Abbreviation | Definition | Abbreviation | Definition |
|---|---|---|---|
| ant | anterior | PA | posteroanterior |
| AP | anteroposterior | PET | positron emission tomography |
| CT | computed tomography | pos | posterior |
| inf | inferior | RLQ | right lower quadrant |
| lat | lateral | RUQ | right upper quadrant |
| LLQ | left lower quadrant | sup | superior |
| LUQ | left upper quadrant | | |

# Chapter Review

*Match the word parts to their definitions.*

## WORD PART DEFINITIONS

| Prefixes |
|----------|
| af- |
| bi- |
| contra- |
| ef- |
| endo- |
| epi- |
| ipsi- |
| meta- |
| uni- |

**Definition**

1. _____ above, upon
2. _____ beyond, change
3. _____ one
4. _____ within
5. _____ two
6. _____ toward
7. _____ same
8. _____ opposite
9. _____ away from

| Combining Forms |
|-----------------|
| anter/o |
| axill/o |
| brachi/o |
| caud/o |
| cephal/o |
| cervic/o |
| corpor/o |
| crani/o |
| cyt/o |
| dextr/o |
| dist/o |
| hist/o |
| infer/o |
| inguin/o |
| lapar/o |
| later/o |
| medi/o |
| poster/o |
| proxim/o |
| super/o |
| sinistr/o |
| thorac/o |
| viscer/o |

**Definition**

10. _____ organ
11. _____ downward
12. _____ front
13. _____ far
14. _____ middle
15. _____ armpit
16. _____ upward
17. _____ near
18. _____ left
19. _____ arm
20. _____ tail
21. _____ abdomen
22. _____ side
23. _____ right
24. _____ back
25. _____ tissue
26. _____ body
27. _____ head
28. _____ skull
29. _____ cell
30. _____ groin
31. _____ neck
32. _____ chest

# WORDSHOP

| Prefixes | Combining Forms | Suffixes |
|---|---|---|
| bi- | abdomin/o | -ad |
| contra- | anter/o | -al |
| hyper- | crani/o | -ar |
| hypo- | cyt/o | -ic |
| in- | dextr/o | -ia |
| inter- | gastr/o | -ior |
| intra- | hist/o | -logy |
| ipsi- | inguin/o | -oid |
| mid- | later/o | -plasm |
| supra- | lumb/o | |
| | pelv/o | |
| | poster/o | |
| | sagitt/o | |
| | super/o | |
| | thorac/o | |

Build the following terms by combining the word parts above. Some word parts may be used more than once. Some may not be used at all. The number in parentheses is the number of word parts needed to correctly build the term.

| Definition | Term |
|---|---|
| 1. pertaining to the middle of the sagittal plane (3) | |
| 2. pertaining to two sides (3) | |
| 3. toward the right (2) | |
| 4. pertaining to back to front (3) | |
| 5. pertaining to the chest (2) | |
| 6. pertaining to the abdomen and pelvis (3) | |
| 7. pertaining to the lower back (2) | |
| 8. pertaining to the opposite side (3) | |
| 9. formation of cells (2) | |
| 10. pertaining to upward (2) | |
| 11. pertaining to above the chest (3) | |
| 12. the study of tissue (2) | |
| 13. pertaining to under the stomach (3) | |
| 14. pertaining to the same side (3) | |
| 15. pertaining to within the skull (3) | |

*Sort the terms below into the correct categories.*

## TERM SORTING

| Organization of the Body | Positional and Directional Terms | Body Cavities and Planes | Abdominal Regions and Quadrants |
|---|---|---|---|
|  |  |  |  |
|  |  |  |  |
|  |  |  |  |
|  |  |  |  |
|  |  |  |  |
|  |  |  |  |
|  |  |  |  |
|  |  |  |  |
|  |  |  |  |
|  |  |  |  |

| | | | |
|---|---|---|---|
| afferent | hilum | nucleus | supine |
| anterior | hypochondriac | organ | system |
| apex | hypogastric | pleural | thoracic |
| coronal | iliac | posterior | transverse |
| cranial | inguinal | prone | umbilical |
| cytoplasm | lateral | sagittal | ventral |
| distal | lumbar | sinus | vestibule |
| efferent | lumen | spinal | viscera |
| epigastric | midsagittal | superior | |

*Replace the highlighted words with the correct terms.*

## TRANSLATIONS

1. Susie was being treated for a cut on the **pertaining to the sole of the foot** surface of her foot and a wart on **the pertaining to the palm** surface of her hand.

2. Maureen located a vein in the **pertaining to the front of the elbow** space of the patient's left arm for a blood draw.

3. The patient described her leg pain as **pertaining to two sides,** although occasionally it seemed to be only on the right.

4. Sam had cancer sores on his **pertaining to the cheek** membrane.

5. The patient had a **process of viewing living tissue that has been removed for the purpose of diagnosis** of a mole that had recently increased in size.

6. The **space within an artery, vein, intestine, or tube** of one of the patient's coronary arteries was completely blocked.

7. The paralyzed patient had fractured one of the bones in his **pertaining to the chest** spine.

8. Nora had a fracture of the **pertaining to far from the origin** phalanx of her right index finger.

9. A tumor growing in the patient's **the space between the lungs** pressed on his esophagus.

10. The damage caused by the patient's right hemispheric stroke was **pertaining to the opposite side.**

11. The patient was in a **lying on one's back** position so that the physician could examine her abdomen.

12. Jeremy complained of pain resulting from a **lateral to the sides of the hypogastric region** hernia.

13. The man had **pertaining to the chest** and **pertaining to the hip** contusions.

14. Mr. Jones had **pertaining to above the stomach** pain.

Alex McConell did not break his wrist playing tennis. No, he tripped and fell leaving the court while trying to answer his cell phone. He broke his fall with his free hand and then landed heavily on his left shoulder. Alex wanted to keep playing, but his partner insisted on taking him to the emergency department at Community Memorial Hospital.

As the doctor on call in the emergency department examines Alex, she observes a moderately distressed young man favoring his left shoulder with extensive soft tissue swelling in the left wrist area. She orders wrist and shoulder x-ray studies because she suspects Alex has a Colles' fracture of the wrist and possibly a shoulder separation.

The radiologic technologist takes posteroanterior, oblique, and lateral x-rays of Alex's left wrist and shoulder. The x-rays show a comminuted fracture of the dorsal aspect of the distal radius (Colles fracture), but the shoulder x-rays are normal.

Alex's wrist is put in a cast with a sling, and he is sent home with directions to take ibuprofen prn (as needed) for his discomfort.

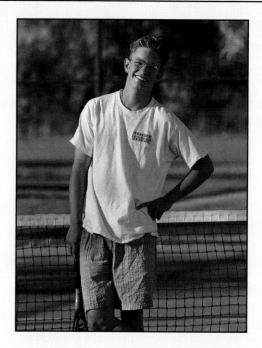

---

McConell, Alexander - 501071 Opened by Morita, Samuel J, MD    _ ⊡ ☒

Task   Edit   View   Time Scale   Options   Help

As Of 10:07

**McConell, Alexander**

Age: 29 years         Sex: Male         Loc: CMHDIC-STL
DOB: 11/06/1982       MRN: 501071       FIN: 5411777

| Reference Text Browser | Form Browser | Medication Profile |

Orders | Last 48 Hours | ED | Lab | **Radiology** | Assessments | Surgery | Clinical Notes | Pt. Info | Pt. Schedule | Task List | I & O | MAR

Flowsheet: Radiology   ▼   ...   Level: Radiology   ▼      ⦿ Table   ○ Group   ○ List

◀ ▶                                                                                  ◀ ▶

Navigator   ☒
✓   Radiology

LEFT WRIST: PA, oblique, and lateral views of the left wrist reveal a transverse fracture of the distal radius, just proximal to the epiphysis. The distal fragment is displaced and angulated posteriorly at approximately 15 degrees. The articular surface of the radius is not involved. There is soft tissue swelling adjacent to the fracture site, particularly on the dorsal aspect. No other abnormalities are noted.

Diagnosis: Colles fracture, left wrist.

PROD   MAHAFC   13 Oct 2011   10:07

## Exercise 18: Radiology Report

*Using the radiology report on p. 58, answer the following questions.*

1. Which end of the radius was fractured? The end closest to the wrist or the end nearest the elbow?

   _____

2. Was the bone displaced backward or forward? _____

3. The term *articular* means "pertaining to the _____ ."

4. What does *dorsal* mean? _____

5. A PA view means _____ .

---

For more interactive learning, go to the Shiland Evolve site, and click on:
- **Whack-A-Word-Part** to review body structure and directional terminology.
- **Wheel of Terminology** and **Word Shop** to practice word building.
- **Tournament of Terminology** to test your knowledge of body structure and directional terminology terms.
- **Terminology Triage** to categorize structural and directional terms. Keep in mind that if you recognize the suffix in each term, you will be able to categorize most of the terms correctly.

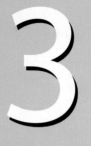

*The leadership instinct you are born with is the backbone. You develop the funny bone and the wishbone that go with it.*
**—Elaine Agather**

## OBJECTIVES

- Recognize and use terms related to the anatomy and physiology of the musculoskeletal system.
- Recognize and use terms related to the pathology
  of the musculoskeletal system.
- Recognize and use terms related to the diagnostic procedures for the musculoskeletal system.
- Recognize and use terms related to the therapeutic interventions for the musculoskeletal system.

# Musculoskeletal System

## CHAPTER AT A GLANCE

*Use this list of key word parts and terms to assess your knowledge. Check off the ones you have mastered.*

### ANATOMY AND PHYSIOLOGY

- [ ] appendicular skeleton
- [ ] articulation
- [ ] axial skeleton
- [ ] bone depression
- [ ] bone process
- [ ] bursa
- [ ] cartilage
- [ ] fascia
- [ ] ligament
- [ ] muscle
- [ ] tendon
- [ ] vertebra

### KEY WORD PARTS

#### PREFIXES
- [ ] dia-
- [ ] dys-
- [ ] endo-, end-
- [ ] epi-
- [ ] inter-
- [ ] peri-
- [ ] syn-

#### SUFFIXES
- [ ] -al
- [ ] -centesis
- [ ] -clasis
- [ ] -desis
- [ ] -graphy
- [ ] -itis
- [ ] -listhesis
- [ ] -lysis
- [ ] -malacia
- [ ] -physis
- [ ] -plasty
- [ ] -scopy
- [ ] -trophy

#### COMBINING FORMS
- [ ] arthr/o
- [ ] burs/o
- [ ] chondr/o
- [ ] cost/o
- [ ] dactyl/o
- [ ] electr/o
- [ ] fasci/o
- [ ] my/o
- [ ] myel/o
- [ ] oste/o
- [ ] plant/o
- [ ] prosthes/o
- [ ] rhabdomy/o
- [ ] spondyl/o
- [ ] syndesm/o
- [ ] tendin/o
- [ ] vertebr/o

## KEY TERMS

- ☐ arthrocentesis
- ☐ arthrodesis
- ☐ arthroplasty
- ☐ arthroscopy
- ☐ bursitis
- ☐ carpal tunnel syndrome (CTS)
- ☐ costochondritis
- ☐ electromyography (EMG)
- ☐ herniated intervertebral disk

- ☐ muscular dystrophy (MD)
- ☐ osteoarthritis (OA)
- ☐ osteoclasis
- ☐ osteomalacia
- ☐ osteomyelitis
- ☐ osteoporosis
- ☐ pathologic fractures
- ☐ plantar fasciitis
- ☐ prosthesis

- ☐ rhabdomyolysis
- ☐ rheumatoid arthritis (RA)
- ☐ spinal stenosis
- ☐ spondylosis
- ☐ spondylolisthesis
- ☐ subluxation
- ☐ syndactyly
- ☐ syndesmoplasty
- ☐ tendinitis

---

**musculoskeletal**
  muscul/o = muscle
  skelet/o = skeleton

**bone** = oste/o, oss/i, osse/o

**joint** = arthr/o, articul/o

**muscle** = muscul/o, my/o, myos/o

**ligament** = ligament/o, syndesm/o

**tendon** = tendin/o, tend/o, ten/o

**fascia** = fasci/o

**cartilage** = chondr/o, cartilag/o

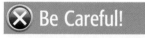 **Be Careful!**

*Do not confuse the combining form **fasci/o**, meaning fascia, with the combining form **faci/o**, meaning face.*

**hematopoiesis**
  hemat/o = blood
  -poiesis = formation

**orthopedist**
  orth/o = straight
  ped/o = child
  -ist = one who specializes

**rheumatology**
  rheumat/o = watery flow
  -logy = study of

**physiatry**
  physi/o = nature
  -iatry = process or treatment

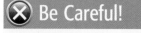 **Be Careful!**

*Don't confuse a **physiatrist** with a **psychiatrist**.*

---

## FUNCTIONS OF THE MUSCULOSKELETAL SYSTEM

The **musculoskeletal** (muss skyoo loh SKELL uh tul) **system (MS)** consists of three interrelated parts: **bones, joints (articulations),** and **muscles.** Bones are connected to one another by fibrous bands of tissue called **ligaments** (LIH gah ments). Muscles are attached to the bone by bands of tissue called **tendons** (TEN duns). The tough fibrous covering of the muscles (and some nerves and blood vessels) is called the **fascia** (FASH ee ah). **Cartilage** (KAR tih lij) is a flexible form of connective tissue that covers the ends of many bones, gives form to the external ear, and tip of the nose, and provides support and protection to many other sites in the body.

Imagine a body without bones and muscles! Where would the organ systems be placed? What would protect the vital organs? And how would a person move? The musculoskeletal system meets these needs by:

1. Acting as a framework for the organ systems
2. Protecting many of the body's organs
3. Providing the organism with the ability to move

Along with these functions, some bones are responsible for storage of minerals (calcium [Ca] and phosphorus [P]) and the continual formation of blood, a process called **hematopoiesis** (hee mah toh poh EE sis), in the bone marrow.

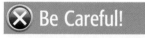 **Be Careful!**    *The combining form **ped/o** can mean child or foot.*

## SPECIALTIES/SPECIALISTS

Orthopedics is the healthcare specialty that deals with the majority of musculoskeletal disorders. Historically, the word **orthopedics** comes from **orth/o** (straight) and **ped/o** (child) because corrective procedures for disorders like knock knees and bowlegs were most successful with the softer bones of children. The specialist is called an **orthopedist.**

**Rheumatology** is a specialty that deals with disorders of connective tissue, including bone and cartilage. The origin of the term is derived from the Greeks who believed that many joint disorders were caused by an effusion (outpouring) of fluid into the joint space. The specialist is called a **rheumatologist**.

**Physiatry,** also called physical medicine, concerns diagnosis and treatment of disease or injury with the use of physical agents such as exercise, heat, massage, and light. The specialist is called a **physiatrist**.

## Exercise 1: Combining Forms for the Musculoskeletal System

*Match the musculoskeletal combining forms with their meanings. More than one answer may be correct.*

____ 1. joint          ____ 5. ligament          A. fasci/o          G. tendin/o

____ 2. bone           ____ 6. fascia            B. hemat/o          H. ligament/o

____ 3. muscle         ____ 7. cartilage         C. oste/o           I. myos/o

____ 4. tendon         ____ 8. blood             D. osse/o           J. articul/o

                                                 E. arthr/o          K. syndesm/o

                                                 F. chondr/o         L. ten/o

*Decode the following terms using your knowledge of musculoskeletal word parts and suffixes learned in Chapter 1.*

9. articular _____

10. tendinous _____

11. muscular _____

12. syndesmal _____

13. chondral _____

14. osseous _____

## ANATOMY AND PHYSIOLOGY

### Bones

#### Types of Bones

Most adult bodies contain 206 bones. These bones are categorized as belonging either to the **axial** (ACK see ul) **skeleton,** which consists of the skull, rib cage, and spine, or the **appendicular** (ap pen DICK yoo lur) **skeleton,** which consists of the shoulder bones, collar bones, pelvic bones, arms, and legs (Fig. 3-1). Human bones appear in a variety of shapes that suit their function in the body. See Fig. 3-1 and the following table for the locations and descriptions of these bones.

**appendicular** = appendic/o

**skeleton** = skelet/o

### Shapes of Human Bones

| Types | Examples |
|---|---|
| long bones | humerus (upper arm bone), femur (thigh bone) |
| short bones | carpal (wrist bone), tarsal (ankle bone) |
| flat bones | sternum (breastbone), scapula (shoulder blade) |
| irregular bones | vertebra (backbone), stapes (a bone of the ear) |
| sesamoid (SEH sah moyd) bones | patella (kneecap) |

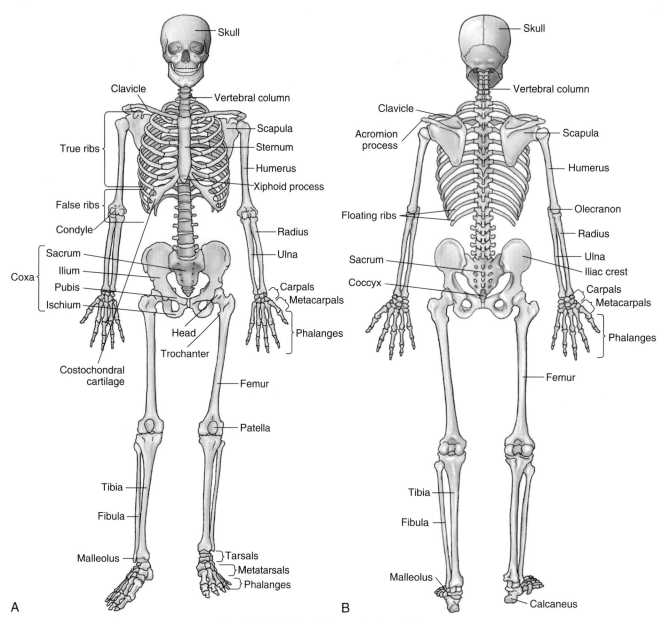

Fig. 3-1 Axial and appendicular skeleton.

**osteocyte**
  oste/o = bone
  -cyte = cell

**osteoblast**
  oste/o = bone
  -blast = embryonic

**osteoclast**
  oste/o = bone
  -clast = breaking down

**bone marrow** = myel/o

**diaphysis**
  dia- = through
  -physis = growth, nature

**epiphysis**
  epi- = above
  -physis = growth, nature

## Bone Structure

All bones are composed of mature bone cells, called **osteocytes** (OS tee oh sytes), and the material between the cells, called the **matrix** (MAY tricks). The matrix stores calcium and phosphorus for the body to use as needed in the form of mineral salts. Other types of bone cells include **osteoblasts,** cells that build bone, and **osteoclasts,** cells that break down bone cells to transform them as needed. The osteocytes and matrix together make up the hard, outer layer of bone known as **compact bone.** Within the compact bony tissue is a second layer of bone tissue called **spongy** or **cancellous** (KAN seh lus) **bone.** This spongy bone is composed of the same osteocytes and matrix, but, as its name implies, it is less dense. Within the spongy layer lie the medullary cavity and the red **bone marrow,** which produces all of the blood cells needed by the body.

Each long bone (Fig. 3-2) is composed mainly of a long shaft called the **diaphysis** (dye AFF ih sis). Each end of the bone is called an **epiphysis** (eh

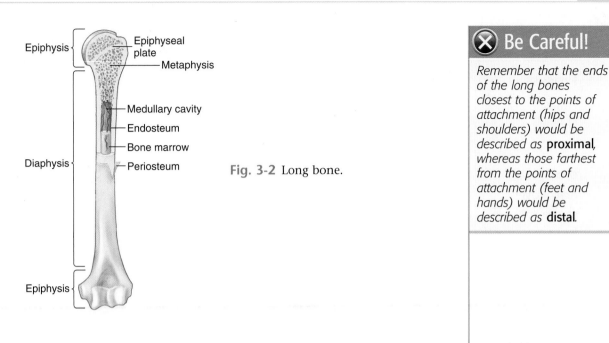

Epiphysis
- Epiphyseal plate
- Metaphysis

Diaphysis
- Medullary cavity
- Endosteum
- Bone marrow
- Periosteum

Epiphysis

**Fig. 3-2** Long bone.

**⊗ Be Careful!**

*Remember that the ends of the long bones closest to the points of attachment (hips and shoulders) would be described as* **proximal***, whereas those farthest from the points of attachment (feet and hands) would be described as* **distal***.*

PIFF ih sis) (*pl.* epiphyses). Underneath the epiphyses are the **epiphyseal** (eh pee FIZZ ee ul) **plates,** the areas where bone growth normally occurs. Around the ages from 16 to 25, the plates close, and bone growth stops. The epiphysis and epiphyseal plates together form the **metaphysis** (meh TAFF ih sis).

   The outer covering of the bone is called the **periosteum** (pair ee OS tee um), and the inner aspect of the bone is known as the **endosteum** (en DOS tee um). These two coverings hold the cells responsible for bone remodeling: osteoblasts and osteoclasts. The shape of a bone enables practitioners to speak very specifically about a particular area on that bone. For instance, any groove, opening, or hollow space is called a **depression.** Depressions provide an entrance and exit for vessels and protection for the organs they hold. Raised or projected areas are called **processes.** These are often areas of attachment for ligaments or tendons. The tables that follow give examples of bone depressions and processes.

**metaphysis**
   meta- = change
   -physis = growth, nature

**periosteum**
   peri- = surrounding
   oste/o = bone
   -um = structure

**endosteum**
   endo- = within
   oste/o = bone
   -um = structure

## Bone Depressions

| Depression | Combining Form | Meaning/Function | Example |
|---|---|---|---|
| **foramen** <br> foh RAY men (*pl.* foramina) | foramin/o | an opening or hole | foramen magnum, mental foramina |
| **fossa** <br> FAH sah (*pl.* fossae) | foss/o | a hollow or depression, especially on the surface of the end of a bone | olecranal fossa |
| **sinus** <br> SYE nus (*pl.* sinuses) | sin/o <br> sinus/o | a cavity or channel lined with a membrane | paranasal sinuses |

## Bone Processes

| Process | Combining Form | Meaning/Function | Example |
|---------|---------------|------------------|---------|
| **condyle**<br>KON dyle | condyl/o | a rounded projection at the end of a bone that anchors the ligaments and articulates with adjacent bones | medial condyle of the femur |
| **crest** | | a narrow elongated elevation | iliac crest |
| **epicondyle**<br>eh pee KON dyle | epicondyl/o | a projection on the surface of the bone above the condyle | lateral epicondyle of the humerus |
| **head** | | a rounded, usually proximal portion of some long bones | femoral head, humeral head |
| **spine** | spin/o | a thornlike projection | spinous process of a vertebra |
| **trochanter**<br>troh KAN tur | trochanter/o | one of two bony projections on the proximal ends of the femurs that serve as points of attachment for muscles | greater trochanter |
| **tubercle**<br>TOO bur kuhl | tubercul/o | a nodule or small raised area | costal tubercle |
| **tuberosity**<br>too bur OSS ih tee | | an elevation or protuberance, larger than a tubercle | ischial tuberosity |

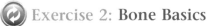 Exercise 2: **Bone Basics**

*Match the bone word parts with their meanings.*

_____  1. myel/o        _____  9. -blast         A. trochanter
                                                 B. foramen, hole
_____  2. -physis       _____  10. epi-          C. above, upon
                                                 D. cell
_____  3. peri-         _____  11. foss/o        E. bone marrow
                                                 F. surrounding, around
_____  4. condyl/o      _____  12. endo-         G. embryonic
                                                 H. spine
_____  5. spin/o        _____  13. trochanter/o  I. breaking down
                                                 J. growth
_____  6. sin/o         _____  14. -cyte         K. hollow, depression
                                                 L. condyle, knob
_____  7. foramin/o     _____  15. -clast        M. within
                                                 N. sinus, cavity
_____  8. -um                                    O. structure

*Fill in the blank.*

16. Osteoblasts _____ bone, whereas osteoclasts _____ bone.

17. The shaft of a long bone is called the _____; the ends of a long bone are called
    _____(plural!).

18. The outer covering of bone is the _____, whereas the inner lining is the
    _____.

19. A foramen, a sinus, and a fossa are examples of bone _____. A condyle, a trochanter,
    and a tuberosity are examples of bone _____.

20. A synonym for a sinus is a/an _____.

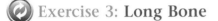 Exercise 3: **Long Bone**

*Label the long bone with the labels provided.*

diaphysis
epiphysis
bone marrow
periosteum
endosteum
medullary cavity
epiphyseal plate

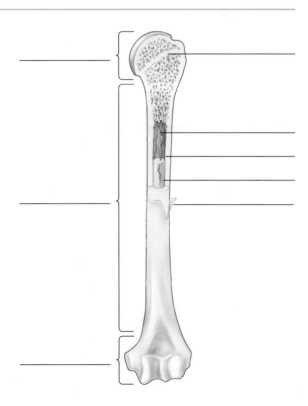

## AXIAL SKELETON

The axial skeleton includes the skull, spine, and rib cage (see Fig. 3-1).

### Skull

skull, cranium = crani/o

face = faci/o

frontal = front/o

parietal = pariet/o

occipital = occipit/o

temporal = tempor/o

mastoid = mastoid/o

ethmoid = ethmoid/o

sphenoid = sphenoid/o

The skull is made up of two parts: the **cranium** (KRAY nee um) that encloses and protects the brain and the **facial bones** (Fig. 3-3).

#### Cranium
**Frontal bone:** Forms the anterior part of the skull and the forehead.
**Parietal** (puh RYE uh tul) **bones:** Form the sides of the cranium.
**Occipital** (ock SIP ih tul) **bone:** Forms the back of the skull. Notable is a large hole at the ventral surface in this bone, the foramen magnum (meaning *large*), which allows brain communication with the spinal cord.
**Temporal** (TEM poor ul) **bones:** Form the lower two sides of the cranium. The **mastoid process** is the posterior part of the bone behind the ear.
**Ethmoid** (EHTH moyd) **bone:** Forms the roof and walls of the nasal cavity.
**Sphenoid** (SFEE noyd) **bone:** Anterior to the temporal bones and the basilar part of the occipital bone.
**Paranasal sinuses:** Air-filled cavities that are named for the bones in which they are located. Each is lined with a mucous membrane (Fig 3-3, *B*).

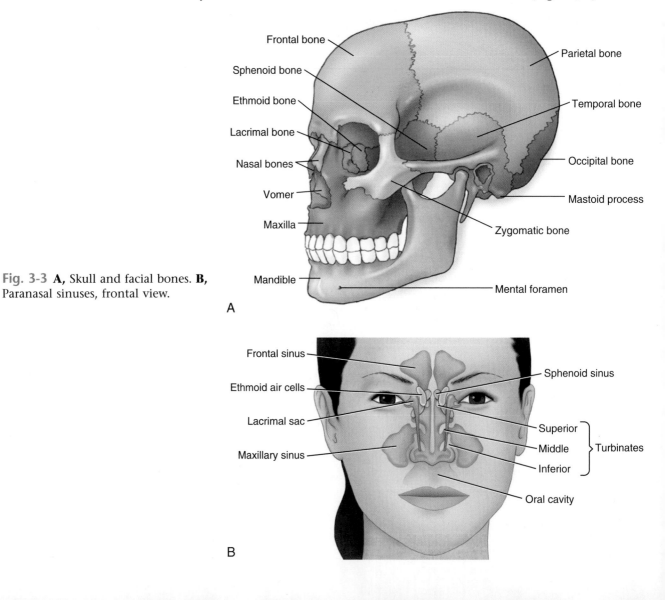

Fig. 3-3 **A,** Skull and facial bones. **B,** Paranasal sinuses, frontal view.

The last three bones of the skull, the ossicles, are tiny bones within the ear. These will be discussed in Chapter 14.

### Facial Bones

Use Fig. 3-3 to locate the names and locations of the majority of the following facial bones:

**Zygoma** (zye GOH mah): Cheekbone. Also called the *zygomatic* (zye goh MAT tick) *bone.*

**Lacrimal** (LACK rih mul) **bones:** Paired bones at the corner of each eye that cradle the tear ducts.

**Maxilla** (MACK sill ah): Upper jaw bone. Also called the **maxillary bone.**

**Mandible** (MAN dih bul): Lower jaw bone. Also called the **mandibular bone.**

**Vomer** (VOH mur): Bone that forms the posterior/inferior part of the nasal septal wall between the nostrils.

**Palatine** (PAL eh tyne) **bones:** Shell-shaped structures that make up part of the roof of the mouth.

**Nasal turbinates (conchae)** (KON kee): Make up part of the interior of the nose.

**Nasal Bones:** Pair of small bones that make up the bridge of the nose.

zygoma = zygom/o, zygomat/o

lacrimal = lacrim/o

maxilla = maxill/o

mandible = mandibul/o

vomer = vomer/o

palatine = palat/o

nasal = nas/o

### Rib Cage

The **ribs** consist of 12 pairs of thin, flat bones attached to the thoracic vertebrae in the back and to **costochondral** (kost toh KON drul) tissue in the front (see Fig. 3-1). The ribs can be categorized as follows:

- True ribs: Seven pairs attached directly to the breastbone (sternum) in the front of the body
- False ribs: Five pairs attached to the sternum by cartilage
- Floating ribs: Two pairs of false ribs not attached in the front of the body at all

In addition to ribs, the rib cage includes the **sternum** (STUR num), also known as the *breastbone.* The sharp point at the most inferior aspect of the sternum is called the **xiphoid** (ZIH foyd) **process.** The combining form xiph/o derives from the Greek word for sword, which the xiphoid resembles.

rib = cost/o

costochondral
  cost/o = rib
  chondr/o = cartilage
  -al = pertaining to

sternum = stern/o

xiphoid = xiph/o

### Spine

The **spinal,** or **vertebral,** column is divided into five regions from the neck to the tailbone. It is composed of 26 bones called the **vertebrae** (VUR teh bray). Fig. 3-4, *A.* The following table lists and illustrates the bones in the spine. Fig. 3-4, *B* illustrates a vertebra with the **laminae** (*sing.* lamina), **spinous transverse processes,** and **facets.** Laminae are thin, platelike arches in the vertebrae. Facets are processes that articulate between vertebrae.

spine = spin/o

vertebra = vertebr/o, spondyl/o

lamina = lamin/o

### Bones of the Spine

| Region | Type and Abbreviation |
|---|---|
| cervical (SUR vih kul) | neck bones (C1-C7) |
| thoracic (thoh RAS ick) | upper back (T1-T12) |
| lumbar (LUM bar) | lower back (L1-L5) |
| sacral (SAY krul) | sacrum (S1-S5) (5 bones, fused) |
| coccygeal (kock sih JEE ul) | coccyx (KOCK sicks) or tailbone |

cervical = cervic/o

thoracic = thorac/o

lumbar = lumb/o

sacral = sacr/o

coccygeal = coccyg/o

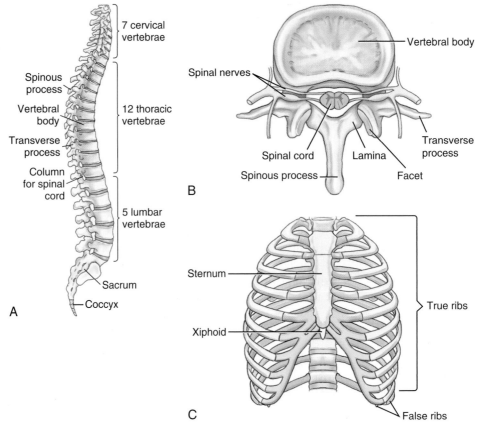

Fig. 3-4 **A**, Spine. **B**, Vertebra. **C**, Ribs.

## Exercise 4: Axial Skeletal Combining Forms

*Match each axial skeletal term with its correct combining form.*

| | | |
|---|---|---|
| ____ 1. cervic/o | ____ 9. zygomat/o | A. lower jaw bone |
| | | B. rib |
| ____ 2. lamin/o | ____ 10. lumb/o | C. backbone |
| | | D. lower back |
| ____ 3. ethmoid/o | ____ 11. mandibul/o | E. cheekbone |
| | | F. roof and walls of nasal cavity |
| ____ 4. chondr/o | ____ 12. coccyg/o | G. cartilage |
| | | H. roof of mouth |
| ____ 5. thorac/o | ____ 13. vertebr/o | I. neck |
| | | J. skull |
| ____ 6. crani/o | ____ 14. palat/o | K. lamina of vertebra |
| | | L. upper jaw bone |
| ____ 7. occipit/o | ____ 15. maxill/o | M. back of skull |
| | | N. chest |
| ____ 8. cost/o | ____ 16. stern/o | O. tailbone |
| | | P. breastbone |

*Decode the following terms below using your knowledge of word parts.*

17. submandibular _____

18. costochondral _____

19. lumbosacral _____

20. thoracic _____

21. substernal _____

### Exercise 5: Bones of the Cranium and Face

*Using the diagram provided below, label the bones of the cranium and face with their anatomic terms and combining forms where appropriate.*

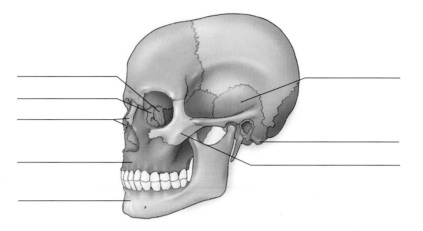

### Exercise 6: Bones of the Spine

*Label the bones of the spine with their anatomic terms and combining forms where appropriate.*

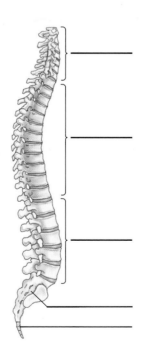

## Exercise 7: Rib Cage

*Label the rib cage with its anatomic terms and combining forms where appropriate.*

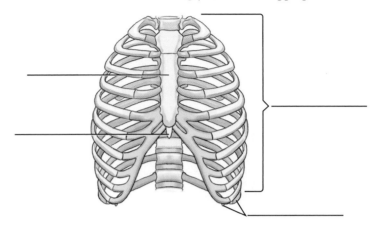

## Exercise 8: Vertebra

*Label the parts of the vertebra with their anatomic terms and combining forms where appropriate.*

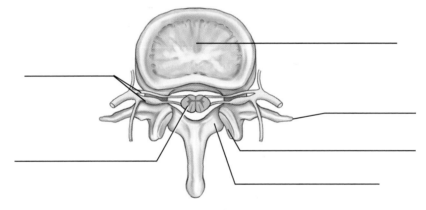

## APPENDICULAR SKELETON

The appendicular skeleton is composed of the upper appendicular and lower appendicular skeletons.

### Upper Appendicular

**scapula** = scapul/o

**clavicle** = clavicul/o, cleid/o

The upper appendicular skeleton (Fig. 3-5) includes the shoulder girdle, which is composed of the **scapula, clavicle,** and **upper extremities.** Refer to Fig. 3-1 for a correlation of each bone's description with its location.

**Scapula** (SKAP yoo lah): The scapulae, or shoulder blades, are flat bones that help to support the arms. The **acromion** (ack ROH mee un) **process** is the lateral protrusion of the scapula that forms the highest point of the shoulder.

**Clavicle** (KLA vih kul): The clavicle, or collarbone, is one of a pair of long, curved horizontal bones that attach to the upper sternum at one end and the acromion process of the scapula at the other. These bones help to stabilize the shoulder anteriorly. A "wishbone" is composed of the fused clavicles of a bird.

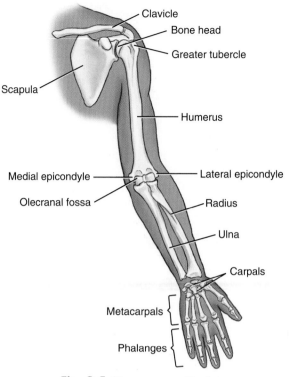

**Fig. 3-5** Upper appendicular.

The upper extremities (see Fig. 3-5) consist of the following:

**Humerus** (HYOO mur us): Upper arm bone.
**Radius** (RAY dee us): Lower lateral arm bone parallel to the ulna. The distal end articulates with the thumb side of the hand.
**Ulna** (UL nuh): Lower medial arm bone. The distal end articulates with the little finger side of the hand. The **olecranon** (oh LECK ruh non) is a proximal projection of the ulna that forms the tip of the elbow. Commonly known as the funny bone, this structure is actually a process.
**Carpus** (KAR pus): One of eight wrist bones.
**Metacarpus** (meh tuh KAR pus): One of the five bones that form the middle part of the hand.
**Phalanx** (FAY lanks): One of the 14 bones that constitute the fingers of the hand, two in the thumb and three in each of the other four fingers (*pl.* phalanges). The three bones in each of the four fingers are differentiated as proximal, medial, and distal. The joints between these are referred to as proximal and distal interphalangeal (PIP, DIP) joints. When one is referring to a whole finger (or toe), the term **digitus** is used.

**humerus** = humer/o
**radius** = radi/o
**ulna** = uln/o
**olecranon** = olecran/o
**carpal** = carp/o
**metacarpal** = metacarp/o
**phalanx** = phalang/o
**digitus** = digit/o, dactyl/o

## Lower Appendicular

The lower half of the appendicular skeleton can be divided into the **pelvis** and the **lower extremities** (Fig. 3-6). The **acetabulum** (*pl.* acetabula) is the socket into which the femoral head fits. The pelvic bones (also called the *pelvic girdle*) consist of the following three bones:

**Ilium** (ILL ee um): The superior and widest bone of the pelvis.
**Ischium** (ISS kee um): The lower portion of the pelvic bone.
**Pubis** (PYOO bis) **or pubic bone:** The lower anterior part of the pelvic bone.

**pelvis** = pelv/i, pelv/o
**ilium** = ili/o
**ischium** = ischi/o
**pubis** = pub/o

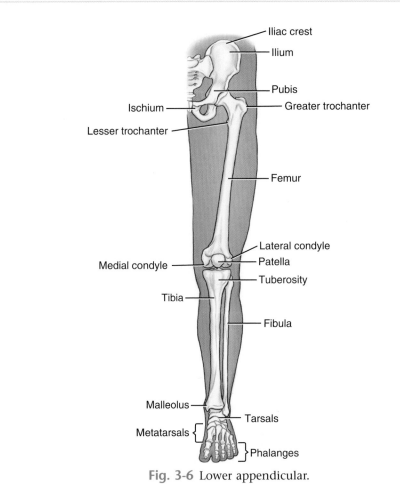

Fig. 3-6 Lower appendicular.

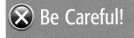 **Be Careful!** *Do not confuse **ilium** with its homonym, **ileum**, which is a part of the digestive system.*

The lower extremities include the following:

**Femur** (FEE mur): Thigh bone, upper leg bone.
**Patella** (puh TELL uh): Kneecap.
**Tibia** (TIB ee uh): Shin bone, lower medial leg bone.
**Fibula** (FIB yuh luh): Smaller, lower lateral leg bone.
**Malleolus** (mah LEE oh lus): Process on the distal ends of tibia and fibula.
**Tarsus** (TAR sus): One of the seven bones of the ankle, hindfoot, and midfoot. The **calcaneus** is the heel bone.
**Metatarsus** (met uh TAR sus): One of the five foot bones between the tarsals and the phalanges.
**Phalanx:** One of 14 toe bones, two in the great toe and three in each of the other four toes.

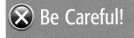 **Be Careful!** *Do not confuse **perone/o**, meaning fibula, and **peritone/o**, meaning the lining of the abdomen.*

**femur** = femor/o

**patella** = patell/o, patell/a

**tibia** = tibi/o

**fibula** = fibul/o, perone/o

**malleolus** = malleol/o

**tarsal** = tars/o

**calcaneus** = calcane/o

**metatarsal** = metatars/o

# Exercise 9: The Appendicular Skeleton

*Match the upper appendicular combining forms with their meanings.*

**Combining Forms**                                    **Upper Appendicular**

____  1. humer/o            ____  6. metacarp/o        A. collarbone, clavicle
                                                       B. wristbone
____  2. scapul/o           ____  7. digit/o           C. finger, toe
                                                       D. one of the finger or toe bones
____  3. uln/o              ____  8. phalang/o         E. lower lateral arm bone
                                                       F. upper arm bone
____  4. olecran/o          ____  9. radi/o            G. lower medial arm bone
                                                       H. elbow
____  5. clavicul/o, cleid/o ____  10. carp/o          I. shoulder blade
                                                       J. hand bone

*Match the lower appendicular combining forms with their meanings.*

**Combining Forms**                                    **Lower Appendicular**

____  11. patell/o          ____  17. pelv/o, pelv/i   K. foot bone
                                                       L. lower portion of pelvic bone
____  12. pub/o             ____  18. ischi/o          M. ankle bone
                                                       N. lower anterior pelvic bone
____  13. metatars/o        ____  19. fibul/o, perone/o O. shin bone
                                                       P. kneecap
____  14. tibi/o            ____  20. femor/o          Q. superior, widest bone of pelvis
                                                       R. processes on distal tibia and fibula
____  15. ili/o             ____  21. tars/o           S. thigh bone
                                                       T. pelvis
____  16. malleol/o         ____  22. calcane/o        U. lower, lateral leg bone
                                                       V. heel bone

*Decode the terms.*

23. interphalangeal _____

24. humeroulnar _____

25. intrapatellar _____

26. femoral _____

27. supraclavicular _____

## Exercise 10: Upper Appendicular Skeleton

*Label the upper appendicular skeleton with its anatomic terms and combining forms where appropriate.*

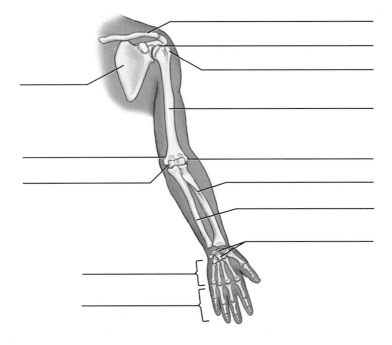

## Exercise 11: Lower Appendicular Skeleton

*Label the lower appendicular skeleton with its anatomic terms and combining forms where appropriate.*

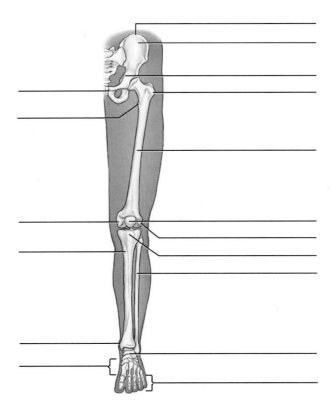

## Joints

Joints, or *articulations* as they are sometimes called, are the parts of the body where two or more bones of the skeleton join. Examples of joints include the knee, which joins the tibia and the femur, and the elbow, which joins the humerus with the radius and ulna. Joints provide **range of motion (ROM),** the range through which a joint can be extended and flexed. Different joints have different ROM, ranging from no movement at all to full range of movement. Categorized by ROM, they are as follows:

**No ROM:** Most **synarthroses** (sin ar THROH sees) are immovable joints held together by fibrous cartilaginous tissue. The suture lines of the skull are examples of synarthroses.

**Limited ROM: Amphiarthroses** (am fee ar THROH sees) are joints joined together by cartilage that are slightly movable, such as the vertebrae of the spine or the pubic bones.

**Full ROM: Diarthroses** (dye ar THROH sees) are joints that have free movement. The most commonly known are ball-and-socket joints (such as the hip) and hinge joints (such as the knees). Other examples of diarthroses include the elbows, wrists, shoulders, and ankles. See Fig. 3-7 for an illustration of a knee joint that shows the bones, muscles, tendons, bursae, synovial membrane, and cavity in the knee.

Diarthroses, or **synovial** (sih NOH vee ul) **joints,** as they are frequently called, are the most complex of the joints. Because these joints help a person move around for a lifetime, they are designed to efficiently cushion the jarring of the bones and to minimize friction between the surfaces of the bones. Many of the synovial joints have **bursae** (BURR see) (*sing.* bursa), which are sacs of fluid that are located between the bones of the joint and the tendons that hold the muscles in place. Bursae help cushion the joints when they move. Synovial joints also have joint capsules that enclose the ends of the bones, a synovial membrane that lines the joint capsules and secretes fluid to lubricate the joint, and articular cartilage that covers and protects the bone. The **menisci** (*sing.* meniscus) consist of crescent-shaped cartilage in the knee joint that additionally cushions the joint. **Ligaments** are strong bands of white fibrous connective tissue that connect one bone to another at the joints.

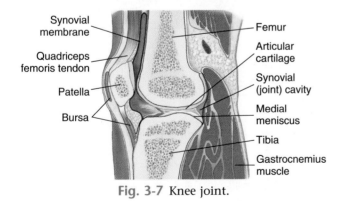

Fig. 3-7 Knee joint.

*Synovial membrane*
*Quadriceps femoris tendon*
*Patella*
*Bursa*
*Femur*
*Articular cartilage*
*Synovial (joint) cavity*
*Medial meniscus*
*Tibia*
*Gastrocnemius muscle*

## Muscles

A **muscle** is a tissue that is composed of cells with the ability to contract and relax. Because of those two specialized actions, the body is able to move. The muscles in the human body are specialized into three different functions:

• **Skeletal muscle** is striated (striped in appearance) and allows the skeleton to move voluntarily

---

**joint** = articul/o, arthr/o

**synarthrosis**
 syn- = together
 arthr/o = joint
 -sis = condition

**amphiarthrosis**
 amphi- = both
 arthr/o = joint
 -sis = condition

**diarthrosis**
 dia- = through
 arthr/o = joint
 -sis = condition

**synovial** = synovi/o

**bursa** = burs/o

**meniscus** = menisc/o

**muscle** = my/o, myos/o, muscul/o

**skeletal muscle** = rhabdomy/o

**smooth muscle** =
leiomy/o

**heart muscle** =
myocardi/o

**tendon** = tend/o,
tendin/o, ten/o

- **Smooth muscle** that is responsible for involuntary movement of the organs
- **Heart muscle** that pumps blood to the circulatory system

Muscles are attached to bones by strong fibrous bands of connective tissue called **tendons.** The bone that is at the end of the attachment that does not move and is nearest to the trunk is termed the *origin* (O); the bone that is at the end that does move and is farthest from the trunk is termed the *insertion (I)*. The function of a muscle is its *action* (A). For example, a flexor muscle bends a joint, and an extensor muscle stretches out a joint. These muscle pairs are termed *antagonistic* muscles. *Synergistic* muscles work together to refine a movement.

The illustrations in Fig. 3-8 show posterior and anterior views of the major skeletal muscles of the body. Although the naming of all the muscles in the body is too much to cover in this text, there are a few helpful conventions that

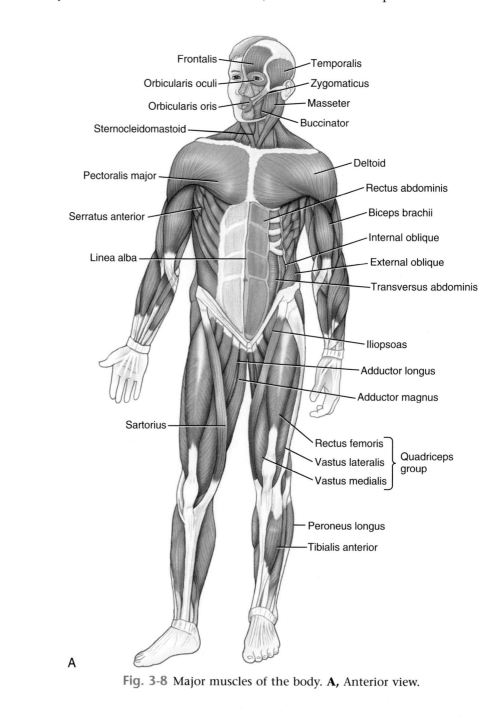

Frontalis
Temporalis
Orbicularis oculi
Zygomaticus
Orbicularis oris
Masseter
Buccinator
Sternocleidomastoid
Deltoid
Pectoralis major
Rectus abdominis
Biceps brachii
Serratus anterior
Internal oblique
External oblique
Linea alba
Transversus abdominis
Iliopsoas
Adductor longus
Adductor magnus
Sartorius
Rectus femoris
Vastus lateralis
Quadriceps group
Vastus medialis
Peroneus longus
Tibialis anterior

A

**Fig. 3-8** Major muscles of the body. **A,** Anterior view.

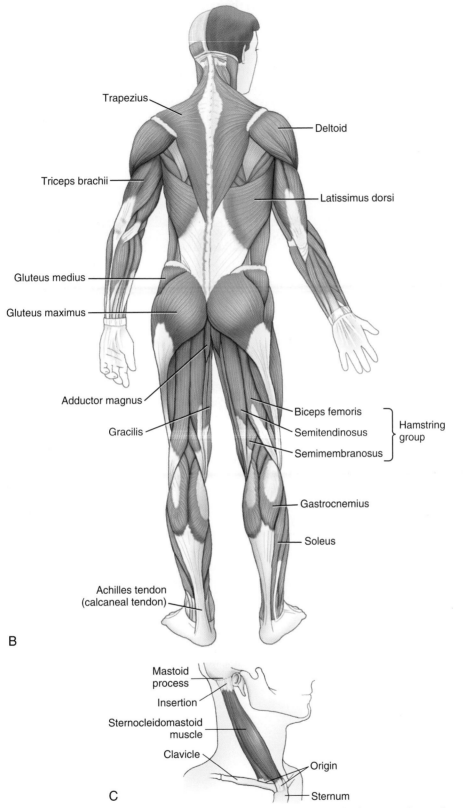

Trapezius

Deltoid

Triceps brachii

Latissimus dorsi

Gluteus medius

Gluteus maximus

Adductor magnus

Biceps femoris

Gracilis

Semitendinosus

Semimembranosus

Hamstring group

Gastrocnemius

Soleus

Achilles tendon (calcaneal tendon)

B

Mastoid process

Insertion

Sternocleidomastoid muscle

Clavicle

Origin

Sternum

C

**Fig. 3-8, cont'd B,** Posterior view. **C,** Close-up of the sternocleidomastoid muscle.

**sternocleidomastoid**
stern/o = sternum
cleid/o = clavicle
mastoid/o = mastoid

can be followed. Refer to the table below for examples of how muscles are named by their location, number of insertions, size, shape, and muscle action. Some muscles get their names from their general location. For instance the pectoris muscle is a large muscle in the chest (pector/o). The final convention is to name a muscle by its origins and insertion. For example, the **sternocleidomastoid** (stur noh kly doh MASS toyd) muscle (Fig. 3-8, *C*) attaches to the sternum, the clavicle, and the mastoid process. Some muscles get their names from their general location. For instance, the pectoralis major is a large muscle in the chest.

## Muscle Naming Conventions

| Naming Device | Name of Muscle | Word Origin | Definition |
|---|---|---|---|
| location | zygomaticus | *zygomatic/o* zygoma<br>*-us* noun ending | Cheek muscle. |
| number of insertions | biceps brachii | *bi-* two<br>**ceps* heads<br>*brachi/o* arm<br>*-i pl.* noun ending | Muscle that flexes upper arm. |
| size | gluteus maximus | *glute/o* buttock<br>*-us* noun ending<br>*maxim/o* large<br>*-us* noun ending | Large buttock muscle. |
| shape | deltoid | *delt/o* triangle<br>*-oid* like | Triangular muscle in upper back. |
| muscle action | adductor longus | *ad-* toward<br>*duct/o* carrying<br>*-or* one who<br>*long/o* long<br>*-us* noun ending | Upper leg muscle that carries one leg back to the midline. |
| origin/insertion | sternocleidomastoid<br>(see Fig. 3-8, *C*) | *stern/o* breastbone<br>*cleid/o* collarbone<br>*mastoid/o* mastoid process | Muscle that originates in the sternum and collarbone and inserts on the mastoid process. |

***ceps** is a variation of **cephal/o,** the combining form for head. These word parts are used for "the head" or the beginning of a structure and also are used for bones (bone heads), as well as muscle heads.

# Exercise 12: Joints and Muscles

*Match the joint and muscle combining forms with their meanings.*

____  1. arthr/o, articul/o      ____  7. my/o, myos/o, muscul/o

____  2. myocardi/o             ____  8. leiomy/o

____  3. delt/o                 ____  9. tendin/o, ten/o, tend/o

____  4. rhabdomy/o             ____ 10. burs/o

____  5. synovi/o               ____ 11. glute/o

____  6. menisc/o

A. smooth muscle
B. triangle
C. sac of fluid to cushion joints
D. skeletal muscle
E. joint
F. crescent-shaped cartilage
G. heart muscle
H. synovial
I. muscle
J. connects bone to muscle
K. buttock

*Build the terms.*

12. pertaining to within the muscle _____

13. pertaining to buttocks _____

14. pertaining to the synovium _____

## Muscle Actions

| | Action | Word Origin | Description |
|---|---|---|---|
| | **extension**<br>ecks TEN shun | *ex-* out<br>*tens/o* stretching<br>*-ion* process of | Process of stretching out; increasing the angle of a joint. |
| | **flexion**<br>FLEK shun | *flex/o* bending<br>*-ion* process of | Process of decreasing the angle of a joint. |
| | **abduction**<br>ab DUK shun | *ab-* away from<br>*duct/o* carrying<br>*-ion* process of | Process of carrying away from the midline. |
| | **adduction**<br>ad DUK shun | *ad-* toward<br>*duct/o* carrying<br>*-ion* process of | Process of carrying toward the midline. |
| | **supination**<br>soo pin NAY shun | | Turning the palm upward. |
| | **pronation**<br>proh NAY shun | | Turning the palm downward. |
| | **dorsiflexion**<br>DOOR sih flek shun | *dors/i* back<br>*flex/o* bending<br>*-ion* process of | Process of bending back. |
| | **plantar flexion**<br>PLAN tar FLEK shun | *plant/o* sole<br>*-ar* pertaining to<br>*flex/o* bending<br>*-ion* process of | Lowering the foot; pointing the toes away from the shin. |

## Muscle Actions—cont'd

| | Action | Word Origin | Description |
|---|---|---|---|
| | **eversion**<br>ee VER shun | *e-* out<br>*vers/o* turning<br>*-ion* process of | Process of turning out. |
| | **inversion**<br>in VER shun | *in-* in<br>*vers/o* turning<br>*-ion* process of | Process of turning in. |
| | **protraction**<br>proh TRAK shun | *pro-* forward<br>*tract/o* pulling<br>*-ion* process of | Process of pulling forward; the forward movement of a muscle. |
| | **retraction**<br>ree TRAK shun | *re-* backward<br>*tract/o* pulling<br>*-ion* process of | Process of backward pulling; the backward movement of a muscle. |
| | **rotation**<br>roh TAY shun | *rot/o* wheel<br>*-ation* process of | Process of a bone turning on its axis (like a wheel). |
| | **circumduction**<br>sir cum DUK shun | *circum-* around<br>*duct/o* carrying<br>*-ion* process of | Process of carrying around; the circular movement of the distal end of a limb around its point of attachment. |

# Exercise 13: Muscle Actions

*Label each illustration with the muscle action indicated.*

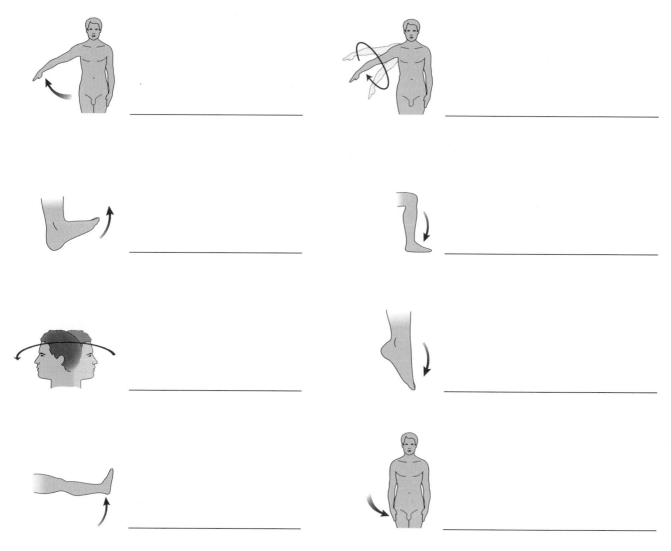

_____

_____

_____

_____

_____

_____

_____

_____

# Exercise 14: Muscle Actions

*Match the muscle action with the correct definition.*

| | |
|---|---|
| ____ 1. plantar flexion | ____ 8. rotation |
| ____ 2. circumduction | ____ 9. supination |
| ____ 3. pronation | ____ 10. eversion |
| ____ 4. inversion | ____ 11. dorsiflexion |
| ____ 5. adduction | ____ 12. abduction |
| ____ 6. extension | ____ 13. flexion |
| ____ 7. protraction | ____ 14. retraction |

A. process of turning in
B. process of bending
C. process of bone turning on its axis
D. process of bending back
E. process of pulling backward
F. turning the palm downward
G. process of carrying away from (the midline)
H. turning the palm upward
I. process of turning out
J. process of pulling forward
K. process of stretching out
L. process of carrying around
M. process of carrying toward (the midline)
N. lowering the foot

You can review the anatomy of the musculoskeletal system by clicking on **Body Spectrum Electronic Anatomy Coloring Book → Muscular** and **Skeletal.**

## Case Study  Dylan Koldmann

Seven-year-old Dylan Koldmann is brought to the ED by his parents for a right arm injury. Dylan had been riding his bike when he attempted to turn a corner, and his bike skidded on some stones. He tried to break his fall with his right hand and arm as his bike went down. He has numerous scrapes on his right hand and palm as well as the outside of his arm, with pieces of stones embedded in the arm and hand. He complains of severe pain in his hand, especially his thumb. He is able to move all of his fingers except the thumb; there is swelling on his palm, and it is worse near his thumb with some bruising. He can move his wrist, elbow, and forearm, but the scrapes make it painful to move.

X-rays of the arm and hand show a Salter-Harris type II fracture of his right thumb. No other fractures are noted on the arm or elbow areas. He is treated for the scratches, and his right hand and forearm are placed in a soft splint.

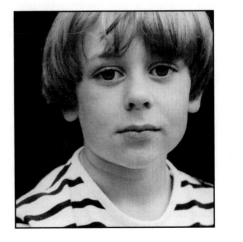

He is given pain medication. Dylan's parents are told to bring him back the next day to see the orthopedist.

## Case Study Dylan Koldmann

KOLDMANN, DYLAN M. - 507940 Opened by Bradley Oppenheimer, MD ⬓ ⬚ ✕

Task   Edit   View   Time Scale   Options   Help

As Of 16:10

| KOLDMANN, DYLAN M. | Age: 7 years | Sex: Male | Loc: ARH |
| | DOB: 01/27/2004 | MRN: 507940 | FIN: 3506004 |

| Reference Text Browser | Form Browser | Medication Profile |

| Orders | Last 48 Hours | ED | Lab | Radiology | Assessments | Surgery | Clinical Notes | Pt. Info | Pt. Schedule | Task List | I & O | MAR |

Flowsheet: ED ▾ ...   Level: ED Record ▾     ⦿ Table ○ Group ○ List

Navigator ✕
✓ ED Record

7-year-old sustained injury to right hand when fell off bike. Pain over thenar eminence. Able to bend at his wrist and flex at his DIP and PIP joints and every digit of the hand with exception of first digit.

Exam of right hand is significant for mild protrusion but no ecchymosis and minimal edema overlying thenar eminence of the right hand. Good wrist mobility. X-ray significant for what appears to be a Salter-Harris fracture of the first metacarpal. Immobile and follow-up tomorrow with Ortho for possible cast.

PROD | MAHAFC | 26 March 2011 | 16:10

## Exercise 15: Emergency Department Report

*Use the emergency department record above to answer the following questions.*

1. Dylan's injury is to the fleshy area of the palm near the thumb, the "thenar eminence." Explain the difference between a DIP (distal interphalangeal joint) and a PIP (proximal interphalangeal) joint.

   _____

2. Not being able to "flex" a body part means one is unable to _____.

3. "First digit, R hand" means _____.

4. The first metacarpal is a bone of the _____.

Click on **Hear It, Spell It** to practice spelling the anatomy and physiology terms you have learned in this chapter.

Practice pronouncing anatomy and physiology terms! Click **Hear It, Say It.**

## Combining and Adjective Forms for the Anatomy of the Musculoskeletal System

| Meaning | Combining Form | Adjective Form |
|---|---|---|
| bone | oste/o, osse/o, oss/i | osseous, osteal |
| bone marrow | myel/o | |
| bursa | burs/o | bursal |
| calcaneus (heel bone) | calcane/o | calcaneal |
| carpal bone | carp/o | carpal |
| cartilage | chondr/o, cartilag/o | cartilaginous, chondral |
| clavicle (collarbone) | clavicul/o, cleid/o | clavicular, cleidal |
| coccyx (tailbone) | coccyg/o | coccygeal |
| condyle | condyl/o | condylar |
| elbow (olecranon) | olecran/o | olecranal |
| epicondyle | epicondyl/o | epicondylar |
| ethmoid | ethmoid/o | ethmoidal |
| fascia | fasci/o | fascial |
| femur (thigh bone) | femor/o | femoral |
| fibula (lower lateral leg bone) | fibul/o, perone/o | fibular, peroneal |
| finger, toe, (whole), digitus | dactyl/o, digit/o | digital |
| foramen | foramin/o | foraminal |
| frontal bone | front/o | frontal |
| humerus (upper arm bone) | humer/o | humeral |
| ilium | ili/o | iliac |
| ischium | ischi/o | ischial |
| jaw | gnath/o | |
| joint (articulation) | arthr/o, articul/o | articular |
| lacrima | lacrim/o | lacrimal |
| lamina | lamin/o | laminar |
| ligament | ligament/o, syndesm/o | ligamentous, syndesmal |
| lower back | lumb/o | lumbar |
| malleolus | malleol/o | malleolar |
| mandible (lower jaw bone) | mandibul/o | mandibular |
| mastoid process | mastoid/o | mastoid |
| maxilla (upper jaw bone) | maxill/o | maxillary |
| meniscus | menisc/o | menisceal |
| metacarpus (hand bone) | metacarp/o | metacarpal |

*Continued*

## Combining and Adjective Forms for the Anatomy of the Musculoskeletal System—cont'd

| Meaning | Combining Form | Adjective Form |
|---|---|---|
| metatarsus (foot bone) | metatars/o | metatarsal |
| muscle | my/o, myos/o, muscul/o | muscular |
| muscle (heart) | myocardi/o, cardiomy/o | myocardial |
| muscle (skeletal) | rhabdomy/o | |
| muscle (smooth) | leiomy/o | |
| neck | cervic/o | cervical |
| occiput | occipit/o | occipital |
| palatine bone | palat/o | palatine |
| parietal bone | pariet/o | parietal |
| patella (kneecap) | patell/o, patell/a | patellar |
| pelvis | pelv/i, pelv/o | pelvic |
| phalanx (one of the bones of the fingers or toes) | phalang/o | phalangeal |
| pubis (pubic bone) | pub/o | pubic |
| radius (lower lateral arm bone) | radi/o | radial |
| rib (costa) | cost/o | costal |
| sacrum | sacr/o | sacral |
| scapula (shoulderblade) | scapul/o | scapular |
| skeleton | skelet/o | skeletal |
| skull (cranium) | crani/o | cranial |
| sole | plant/o | plantar |
| sphenoid | sphenoid/o | sphenoidal |
| spinal column, spine | spin/o, rachi/o, vertebr/o | spinal, vertebral, rachial |
| sternum, breastbone | stern/o | sternal |
| tarsus (anklebone) | tars/o | tarsal |
| temporal bone | tempor/o | temporal |
| tendon | tendin/o, tend/o, ten/o | tendinous |
| thorax (chest) | thorac/o | thoracic |
| tibia (shinbone) | tibi/o | tibial |
| ulna | uln/o | ulnar |
| vertebra (backbone) | vertebr/o, spondyl/o | vertebral |
| vomer | vomer/o | |
| xiphoid process | xiph/o | xiphoid |
| zygoma (cheekbone) | zygomat/o | zygomatic |

## Prefixes for the Anatomy of the Musculoskeletal System

| Prefix | Meaning |
|---|---|
| ab- | away from |
| ad- | toward |
| amphi- | both |
| bi- | two |
| circum- | around |
| dia- | through, complete |
| endo-, end- | within |
| epi- | above, upon |
| ex-, e- | out |
| in- | in |
| inter- | between |
| intra- | within |
| peri- | surrounding, around |
| pro- | forward |
| re- | back |
| syn- | together, joined |

## Suffixes for the Anatomy of the Musculoskeletal System

| Suffix | Meaning |
|---|---|
| -ar, -al, -ic, -ous, -eal | pertaining to |
| -blast | embryonic |
| -clast | breaking down |
| -cyte | cell |
| -oid | full of, like |
| -physis | growth |
| -poiesis | formation |
| -sis | condition |
| -um | structure |

# PATHOLOGY

## Terms Related to Congenital Conditions

| Term | Word Origin | Definition |
|---|---|---|
| **achondroplasia**<br>a kon droh PLAY zha | *a-* without<br>*chondr/o* cartilage<br>*-plasia* condition of development | Disorder of the development of cartilage at the epiphyses of the long bones and skull, resulting in dwarfism. |
| **muscular dystrophy**<br>MUSS kyoo lur<br>DISS troh fee | *muscul/o* muscle<br>*-ar* pertaining to<br>*dys-* bad, abnormal<br>*-trophy* process of nourishment, development | Group of disorders characterized as an inherited progressive atrophy of skeletal muscle without neural involvement (Fig. 3-9). |

*Continued*

## Terms Related to Congenital Conditions—cont'd

| Term | Word Origin | Definition |
| --- | --- | --- |
| polydactyly<br>pall ee DACK tih lee | *poly-* many, much<br>*dactyl/o* fingers, toes<br>*-y* process of | Condition of more than five fingers or toes on each hand or foot (Fig. 3-10, *A*). |
| spina bifida occulta<br>SPY nah<br>BIFF ih dah<br>ah KULL tah | *spin/o* spine<br>*bi-* two<br>*-fida* to split<br>*occulta* hidden | Congenital malformation of the bony spinal canal without involvement of the spinal cord. |
| syndactyly<br>sin DACK tih lee | *syn-* joined, together<br>*dactyl/o* fingers, toes<br>*-y* process of | Condition of the joining of the fingers or toes, giving them a webbed appearance (Fig. 3-10, *B*). |
| talipes<br>TALL ih peez | | Deformity resulting in an abnormal twisting of the foot. Also called **clubfoot** (Fig. 3-11). May also be acquired. |
| torticollis<br>tore tih KOLL lis | *tort/i* twist<br>*coll/o* neck<br>*-is* noun ending | Prolonged congenital or acquired condition that manifests itself as a contraction of the muscles of the neck. Also called **wryneck**. |

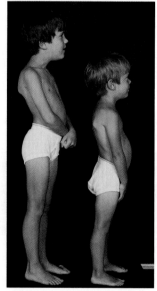

Fig. 3-9 Muscular dystrophy. These brothers show typical stance, lumbar lordosis, and forward thrusting of the abdomen.

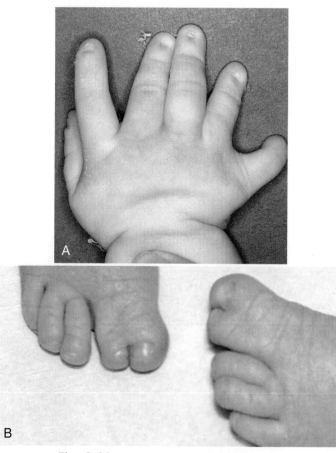

Fig. 3-10 **A,** Polydactyly. **B,** Syndactyly.

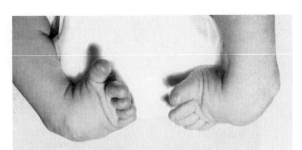

**Fig. 3-11** Talipes.

## Exercise 16: Congenital Disorders

*Match the congenital disorder with its description.*

____ 1. muscular dystrophy     ____ 3. talipes

____ 2. torticollis     ____ 4. spina bifida occulta

A. wryneck
B. progressive muscle weakening without involvement of nerves
C. clubfoot
D. malformation of the spinal canal

*Build the terms.*

5. Process of joined fingers/toes _____

6. Condition of development without cartilage _____

7. Process of many fingers/toes _____

### Terms Related to Bone Disease

| Term | Word Origin | Definition |
| --- | --- | --- |
| **osteodynia**<br>ahs tee oh DIN ee ah | *oste/o* bone<br>*-dynia* pain | Bone pain. |
| **osteitis deformans**<br>ahs tee EYE tis<br>dee FOR menz | *oste/o* bone<br>*-itis* inflammation<br>*deformans* misshapen | Misshaped bone resulting from inflammation. Also known as **Paget disease**. |
| **osteomalacia**<br>ahs tee oh mah LAY sha | *oste/o* bone<br>*-malacia* softening | Softening of bone caused by loss of minerals from the bony matrix as a result of vitamin D deficiency. When osteomalacia occurs in childhood, it is called **rickets**. |
| **osteomyelitis**<br>ahs tee oh mye eh LYE tis | *oste/o* bone<br>*myel/o* bone marrow<br>*-itis* inflammation | Inflammation of the bone and bone marrow. |
| **osteoporosis**<br>ahs tee oh poor OH sis | *oste/o* bone<br>*por/o* passage<br>*-osis* abnormal condition | Loss of bone mass, which results in the bones being fragile and at risk for fractures (Fig. 3-12). **Osteopenia** refers to a less severe bone mass loss. (-penia = deficiency) |

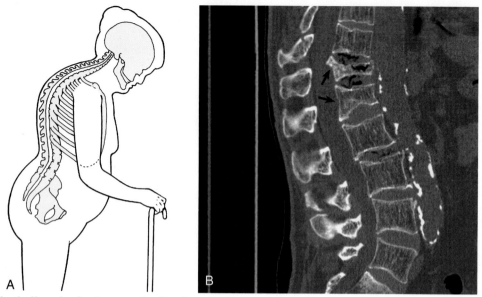

**Fig. 3-12 A,** The hallmark of osteoporosis: the dowager hump. Affected persons lose height, have a bent spine, and appear to sink into their hips. **B,** X-ray showing a compression fracture of T12 and L1 subsequent to osteoporosis.

## Terms Related to Chondropathies

| Term | Word Origin | Definition |
|------|-------------|------------|
| **chondromalacia**<br>kon droh mah LAY see ah | *chondr/o* cartilage<br>*-malacia* softening | Softening of the cartilage. |
| **costochondritis**<br>kahs toh kon DRY tis | *cost/o* rib<br>*chondr/o* cartilage<br>*-itis* inflammation | Inflammation of the cartilage of the ribs. |

## Terms Related to Arthropathies and Related Disorders

| Term | Word Origin | Definition |
|------|-------------|------------|
| **arthrosis**<br>ar THROH sis | *arthr/o* joint<br>*-osis* abnormal condition | Abnormal condition of a joint; may be **hemarthrosis, hydrarthrosis,** or **pyarthrosis** (blood, fluid, or pus respectively, in a joint cavity). |
| **Baker cyst**<br>BAY kur sist | *cyst/o* sac, bladder | Cyst of synovial fluid in the popliteal area of leg; often associated with rheumatoid arthritis. |
| **bunion**<br>BUN yun | *bunion/o* bunion | Fairly common, painful enlargement and inflammation of the first metatarsophalangeal joint (the base of the great toe). |
| **bursitis**<br>bur SYE tis | *burs/o* bursa<br>*-itis* inflammation | Inflammation of a bursa. |
| **carpal tunnel syndrome (CTS)**<br>KAR pul<br>TUN ul | *carp/o* wrist bone<br>*-al* pertaining to<br>*syn-* joined together<br>*-drome* to run | Compression injury that manifests itself as fluctuating pain, numbness, and paresthesias of the hand caused by compression of the median nerve at the wrist (Fig. 3-13). |

## Terms Related to Arthropathies and Related Disorders—cont'd

| Term | Word Origin | Definition |
|------|-------------|------------|
| **crepitus**<br>KREP ih tus | *crepit/o* crackling<br>*-us* thing | Crackling sound heard in joints. |
| **osteoarthritis (OA)**<br>ahs tee oh arth RYE tis | *oste/o* bone<br>*arthr/o* joint<br>*-itis* inflammation | Joint disease characterized by degenerative articular cartilage and a wearing down of the bones' edges at a joint; considered a "wear and tear" disorder. Also called **degenerative joint disease** (DJD) (Fig. 3-14). |
| **osteophytosis**<br>ahs tee oh fye TOH sis | *oste/o* bone<br>*phyt/o* growth nature<br>*-osis* abnormal condition | Abnormal bone growth in a joint. **Heberden nodes** are osteophytes of the interphalangeal joints in rheumatoid arthritis (Fig. 3-15). |
| **rheumatoid arthritis (RA)**<br>ROO mah toyd<br>arth RYE tis | *rheumat/o* watery flow<br>*-oid* full of, like<br>*arthr/o* joint<br>*-itis* inflammation | Inflammatory joint disease believed to be autoimmune in nature; occurs in a much younger population (ages 20 to 45) than OA (Fig. 3-15). |
| **scleroderma**<br>SKLAIR oh dur mah | *scler/o* hard<br>*derm/o* skin<br>*-a* noun ending | Connective tissue disorder that causes hardening and thickening of the skin. |
| **systemic lupus erythematosus (SLE)**<br>siss TEM ick LOO pus<br>eh rith mah TOH sis | *system/o* system<br>*-ic* pertaining to<br>*erythemat/o* red<br>*-ous* pertaining to | Chronic, systemic inflammation of unknown etiology (cause). Characterized by distinctive red, butterfly-like rash on nose and cheeks. Also called **disseminated lupus erythematosus** (DLE) (Fig. 3-16). |
| **temporomandibular joint disorder (TMJ)**<br>tem pore oh man DIB byoo lur | *tempor/o* temporal bone<br>*mandibul/o* lower jaw<br>*-ar* pertaining to | Dysfunctional temporomandibular joint, accompanied by gnathalgia, or jaw pain. |
| **tendinitis**<br>ten din EYE tis | *tendin/o* tendon<br>*-itis* inflammation | Inflammation of a tendon. |

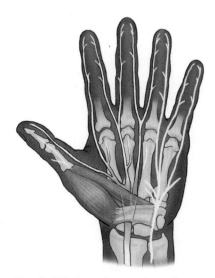

Fig. 3-13 Carpal tunnel syndrome.

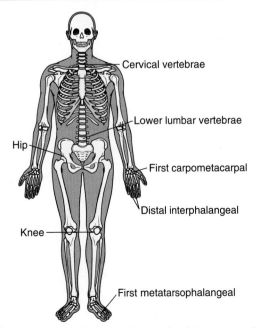

Cervical vertebrae

Lower lumbar vertebrae

Hip

First carpometacarpal

Distal interphalangeal

Knee

First metatarsophalangeal

Fig. 3-14 Joints most frequently involved in osteoarthritis.

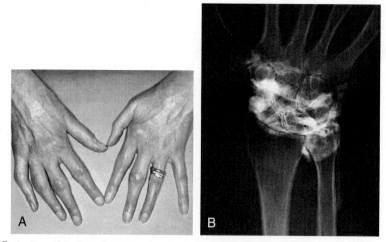

Fig. 3-15 **A,** Bouchard nodes seen in rheumatoid arthritis of the hands. Moderate involvement. **B,** Arthrogram of wrist showing RA and resultant osteophytosis.

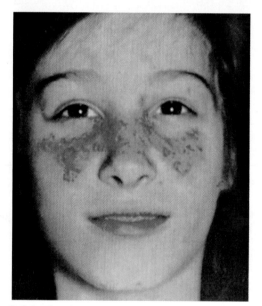

Fig. 3-16 The characteristic butterfly-like rash of SLE.

## Exercise 17: Bone, Cartilage, and Joint Disorders

*Match the bone, cartilage, or joint disorders with their definitions.*

____ 1. chondromalacia

____ 2. crepitus

____ 3. bunion

____ 4. TMJ

____ 5. osteitis deformans

____ 6. rheumatoid arthritis

____ 7. costochondritis

____ 8. Baker cyst

____ 9. osteoarthritis

____ 10. osteomyelitis

____ 11. carpal tunnel syndrome

____ 12. osteophytosis

A. softening of the cartilage
B. inflammation of the bone and bone marrow
C. crackling sound in a joint
D. autoimmune inflammatory joint disease
E. compression injury of median nerve of wrist
F. enlargement of first metatarsophalangeal joint
G. also known as Paget disease
H. degenerative joint disease
I. fluid-filled sac behind knee
J. inflammation of cartilage of ribs
K. abnormal bony growths around joints
L. dysfunctional joint in jaw bone

*Build the terms.*

13. pain in a bone _____

14. inflammation of a bursa _____

15. inflammation of a tendon _____

16. abnormal condition of passages in bone _____

17. softening of bone _____

## Spinal Malcurvatures

Back pain accounts for the greatest number of musculoskeletal complaints in the United States. In healthcare terminology, those complaints are classified as **dorsalgia** (door SAL zsa) (**dors/o** = back + **-algia** = pain), upper back pain, and **lumbago** (lum BAY goh) (**lumb/o** = lumbar + **-ago** = disease), lower back pain.

The spine has natural curves that allow support and flexibility; however, sometimes these curves become exaggerated and cause pain and disfigurement. The following are the most common types of disorders and malcurvatures of the spine. Occasionally, combinations of these disorders occur.

### Terms Related to Deforming Dorsopathies and Spondylopathies

| Term | Word Origin | Definition |
|------|-------------|------------|
| ankylosing spondylitis<br>ang kih LOH sing<br>spon dill LYE tis | *ankyl/o* stiffening<br>*spondyl/o* vertebra<br>*-itis* inflammation | Chronic inflammatory disease of idiopathic origin, which causes a fusion of the spine. |
| herniated intervertebral disk | *inter-* between<br>*vertebr/o* vertebra<br>*-al* pertaining to | Protrusion of the central part of the disk that lies between the vertebrae, resulting in compression of the nerve root and pain. |
| kyphosis<br>kye FOH sis | *kyph/o* round back<br>*-osis* abnormal condition | Extreme posterior curvature of the thoracic area of the spine (Fig. 3-17A). |
| lordosis<br>lore DOH sis | *lord/o* swayback<br>*-osis* abnormal condition | Swayback; exaggerated anterior curve of the lumbar vertebrae (lower back) (Fig. 3-17, *B*). |
| scoliosis<br>skoh lee OH sis | *scoli/o* curvature<br>*-osis* abnormal condition | Lateral S curve of the spine that can cause an individual to lose inches in height (Fig. 3-17, *C*). |
| spinal stenosis<br>SPY nul<br>steh NOH sis | *spin/o* spine<br>*-al* pertaining to<br>*stenosis* abnormal condition of narrowing | Abnormal condition of narrowing of the spinal canal with attendant pain, sometimes caused by osteoarthritis or spondylolisthesis (Fig. 3-18). |
| spondylolisthesis<br>spon dih loh liss THEE sis | *spondyl/o* vertebra<br>*-listhesis* slipping | Condition resulting from the partial forward dislocation of one vertebra over the one beneath it. |
| spondylosis<br>spon dih LOH sis | *spondyl/o* vertebra<br>*-osis* abnormal condition | An abnormal condition characterized by stiffening of the vertebral joints. |

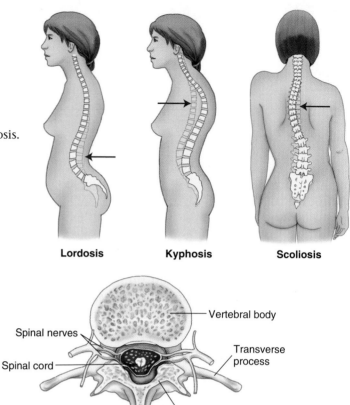

Fig. 3-17 **A,** Kyphosis, **B,** Lordosis, **C,** Scoliosis.

**Lordosis**  **Kyphosis**  **Scoliosis**

Fig. 3-18 Spinal stenosis. Bony overgrowth has narrowed the spinal canal and pinched the spinal nerves. Compare with normal vertebra in Fig. 3-4B.

Vertebral body

Spinal nerves

Transverse process

Spinal cord

Spinous process

Lamina

## Terms Related to Muscle Disorders

| Term | Word Origin | Definition |
|---|---|---|
| **contracture**<br>kun TRACK chur | *con-* together<br>*tract/o* pulling<br>*-ure* condition | Chronic fixation of a joint in flexion (such as a finger) caused by atrophy and shortening of muscle fibers after a long period of disuse. |
| **fibromyalgia**<br>fye broh mye AL jah | *fibr/o* fiber<br>*my/o* muscle<br>*-algia* pain | Disorder characterized by musculoskeletal pain, fatigue, muscle stiffness and spasms, and sleep disturbances. |
| **myasthenia gravis**<br>mye ah STHEE nee ah GRAV us | *my/o* muscle<br>*a-* without, no<br>*-sthenia* condition of strength<br>*gravis* severe | Usually severe condition characterized by fatigue and progressive muscle weakness, especially of the face and throat. |
| **plantar fasciitis**<br>plan tur<br>fass ee EYE tis | *plant/o* sole<br>*-ar* pertaining to<br>*fasci/o* fascia<br>*-itis* inflammation | Inflammation of the fascia on the sole of the foot. |
| **polymyositis**<br>pahl ee mye oh SYE tis | *poly-* many<br>*myos/o* muscle<br>*-itis* inflammation | Chronic, idiopathic inflammation of a number of voluntary muscles. |
| **postlaminectomy syndrome**<br>post lam in ECK tuh mee | *post-* after<br>*lamin/o* lamina<br>*-ectomy* removal | Group of symptoms that occur together after the removal of a lamina to correct a spinal disorder. |
| **rhabdomyolysis**<br>rab doh mye AL ih sis | *rhabdomy/o* striated muscle<br>*-lysis* breakdown, destruction | Breakdown of striated/skeletal muscle. |

## Exercise 18: Spinal and Muscle Disorders

*Match the muscle and spinal disorders with their definitions.*

____ 1. ankylosing
     spondylitis

____ 2. spinal stenosis

____ 3. herniated
     intervertebral disk

____ 4. plantar fasciitis

____ 5. postlaminectomy
     syndrome

____ 6. lumbago

____ 7. contracture

____ 8. fibromyalgia

____ 9. lordosis

____ 10. scoliosis

____ 11. dorsalgia

____ 12. myasthenia
      gravis

A. upper back pain
B. inflammation of the fascia of the foot
C. chronic flexion of a joint caused by muscle
   atrophy
D. muscle disorder characterized by
   musculoskeletal pain, fatigue, and sleep
   disorders
E. lateral S curve of the spine
F. protrusion of the central part of the vertebral
   disk
G. narrowing of the spinal canal
H. chronic inflammatory disease of idiopathic
   origin, which causes fusion of the spine
I. usually severe disease characterized by
   muscular weakness
J. symptoms that occur after removal of the
   lamina
K. swayback
L. lower back pain

*Build the terms.*

13. condition of slipping of the vertebrae _____

14. abnormal condition of the vertebra _____

15. abnormal condition of curvature _____

16. pertaining to inflammation of the fascia of the sole _____

17. breakdown of striated muscle _____

18. inflammation of many muscles _____

## Trauma

### Fractures

Put simply, a fracture is a broken bone. However, there are a number of types of breaks, each with its own name. Most fractures occur as a result of trauma, but some can result from an underlying disease, such as osteoporosis or cancer; these **pathologic fractures** are also sometimes called *spontaneous fractures*. All fractures may be classified as simple (closed) or compound (open) fractures. The break in a simple fracture does not rupture the skin, but a compound fracture splits open the skin, which allows more opportunity for infection to take place. See the following table for different types of fractures.

### Sprain/Strain and Dislocation/Subluxation

A **sprain** is a traumatic injury to a joint involving the ligaments. Swelling, pain, and discoloration of the skin may be present. The severity of the injury is measured in grades. **A strain** is a lesser injury, usually described as overuse or overstretching of a muscle or tendon.

A bone that is completely out of its place in a joint is called a **dislocation.** If the bone is partially out of the joint, it is considered to be a **subluxation** (sub luck SAY shun). This can be a congenital or an acquired condition.

**Compartment syndrome** is a potentially serious medical condition that is a result of swelling within the fascia. The increased pressure limits the blood supply, which in turn may lead to nerve and muscle damage.

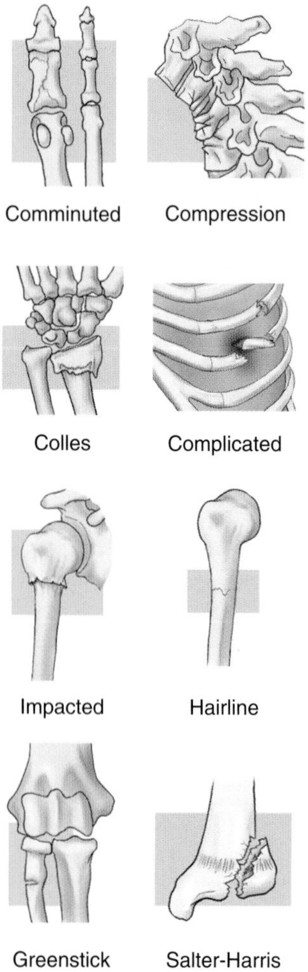

Comminuted    Compression

Colles    Complicated

Impacted    Hairline

Greenstick    Salter-Harris

**Fig. 3-19** Fractures.

| Terms Related to Trauma | |
|---|---|
| **Type** | **Definition** |
| **FRACTURES** (Fig. 3-19) | |
| Colles | Fracture at distal end of the radius at the epiphysis. Often occurs when patient has attempted to break his/her fall. |
| comminuted | Bone is crushed and/or shattered into multiple pieces. |
| complicated | Bone is broken and pierces an internal organ. |
| compression | Fractured area of bone collapses on itself. |
| greenstick | Partially bent and partially broken. Relatively common in children. |
| hairline | Minor fracture appearing as a thin line on x-ray. May not extend through bone. |
| impacted | Broken bones with ends driven into each other. |
| Salter Harris | Fracture of epiphyseal plate in children. |
| **OTHER TRAUMA** (Figs. 3-20 and 3-21) | |
| dislocation | Bone that is completely out of its joint socket. |
| subluxation | Partial dislocation. |
| sprain | Traumatic injury to ligaments of a joint, including tearing of a ligament. |
| strain | Overstretching of muscle or a tendon. |

All fracture examples are coded as closed fractures.

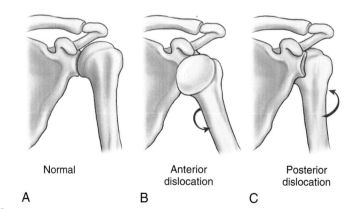

Normal          Anterior dislocation          Posterior dislocation

A          B          C

**Fig. 3-20  A,** Normal shoulder. Dislocated shoulder, anterior **(B)** and posterior **(C).**

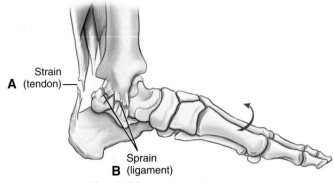

Fig. 3-21 **A,** Strain **B,** sprain.

## Exercise 19: **Fractures**

*Match the fractures with their definitions.*

_____ 1. complicated        _____ 6. simple/closed

_____ 2. greenstick         _____ 7. compound/open

_____ 3. Colles             _____ 8. hairline

_____ 4. impacted           _____ 9. pathologic

_____ 5. comminuted

A. broken bone pierces internal organ.
B. broken bone pierces skin.
C. spontaneous fracture as a result of disease.
D. bone is partially bent and partially broken.
E. bone is broken, skin is closed.
F. distal end of radius is broken.
G. ends of broken bone are driven into each other.
H. fracture appears as a line on the bone and fracture may not be completely through bone.
I. bone is crushed.

## Exercise 20: **Other Trauma**

1. A partial displacement of a bone at a joint is a _____; full displacement is a

   _____.

2. An injury that can be described in grades and involves the soft tissue of a joint is a

   _____.

3. An overstretching of a muscle is a _____.

4. Swelling within the confines of a muscle fascia can lead to _____.

## Terms Related to Benign Neoplasms

| Term | Word Origin | Definition |
|------|-------------|------------|
| **chondroma** <br> kon DROH mah | *chondr/o* cartilage <br> *-oma* tumor, mass | Benign tumor of the cartilage, usually occurring in children and adolescents. |
| **exostosis** <br> eck sahs TOH sis | *ex-* out <br> *oste/o* bone <br> *-osis* abnormal condition | Abnormal condition of bony growth. Also called **hyperostosis** and **osteochondroma**. |
| **leiomyoma** <br> lye oh mye OH mah | *leiomy/o* smooth muscle <br> *-oma* tumor, mass | Benign tumor of smooth muscle. The most common leiomyoma is in the uterus and is termed a fibroid. |
| **osteoma** <br> ahs tee OH mah | *oste/o* bone <br> *-oma* tumor, mass | Benign bone tumor, usually of compact bone. |
| **rhabdomyoma** <br> rab doh mye OH mah | *rhabdomy/o* skeletal muscle <br> *-oma* tumor, mass | Benign tumor of striated/voluntary/skeletal muscle. |

## Terms Related to Malignant Neoplasms

| Term | Word Origin | Definition |
|------|-------------|------------|
| **chondrosarcoma** <br> kon droh sar KOH mah | *chondr/o* cartilage <br> *-sarcoma* connective tissue cancer | Malignant tumor of the cartilage. Occurs most frequently in adults (Fig. 3-22). |
| **leiomyosarcoma** <br> lye oh mye oh sar KOH mah | *leiomy/o* smooth muscle <br> *-sarcoma* connective tissue cancer | Malignant tumor of smooth muscle. Most commonly appearing in the uterus. |
| **osteosarcoma** <br> ahs tee oh sar KOH mah | *oste/o* bone <br> *-sarcoma* connective tissue cancer | Malignant tumor of bone. Also called **Ewing sarcoma**. Most common children's bone cancer. |
| **rhabdomyosarcoma** <br> rab doh mye oh sar KOH mah | *rhabdomy/o* skeletal muscle <br> *-sarcoma* connective tissue cancer | Highly malignant tumor of skeletal muscle. Also called **rhabdosarcoma** or **rhabdomyoblastoma**. |

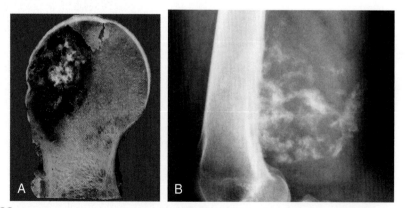

**Fig. 3-22 A,** Chondrosarcoma of femur. **B,** X-ray showing prominent dense calcification in a large neoplastic mass.

## Exercise 21: Neoplasms

*Match the neoplasms with their definitions.*

____ 1. rhabdomyosarcoma      ____ 3. leiomyosarcoma

____ 2. osteosarcoma      ____ 4. chondrosarcoma

A. connective tissue cancer of bone
B. connective tissue cancer of cartilage
C. connective tissue cancer of skeletal muscle
D. connective tissue cancer of smooth muscle

*Build the term.*

5. benign tumor of skeletal muscle _____

6. benign bone tumor _____

7. benign tumor of smooth muscle _____

8. benign tumor of cartilage _____

9. an abnormal condition of out(growth) of bone _____

Click on **Hear It, Spell It** to practice spelling the pathology terms you have learned in this chapter. To see how well you can pronounce the pathology terms in the chapter, click on **Hear It, Say It.**

## *Case Study* Jean Herold

Jean Herold is a 54-year-old nurse's aide who exercises three to four times a week at her local fitness center. As she is leaving the center one night, she slips on some ice and falls heavily on her right upper arm and shoulder. Jean drove herself home but spends the night in a great deal of pain, and the next day her friend drives her to the hospital. She has x-rays and a CT scan of her right arm and shoulder. She is diagnosed with a fracture to the top of her upper arm bone and is given pain and nausea medication. She is admitted to the hospital and has surgery the next day.

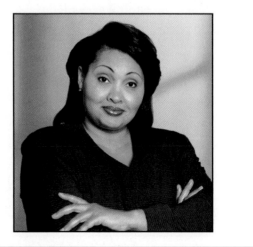

## *Case Study* Jean Herold

Herold, Jean F - 12438 Opened by Landrey, Melissa, PA

Task  Edit  View  Time Scale  Options  Help

**Herold, Jean F**

Age: 54 years
DOB: 07/23/1957

Sex: Female
MRN: 12438

Loc: AR-OC
FIN: 8425633

Reference Text Browser | Form Browser | Medication Profile

Orders | Last 48 Hours | ED | Lab | Radiology | **Assessments** | Surgery | Clinical Notes | Pt. Info | Pt. Schedule | Task List | I & O | MAR

Flowsheet: Assessments      ...      Level: History & Physical         ● Table  ○ Group  ○ List

Navigator

✓  History & Physical

| | |
|---|---|
| CHIEF COMPLAINT: | Right shoulder pain/fracture |
| HISTORY OF PRESENT ILLNESS: | Patient is a 54-year-old female who works as a health-care worker. While out exercising last night, she fell on her right shoulder. She has a comminuted fracture of the proximal humerus involving the humeral head, extending into the joint space. Admitted for observation and analgesia. CT of shoulder reveals the need for a humeral prosthesis. Some discomfort with deep inspiration. Unclear whether this is in the shoulder or possible right chest wall. |
| PAST MEDICAL HISTORY: | Cholecystectomy 1986. ORIF left forearm, fracture same forearm, age 9. Has some dependent edema and takes Lasix 80 mg daily for it. Does not wear compression stockings as they make her feet feel cold. Also diagnosis of fibromyalgia. |
| FAMILY HISTORY: | Mother died age 64 post surgical pulmonary embolus. |
| REVIEW OF SYSTEMS: | Negative. |
| PHYSICAL EXAM: | Pleasant, uncomfortable, overweight female appearing her stated age and in no distress. HEENT normal, neck supple, thyroid normal. No JVD, carotids normal. Lungs decreased breath sounds at bases. Heart regular rate and rhythm. Extremities: normal range of motion of lower extremities. Motor sensory deep tendon reflexes are normal in arm. Trace pretibial edema bilaterally without venostasis changes. Excellent peripheral pulses. Cannot adduct her arm and shoulder without pain. |
| IMAGING: | X-ray of shoulder and CT show comminuted fracture. |
| ASSESSMENT: | Comminuted right proximal humeral fracture involving humeral head. |
| PLAN: | Admit for analgesia, IV fluids. Has a little nausea probably from analgesics. Won't have surgery until tomorrow. Preoperative labs, EKG, and chest x-ray will be obtained before that time. |

PROD | MAHAFC | 22 Jan 2012 | 09:19

## Exercise 22: Admission Record

*Using the admission record on p. 102, answer the following questions:*

1. Which bone did she break while exercising? Give both the medical term and the common name.

   _____

2. Did she fracture the area *closest to her shoulder* or *farthest from her shoulder?* Underline one.

3. Describe the type of fracture sustained. _____

4. What other MS disorder does she currently have? _____

5. What does "cannot adduct her arm and shoulder without pain" mean? _____

## Age Matters

### Pediatrics

As can be seen from our table of congenital disorders, there are several musculoskeletal conditions that a child may be born with: achondroplasia, muscular dystrophy, two disorders of the phalanges (syndactyly and polydactyly), spina bifida occulta, talipes, and congential torticollis. Although not exclusive to childhood, pediatric statistics reveal high numbers of children treated each year for the effects of physical trauma. Fractures are common: beginning with clavicular fractures (the result of birth trauma) to fractures of the arms (humerus, radius, and ulna) and the legs (femur, tibia, and fibula). Sprains, strains, dislocations, and subluxations are other pediatric diagnoses that appear with regularity for this system.

### Geriatrics

Statistics collected on the geriatric population of patients also report a high number of fractures. These, however, are mainly fractures of the hip and femur and are often preceded by bone loss caused by osteoporosis or cancer. Osteoarthritis, often referred to as "wear and tear disease," is another disorder that afflicts many patients as they age. The high number of total knee replacement surgeries today are often the result of this disease.

You can review the pathology terms you've learned in this chapter by playing **Medical Millionaire.**

## DIAGNOSTIC PROCEDURES

### Terms Related to Imaging

| Term | Word Origin | Definition |
|---|---|---|
| arthrography<br>ar THRAH gruh fee | *arthr/o* joint<br>*-graphy* process of recording | X-ray recording of a joint. |
| arthroscopy<br>ar THRAHS kuh pee | *arthr/o* joint<br>*-scopy* process of viewing | Visual examination of a joint, accomplished by use of an arthroscope (Fig. 3-23). |
| computed tomography (CT) scan | *tom/o* section<br>*-graphy* process of recording | Imaging technology that records transverse planes of the body for diagnostic purposes. |

## Terms Related to Imaging—cont'd

| Term | Word Origin | Definition |
|------|-------------|------------|
| **DEXA scan**<br>DECK suh | | Dual energy x-ray absorptiometry, a procedure that measures the density of bone at the hip and spine. Also called **bone mineral density studies** (Fig. 3-24). |
| **electromyography (EMG)**<br>ee leck troh mye AH gruh fee | *electr/o* electricity<br>*my/o* muscle<br>*-graphy* process of recording | Procedure that records the electrical activity of muscles. |
| **magnetic resonance imaging (MRI)** | | Procedure that uses magnetic properties to record detailed information about internal structures. |
| **myelogram**<br>MYE eh loh gram | *myel/o* spinal cord<br>*-gram* record, recording | X-ray of spinal canal done after injection of contrast medium. |
| **x-ray (radiograph)** | | Imaging technique using electromagnetic radiation for recording internal structures. |

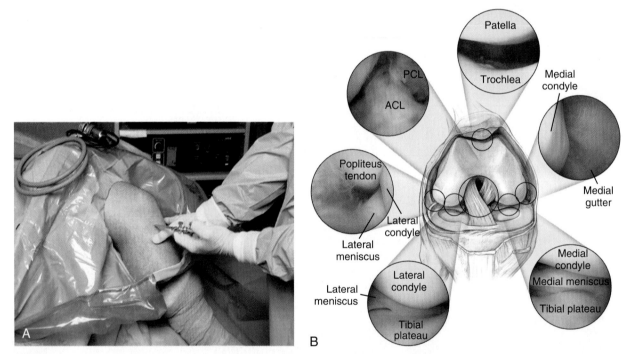

**Fig. 3-23 A,** Arthroscopy of the knee. **B,** Knee structures that can be seen during arthroscopy at six different points (circles).

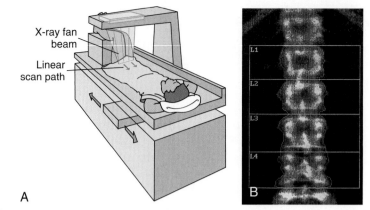

X-ray fan
beam

Linear
scan path

A

B

**Fig. 3-24** Dual energy x-ray absorptiometry (DEXA). **A,** DEXA system. **B,** Scan of lumbar vertebrae.

## Other Diagnostic Tests

| Term | Word Origin | Definition |
|------|-------------|------------|
| **goniometry** <br> goh nee AH meh tree | *goni/o* angle <br> *-metry* process of measuring | The process of measuring a joint's range of motion. The instrument used is called a **goniometer** (Fig. 3-25). |
| **Phalen test** <br> FAY lin | | A diagnostic test where the back (dorsal surfaces) of the patient's hands are pressed together to elicit the symptoms of carpal tunnel syndrome. |
| **range-of-motion testing (ROM)** | | An assessment of the degree to which a joint can be extended and flexed. |
| **rheumatoid factor test** <br> ROO mah toyd | *rheumat/o* watery flow <br> *-oid* resembling | Lab test that looks for **rheumatoid factor** (RF) present in the blood of those who have rheumatoid arthritis. |
| **serum calcium (Ca)** | | Test to measure the amount of calcium in the blood. |

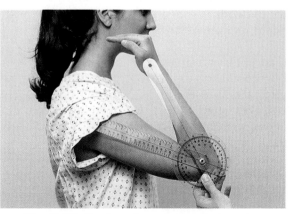

**Fig. 3-25** Goniometry using a goniometer.

## Exercise 23: Diagnostic Procedures

*Match the diagnostic tests to their definitions.*

____ 1. MRI          ____ 5. RF          A. test for rheumatoid arthritis

B. imaging technique using electromagnetic radiation

____ 2. DEXA scan    ____ 6. serum calcium    C. imaging of a plane of the body

D. blood test for Ca

____ 3. x-ray        ____ 7. EMG          E. test to measure bone density, using dual energy x-ray

____ 4. ROM          ____ 8. CT scan      F. imaging using magnetic resonance

G. range of motion

H. electromyography

*Build the terms.*

9. Process of viewing a joint _____

10. Process of recording a joint _____

11. Process of recording the electrical (activity) of a muscle _____

12. Process of recording the spinal cord _____

## THERAPEUTIC INTERVENTIONS

### Setting Fractures

Broken bones must be "set"—that is, aligned and immobilized; the most common method is with a plaster cast. If a bone does not mend and realign correctly, it is said to be a **malunion.** If no healing takes place, it is a **nonunion.** A piece of bone that does not have a renewed blood supply will die; this tissue then is called a **sequestrum** (seh KWES trum). Removal of dirt, damaged tissue, or foreign objects from a wound is one of the first steps in repairing an open fracture. This removal of debris is called **débridement** (de breed MON). Methods of fixation and alignment are described as follows:

**External fixation (EF):** Noninvasive stabilization of broken bones in which no opening is made in the skin; instead, the stabilization takes place mainly through devices external to the body that offer traction (Fig. 3-26, *A*).

**Internal fixation (IF):** Stabilization of broken bones in their correct position, using pins, screws, plates, and so on, which are fastened to the bones to maintain correct alignment (Fig. 3-26, *B*).

**Reduction:** Alignment and immobilization of the ends of a broken bone. Also referred to as **manipulation.** *Open reduction* (OR) requires incision of the skin; *closed reduction* (CR) does not require incision.

Click on **Animations** to view animations of an open reduction internal fixation (ORIF) of an ankle fracture and a closed reduction (CR) and pinning of a hip fracture.

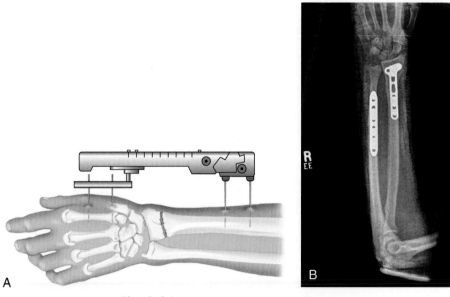

Fig. 3-26 Fixation. **A,** External. **B,** Internal.

## Terms Related to Therapeutic Interventions

| Term | Word Origin | Definition |
|---|---|---|
| **amputation**<br>am pyoo TAY shun | | Removal of a limb when there are no feasible options to save it. |
| **arthrocentesis**<br>ar throh sen TEE sis | *arthr/o* joint<br>*-centesis* surgical puncture | Surgical puncture of a joint to remove fluid. |
| **arthrodesis**<br>ar throh DEE sis | *arthr/o* joint<br>*-desis* binding | Binding or stabilization of a joint by operative means. |
| **arthroplasty**<br>ar throh plas tee | *arthr/o* joint<br>*-plasty* surgical repair | General term meaning surgical repair of a joint. |
| **bunionectomy**<br>bun yun ECK tuh mee | *bunion/o* bunion<br>*-ectomy* excision, resection | Removal of a bunion (Fig. 3-27). |
| **kyphoplasty**<br>KYE foh plas tee | *kyph/o* round back<br>*-plasty* surgical repair | Minimally invasive procedure designed to address the pain of fractured vertebrae resulting from osteoporosis or cancer (Fig. 3-28). A balloon is used to inflate the area of fracture before a cementlike substance is injected. The substance hardens rapidly, and pain relief is immediate in most patients. |
| **laminectomy**<br>lam ih NECK tuh mee | *lamin/o* lamina<br>*-ectomy* excision, resection | Removal of the bony arches of one or more vertebrae to relieve compression of the spinal cord (Fig. 3-29). |
| **meniscectomy**<br>men iss ECK tuh mee | *menisc/o* meniscus<br>*-ectomy* removal | Removal of a meniscus such as in the knee. |
| **myorrhaphy**<br>mye ORE rah fee | *my/o* muscle<br>*-rrhaphy* suture | Suture of a muscle. |

*Continued*

## Terms Related to Therapeutic Interventions—cont'd

| Term | Word Origin | Definition |
|------|-------------|------------|
| **operative ankylosis**<br>AH pur ah tiv<br>ang kih LOH sis | *ankyl/o* stiffening<br>*-osis* abnormal condition | Procedure used in the treatment of spinal fractures or after diskectomy or laminectomy for the correction of a herniated vertebral disk; also used to describe surgical fixation of a joint. Also called **arthrodesis**. |
| **osteoclasis**<br>AHS tee oh klay sis | *oste/o* bone<br>*-clasis* intentional breaking | Refracture of a bone; usually done if a bone has a malunion. |
| **osteoplasty**<br>AHS tee oh plas tee | *oste/o* bone<br>*-plasty* surgical repair | Surgical repair of a bone. |
| **prosthesis**<br>prahs THEE sis | *prosth/o* addition<br>*-is* thing | An artificial body part that is constructed to replace missing limbs, eyes, and other body parts (*pl.* prostheses). |
| **spondylosyndesis**<br>spon dih loh sin DEE sis | *spondyl/o* vertebra<br>*syn-* together<br>*-desis* binding | Fixation of an unstable segment of the spine by skeletal traction, immobilization of the patient in a body cast, or stabilization with a bone graft or synthetic device. Also called **spinal fusion** and **spondylodesis**. |
| **syndesmoplasty**<br>sin DEZ moh plas tee | *syndesm/o* ligament<br>*-plasty* surgical repair | Surgical repair of a ligament. |
| **tenomyoplasty**<br>ten oh MYE oh plas tee | *ten/o* tendon<br>*my/o* muscle<br>*-plasty* surgical repair | Surgical repair of a muscle and a tendon. |
| **total hip replacement (THR)** | | Replacement of the femoral head and the acetabulum of the hip with either plastic or metal appliances. |
| **total knee replacement (TKR)** | | Extensive surgical procedure that involves the replacement of the entire knee joint, either unilaterally or bilaterally (Fig. 3-30). |
| **traction** | *tract/o* pulling<br>*-ion* process of | The process of pulling a body part into correct alignment, as to correct a dislocation. |

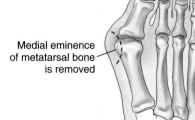

Medial eminence of metatarsal bone is removed

**Fig. 3-27** Bunionectomy.

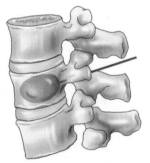

**Fig. 3-28** Kyphoplasty.

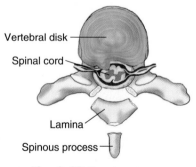

Vertebral disk

Spinal cord

Lamina

Spinous process

**Fig. 3-29** Laminectomy.

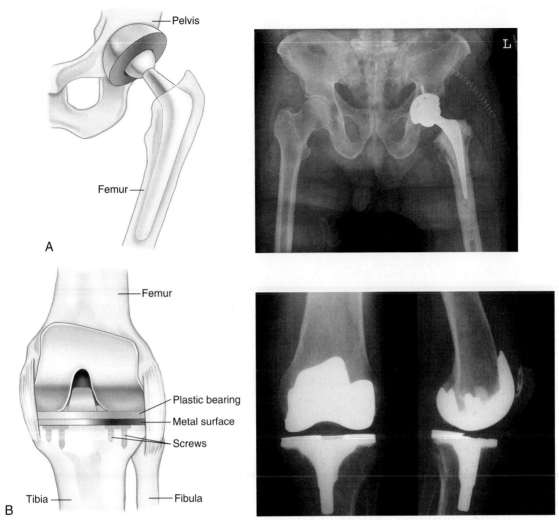

**Fig. 3-30 A,** Total hip replacement (THR). **B,** Total knee replacement (TKR).

## Exercise 24: Therapeutic Interventions

*Match the therapeutic terms with their definitions.*

_____ 1. débridement _____ 6. arthrodesis

_____ 2. open reduction _____ 7. prosthesis

_____ 3. amputation _____ 8. spondylosyndesis

_____ 4. myorrhaphy _____ 9. arthrocentesis

_____ 5. osteoclasis _____ 10. closed reduction

A. suture of muscle
B. intentional fracture of bone
C. alignment of ends of bone with incision
D. alignment of ends of bone without incision
E. surgical puncture of a joint
F. artificial body part
G. removal of a limb
H. removal of debris
I. spinal fusion
J. fixation of a joint

*Build a term that means:*

11. surgical repair of a joint _____

12. intentional breaking of a bone _____

13. excision of a bunion _____

14. surgical repair of a tendon and muscle _____

15. removal of a meniscus _____

16. surgical repair of a ligament _____

## PHARMACOLOGY

**analgesics:** Reduce pain. Examples include morphine (MS Contin), hydrocodone (Vicodin or Lortab, in combination with acetaminophen), acetaminophen (Tylenol), and NSAIDs such as naproxen (Anaprox).

**antiinflammatories:** Used to reduce inflammation and pain. Examples
include steroidal and nonsteroidal antiinflammatory drugs (NSAIDs). Pred-
nisolone (Delta-Cortef) is an example of a steroid; ibuprofen (Advil, Motrin)
and celecoxib (Celebrex) are examples of NSAIDs.

**antirheumatics:** Manage symptoms of rheumatoid arthritis. Methotrexate,
hydroxychloroquine (Plaquenil), and gold sodium thiomalate (Myochrysine)
are common examples.

**bisphosphonates:** Prevent and sometimes reverse bone loss to treat diseases
such as osteoporosis, Paget disease, or bone cancer. Examples include alen-
dronate (Fosamax) and zoledronic acid (Zometa).

**disease-modifying antirheumatic drugs (DMARDs):** Slow progression of
rheumatoid arthritis while also reducing signs and symptoms. Examples
include leflunomide (Arava), etanercept (Enbrel), and infliximab (Remicade).

**muscle relaxants:** Relieve pain caused by muscle spasms by relaxing the skeletal muscles. Examples include cyclobenzaprine (Flexeril) and metaxalone
(Skelaxin).

## Exercise 25: Pharmacology

1. What class of drugs may prevent osteoporosis? _____.

2. Rheumatoid arthritis progression may be treated with _____.

3. NSAIDs are used to treat what kinds of symptoms? _____

4. _____ are used to treat muscle spasms.

Click on **Hear It, Spell It** to practice spelling the diagnostic and therapeutic terms you have learned in this chapter.
To hear how well you pronounce the terms in the chapter, click on **Hear It, Say It.**

## Abbreviations

| Abbreviation | Meaning | Abbreviation | Meaning |
|---|---|---|---|
| A | action | MRI | magnetic resonance imaging |
| C1-C7 | first cervical through seventh cervical vertebrae | MS | musculoskeletal |
| | | NSAIDs | nonsteroidal anti-inflammatory drugs |
| CR | closed reduction | | |
| CREF | closed reduction external fixation | O | origin |
| CT | computed tomography | OA | osteoarthritis |
| CTS | carpal tunnel syndrome | OR | open reduction |
| D1-D12 | first dorsal through twelfth dorsal vertebrae | ORIF | open reduction internal fixation |
| | | PIP | proximal interphalangeal joint |
| DEXA, DXA | dual energy x-ray absorptiometry | RA | rheumatoid arthritis |
| DIP | distal interphalangeal joint | RF | rheumatoid factor |
| DJD | degenerative joint disease | ROM | range of motion |
| EF | external fixation | S1-S5 | first sacral through fifth sacral segments |
| EMG | electromyography | | |
| Fx, # | fracture | SLE | systemic lupus erythematosus |
| I | insertion | T1-T12 | first thoracic through twelfth thoracic vertebrae |
| L1-L5 | first lumbar through fifth lumbar vertebrae | | |
| | | THR | total hip replacement |
| MD | muscular dystrophy | TKR | total knee replacement |

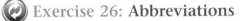

## Exercise 26: **Abbreviations**

*Explain the meanings of the abbreviations used in the following examples.*

1. Greta is an 83-year-old white female with a compression Fx of L5.

   _____

2. The patient had been self-medicating her OA with NSAIDs.

   _____

3. Bursitis caused a limited ROM of the shoulder joint for Paul.

   _____

4. Which of the following is not an imaging procedure—CT, CTS, MRI?

   _____

# Chapter Review

*Match the word parts to their definitions.*

## WORD PART DEFINITIONS

| Prefix/Suffix |
|---|
| *-centesis* |
| *-clasis* |
| *-desis* |
| *-listhesis* |
| *-malacia* |
| *-osis* |
| *peri-* |
| *-physis* |
| *-plasia* |
| *syn-* |

**Definition**

1. _____ binding
2. _____ condition of development
3. _____ surgical puncture
4. _____ together, joined
5. _____ softening
6. _____ slipping
7. _____ surrounding, around
8. _____ intentional breaking
9. _____ growth
10. _____ abnormal condition

| Combining Form |
|---|
| *arthr/o* |
| *carp/o* |
| *cervic/o* |
| *chondr/o* |
| *cleid/o* |
| *coccyg/o* |
| *cost/o* |
| *dactyl/o* |
| *femor/o* |
| *gnath/o* |
| *humer/o* |
| *mandibul/o* |
| *my/o* |
| *myel/o* |
| *olecran/o* |
| *oste/o* |
| *patell/a* |
| *phalang/o* |
| *rhabdomy/o* |
| *scapul/o* |
| *spondyl/o* |
| *zygomat/o* |

**Definition**

11. _____ collarbone
12. _____ bone
13. _____ jaw (entire)
14. _____ skeletal muscle
15. _____ upper arm bone
16. _____ wrist
17. _____ cheekbone
18. _____ thigh bone
19. _____ neck
20. _____ vertebra
21. _____ cartilage
22. _____ spinal cord
23. _____ finger/toe (whole)
24. _____ finger/toe bone
25. _____ rib
26. _____ muscle
27. _____ elbow
28. _____ tailbone
29. _____ kneecap
30. _____ joint
31. _____ lower jaw
32. _____ shoulder blade

# WORDSHOP

| Prefixes | Combining Forms | Suffixes |
|----------|-----------------|----------|
| a- | arthr/o | -desis |
| an- | chondr/o | -itis |
| inter- | cost/o | -lysis |
| peri- | dactyl/o | -malacia |
| poly- | my/o | -oma |
| syn- | myos/o | -osis |
|  | oste/o | -plasia |
|  | phyt/o | -plasty |
|  | rhabdomy/o | -rrhaphy |
|  | spin/o | -um |
|  | spondyl/o | -y |
|  | syndesm/o |  |
|  | ten/o |  |

*Build the following terms by combining the word parts above. Some word parts may be used more than once. Some may not be used at all. The number in parentheses indicates the number of word parts needed.*

| Definition | Term |
|------------|------|
| 1. structure surrounding bone (3) | |
| 2. inflammation of many muscles (3) | |
| 3. inflammation surrounding a joint (3) | |
| 4. softening of the cartilage (2) | |
| 5. condition of many fingers/toes (3) | |
| 6. destruction of skeletal muscle (2) | |
| 7. abnormal condition of bone growth (3) | |
| 8. binding of a joint (2) | |
| 9. suture of a muscle (2) | |
| 10. condition of joined fingers/toes (3) | |
| 11. tumor of cartilage (2) | |
| 12. binding of vertebrae together (3) | |
| 13. surgical repair of a ligament (2) | |
| 14. no formation of cartilage (3) | |
| 15. surgical repair of a tendon and a muscle (3) | |

*Sort the terms below into the correct categories.*

## TERM SORTING

| Anatomy and Physiology | Pathology | Diagnostic Procedures | Therapeutic Interventions |
|---|---|---|---|
| | | | |
| | | | |
| | | | |
| | | | |
| | | | |
| | | | |
| | | | |
| | | | |
| | | | |
| | | | |

| | | | |
|---|---|---|---|
| arthrocentesis | CTS | MRI | radius |
| arthrodesis | DEXA | myelogram | ROM |
| arthrography | diaphysis | myorrhaphy | serum calcium |
| arthroscopy | digitus | osteoclasis | spondylolisthesis |
| arthrosis | EMG | osteomyelitis | sternum |
| articulation | goniometry | osteoplasty | syndactyly |
| bunion | humerus | osteoporosis | tendinitis |
| bursitis | laminectomy | osteosarcoma | tenomyoplasty |
| cartilage | ligament | Phalen test | TKR |
| costa | meniscectomy | prosthesis | ulna |

*Replace the highlighted words with the correct terms.*

## TRANSLATIONS

1. Ms. Alston was diagnosed with **softening of the cartilage** of her knee and a **cyst of synovial fluid in the popliteal area of her leg.**

2. After a crushing injury to her leg, the physician performed **removal of the limb** and replaced it with a/an **artificial body part.**

3. The surgeon performed a **suture of a muscle** to correct Mr. Adams' injury.

4. The patient had a **surgical puncture of a joint** to correct **an abnormal condition of blood in the joint** of Jason's left hip.

5. Dr. Matthews performed **an alignment and immobilization** of the right **collarbone** of 5-year-old Caitlin, who had fallen while jumping on her bed.

6. The student had a **diagnostic test where the dorsal surfaces of the hands are pressed together** to diagnose **compression injury of the median nerve at the wrist.**

7. Sarah Henderson had **abnormal bone growths** in the **joints between the bones of her fingers.**

8. The patient had **an extreme posterior curvature of the thoracic area of the spine** that was a result of her **loss of bone mass.**

9. The patient was admitted for **inflammation of the bone and bone marrow** of his **lower lateral arm bone.**

10. The patient complained of **inflammation of the fascia on the sole of the foot** and **inflammation of a tendon.**

11. **A procedure that records the electrical activity of muscles** was used to confirm the child's **group of disorders characterized as an inherited progressive atrophy of skeletal muscle.**

12. An x-ray revealed a **partially bent and partially broken** fracture of the child's right **upper arm bone.**

13. The baby was diagnosed with **condition of more than five fingers on her hand** and **condition of the joining of the toes.**

14. Mrs. Anderhub had **a removal of a bunion** to correct her **painful enlargement and inflammation of the first metatarsophalangeal joint.**

Ms. Auden has been experiencing pain in her knees for several years, a common symptom of osteoarthritis, also called "the wear-and-tear" disease. She has been taking an assortment of medications, but because she has stomach irritation with these drugs, she sought help from an acupuncturist recommended by a friend. Unfortunately, this has not relieved her pain.

Ms. Auden undergoes arthroscopy, which shows extensive deterioration of the joint. After reviewing the results of the arthroscopy, x-rays, and an MRI, her orthopedic surgeon advises a TKR. Ms. Auden is nervous but decides she can no longer put up with the pain. She agrees to have the surgery.

Ms. Auden has her TKR done 2 weeks after her appointment. Immediately after surgery, a compression bandage is attached to completely immobilize her knee in extension. By the time she goes home from the hospital, this is removed and replaced by a plastic shell. Almost

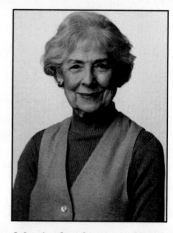

immediately, Ms. Auden begins physical therapy to strengthen the joint muscles and give the new joint mobility. At-home exercises include ROM exercises, muscle strengthening, and stationary bicycling. Her recovery time takes several weeks, but on follow-up she says, "I just wish I had done this sooner!"

---

Auden, Evelyn E - 29202 Opened by Chong, Mae-Li (surgeon)

Task   Edit   View   Time Scale   Options   Help

As Of 11:11

**Auden, Evelyn E**

| Age: 72 years | Sex: Female | Loc: ARH-ANC |
| DOB: 09/02/1939 | MRN: 29202 | FIN: 8425633 |

Reference Text Browser | Form Browser | Medication Profile

Orders | Last 48 Hours | ED | Lab | Radiology | Assessments | **Surgery** | Clinical Notes | Pt. Info | Pt. Schedule | Task List | I & O | MAR

Flowsheet: Surgery      Level: Operative Report      ● Table  ○ Group  ○ List

Navigator
✓ Operative Report

Preoperative Diagnosis: Degenerative Joint
   Disease, Right Knee
Postoperative Diagnosis: Degenerative Joint
   Disease, Right Knee
Name of Operation: Total Knee Replacement

Components: Zimmer NextGen LPS
Femur: size G
Tibia: 6
Articulating Surface: 10 mm
Patella: 38

Anesthesia: Spinal
Estimated Blood Loss: 150 cc
Antibiotics: Vancomycin 1 gm
Tourniquet: 350 mmHg
Complications: none

**Procedure**
The patient was properly identified in the OR, and the leg was prepped and draped in the routine fashion. The leg was exsanguinated, and the tourniquet inflated. A standard anterior approach was made along with the median parapatellar arthrotomy. The patella was everted. The fat pad was partially removed, the knee flexed, and all joint surfaces prepared in the conventional manner to the size needed. The surfaces were prepared with pulse irrigating system followed by antibiotic irrigation. They were then dried. All components were cemented simultaneously. Any excess cement was removed with curettes and/or osteotomes.
   The knee was placed in full extension, if not slight hyperextension, while the cement cured. The patient tolerated the procedure well and left the operating room in stable condition.

PROD | MAHAFC | 12 April 2012 | 11:11

## Operative Report

1. A synonym for the preoperative diagnosis of degenerative joint disease is _____.

2. An "anterior approach" to the knee would be through which part of the knee?

   _____

3. What is the patella? _____

4. To what does the term parapatellar refer? _____

5. What is an arthrotomy? _____

6. If the patella was everted, how would it be placed? _____

7. What is an osteotome? _____

8. What would hyperextension be? _____

For more interactive learning go to the Shiland Evolve site and click on:
- **Whack-A-Word-Part** to review musculoskeletal word parts.
- **Wheel of Terminology** and **Word Shop** to practice building musculoskeletal terms.
- **Tournament of Terminology** to test your knowledge of the musculoskeletal system.
- **Terminology Triage** to sort musculoskeletal terms into categories.

# 4

*Genius is one percent inspiration and ninety-nine percent perspiration.*
**—Thomas Edison**

## OBJECTIVES

- Recognize and use terms related to the anatomy and physiology of the integumentary system.
- Recognize and use terms related to the pathology of the integumentary system.
- Recognize and use terms related to the diagnostic procedures for the integumentary system.
- Recognize and use terms related to the therapeutic interventions for the integumentary system.

# Integumentary System

## CHAPTER AT A GLANCE

*Use this list of key word parts and terms to assess your knowledge. Check off the ones you have mastered.*

### ANATOMY AND PHYSIOLOGY

- [ ] dermis
- [ ] epidermis
- [ ] eponychium
- [ ] hair follicle
- [ ] nail bed
- [ ] nail body
- [ ] nail root
- [ ] sebaceous glands
- [ ] subcutaneous tissue
- [ ] sudoriferous glands

### KEY WORD PARTS

**PREFIXES**
- [ ] an-
- [ ] crypt-
- [ ] epi-
- [ ] hyper-
- [ ] intra-
- [ ] par-
- [ ] sub-
- [ ] trans-

**SUFFIXES**
- [ ] -cide
- [ ] -ectomy
- [ ] -itis
- [ ] -lytic
- [ ] -oma
- [ ] -osis
- [ ] -plasty

**COMBINING FORMS**
- [ ] cutane/o
- [ ] dermat/o, derm/o
- [ ] follicul/o
- [ ] hidr/o
- [ ] kerat/o
- [ ] melan/o
- [ ] myc/o
- [ ] onych/o
- [ ] pedicul/i
- [ ] rhytid/o
- [ ] seb/o
- [ ] trich/o
- [ ] ungu/o

### KEY TERMS

- [ ] alopecia
- [ ] anhidrosis
- [ ] curettage
- [ ] débridement
- [ ] decubitus ulcer
- [ ] dermatoplasty
- [ ] ecchymosis
- [ ] eczema
- [ ] escharotomy
- [ ] folliculitis
- [ ] hematoma
- [ ] herpes simplex virus (HSV)
- [ ] hypertrichosis
- [ ] intradermal (ID)
- [ ] keratolytic
- [ ] melanoma
- [ ] nevus
- [ ] onychocryptosis
- [ ] onychomycosis
- [ ] paronychia
- [ ] pediculicide
- [ ] rhytidectomy
- [ ] seborrhea
- [ ] subcutaneous
- [ ] subungual
- [ ] tinea pedis
- [ ] transdermal
- [ ] tuberculosis (TB) skin tests
- [ ] verruca

**skin** = derm/o, dermat/o, cut/o, cutane/o

**hair** = trich/o, pil/o

**nail** = onych/o, ungu/o

**oil, sebum** = seb/o, sebac/o

**sweat** = hidr/o, sudor/i

## FUNCTIONS OF THE INTEGUMENTARY SYSTEM

The most important function of the **skin** (integument) is that it acts as the first line of defense in protecting the body from disease by providing an external barrier. It also helps regulate the temperature of the body, provides information about the environment through the sense of touch, assists in the synthesis of vitamin D (essential for the normal formation of bones and teeth), and helps eliminate waste products from the body. It is the largest organ of the body and accomplishes its diverse functions with assistance from its accessory structures, which include the **hair, nails**, and two types of **glands: sebaceous (oil)** and **sudoriferous (sweat).** Any impairment of the skin has the potential to lessen its ability to carry out these functions, which can lead to disease.

## SPECIALTIES/SPECIALISTS

The study of the skin, hair, and nails is called dermatology. A **dermatologist** is one who specializes in this area.

## ANATOMY AND PHYSIOLOGY

### Skin

The skin is composed of two layers: the **epidermis** (eh pih DUR mis), which forms the outermost layer, and the **dermis** or **corium** (KORE ee um), the inner layer (Fig. 4-1). The dermis is attached to a layer of connective tissue called the **hypodermis** or the **subcutaneous** (sub kyoo TAY nee us) layer, which is mainly composed of fat (adipose tissue).

**epidermis**
   epi- = above, upon
   derm/o = skin
   -is = structure

**hypodermis**
   hypo- = under, below
   derm/o = skin
   -is = structure

**subcutaneous**
   sub- = under, below
   cutane/o = skin
   -ous = pertaining to

**fat** = adip/o

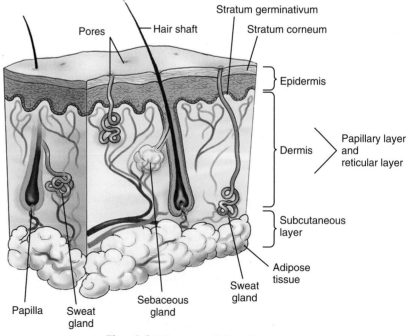

Fig. 4-1 Diagram of the skin.

### Epidermis

The top layer, the epidermis, is composed of several different layers, or strata, (*sing.* stratum) of epithelial (eh pih THEE lee ul) tissue. Epithelial tissue covers many of the external and internal surfaces of the body. Because the type of epithelial tissue that covers the body has a microscopic **scaly** appearance, it is referred to as **stratified squamous epithelium** (SKWAY muss eh pih THEE lee um) (squamous means scaly).

Although there is a limited blood supply to the epidermis (it is **avascular** [a VAS kyoo lur]—that is, it contains no blood vessels), constant activity is taking place. New skin cells are formed in the **basal** (BAY sul) (bottom) layer of the epidermis, the **stratum germinativum** (STRAY tum jur mih nuh TIH vum). This layer is also the site where **melanin** (pigment) is produced by cells called **melanocytes.** When the skin is exposed to ultraviolet light, the melanocytes secrete more melanin. Birthmarks, age spots, and freckles result from the clumping of melanin. Individuals have different skin colors because of varying numbers of melanocytes in the basal layer of the skin. The new cells move outward toward the **stratum corneum** (top layer). During the transition from the lowest layer to the outer layer, these cells are then called **keratinocytes** because they are filled with **keratin** (KAIR ah tin), which is a hard protein material. The nature of the keratin adds to the protective nature of the skin, giving it a waterproof property that helps retain moisture within the body.

### Dermis

The **dermis,** or corium, is the thick, underlying layer of the skin that is composed of vascular connective tissue arranged in two layers. The papillary layer is the upper thin layer composed of fibers made from protein and collagen that serves to regulate blood flow through its extensive vascular supply. The reticular layer is the lower, thicker layer, which also is composed of collagen fibers. This layer holds the **hair follicles, sweat,** and **sebaceous glands,** the glands that produce oil.

## Accessory Structures

### Glands

The **sudoriferous** (soo dur IF uh rus), or sweat, glands are located in the dermis and provide one means of thermoregulation for the body. They secrete sweat through tiny openings in the surface of the skin called **pores.** The secretion of sweat is called **perspiration.** These glands are present throughout the body but are especially abundant in the following areas: the soles of the feet, the palms of the hands, the armpits or axillae (*sing.* axilla), the upper lip, and the forehead.

The sebaceous (seh BAY shus) glands secrete an oily, acidic substance called **sebum** (SEE bum), which helps to lubricate hair and the surface of the skin. The acidic nature of sebum is key in inhibiting the growth of bacteria.

### Hair

Hair has its roots in the dermis; these roots, together with their coverings, are called **hair follicles** (FALL ih kuls). The visible part is called the hair **shaft.** Underneath the follicle is a nipple-shaped structure that encloses the capillaries called the **papilla** (pah PILL ah) (*pl.* papillae). Epithelial cells on top of the papilla are responsible for the formation of the hair shaft. When these cells die, hair can no longer regenerate, and hair loss occurs. The main function of hair is to assist in thermoregulation by holding heat near the body. When cold, hair stands on end, holding a layer of air as insulation near the body (piloerection).

### Nails

Nails cover and thus protect the dorsal surfaces of the distal bones of the fingers and toes (Fig. 4-2). The part that is visible is the **nail body** (also called the nail

---

**scaly** = squam/o

**keratinocyte**
  kerat/o = hard, horny
  -in = substance
  -cyte = cell

**avascular**
  a- = without
  vascul/o = vessel
  -ar = pertaining to

**basal** = bas/o

**melanocyte**
  melan/o = black
  -cyte = cell

**sudoriferous**
  sudor/i = sweat
  -ferous = pertaining to carrying

**sebaceous**
  sebac/o = oil
  -ous = pertaining to

**sebum** = seb/o

**hair** = trich/o, pil/o

**follicle** = follicul/o

**papilla** = papill/o

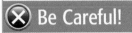 **Be Careful!**

*Don't confuse* **strata,** *meaning layers, with* **striae,** *meaning stretch marks.*

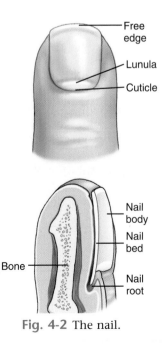

Fig. 4-2 The nail.

**eponychium**
   epi- = above
   onych/o = nail
   -ium = structure

**paronychium**
   par- = near
   onchy/o = nail
   -ium = structure

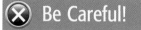 **Be Careful!**

Don't confuse **papill/o**, meaning papilla or "nipple" and **papul/o**, which means pimple.

plate), whereas the **nail root** is in a groove under a small fold of skin at the base of the nail. The **nail bed** is the highly vascular tissue under the nail that appears pink when the blood is oxygenated or blue/purple when it is oxygen deficient. The moonlike white area at the base of the nail is called the **lunula** (LOON yoo lah), beyond which new growth occurs. The small fold of skin above the lower part of the nail is called the **cuticle** (KYOO tih kul) or **eponychium** (eh puh NICK ee um). The **paronychium** (pair ih NICK ee um) is the fold of skin that is near the sides of the nail.

You can review the anatomy of the integumentary system by clicking on **Body Spectrum Electronic Anatomy Coloring Book → Integumentary.**

## Exercise 1: Anatomy and Physiology

*Match the integumentary term to its combining form.*

____ 1. follicle

____ 2. fat

____ 3. black

____ 4. scaly

____ 5. sweat

____ 6. hard, horny

____ 7. skin

____ 8. oil, sebum

____ 9. hair

____10. nail

A. squam/o
B. follicul/o
C. trich/o, pil/o
D. sudor/i, hidr/o
E. kerat/o
F. melan/o
G. derm/o, cutane/o
H. adip/o
I. sebac/o, seb/o
J. onych/o, ungu/o

*Decode the terms:*

11. avascular _____

12. subungual _____

13. hypodermic _____

## Exercise 2: **The Skin**

*Label the structures of the skin with their anatomic terms and combining forms where appropriate.*

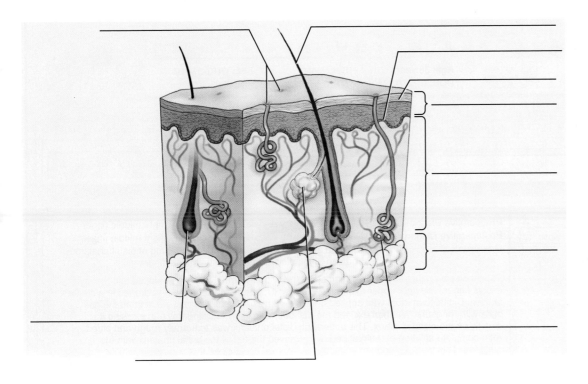

---

## Case Study  *Todd Feldman*

Todd Feldman is a 38-year-old carpenter. One day, he is working on a house when he accidentally hits the middle finger of his right hand with his hammer. It swells immediately and is very painful. He goes to the ED to have it checked out. The ED doctor orders an x-ray, which shows that the top of the finger is crushed. The nail is also damaged. A hand surgeon examines Todd and tells him that he needs surgery on his finger to remove the nail and the tip of the bone.

Surgery is scheduled for the next day and proceeds without incident. He is sent home with instructions for wound care and dressings. Six months later, Todd's nail has grown back partially and he has regained full dexterity of the finger.

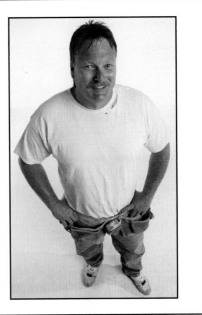

*Case Study* Todd Feldman

Feldman, Todd T - 555422 Opened by Dover, Scott MD    ⬜ ⬜ ✕

Task   Edit   View   Time Scale   Options   Help

As Of 16:24

| Feldman, Todd T | Age: 38 years | Sex: Male | Loc: WHC-SMMC |
| | DOB: 01/27/1974 | MRN: 555422 | FIN: 3506004 |

Reference Text Browser | Form Browser | Medication Profile

Orders | Last 48 Hours | ED | Lab | Radiology | Assessments | **Surgery** | Clinical Notes | Pt. Info | Pt. Schedule | Task List | I & O | MAR

Flowsheet: Surgery ▼ ...   Level: Operative Report ▼    ● Table  ○ Group  ○ List

Navigator    ✕
✓  Operative Report

| Preoperative Diagnosis: | Nail bed deformity and nail plate deformity, right middle finger |
| Postoperative Diagnosis: | Nail bed deformity and nail plate deformity, right middle finger |
| Operation: | Nail bed and nail plate ablation and shortening of distal phalanx and primary flap coverage, tip, right middle finger |

Patient was brought into the operating suite and middle carpal block was induced into the right middle finger. The right upper extremity was then prepped with Betadine and draped in a sterile fashion. Digital tourniquet was applied and with 43 magnification loupes, we ablated the nail plate with rongeurs. We then excised the nail bed, elliptically excising this and excising it directly off the distal phalanx. The underlying distal phalanx was extremely rough and pitted. After complete ablation of the nail bed, we removed the tuft of the distal phalanx with the rongeurs. This freed up enough volar skin so that we could close this flap primarily. We sutured this with 5-0 nylon and then excised dog ears on both radial and ulnar sides and closed with 5-0 nylon suture. Appearance was excellent. Xeroform was applied, the digital tourniquet was removed, and good circulation returned to the finger. Tube gauze dressing was then applied.

Patient will be dismissed as an outpatient and arrangements made for follow-up in 2 weeks for suture removal.

PROD | MAHAFC | 30 Dec 2012 | 16:24

## Exercise 3: Operative Report

*Using the above operative report, answer the following questions:*

1. What are the two structures, nail bed and nail plate, that are being removed (ablated)? _____

_____

2. Where is the "volar skin" located? (Refer to Chapter 2 if you've forgotten.) _____

3. What is a "digital tourniquet," and why do you think it was used? _____

4. From your knowledge of the anatomy of a nail, what, if any, parts of the nail do you think remain?

_____

Click on **Hear It, Spell It** to practice spelling the anatomy and physiology terms that you have learned in this chapter. To practice pronouncing anatomy and physiology terms, click on **Hear It, Say It.**

## Combining and Adjective Forms for the Anatomy of the Integumentary System

| Meaning | Combining Form | Adjective Form |
|---|---|---|
| base, bottom | bas/o | basal |
| black, dark | melan/o | melanotic |
| fat | adip/o | adipose |
| follicle | follicul/o | follicular |
| gland | aden/o | adenal |
| hair | trich/o, pil/o | pilar |
| hard, horny | kerat/o | keratic |
| nail | onych/o, ungu/o | ungual, onychial |
| papilla | papill/o | papillary |
| scaly | squam/o | squamous |
| sebum, oil | seb/o, sebac/o | sebaceous |
| skin | derm/o, dermat/o, cut/o, cutane/o | cutaneous, dermic, dermatic |
| sudoriferous gland | hidraden/o | |
| sweat | hidr/o, sudor/i | hidrotic, sudorous |
| vessel | vascul/o | vascular |

## Prefixes for the Anatomy of the Integumentary System

| Prefix | Meaning |
|---|---|
| a- | no, not, without |
| epi- | above |
| hypo-, sub- | under, below |

## Suffixes for the Anatomy of the Integumentary System

| Suffix | Meaning |
|---|---|
| -al, -ar, -ous, -ic | pertaining to |
| -cyte | cell |
| -ferous | pertaining to carrying |
| -is | structure |

## PATHOLOGY

### Skin Lesions

A skin **lesion** (LEE zhun) is any visible, localized abnormality of skin tissue. It can be described as either primary or secondary. **Primary lesions** (Fig. 4-3) are early skin changes that have not yet undergone natural evolution or change caused by manipulation. **Secondary lesions** (Fig. 4-4) are the result of natural evolution or manipulation of a primary lesion.

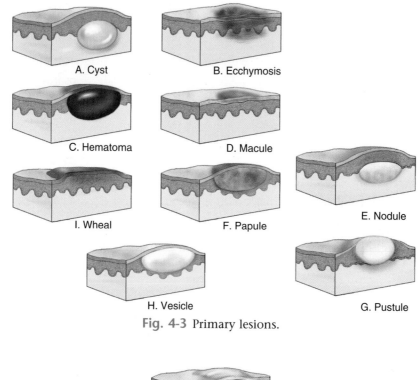

Fig. 4-3 Primary lesions.

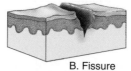

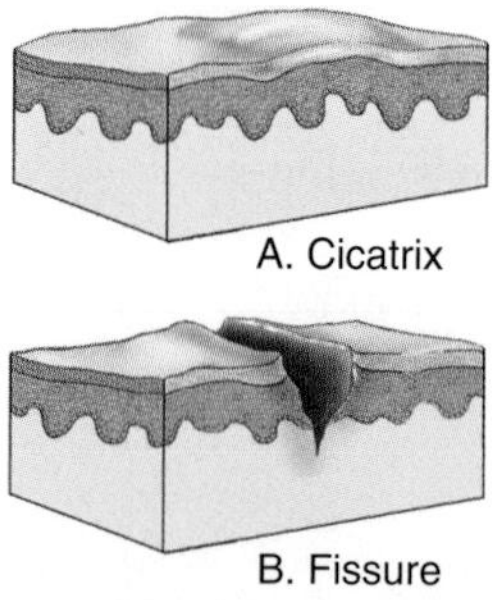

Fig. 4-4 Secondary lesions.

## Terms Related to Primary Skin Lesions

| Term | Word Origin | Definition |
|---|---|---|
| **cyst**<br>sist | *cyst/o* sac, bladder | Nodule filled with a semisolid material, such as a keratinous or sebaceous cyst (see Fig. 4-3, *A*). |
| **ecchymosis**<br>**(pl. ecchymoses)**<br>eck ih MOH sis | *ec-* out<br>*chym/o* juice<br>*-osis* abnormal condition | Hemorrhage or extravasation (leaking) of blood into the subcutaneous tissue. The resultant darkening is commonly described as a **bruise** (see Fig. 4-3, *B*). |

## Terms Related to Primary Skin Lesions—cont'd

| Term | Word Origin | Definition |
|---|---|---|
| hematoma<br>hee mah TOH mah | *hemat/o* blood<br>*-oma* mass | Collection of extravasated blood trapped in the tissues and palpable to the examiner, such as on the ear. (see Fig. 4-3, *C*). |
| macule<br>MACK yool | *macul/o* spot | Flat blemish or discoloration less than 1 cm, such as a freckle, port-wine stain, or tattoo (see Fig. 4-3, *D*). |
| nodule<br>NOD yool | *nod/o* knot<br>*-ule* small | Palpable, solid lesion less than 2 cm, such as a very small lipoma (see Fig. 4-3, *E*). |
| papule<br>PAP yool | *papul/o* pimple | Raised solid skin lesion raised less than 1 cm, such as a pimple (see Fig. 4-3, *F*). |
| patch | | Large, flat, nonpalpable macule, larger than 1 cm. |
| petechia (*pl.* petechiae)<br>peh TEEK ee ah | | Tiny ecchymosis within the dermal layer. |
| plaque<br>plack | | Raised plateaulike papule greater than 1 cm, such as a psoriatic lesion or seborrheic keratosis. |
| purpura<br>PUR pur ah | *purpur/o* purple<br>*-a* noun ending | Massive hemorrhage into the tissues under the skin. |
| pustule<br>PUS tyool | *pustul/o* pustule | Superficial, elevated lesion containing pus that may be the result of an infection, such as acne (see Fig. 4-3, *G*). |
| telangiectasia<br>tell an jee eck TAY zsa | *tel/e* far<br>*angi/o* vessel<br>*-ectasia* dilation | Permanent dilation of groups of superficial capillaries and venules. |
| tumor<br>TOO mur | | Nodule more than 2 cm; any mass or swelling, including neoplasms. |
| vesicle<br>VESS ih kul | *vesicul/o* blister or small sac | Circumscribed, elevated lesion containing fluid and smaller than ½ cm, such as an insect bite. If larger than ½ cm, it is termed a **bulla.** Commonly called a **blister.** (see Fig. 4-3, *H*). |
| wheal<br>wheel | | Circumscribed, elevated papule caused by localized edema, which can result from a bug bite. **Urticaria,** or **hives,** results from an allergic reaction. |

## Terms Related to Secondary Skin Lesions

| Term | Word Origin | Definition |
|---|---|---|
| atrophy<br>AT troh fee | *a-* no, not, without<br>*troph/o* development<br>*-y* process | Paper-thin, wasted skin often occurring in the aged or as stretch marks (**striae,** STRY ay) from rapid weight gain. |
| cicatrix (*pl.* cicatrices)<br>SICK ah tricks | | A **scar**—an area of fibrous tissue that replaces normal skin after destruction of some of the dermis (see Fig. 4-4, *A*). |
| eschar<br>ES kar | *eschar/o* scab | Dried serum, blood, and/or pus. May occur in inflammatory and infectious diseases, such as impetigo, or as the result of a burn. Also called a **scab.** |

*Continued*

## Terms Related to Secondary Skin Lesions—cont'd

| Term | Word Origin | Definition |
|------|-------------|------------|
| **fissure** FISH ur | | Cracklike lesion of the skin, such as an anal fissure (see Fig. 4-4, *B*). |
| **keloid** KEE loyd | | Type of scar that is an overgrowth of tissue at the site of injury in excess of the amount of tissue necessary to repair the wound. The extra tissue is partially due to an accumulation of collagen at the site (Fig. 4-5). |
| **ulcer** UL sur | | Circumscribed craterlike lesion of the skin or mucous membrane resulting from **necrosis** (neck KROH sis), or tissue death, that can accompany an inflammatory, infectious, or malignant process. An example is a **decubitus ulcer** (deh KYOO bih tus) seen sometimes in bedridden patients (see Fig 4-16). |

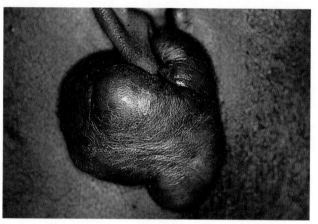

**Fig. 4-5** Keloid caused by ear piercing.

## Exercise 4: Skin Lesions

*Match the primary lesions with their definitions.*

____ 1. vesicle     ____ 4. ecchymosis

____ 2. papule      ____ 5. macule

____ 3. wheal       ____ 6. pustule

A. extravasated blood into subcutaneous tissue caused by trauma
B. flat blemish or discoloration
C. circumscribed, raised papule
D. superficial, elevated lesion containing pus
E. circumscribed, raised lesion containing fluid
F. solid, raised skin lesion

*Match the smaller version of a primary skin lesion with the larger version.*

____ 7. petechia     ____10. macule

____ 8. vesicle      ____11. nodule

____ 9. papule

A. plaque
B. tumor
C. ecchymosis
D. bulla
E. patch

*Match the secondary lesions with their definitions.*

____12. ulcer          ____15. atrophy          A. paper-thin, wasted skin
                                                B. scab
____13. cicatrix       ____16. eschar           C. cracklike lesion
                                                D. circumscribed, craterlike
____14. fissure                                    lesion
                                                E. scar

## Terms Related to Dermatitis and Bacterial Infections

| Term | Word Origin | Definition |
|------|-------------|------------|
| **atopic dermatitis**<br>a TOP ick<br>dur mah TYE tis | *a-* no, not, without<br>*top/o* place, location<br>*-ic* pertaining to<br>*dermat/o* skin<br>*-itis* inflammation | Chronic, pruritic superficial inflammation of the skin usually associated with a family history of allergic disorders. |
| **cellulitis**<br>sell yoo LYE tis | *cellul/o* cell<br>*-itis* inflammation | Diffuse, spreading, acute inflammation within solid tissues. The most common cause is a *Streptococcus pyogenes* infection (Fig. 4-6). |
| **contact dermatitis** | *dermat/o* skin<br>*-itis* inflammation | Irritated or allergic response of the skin that can lead to an acute or chronic inflammation (Fig. 4-7). |
| **eczema**<br>ECK suh muh | | Superficial inflammation of the skin, characterized by vesicles, weeping, and pruritus. Also called **dermatitis.** |
| **folliculitis**<br>foh lick yoo LYE tis | *follicul/o* follicle<br>*-itis* inflammation | Inflammation of the hair follicles, which may be superficial or deep, acute or chronic. |
| **furuncle**<br>FYOOR ung kul | | Localized, suppurative staphylococcal skin infection originating in a gland or hair follicle and characterized by pain, redness, and swelling. If two or more furuncles are connected by subcutaneous pockets, it is termed a **carbuncle** (Fig. 4-8). |

*Continued*

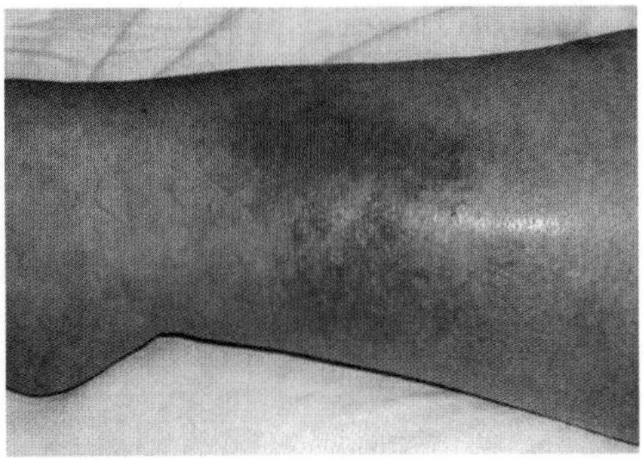

Fig. 4-6 Cellulitis of the lower leg.

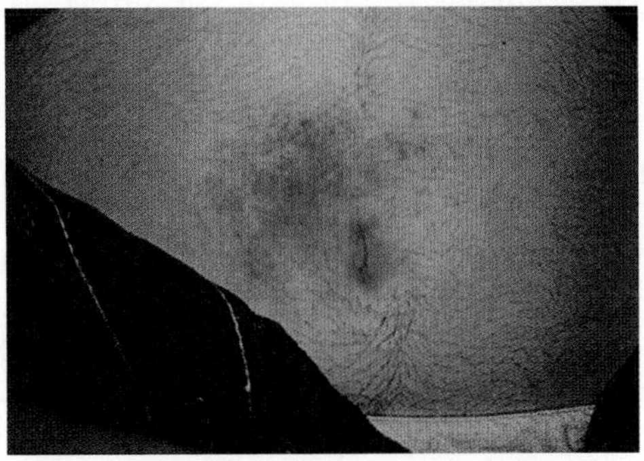

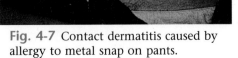

Fig. 4-7 Contact dermatitis caused by allergy to metal snap on pants.

### Terms Related to Dermatitis and Bacterial Infections—cont'd

| Term | Word Origin | Definition |
|---|---|---|
| **impetigo**<br>im peh TYE goh | | Superficial vesiculopustular skin infection, normally seen in children, but possible in adults (Fig. 4-9). |
| **pilonidal cyst**<br>pye loh NYE duhl | *pil/o* hair<br>*nid/o* nest<br>*-al* pertaining to | Growth of hair in a cyst in the sacral region. |
| **pruritus**<br>proo RYE tuss | | Itching. |
| **seborrheic dermatitis**<br>seh boh REE ick | *seb/o* sebum<br>*-rrheic* pertaining to discharge<br>*dermat/o* skin<br>*-itis* inflammation | Inflammatory scaling disease of the scalp and face. In newborns, this is known as **cradle cap.** |

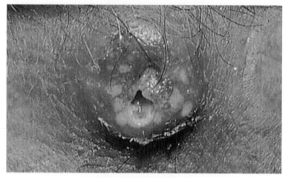

Fig. 4-8 Furuncle.

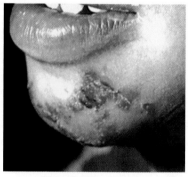

Fig. 4-9 Impetigo.

## Exercise 5: Dermatitis and Bacterial Infections

*Fill in the blank.*

1. Another term for dermatitis is _____.

2. A chronic, pruritic superficial inflammation of the skin associated with a family history of allergic disorders is called _____.

3. An irritated or allergic response of the skin that can lead to an acute or chronic inflammation is called

_____.

4. An inflammatory scaling disease of the scalp and face is termed _____.

5. A superficial vesiculopustular skin infection normally seen in children is called _____.

6. A localized, suppurative staphylococcal skin infection in a gland or hair follicle is called a

_____.

7. Growth of hair in a cyst in the sacral region of the skin is a _____.

*Build the terms.*

8. inflammation of the hair follicles _____

9. inflammation of the (skin) cells _____

## Terms Related to Yeast and Fungal Infections

| Term | Word Origin | Definition |
|---|---|---|
| **candidiasis**<br>kan dih DYE ah sis | | Yeast infection in moist, occluded areas of the skin (armpits, inner thighs, underneath pendulous breasts) and mucous membranes. Also called **moniliasis** (mah nih LYE ah sis). |
| **dermatomycosis**<br>dur muh toh mye KOH sis | *dermat/o* skin<br>*myc/o* fungus<br>*-osis* abnormal condition | Fungal infection of the skin. Also called **dermatophytosis.** |
| **tinea capitis**<br>TIN ee ah<br>KAP ih tis | *capit/o* head<br>*-is* structure | Fungal infection of the scalp; also known as **ringworm.** |
| **tinea corporis**<br>TIN ee ah<br>KOR poor is | *corpor/o* body<br>*-is* structure | Ringworm of the body, manifested by pink to red papulosquamous annular (ringlike) plaques with raised borders; also known as **ringworm** (Fig. 4-10). |
| **tinea cruris**<br>TIN ee ah<br>KROO ris | *crur/o* leg<br>*-is* structure | A fungal infection that occurs mainly on external genitalia and upper legs in males, particularly in warm weather; also known as **jock itch.** |
| **tinea pedis**<br>TIN ee ah<br>PEH dis | *ped/o* foot<br>*-is* structure | Fungal infection of the foot; also known as **athlete's foot.** |

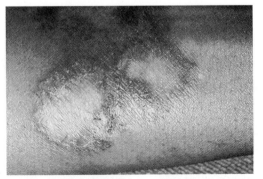

**Fig. 4-10** Tinea corporis.

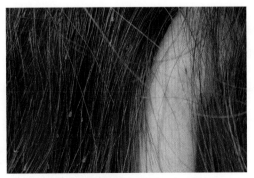

**Fig. 4-11** Lice in hair (pediculosis).

## Terms Related to Parasitic Infestations

| Term | Word Origin | Definition |
| --- | --- | --- |
| **pediculosis**<br>peh dick yoo LOH sis | *pedicul/i* lice<br>*-osis* abnormal condition | Parasitic infestation with lice, involving the head, body, or genital area (Fig. 4-11). |
| **scabies**<br>SKAY bees | | Parasitic infestation caused by mites; characterized by pruritic papular rash. |

## Terms Related to Viral Infections

| Term | Word Origin | Definition |
| --- | --- | --- |
| **exanthematous diseases**<br>eks an THEM ah tus | *exanthemat/o* rash<br>*-ous* pertaining to | Generally, viral diseases characterized by a specific type of rash **(exanthem).** The main ones are measles, rubella, fifth disease, roseola, and chickenpox. |
| **herpes simplex virus (HSV)**<br>HUR peez<br>SIM plecks | | Viral infection characterized by clusters of small vesicles filled with clear fluid on raised inflammatory bases on the skin or mucosa. HSV-1 causes fever blisters (**herpetic stomatitis**) and **keratitis,** an inflammation of the cornea. HSV-2 is more commonly known as **genital herpes.** |
| **herpes zoster**<br>HUR peez<br>ZAH stur | | Acute, painful rash caused by reactivation of the latent varicella-zoster virus. Also known as **shingles** (Fig. 4-12). |
| **verruca** (*pl.* **verrucae**)<br>veh ROO kah | | Common, contagious epithelial growths usually appearing on the skin of the hands, feet, legs, and face; can be caused by any of 60 types of the human papillomavirus (HPV) (Fig. 4-13). Also called **warts.** |

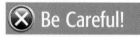 **Be Careful!**

*The combining form **stomat/o** in the term stomatitis means mouth, not stomach.*

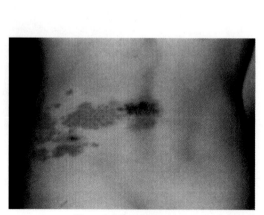
Fig. 4-12 Herpes zoster.

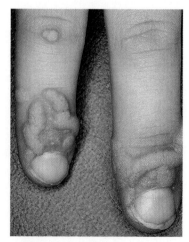
Fig. 4-13 Verrucae (warts).

## ⟳ Exercise 6: Yeast, Fungal, Parasitic, and Viral Infections

*Match these fungal or yeast infections with their definitions or synonyms.*

____ 1. athlete's foot      ____ 5. rash

____ 2. ringworm of scalp    ____ 6. ringworm of body

____ 3. moniliasis        ____ 7. shingles

____ 4. jock itch        ____ 8. warts

A. tinea corporis
B. tinea cruris
C. tinea capitis
D. tinea pedis
E. verrucae
F. candidiasis
G. herpes zoster
H. exanthem

*Build the term.*

9. infestation with lice _____.

10. virus causing stomatitis _____.

11. infestation with mites _____.

12. fungal infection of the skin _____.

## Terms Related to Disorders of Hair Follicles and Sebaceous Glands

| Term | Word Origin | Definition |
| --- | --- | --- |
| **acne vulgaris**<br>ACK nee<br>vul GARE us | *vulgar/o* common<br>*-is* noun ending | Inflammatory disease of the sebaceous glands characterized by papules, pustules, inflamed nodules, and **comedones** (kah mih DOH neez) (*sing.* comedo), which are plugs of sebum that partially or completely block a pore. Blackheads are open comedones, and whiteheads are closed comedones. |
| **alopecia**<br>al oh PEE shee ah | | Hair loss, resulting from genetic factors, aging, or disease (Fig. 4-14). |
| **hypertrichosis**<br>hye pur trih KOH sis | *hyper-* excessive<br>*trich/o* hair<br>*-osis* abnormal condition | Abnormal excess of hair; also known as **hirsutism** (HER soo tih zum). |
| **keratinous cyst**<br>kur AT tin us | *kerat/o* hard, horny<br>*-in* substance<br>*-ous* pertaining to | Benign cavity lined by keratinizing epithelium and filled with sebum and epithelial debris. Also called a **sebaceous cyst.** |
| **milia**<br>MILL ee ah | | Tiny superficial keratinous cysts caused by clogged oil ducts. |

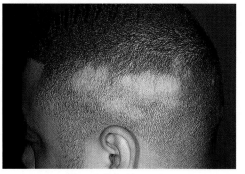

Fig. 4-14 Alopecia.

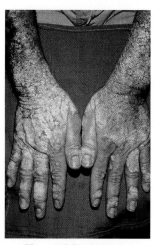

Fig. 4-15 Psoriasis.

## Term Related to Scaling Papular Diseases

| Term | Word Origin | Definition |
|---|---|---|
| **psoriasis**<br>sur EYE ah sis | | Common chronic skin disorder characterized by circumscribed, salmon-red patches covered by thick, dry, silvery scales that are the result of excessive development of epithelial cells (Fig. 4-15). |

## Terms Related to Cornification and Pressure Injuries

| Term | Word Origin | Definition |
|---|---|---|
| **callus**<br>KAL us | | Common painless thickening of the stratum corneum at locations of external pressure or friction. |
| **corn** | | Horny mass of condensed epithelial cells overlying a bony prominence as the result of pressure or friction; also referred to as a **clavus** (KLA vus). |
| **decubitus ulcer**<br>deh KYOO bih tus | | Inflammation, ulcer, or sore in the skin over a bony prominence. Most often seen in aged, debilitated, cachectic (wasted), or immobilized patients; pressure sores or ulcers are graded by stages of severity. The highest stage, stage 4, involves muscles, fat, and bone. Also known as a **bedsore, pressure ulcer,** or **pressure sore** (Fig. 4-16). |
| **ichthyosis**<br>ick thee OH sis | *ichthy/o* fish<br>*-osis* abnormal condition | Category of dry skin that has the scaly appearance of a fish. It ranges from mild to severe. The mild form is known as **xeroderma** (zir uh DUR mah). Xer/o means "dry." |

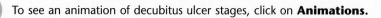

To see an animation of decubitus ulcer stages, click on **Animations.**

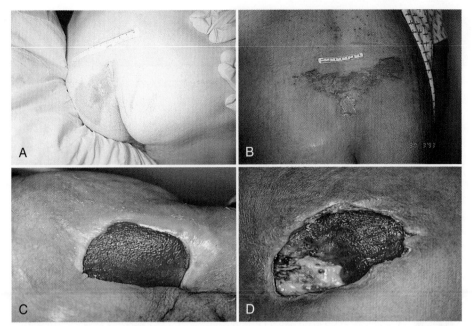

Fig. 4-16 **A,** Stage 1 decubitus ulcer. **B,** Stage 2 decubitus ulcer. **C,** Stage 3 decubitus ulcer. **D,** Stage 4 decubitus ulcer.

## Exercise 7: Disorders of Hair Follicles and Sebaceous Glands, Scaling Papular Diseases, and Pressure Injuries

*Fill in the blanks with the correct terms from the list below.*

**acne vulgaris, alopecia, clavus, decubitus ulcer, hypertrichosis, keratinous cyst, milia, pressure sore, psoriasis, xeroderma**

1. What is a disorder of circumscribed salmon-red patches covered with thick, silvery scales?_____

_____

2. What is another name for hirsutism? _____

3. What is the term for hair loss? _____

4. What is the term for a benign cavity filled with sebum and epithelial debris and lined with keratinized

   epithelium? _____

5. What is the common inflammatory disease of the sebaceous glands characterized by comedones,

   papules, pustules, and inflamed nodules? _____

6. What is another term for a corn? _____

7. What are two alternative terms for bedsores? _____

8. What are tiny, superficial keratinous cysts? _____

9. What is the term for mildly dry skin?_____

## Terms Related to Pigmentation Disorders

| Term | Word Origin | Definition |
|------|-------------|------------|
| albinism<br>AL bih niz um | *albin/o* white<br>*-ism* condition | Complete lack of melanin production by existing melanocytes, resulting in pale skin, white hair, and pink irides (*sing.* iris). |
| dyschromia<br>diss KROH mee ah | *dys-* abnormal<br>*chrom/o* color<br>*-ia* condition | Abnormality of skin pigmentation. **Hyperchromia** is abnormally increased pigmentation. **Hypochromia** is abnormally decreased pigmentation. |
| vitiligo<br>vih tih LYE goh | | Benign acquired disease of unknown origin, consisting of irregular patches of various sizes lacking in pigment (Fig. 4-17). |

### ⊗ Be Careful!

**Hidr/o** *with an i means sweat;* **hydr/o** *with a y means water. Both are pronounced HYE droh.*

### ⊗ Be Careful!

*Don't confuse* **milia**, *a condition resulting from oil-filled ducts, with* **miliaria**, *a condition resulting from sweat-filled ducts.*

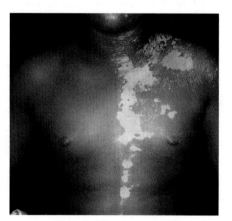

Fig. 4-17 Vitiligo.

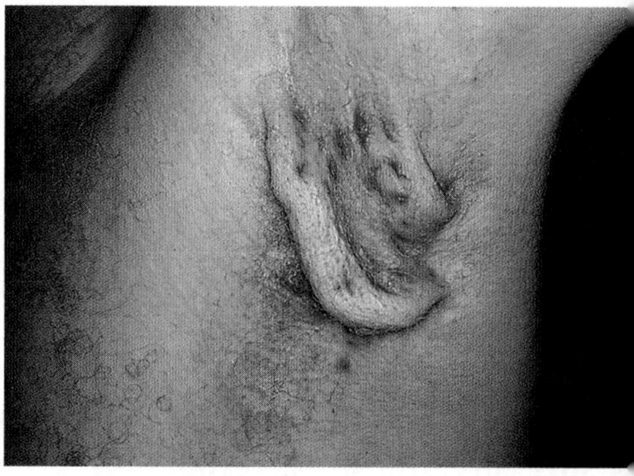

Fig. 4-18 Hidradenitis.

## Terms Related to Disorders of Sweating

| Term | Word Origin | Definition |
|------|-------------|------------|
| anhidrosis<br>an hye DROH sis | *an-* no, not, without<br>*hidr/o* sweating<br>*-osis* abnormal condition | A condition in which a person produces little or no sweat. |
| hidradenitis<br>hye drah din EYE tis | *hidraden/o* sweat gland<br>*-itis* inflammation | Inflammation of the sweat glands (Fig. 4-18). |
| hyperhidrosis<br>hye pur hye DROH sis | *hyper-* excessive<br>*hidr/o* sweat<br>*-osis* abnormal condition | Excessive perspiration caused by heat, strong emotion, menopause, hyperthyroidism, or infection. |
| miliaria<br>mill ee AIR ee uh | | Minute vesicles and papules, often with surrounding **erythema** (redness), caused by occlusion of sweat ducts during times of exposure to heat and high humidity. |

## Exercise 8: Pigmentation Disorders and Disorders of Sweating

*Build the terms.*

1. abnormal condition of excessive sweat _____

2. abnormal condition of pigmentation _____

3. inflammation of the sweat glands _____

4. abnormal condition of no sweat _____

*Fill in the blank.*

5. An acquired disorder of irregular patches of various sizes lacking in pigment is _____.

6. A patient whose body produces no melanin has a condition of _____.

7. Minute vesicles and papules caused by occlusion of sweat ducts are called _____.

## Terms Related to Disorders of the Nails

| Term | Word Origin | Definition |
|------|-------------|------------|
| onychia<br>oh NIK ee ah | *onych/o* nail<br>*-ia* condition | Inflammation of the fingernail. Also called **onychitis.** |
| onychocryptosis<br>on ik oh krip TOH sis | *onchy/o* nail<br>*crypt-* hidden<br>*-osis* abnormal condition | Abnormal condition of hidden (ingrown) nail. |
| onycholysis<br>on ih KAHL ih sis | *onych/o* nail<br>*-lysis* loosening | Separation of the nail plate from the nail bed (Fig. 4-19). |
| onychomalacia<br>on ik oh mah LAY shah | *onych/o* nail<br>*-malacia* softening | Softening of the nails. |
| onychomycosis<br>on ik oh my KOH sis | *onych/o* nail<br>*myc/o* fungus<br>*-osis* abnormal condition | Abnormal condition of nail fungus. Also called **tinea unguium** (see Fig. 4-20). |
| paronychia<br>pair uh NIK ee ah | *par-* beside, near<br>*onych/o* nail<br>*-ia* condition | Infection of the skin beside the nail. |

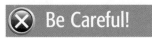

**Be Careful!**

Paronychium *is the structure that surrounds the nail.* Paronychia *is an infection of the nail.*

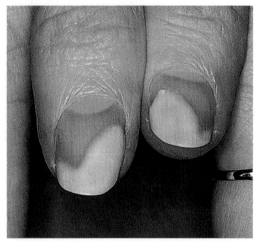

Fig. 4-19 Onycholysis.

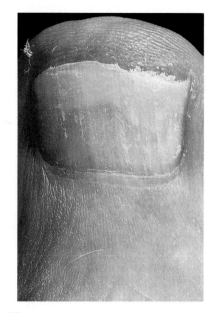

Fig. 4-20 Onychomycosis (tinea unguium). Early changes show subungual debris at the distal end of the nail plate.

 Exercise 9: **Disorders of the Nails**

*Match the word parts to their definitions.*

____ 1. loosening        ____ 4. softening          A. -ia
                                                     B. crypt-
____ 2. fungus           ____ 5. condition          C. -lysis
                                                     D. myc/o
____ 3. hidden                                       E. -malacia

*Build the terms.*

6. softening of the nail _____

7. abnormal condition of fungus of the nail _____

8. abnormal condition of hidden nail _____

9. loosening of the nail _____

### Burns

Burns are injuries to tissues that result from exposure to thermal, chemical, electrical, or radioactive agents. They may be classified into four different degrees of severity, depending on the layers of the skin that are damaged. Coders must categorize burns higher than second degree according to the "rule of nines" (Fig. 4-21) that divides the body into percentages that are, for the most part, multiples of nine: the head and neck equal 9%, each upper limb 9%, each lower limb 18%, the front and back of the torso 36%, and the genital area 1%. Fig. 4-22 is an illustration of the different degrees of burns.

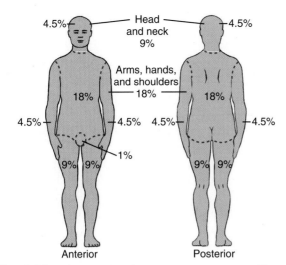

Fig. 4-21 Rule of nines for estimating extent of burns.

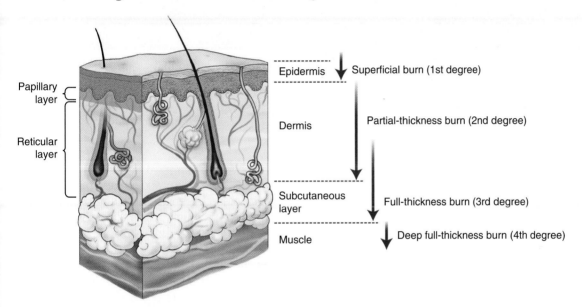

Fig. 4-22 Degrees of burns and depth of tissue involvement.

- **Superficial burn:** burn in which only the first layer of the skin, the epidermis, is damaged; also known as a *first-degree burn*. Characterized by redness (erythema), tenderness, and hyperesthesia, with no scar development.
- **Partial-thickness burn:** burn in which only the first and second layers of the skin (epidermis and part of the dermis) are affected; sometimes called a *second-degree burn*. If the burn extends to the papillary level, it is classified as a *superficial partial-thickness burn*. If it extends farther, to the reticular layer, it is classified as a *deep partial-thickness burn*. Characterized by redness, blisters, and pain, with possible scar development.
- **Full-thickness burn:** burn that damages the epidermis, dermis, and subcutaneous tissue; also known as a *third-degree burn*. Pain is not present because the nerve endings in the skin have been destroyed. Skin appearance may be deep red, pale gray, brown, or black. Scar formation is likely.
- **Deep full-thickness burn:** although not a universally accepted category, some burn specialists use this category to describe a rare burn that extends beyond the subcutaneous tissue into the muscle and bone. Also called a *fourth-degree burn*.

## ⟳ Exercise 10: Burns

*Match the characteristics of the burns listed with their degree.*

____ 1. superficial

____ 2. partial thickness

____ 3. full thickness

____ 4. deep full thickness

A. Ironing a blouse for work, Rhonda burned her hand, resulting in blisters and erythema.

B. John suffered burns over two thirds of his body with many areas of tissue burned to the bone.

C. Because Kristin forgot to reapply her sunblock, she sustained a sunburn that resulted in painful reddened skin.

D. Smoking in bed resulted in burns that destroyed the epidermis and dermis and extended through the hypodermis on the victim's chest and shoulders.

## Terms Related to Benign (Noncancerous) Skin Growths

| Term | Word Origin | Definition |
|---|---|---|
| **angioma** <br> an jee OH mah | *angi/o* vessel <br> *-oma* tumor, mass | Localized vascular lesion that includes hemangiomas (Fig. 4-23), vascular nevi, and lymphangiomas. |
| **dermatofibroma** <br> dur mat toh fye BROH mah | *dermat/o* skin <br> *fibr/o* fiber <br> *-oma* tumor, mass | Fibrous tumor of the skin that is painless, round, firm, and usually found on the extremities. |
| **dysplastic nevus** (*pl.* nevi) <br> dis PLAS tick NEE vus | *dys-* abnormal <br> *plast/o* formation <br> *-ic* pertaining to <br> *nev/o* birthmark <br> *-us* structure, thing | A nevus is a pigmented lesion often present at birth. It is also called a **mole.** Various abnormal changes of a pigmented congenital skin blemish give rise to concern for progression to malignancy. Changes of concern are categorized as ABCDE. <br> **a**symmetry <br> **b**orders, irregular <br> **c**olors, changes or uneven pigmentation <br> **d**iameter, increasing size or >6 mm <br> **e**levation |
| **lipoma** <br> lih POH mah | *lip/o* fat <br> *-oma* tumor, mass | Fatty tumor that is a soft, movable, subcutaneous nodule (Fig. 4-24). |
| **seborrheic keratosis** <br> seh boh REE ick <br> kair ah TOH sis | *seb/o* sebum <br> *-rrheic* pertaining to discharge <br> *kerat/o* hard, horny <br> *-osis* abnormal condition | Benign, circumscribed, pigmented, superficial warty skin lesion. An **actinic keratosis** is a lesion caused by sun exposure. |
| **skin tags** | | Small, soft, pedunculated (with a stalk) lesions that are harmless outgrowths of epidermal and dermal tissue, usually occurring on the neck, eyelids, armpits, and groin; usually occur in multiples. Also known as **acrochordons** (ack roh KORE dons). |

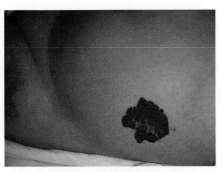

Fig. 4-23 Hemangioma.

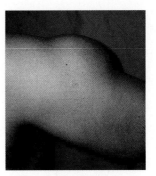

Fig. 4-24 Lipoma.

## Exercise 11: Benign Skin Growths

*Matching the benign skin growths to their definitions.*

____ 1. pigmented lesion

____ 2. acrochordon

____ 3. fatty tumor

____ 4. benign warty skin lesion

____ 5. vascular nevus

A. skin tag
B. lipoma
C. seborrheic keratosis
D. mole
E. angioma

*Decode the terms.*

6. dermatofibroma _____

7. angioma _____

8. seborrheic keratosis _____

## Terms Related to Malignant Neoplasms

| Term | Word Origin | Definition |
|---|---|---|
| **basal cell carcinoma (BCC)** BAY suhl kar sih NOH mah | *bas/o* base *-al* pertaining to *carcinoma* cancer of epithelial origin | The most common form of skin cancer, it originates in the basal layer of the epidermis. It usually occurs on the face as a result of sun exposure and rarely metastasizes (spreads to distant sites). |
| **Kaposi sarcoma (KS)** KAP uh see sar KOH mah | *sarcoma* connective tissue cancer | A rare form of skin cancer that takes the form of red/blue/brown/purple nodules, usually on the extremities. One form appears most often in patients with deficient immune systems, such as AIDS. |
| **malignant melanoma** mell uh NOH mah | *melan/o* black, dark *-oma* tumor, mass | This cancerous tumor arises from mutated melanocytes. This particular cancer is the leading cause of death from all skin diseases (Fig. 4-25). |
| **squamous cell carcinoma (SCC)** SKWAY muss | *squam/o* scaly *-ous* pertaining to *carcinoma* cancer of epithelial origin | The second most common type of skin cancer, also caused by sun exposure, but developing from squamous cells (Fig. 4-26). |

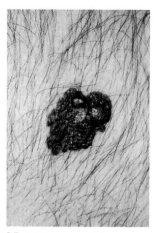

Fig. 4-25 Malignant melanoma on arm.

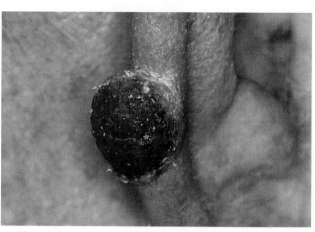

Fig. 4-26 Squamous cell carcinoma on the ear.

## Exercise 12: Malignant Neoplasms

*Match the malignant neoplasms to their definitions.*

_____ 1. squamous cell carcinoma

_____ 2. Kaposi sarcoma

_____ 3. basal cell carcinoma

_____ 4. malignant melanoma

A. most common type of skin cancer, derived from base level of epidermis; rarely metastasizes
B. cancer arising from mutated pigment cells
C. malignancy of squamous skin cells
D. rare form of skin cancer that appears most often in patients with deficient immune systems, such as AIDS.

Click on **Hear It, Spell It** to practice spelling the pathology terms you have learned in this chapter. To see how well you can pronounce the pathology terms in this chapter, click on **Hear It, Say It.**

## *Age Matters*

### Pediatrics

Children routinely appear at physician offices with skin disorders. Some of the most common are impetigo, acne, seborrheic dermatitis, cellulitis, and pediculosis. Although none of these are serious disorders, impetigo and pediculosis are highly contagious. Also seen are the different degrees of burns, usually accidental, but potentially life threatening.

### Geriatrics

Elderly patients have a completely different set of diagnoses. The disorders categorized as those related to cornification, especially corns and calluses, are seen routinely in medical offices. These masses or thickenings of the skin are formed as a defensive response to constant friction, usually within shoes. Pressure sores (also called bedsores or decubitus ulcers) are seen most often in bed-ridden patients whose skin may already be atrophied and thin. Eczema, actinic keratoses, cellulitis, and fungal infections are also common complaints. The last category of skin disorders often seen in the elderly is the area of neoplasms. Although younger patients with skin cancers are often seen, older patients, by definition, have had a longer time to be exposed to the sun and develop malignancies.

## DIAGNOSTIC PROCEDURES

### Terms Related to Biopsies

| Term | Word Origin | Definition |
|---|---|---|
| excisional biopsy | | Biopsy in which the entire tumor may be removed with borders as a means of diagnosis and treatment. |
| exfoliation<br>ecks foh lee A shun | | Scraping or shaving off samples of friable (easily crushed) lesions for a laboratory examination called **exfoliative cytology.** |
| incisional biopsy | | Biopsy in which larger tissue samples may be obtained by excising a wedge of tissue and suturing the incision. |
| needle aspiration | | Aspiration of fluid from lesions to obtain samples for culture and examination. |
| punch biopsy | | Biopsy in which a tubular punch is inserted through to the subcutaneous tissue, and the tissue is cut off at the base (Fig. 4-27). |

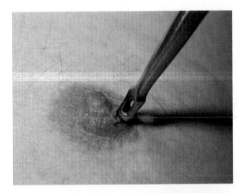

**Fig. 4-27** Punch biopsy.

### Terms Related to Laboratory Tests

| Term | Word Origin | Definition |
|---|---|---|
| bacterial analyses | | Culture and serology of lesions to help diagnose such disorders as impetigo. |
| fungal tests | | Cultures of scrapings of lesions used to identify fungal infections, such as tinea pedis, tinea capitis, and tinea cruris. |
| sweat tests | | Laboratory test for abnormally high levels of sodium and chloride present in the perspiration of persons with cystic fibrosis. |
| tuberculosis (TB) skin tests | | Intradermal test (e.g., Mantoux test) using purified protein derivative (PPD) to test for either dormant or active tuberculosis; much more accurate test than the multiple puncture tine test, which had been used for screening purposes (Fig 4-28). |
| Tzanck test<br>tzahnk | | Microscopic examination of lesions for the purpose of diagnosing herpes zoster and herpes simplex. |
| viral culture | | Sampling of vesicular fluid for the purpose of identifying viruses. |

*Continued*

## Terms Related to Laboratory Tests—cont'd

| Term | Word Origin | Definition |
|------|-------------|------------|
| Wood's light examination | | Method used to identify a variety of skin infections through the use of a Wood's light, which produces ultraviolet light; tinea capitis and pseudomonas infections in burns are two of the disorders it can reveal (Fig. 4-29). |
| wound and abscess cultures | | Lab samplings that can identify pathogens in wounds, such as diabetic or decubitus ulcers, postoperative wounds, or abscesses. |

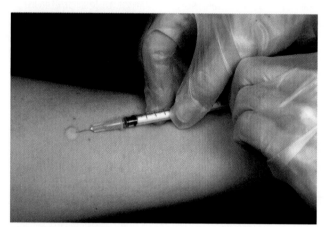

Fig. 4-28 Mantoux test. The technician is in the process of correctly placing a Mantoux tuberculin skin test in the recipient's forearm, which will cause a 6 mm to 10 mm wheal, i.e., a raised area of skin surface, to form at the injection site.

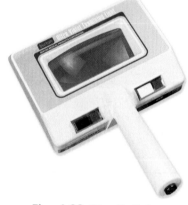

Fig. 4-29 Wood's light.

## Exercise 13: Diagnostic Procedures

*Fill in the blanks with the correct terms from the list below.*

**excisional, exfoliation, incisional, needle aspiration, punch**

1. An entire tumor is removed in a/an_____biopsy.

2. Fluid from a lesion is aspirated to obtain samples for culture in a/an_____biopsy.

3. A wedge of tissue is removed and the incision is sutured in a/an_____biopsy.

4. Samples of friable lesions are scraped or shaved off in_____.

5. A cylindrical punch is inserted into the subcutaneous tissue layer, and the tissue is cut off at the base

   in a/an_____biopsy.

*Match the following disorders with the tests that may be used to diagnose them.*

____ 6. ringworm

____ 7. impetigo

____ 8. cystic fibrosis

____ 9. tuberculosis

____10. herpes zoster, herpes simplex

____11. tinea capitis, pseudomonas

____12. bedsore, infection

A. Wood's light examination
B. Mantoux test
C. bacterial analysis
D. wound abscess culture
E. sweat test
F. fungal test
G. Tzanck test

## Case Study  *Angelina Herrara*

Angelina Herrara, a 9-year-old female, is brought to the Community Health Clinic by her mother. Angelina had a fever of 102° F for 2 days, and when it broke, her mother noticed that Angelina had a rash on her arms and legs. By nighttime, it had spread to her chest and back, and she was very irritable. Mom tells the practitioner that her daughter was starting to scratch the rash, and that she has seen some small blisters.

The practitioner questions Angelina's mother to find out how the rash started; she states that she has not changed any of her soaps, lotions, laundry products, or clothes. They do not have any pets except fish. She has not eaten any new foods, nor has she been outside.

As he examines Angelina, he notes that the rash is worse at her elbows and knees and between her legs, with reddened skin and a

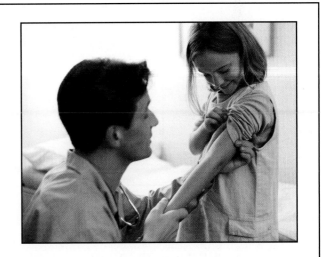

scattering of clear blisters. Angelina is diagnosed with a rash caused by a virus. She is prescribed Benadryl for the itching and a steroid cream. In 3 days, the rash resolves.

*Case Study* Angelina Herrara

---

**HERRARA, ANGELINA S - 77603**                                    ⬛ ⬛ ❎

Task   Edit   View   Time Scale   Options   Help

🛠 🔧 ← → 🔥 🔥 🔲 🔲 🔄 🔼 ⬛ 🔲 🖥 💾 📋 🔗 🖨 ⁉ 📃 ◀    As Of 9:35    📊 🔍 📋

**HERRARA, ANGELINA S.**          Age: 9 years        Sex: Female      Loc: SMOC
                                   DOB: 03/20/2003     MRN: 77603       FIN: 201376

| Reference Text Browser | Form Browser | Medication Profile |

Orders | Last 48 Hours | ED | Lab | Radiology | **Assessment** | Surgery | Clinical Notes | Pt. Info | Pt. Schedule | Task List | I & O | MAR

Flowsheet: Assessment ▼ ... Level: History and Physical ▼     ⦿ Table   ○ Group   ○ List

◀ ▶                                                                    ◀ ▶

| Navigator          ❎ |
| ✔ History and Physical |

Patient presents for her initial evaluation complaining of severe pruritic rash on her left and right antecubital fossa ×4 days. Mother reports the rash began on her daughter's arms but has also erupted on her forearms and lower extremities. Also has multiple lesions across her chest. Mother denies any new lotions, soaps, detergents, clothes, pets. No different foods or exposure to poison ivy. Has no previous history of dermatitis.

Denies current fever, chills; other than rash all other systems are unremarkable.

PHYSICAL EXAMINATION:   Diffuse vesicular lesions across the upper torso, forearms, and thighs.
Erythematous area of vesicular lesions in her right and left popliteal fossa.
Vesicular diffuse lesions, cause unclear.

DIAGNOSIS:              Most likely this represents a viral exanthem.
TREATMENT:              She is given topical hydrocortisone cream and advised to use Benadryl for itching.

PROD  MAHAFC  28 March 2012  9:35

---

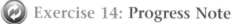

**Exercise 14: Progress Note**

*Review the progress note above and answer the following questions:*

1. How do we know that her rash is itchy?

   _____

2. What phrase tells us that she has had no skin inflammations diagnosed in the past?

   _____

3. What characteristic would "vesicular" lesions have?

   _____

4. "Exanthem" is a medical term for what?

   _____

## THERAPEUTIC INTERVENTIONS

### Terms Related to Grafting Techniques and Other Therapies

| Term | Word Origin | Definition |
|------|-------------|------------|
| **allograft**<br>AL oh graft | *all/o* other | Harvest of skin from another human donor for temporary transplant until an autograft is available. Also called a **homograft.** |
| **autograft**<br>AH toh graft | *auto-* self | Harvest of the patient's own skin for transplant (Fig. 4-30). |
| **dermatome**<br>DUR mah tohm | *dermat/o* skin<br>*-tome* instrument to cut | Instrument used to remove split-skin grafts (Fig. 4-31). |
| **flap** | | Section of skin transferred from one location to an immediately adjacent one. Also called a **skin graft.** |
| **laser therapy** | | Procedure to repair or destroy tissue, particularly in the removal of tattoos, warts, port wine stains, and psoriatic lesions. |
| **occlusive therapy** | *occlus/o* to close<br>*-ive* pertaining to | Use of a nonporous occlusive dressing to cover a treated area to enhance the absorption and effectiveness of a medication; used to treat psoriasis, lupus erythematosus, and chronic hand dermatitis. |
| **Psoralen plus ultraviolet A (PUVA) therapy**<br>SORE ah lin | | Directing a type of ultraviolet light (UV) onto psoriatic lesions. |
| **skin grafting (SG)** | | Skin transplant performed when normal skin cover has been lost as a result of burns, ulcers, or operations to remove cancerous tissue. |
| **full-thickness graft** | | Free skin graft in which full portions of both the epidermis and the dermis are used. |
| **split-thickness skin graft (STSG)** | | Skin graft in which the epidermis and parts of the dermis are used. |
| **xenograft**<br>ZEE noh graft | *xen/o* foreign | Temporary skin graft from another species, often a pig, used until an autograft is available. Also called a **heterograft.** |

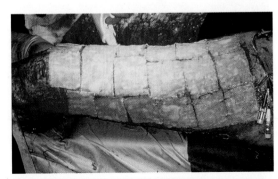

Fig. 4-30 Epithelial autografts. Thin sheets of skin are attached to gauze backing.

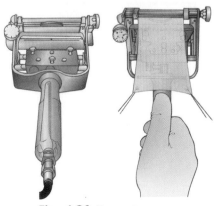

Fig. 4-31 Dermatome.

## Terms Related to Tissue Removal

| Term | Word Origin | Definition |
|------|-------------|------------|
| **cauterization**<br>kah tur ih ZAY shun | *cauter/i* burn<br>*-zation* process of | Destruction of tissue by burning with heat. |
| **cryosurgery**<br>KRY oh sur juh ree | *cry/o* extreme cold | Destruction of tissue through the use of extreme cold, usually liquid nitrogen. |
| **curettage**<br>kyoo ruh TAJZ | | Scraping of material from the wall of a cavity or other surface to obtain tissue for microscopic examination; this is done with an instrument called a **curette** (Fig. 4-32). |
| **débridement**<br>dah breed MON | | First step in wound treatment, involving removal of dirt, foreign bodies (FB), damaged tissue, and cellular debris from the wound or burn to prevent infection and to promote healing. |
| **escharotomy**<br>ess kar AH tuh mee | *eschar/o* scab<br>*-tomy* incision | Surgical incision into necrotic tissue resulting from a severe burn. This may be necessary to prevent edema leading to ischemia (loss of blood flow) in underlying tissue. |
| **incision and drainage (I&D)** | | Cutting open and removing the contents of a wound, cyst, or other lesion. |
| **Mohs surgery**<br>MOHZ | | Repeated removal and microscopic examination of layers of a tumor until no cancerous cells are present (Fig. 4-33). |
| **shaving (paring)** | | Slicing of thin sheets of tissue to remove lesions. |

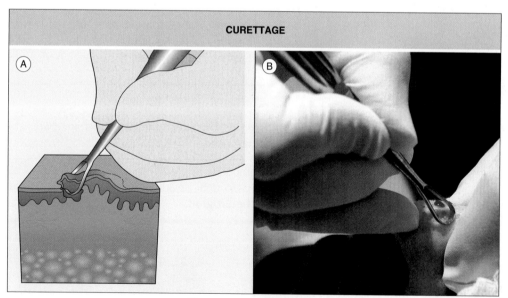

**CURETTAGE**

**Fig. 4-32** Curettage.

## Terms Related to Cosmetic Procedures

| Term | Word Origin | Definition |
|------|-------------|------------|
| blepharoplasty<br>BLEF ar oh plas tee | *blephar/o* eyelid<br>*-plasty* surgical repair | Surgical repair of the eyelid. |
| chemical peel | | Use of a mild acid to produce a superficial burn; normally done to remove wrinkles (Fig. 4-34). |
| dermabrasion<br>dur mah BRAY zhun | *derm/o* skin<br>*-abrasion* scraping of | Surgical procedure to resurface the skin; used to remove acne scars, nevi, wrinkles, and tattoos. |
| dermatoplasty<br>DUR mat tuh plas tee | *dermat/o* skin<br>*-plasty* surgical repair | Transplant of living skin to correct effects of injury, operation, or disease. |

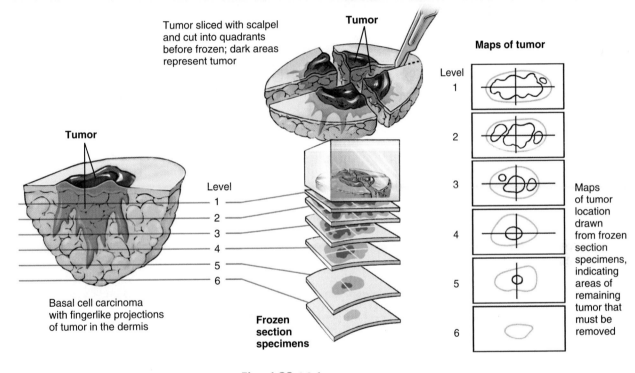

Tumor sliced with scalpel and cut into quadrants before frozen; dark areas represent tumor

Tumor

Maps of tumor

Tumor

Level 1
2
3
4
5
6

Basal cell carcinoma with fingerlike projections of tumor in the dermis

Frozen section specimens

Level 1
2
3
4
5
6

Maps of tumor location drawn from frozen section specimens, indicating areas of remaining tumor that must be removed

Fig. 4-33 Mohs surgery.

## Terms Related to Cosmetic Procedures—cont'd

| Term | Word Origin | Definition |
|------|-------------|------------|
| lipectomy<br>lih PECK tuh mee | *lip/o* fat<br>*-ectomy* removal | Removal of fatty tissue. |
| liposuction<br>LYE poh suck shun | *lip/o* fat | Technique for removing adipose tissue with a suction pump device (Fig 4-35). |
| rhytidectomy<br>rih tih DECK tuh mee | *rhytid/o* wrinkle<br>*-ectomy* removal | Surgical operation to remove wrinkles. Commonly known as a "face-lift." |

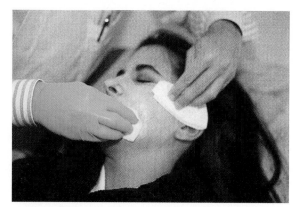

Fig. 4-34 Application of a chemical peel.

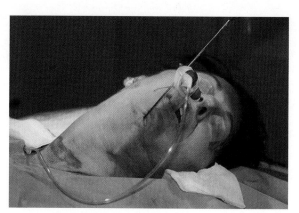

Fig. 4-35 Liposuction of the neck.

## Exercise 15: Therapeutic Interventions

1. Explain the differences among the following:

   A. autograft _____

   B. allograft _____

   C. xenograft _____

2. Which type of graft includes the epidermis and the dermis? _____

3. What instrument is used to cut skin for grafting? _____

*Fill in the blanks with the correct terms from the list below.*

**cauterization, cryosurgery, curettage, débridement, incision and drainage, laser therapy, occlusive therapy, shaving, Mohs surgery**

4. _____ is used to destroy tattoos.

5. Removing dirt, foreign bodies, damaged tissue, and cellular debris from a wound is called

   _____.

6. The destruction of tissue by burning with heat is called _____.

7. The destruction of tissue through the use of extreme cold is called _____.

8. Scraping of material from the wall of a cavity is called _____.

9. I&D is _____.

10. Another term for paring is _____.

11. Use of a dressing to cover a treated area is called _____.

12. Removal of a tumor by layers is called _____.

*Build the term.*

13. removal of wrinkles _____

14. removal of fat _____

15. surgical repair of the eyelid _____

16. scraping of skin _____

17. surgical repair of the skin _____

## PHARMACOLOGY

### Routes of Administration

Several medications are administered on, within, or through the skin. The most common of these routes of administration include the following:

**hypodermic (H):** general term that refers to any injection under the skin.
**intradermal (ID):** route of injection within the dermis (Fig. 4-36, *A*). Also called **intracutaneous.**
**subcutaneous:** route of injection into the fat layer beneath the skin (Fig. 4-36, *B*).
**topical:** type of drug applied directly onto the skin as a cream, gel, lotion, or ointment.
**transdermal therapeutic system (TTS):** use of a transdermal patch; involves placing medication in a gel-like material that is applied to the skin, allowing for a specified timed release of the medicine (Fig. 4-37). Examples are nitroglycerin for angina pectoris and the nicotine patch (NicoDerm) for smoking cessation.

**hypodermic**
hypo = under
derm/o = skin
-ic = pertaining to

**intradermal**
intra- = within
derm/o = skin
-al = pertaining to

**subcutaneous**
sub- = under
cutane/o = skin
-ous = pertaining to

**transdermal**
trans- = through
derm/o = skin
-al = pertaining to

Click on **Hear It, Spell It** to practice spelling the diagnostic and therapeutic terms you have learned in this chapter. To practice pronouncing these terms correctly, click on **Hear It, Say It.**

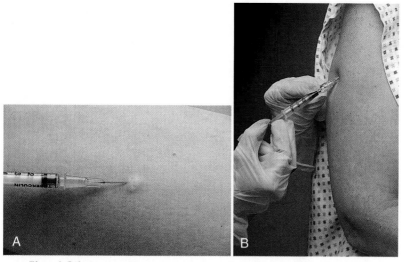

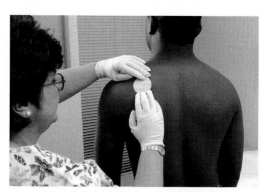

Fig. 4-36 **A,** Intradermal injection. **B,** Subcutaneous injection.

Fig. 4-37 Transdermal patch.

## Dermatologic Drugs

### *Traditional Pharmacology*

**anesthetic**
an- = not, without
-esthetic = pertaining to feeling
anti- = against

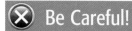

**Be Careful!**

ID *means intradermal;* I&D *means incision and drainage.*

**anesthetic agents:** reduce pain and discomfort; some can be given topically on an affected area. Examples include lidocaine (Solarcaine) and benzocaine (Orajel).

**antibacterials:** prevent and treat bacterial growth. Topical agents such as erythromycin (Ery 2% Pads) and clindamycin (Benzaclin) are used to treat acne. Triple antibiotic ointment (bacitracin, polymixin B, and neomycin), silver sulfadiazine (Silvadene), and mupirocin (Bactroban) are used to prevent and treat skin or wound infections. Oral agents for the treatment of acne include erythromycin (Ery-Tab), tetracycline (Sumycin), and minocycline (Minocin).

**antifungals:** treat fungal infections. Topical agents include nystatin (Nystat), butenafine (Lotrimin Ultra), ciclopirox (Loprox), and econazole (Spectazole).

**antihistamines:** lessen itching by reducing an allergic response. Diphenhydramine (Benadryl) is available in oral and topical formulations. Other oral agents include chlorpheniramine (Chlor-Trimeton), cetirizine (Zyrtec), and loratadine (Claritin).

**antiinflammatories:** reduce inflammation and pain. Oral agents include prednisone and aspirin; topical agents include hydrocortisone (Cortizone), fluocinonide (Lidex), and triamcinolone (Kenalog).

**antipsoriatics:** treat psoriasis. Examples include anthralin (Drithocreme) and calcipotriene (Dovonex).

**antiseptics:** topical agents used to prevent infection by destroying microbials. Examples include iodine and chlorhexidine (Peridex).

**antivirals:** reduce the effect of viruses. Examples include valacyclovir (Valtrex) and acyclovir (Zovirax) for the treatment of herpes simplex virus (cold sores or genital herpes) and herpes zoster (shingles).

**emollients (ih MOLL yents):** topical substances that soften the skin. Examples include mineral oil, lanolin, cetyl alcohol, and stearyl alcohol. A well-known product containing emollients is Lubriderm.

**immunomodulators** or **immunosuppressants:** agents that suppress the body's immune system. Topical agents such as pimecrolimus (Elidel) and tacrolimus (Protopic) are used to treat atopic dermatitis and eczema.

**keratolytics (kair ah toh LIT icks):** topical substances used to break down hardened skin and shed the top layer of dead skin to treat warts, calluses, corns, acne, rosacea, and psoriasis. Examples include salicylic acid, cantharidin, benzoyl peroxide (Benzac, Oxy10), and podofilox (Condylox).

**pediculicides:** destroy lice. Examples include malathion (Ovide), lindane (Kwell), and permethrin (Nix).

**protectives:** topicals with sun protection factors (SPFs) that protect the skin against ultraviolet A and B in sunlight. A wide variety of these are available OTC.

**retinoids:** derived from vitamin A; alters the growth of the top layer of skin and may be used to treat acne, reduce wrinkles, and treat psoriasis. Examples include tretinoin (Retin-A), isotretinoin (Accutane), and tazarotene (Tazorac).

**scabicides:** destroy mites and scabies. Examples include lindane (Kwell), permethrin (Elimite), and crotamiton (Eurax).

**keratolytics**
kerat/o = hard, horny
-lytic = pertaining to breaking down

**pediculicide**
pedicul/i = lice
-cide = killing

**scabicides**
scab/i = mites
-cide = killing

## Complementary and Alternative Methods of Treatment

**herbal medicine:** drugs from minimally altered plant sources, such as aloe vera (to treat sunburn and stomach ulcers) or tea tree oil (used for its antibacterial, antiviral, and antifungal properties to treat boils, wound infections, and acne). Also, therapeutic use of essential oils is helpful in treating dry flaky skin, decubitus ulcers, diabetic ulcers, herpes zoster, and herpes simplex type 1.

## Exercise 16: Pharmacology

*Fill in the blanks.*

1. Medication injected "within the dermis" is given by the _____ route.

2. Medications applied directly to the skin are given by the _____ route.

3. A general term meaning *under the skin* is _____.

4. Medications delivered via a patch through the skin are given by _____.

5. Medication applied to an affected area to reduce pain and discomfort is called a/an

   _____.

6. A topical agent that breaks down hardened skin is called a _____.

7. Medications that treat fungal skin infections are called _____.

8. Medications that target bacteria are called _____.

9. Scabies and mites can be killed by using a _____.

10. Two types of medications that may be used to treat a painful inflammation of the skin are

    _____ and _____.

*Match the following pharmaceutical agents with their actions.*

____11.  softens the skin

____12.  alters the growth of the outer layer of skin

____13.  lessens itching

____14.  prevents infection

____15.  treats herpes simplex virus

____16.  treats lice

____17.  suppresses the immune system

A.  antihistamine
B.  antiseptic
C.  retinoid
D.  emollient
E.  antiviral
F.  immunomodulator
G.  pediculicide

## Abbreviations

| Abbreviation | Meaning | Abbreviation | Meaning |
|---|---|---|---|
| BCC | basal cell carcinoma | ID | intradermal |
| Bx | biopsy | KS | Kaposi sarcoma |
| Decub | pressure ulcer | PPD | purified protein derivative |
| FB | foreign body | PUVA | Psoralen plus ultraviolet A |
| H | hypodermic | SCC | squamous cell carcinoma |
| HPV | human papillomavirus | SG | skin graft |
| HSV-1 | herpes simplex virus 1 | STSG | split-thickness skin graft |
| HSV-2 | herpes simplex virus 2 | TB | tuberculosis |
| I&D | incision and drainage | TTS | transdermal therapeutic system |

# Exercise 17: Abbreviations

*Write the abbreviation for each of the following.*

1. route of administration within the dermis: _____

2. radiation from sunlight: _____

3. skin graft: _____

4. pressure ulcer: _____

5. example of material removed from a wound during débridement: _____

6. incision and drainage: _____

7. biopsy: _____

8. purified protein derivative: _____

9. patch to deliver medicine: _____

10. tuberculosis: _____

# Chapter Review

Match the word parts to their definitions.

## WORD PART DEFINITIONS

| Prefix/Suffix |
| --- |
| -cide |
| crypt- |
| hyper- |
| intra- |
| -itis |
| -lytic |
| -osis |
| par- |
| sub- |
| trans- |

**Definition**

1. _____ excessive
2. _____ abnormal condition
3. _____ through
4. _____ within
5. _____ kill
6. _____ under
7. _____ hidden
8. _____ inflammation
9. _____ near
10. _____ pertaining to destruction

| Combining Form |
| --- |
| adip/o |
| chrom/o |
| cutane/o |
| eschar/o |
| exanthemat/o |
| follicul/o |
| hemat/o |
| hidraden/o |
| hidr/o |
| kerat/o |
| macul/o |
| melan/o |
| myc/o |
| onych/o |
| papul/o |
| pedicul/o |
| pil/o |
| rhytid/o |
| seb/o |
| squam/o |
| vascul/o |
| xen/o |

**Definition**

11. _____ sweat
12. _____ black, dark
13. _____ nail
14. _____ color
15. _____ wrinkle
16. _____ follicle
17. _____ vessel
18. _____ papule, pimple
19. _____ macule
20. _____ blood
21. _____ foreign
22. _____ rash
23. _____ hard, horny
24. _____ sweat gland
25. _____ skin
26. _____ lice
27. _____ oil
28. _____ scab
29. _____ scaly
30. _____ hair
31. _____ fat
32. _____ fungus

# WORDSHOP

| Prefixes | Combining Forms | Suffixes |
|----------|-----------------|----------|
| a- | blephar/o | -ectomy |
| an- | chrom/o | -desis |
| dys- | crypt/o | -ia |
| hyper- | cutane/o | -ic |
| hypo- | dermat/o | -itis |
| par- | fibr/o | -lysis |
| sub- | follicul/o | -malacia |
| trans- | hidr/o | -oma |
|  | myc/o | -osis |
|  | onych/o | -ous |
|  | rhytid/o | -plasty |
|  | seb/o | -rrheic |
|  | trich/o | -y |
|  | troph/o |  |

*Build the following terms by combining the word parts above. Some word parts may be used more than once. Some may not be used at all. The number in parentheses is the number of word parts needed to build the term.*

| Definition | Term |
|------------|------|
| 1. abnormal condition of excessive hair (3) | |
| 2. condition of no development (3) | |
| 3. removal of wrinkle (2) | |
| 4. pertaining to a discharge of oil (2) | |
| 5. condition of near the nail (3) | |
| 6. abnormal condition of no sweat (3) | |
| 7. surgical repair of the eyelids (2) | |
| 8. softening of the nails (2) | |
| 9. inflammation of a hair follicle (2) | |
| 10. condition of abnormal color (3) | |
| 11. pertaining to under the skin (3) | |
| 12. abnormal condition of fungus of the skin (3) | |
| 13. fibrous tumor of the skin (3) | |
| 14. destruction/loosening of a nail (2) | |
| 15 abnormal condition of "hidden" nail (3) | |

Sort the terms below into the correct categories.

## TERM SORTING

| Anatomy and Physiology | Pathology | Diagnostic Procedures | Therapeutic Interventions |
|---|---|---|---|
| | | | |
| | | | |
| | | | |
| | | | |
| | | | |
| | | | |
| | | | |
| | | | |
| | | | |
| | | | |

allograft

alopecia

bacterial analysis

blepharoplasty

cauterization

curettage

débridement

dermabrasion

dermatomycosis

dermatoplasty

epidermis

eponychium

escharotomy

excisional Bx

ecchymosis

eczema

follicle

hyperhidrosis

lunula

Mantoux test

melanocyte

onychomycosis

papilla

perspiration

plaque

punch biopsy

rhytidectomy

sebaceous gland

sebum

strata

tinea pedis

Tzanck test

verruca

vesicle

Wood's light

xenograft

*Replace the underlined text with the correct terms.*

## TRANSLATIONS

1. John was treated for **athlete's foot** after a positive fungal test.

2. Mr. Hassan complained of intense **itching** caused by **parasitic infestation caused by mites.**

3. Melanie said she had **an abnormal condition of excessive perspiration** as the reason for her appointment with her physician.

4. Stephanie went to see her podiatrist to treat her **ingrown toe nail** and asked if he could also treat the **infection beside her nail.**

5. Josh developed an **overgrowth of tissue** where his ear was pierced.

6. When Mia developed **a superficial vesicopustular skin infection,** her mom noticed small **raised solid skin lesions** as well as **tiny blisters** that were characteristic of the disorder.

7. When Laura came home with **an infestation of lice,** her doctor treated it with a **medication that kills lice.**

8. The patient was treated for **an inflammatory disease of the sebaceous glands** with a **drug derived from vitamin A.**

9. The patient was prescribed **topical substances that soften the skin** for her **dry skin.**

10. The patient had **a contagious epithelial growth caused by HPV** on his hand removed with **destruction of tissue through the use of extreme cold.**

11. The burn patient was in for **surgical incision into necrotic tissue** and a consultation for a possible **harvest of skin from another human donor for temporary transplant.**

12. Mrs. Mooreland had **a surgical operation to remove wrinkles** and **a surgical repair of the eyelids.**

13. Mr. Kleinfelter was hospitalized for **a sore in the skin over a bony prominence.**

# *Case Study*  Ben Warner

Eleven-month-old Ben Warner was enjoying himself as he practiced walking in his family's living room. His training circuit consisted of pulling up on the coffee table, edging around to the side near the couch, and then launching himself for a wobbly step before collapsing on the carpet. Unfortunately, Ben's dad left his newspaper and a fresh cup of hot coffee on the table when he went to answer the phone. It only took seconds for Ben to pull the newspaper and coffee onto himself, and his resulting howls brought his father running back to find his little boy with a nasty burn on his arm. Ben was taken to the emergency department (ED) of their local hospital.

The coffee that scalded Ben caused a mottled, sensitive, and painful area on his arm that soon developed a large blister. He was diagnosed as having a second-degree burn. His dad was told that he would need to try to keep Ben from picking at the blister because patients with this type of burn are at risk for developing scar tissue.

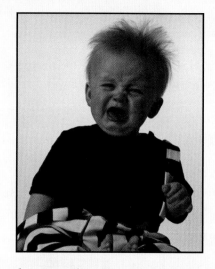

Before leaving the ED, Ben's forearm was treated with Silvadene cream, an antibiotic, and was covered with a loose dressing. His dad was advised to keep the burn covered with sterile bandages and to return in a week to have it checked.

---

WARNER, BENJAMIN R - 607231 Opened by O'BRIAN, JENNIFER A.     — ⬜ ✕

Task   Edit   View   Time Scale   Options   Help

As Of 07:08

**WARNER, BENJAMIN R**          Age: 11 months          Sex: Male          Loc: WHC-SMMC
                               DOB: 01/20/2011         MRN: 607231         FIN: 3506004

| Reference Text Browser | Form Browser | Medication Profile |

| Orders | Last 48 Hours | ED | Lab | Radiology | Assessment | Surgery | Clinical Notes | Pt. Info | Pt. Schedule | Task List | I & O | MAR |

Flowsheet: ED          Level: ED record          ⦿ Table  ○ Group  ○ List

**Navigator**  ✕
✓   ED record

Chief Complaint:  Second-degree burns on forearm of 11-month-old male.
Father states that child pulled hot coffee off table onto arm. Denies other injuries.

**Physical Exam:**
*HEENT:* Oropharynx pink and moist, neck supple without adenopathy; no evidence of burns found on face.
*CV:* RRR with no murmur.
*Lungs:* Clean bilaterally without adventitious sounds.
*ABD:* BS throughout, no organomegaly.
*Skin:* Large area of erythematous skin involving the back of the right hand and extending down the forearm in a splattering pattern. Tissue blanched well with good capillary refill. A large vesicle that had formed on the dorsal side of the hand broke during examination.
*Assessment:* Superficial partial-thickness burn of the right hand/forearm less than 10%.
*Treatment:* Wound cleansed with cool sterile water and dressed with Silvadene cream and a telfa dressing. Children's Tylenol administered with homecare discharge. Dressing instructions given.

PROD  MAHAFC     22 Dec 2011     07:08

### ⊘ ED Record

1. What type of burn is described?

   A. superficial

   B. partial thickness

   C. full thickness

2. What are the characteristics that make this a second-degree burn?

   _____

3. Ben's burn produced a large vesicle. What is a vesicle?

   _____

---

For more interactive learning, go to the Shiland Evolve site and click on:
- **Whack a Word Part** to review integumentary word parts.
- **Wheel of Terminology** and **Word Shop** to practice word building.
- **Tournament of Terminology** to test your knowledge of integumentary terms.
- **Terminology Triage** to practice sorting integumentary terms.

# 5

*Anybody who believes that the way to a man's heart is through his stomach flunked geography.*
—**Robert Byrne**

## OBJECTIVES

- Recognize and use terms related to the anatomy and physiology of the gastrointestinal system.
- Recognize and use terms related to the pathology of the gastrointestinal system.
- Recognize and use terms related to the diagnostic procedures for the gastrointestinal system.
- Recognize and use terms related to the therapeutic interventions for the gastrointestinal system.

# Gastrointestinal System

## CHAPTER AT A GLANCE

*Use this list of key terms and word parts to assess your knowledge. Check off the ones you have mastered.*

### ANATOMY AND PHYSIOLOGY

- ☐ alimentary canal
- ☐ anus
- ☐ appendix
- ☐ cecum
- ☐ colon
- ☐ defecation
- ☐ deglutition
- ☐ digestion
- ☐ esophagus
- ☐ gallbladder
- ☐ large intestine
- ☐ liver
- ☐ mastication
- ☐ oral cavity
- ☐ pancreas
- ☐ peristalsis
- ☐ pylorus
- ☐ rectum
- ☐ sigmoid colon
- ☐ small intestine
- ☐ stomach

### KEY WORD PARTS

**PREFIXES**
- ☐ a-
- ☐ dia-
- ☐ dys-
- ☐ endo-
- ☐ peri-
- ☐ re-

**SUFFIXES**
- ☐ -chezia
- ☐ -ectomy
- ☐ -emesis
- ☐ -flux
- ☐ -itis
- ☐ -pepsia
- ☐ -phagia
- ☐ -rrhaphy
- ☐ -rrhea
- ☐ -scopy
- ☐ -stalsis
- ☐ -stomy
- ☐ -tresia

**COMBINING FORMS**
- ☐ append/o, appendic/o
- ☐ cholecyst/o
- ☐ col/o, colon/o
- ☐ dent/i, odont/o
- ☐ enter/o
- ☐ esophag/o
- ☐ gastr/o
- ☐ hemat/o
- ☐ hepat/o
- ☐ herni/o
- ☐ or/o
- ☐ pancreat/o
- ☐ proct/o
- ☐ py/o
- ☐ pylor/o

### KEY TERMS

- ☐ anastomosis
- ☐ appendicitis
- ☐ barium enema
- ☐ cholecystectomy
- ☐ colonoscopy
- ☐ colostomy
- ☐ diarrhea
- ☐ diverticulosis
- ☐ dyspepsia
- ☐ dysphagia
- ☐ endoscopy
- ☐ esophageal atresia
- ☐ gastroenteritis
- ☐ gastroesophageal reflux disease (GERD)
- ☐ hematemesis
- ☐ hematochezia
- ☐ hemoccult test
- ☐ hemorrhoid
- ☐ hepatitis
- ☐ herniorrhaphy
- ☐ ileus
- ☐ inguinal hernia
- ☐ melena
- ☐ periodontal disease
- ☐ polyp
- ☐ pyloric stenosis
- ☐ pyorrhea

gastrointestinal
gastr/o = stomach
intestin/o = intestines
-al = pertaining to

abdomen = abdomin/o,
lapar/o, celi/o

mucus, mucosa =
mucos/o, myx/o

peristalsis
peri- = surrounding
-stalsis = contraction

gastroenterologist
gastr/o = stomach
enter/o = small intestine
-logist = one who
specializes

exodontist
exo- = outside
odont/o = teeth
-ist = one who
specializes

peri- = surrounding

ped/o = child

orth/o = straight

prosth/o = addition

proct/o = rectum and
anus

## FUNCTIONS OF THE GASTROINTESTINAL SYSTEM

The digestive system (Fig. 5-1) provides the nutrients needed for cells to replicate themselves continually and build new tissue. This is done through several distinct processes: **ingestion,** the intake of food; **digestion,** the breakdown of food; **absorption,** the process of extracting nutrients; and **elimination,** the excretion of any waste products. Other names for this system are the **gastrointestinal (GI) tract,** which refers to the two main parts of the system, and the **alimentary** (al in MEN tair ee) **canal,** which refers to the tubelike nature of the digestive system, starting at the mouth and continuing in varying diameters to the anus.

The digestive system begins in the oral cavity, progresses through the mediastinum and the **abdominal** and pelvic cavities, and finally exits at the anus. The stomach and intestines lie within the peritoneal cavity and are attached to the body wall by a rich vascular membrane termed the mesentery. Internally, the alimentary canal is composed of three layers, or tunics. The inner layer is the tunica **mucosa,** which secretes gastric juices, absorbs nutrients, and protects the tissue through the production of mucus. The submucosa, the next tunic, holds the blood, lymphatic, and nervous tissue. The deepest layer is the tunica muscularis, which contracts and relaxes around the tube in a wavelike movement termed **peristalsis,** to move food through the tract.

## SPECIALTIES/SPECIALISTS

The main digestive system specialty is called **gastroenterology,** and the specialist is called a **gastroenterologist. Proctologists** treat disorders of the rectum and anus.

While **dentists** diagnose and treat disorders of the teeth, there are subspecialists who extract **(exodontists)** and straighten **(orthodontists)** teeth, as well as those who treat children **(pedodontists),** gum disorders **(periodontists)** and replace missing teeth **(prosthodontists).**

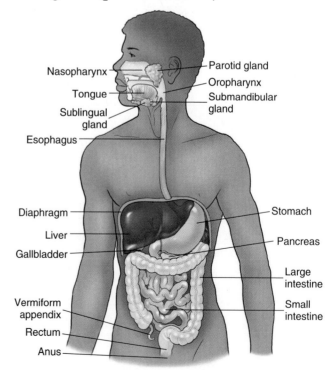

Fig. 5-1 The gastrointestinal system.

## ANATOMY AND PHYSIOLOGY

### Oral Cavity

Food normally enters the body through the mouth, or **oral cavity** (Fig. 5-2, *A*). The function of this cavity initially is to break down the food mechanically by chewing **(mastication)** and lubricate the food to make swallowing **(deglutition** dee gloo TIH shun) easier.

The oral cavity begins at the **lips,** the two fleshy structures surrounding its opening. The inside of the mouth is bounded by the **cheeks,** the **tongue** at the floor, and an anterior **hard palate** (PAL it) and posterior **soft palate,** which form the roof of the mouth. The upper and lower jaws hold 32 permanent **teeth** that are set in the flesh of the **gums.** The **uvula** (YOO vyoo lah) is the tag of flesh that hangs down from the medial surface of the soft palate. The three pairs of **salivary** (SAL ih vair ee) **glands** provide **saliva,** a substance that moistens the oral cavity, initiates the digestion of starches, and aids in chewing and swallowing. The glands are named for their locations: **parotid** (pair AH tid), near the ear; **submandibular** (sub man DIB yoo lur), under the lower jaw; and **sublingual** (sub LEENG gwul), under the tongue. The upper jaw is called the **maxilla,** and the lower is called the **mandible.**

### Throat

The throat, or **pharynx** (FAIR inks), is a tube that connects the oral cavity with the esophagus. It can be divided into three main parts: the nasopharynx, the oropharynx, and the hypopharynx. The **nasopharynx** (nay soh FAIR inks) is the most superior part of the pharynx, located behind the nasal cavity. The **oropharynx** (oh roh FAIR inks) is the part of the throat directly adjacent to the oral cavity, and the **hypopharynx** (hye poh FAIR inks) (also called the **laryngopharynx**) is the part of the throat directly below the oropharynx (Fig. 5-2, *B*).

| |
|---|
| **mouth, oral cavity** = or/o, stomat/o, stom/o |
| **lips** = cheil/o, labi/o |
| **cheek** = bucc/o |
| **tongue** = gloss/o, lingu/o |
| **palate** = palat/o |
| **teeth** = dent/i, odont/o |
| **gums** = gingiv/o |
| **salivary gland** = sialaden/o |
| **saliva** = sial/o |
| **parotid**<br> par- = near<br> ot/o = ear<br> -id = pertaining to |
| **submandibular**<br> sub- = under<br> mandibul/o = lower jaw, mandible<br> -ar = pertaining to |
| **sublingual**<br> sub- = under<br> lingu/o = tongue<br> -al = pertaining to |
| **upper jaw** = maxill/o |
| **lower jaw** = mandibul/o |
| **throat, pharynx** = pharyng/o |
| **nasopharynx**<br> nas/o = nose<br> pharyng/o = throat, pharynx |
| **below** = hypo- |
| **larynx, voicebox** = laryng/o |

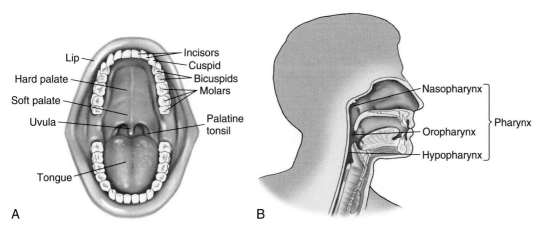

A — Lip, Hard palate, Soft palate, Uvula, Tongue, Incisors, Cuspid, Bicuspids, Molars, Palatine tonsil

B — Nasopharynx, Oropharynx, Hypopharynx, Pharynx

Fig. 5-2 **A,** The oral cavity. **B,** The pharynx.

**esophagus** = esophag/o

**bolus** = bol/o

## Esophagus

The **esophagus** (eh SAH fah gus) is a muscular, mucus-lined tube that extends from the throat to the stomach. It carries a masticated lump of food, a **bolus** (BOH lus), from the oral cavity to the stomach by means of peristalsis. The glands in the lining of the esophagus produce mucus, which aids in lubricating and easing the passage of the bolus to the stomach. The muscle that must relax before the food enters the stomach is known by three names: the **lower esophageal** (eh sah fah JEE ul) **sphincter** (SFINK tur) **(LES),** the **gastroesophageal sphincter,** or the **cardiac sphincter,** which gets its name because of its proximity to the heart. Sphincters are ringlike muscles that appear throughout the digestive and other body systems.

 Exercise 1: **Oral Cavity, Throat, and Esophagus**

*Match the combining forms with the following definitions. There may be more than one combining form for a given definition.*

____  1. teeth

____  2. gums

____  3. roof of mouth

____  4. tongue

____  5. mouth

____  6. lips

____  7. cheek

____  8. salivary gland

____  9. saliva

____  10. throat

____  11. esophagus

A. esophag/o
B. bucc/o
C. cheil/o
D. or/o, stom/o, stomat/o
E. lingu/o
F. palat/o
G. labi/o
H. gingiv/o
I. gloss/o
J. sial/o
K. stomat/o
L. pharyng/o
M. dent/i, odont/o
N. sialaden/o

*Decode the following terms using your knowledge of gastrointestinal word parts.*

12. perioral _____

13. gingival _____

14. periodontal _____

15. submandibular _____

16. nasopharyngeal _____

## Exercise 2: Oral Cavity, Throat, and Esophagus

*Label the figure below with the correct anatomic terms and combining forms where appropriate.*

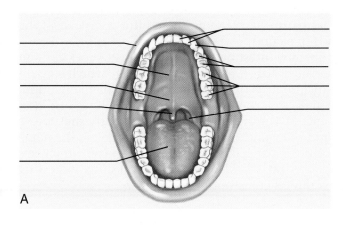

A

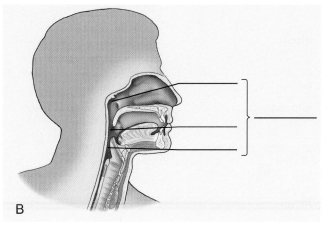

B

## Stomach

The **stomach,** where digestion begins, is an expandable vessel, which is divided into three sections: the top, or **fundus** (FUN dus); the **body;** and the muscle between the stomach and first part of the small intestine, or **pylorus** (pye LORE us) (also called the **gastric antrum**) (Fig. 5-3). The portion of the stomach that surrounds the esophagogastric connection is the **cardia** (KAR dee ah). The **fundus** is the area of the stomach that abuts the diaphragm. This section of the stomach has no acid-producing cells, unlike the remainder of the stomach. The body, or **corporis,** is the central part of the stomach, and the pylorus (*pl.* pylori) is at the distal end of the stomach, where the small intestine begins. A small muscle, the **pyloric sphincter,** regulates the gentle release of food from the stomach into the small intestine. When the stomach is empty, it has an appearance of being lined with many ridges. These ridges, or wrinkles, are called **rugae** (ROO jee) (*sing.* ruga).

The function of the stomach is to temporarily store the chewed food that it receives from the esophagus. This food is mixed with gastric juices and hydrochloric acid to further the digestive process chemically. This mixture is called **chyme** (kyme). The smooth muscles of the stomach contract to aid in the mechanical digestion of the food. A continual coating of mucus protects the stomach and the rest of the digestive system from the acidic nature of the gastric juices.

| | |
|---|---|
| **stomach** = gastr/o | |
| **fundus** = fund/o | |
| **body, corporis** = corpor/o | |
| **pylorus** = pylor/o | |
| **rugae** = rug/o | |

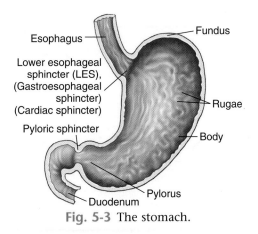

**Fig. 5-3** The stomach.

| |
|---|
| **small intestine** = enter/o |
| **duodenum** = duoden/o |
| **lumen** = lumin/o |
| **jejunum** = jejun/o |
| **ileum** = ile/o |
| **fold, plica** = plic/o |
| **villus** = vill/o |
| **lipid, fat** = lipid/o, lip/o |
| **large intestine, colon** = col/o, colon/o |

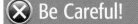

> ### ✖ Be Careful!
>
> *The combining form* **gastr/o** *refers only to the stomach. The combining forms* **abdomin/o,** **lapar/o,** *and* **celi/o** *refer to the abdomen.*

**ileocecal**
    ile/o = ileum
    cec/o = cecum
    -al = pertaining to

**cecum** = cec/o

**appendix** = appendic/o, append/o

**feces** = fec/a

**sigmoid colon** = sigmoid/o

**rectum, straight** = rect/o

**anus** = an/o

**rectum and anus** = proct/o

> ### ✖ Be Careful!
>
> *Don't confuse the term* **ilium,** *meaning part of the hip bone, with* **ileum,** *meaning part of the small intestine.*

## Small Intestine

Once the chyme has been formed in the stomach, the pyloric sphincter relaxes a bit at a time to release portions of it into the first part of the **small intestine,** called the **duodenum** (doo AH deh num). The small intestine gets its name, not because of its length (it is about 20 feet long), but because of the diameter of its **lumen** (LOO mun) (a tubular cavity within the body). The second section of the small intestine is the **jejunum** (jeh JOO num) and the distal part of the small intestine is the **ileum** (ILL ee um).

Multiple circular folds in the small intestines, called **plicae** (PLY see), contain thousands of tiny projections called **villi** (VILL eye) (*sing.* villus), which contain blood capillaries that absorb the products of carbohydrate and protein digestion. The villi also contain lymphatic vessels, known as **lacteals** (LACK tee uls), that absorb **lipid** (LIH pid) substances from the chyme. A lipid is a fatty substance.

The suffix -*ase* is used to form the name of an enzyme. It is added to the name of the substance upon which the enzyme acts: for example, **lipase,** which acts on lipids, or amylase, which acts on starches. -*ose* is a chemical suffix indicating that a substance is a carbohydrate, such as *glucose.*

## Large Intestine

In contrast to the small intestine, the **large intestine** or **colon** (Fig. 5-4) is only about 5 feet long, but it is much wider in diameter. The primary function of the large intestine is the elimination of waste products from the body. Some synthesis of vitamins occurs in the large intestine, but unlike the small intestine, the large intestine has no villi and is not well suited for absorption of nutrients. The **ileocecal** (ILL ee oh SEE kul) valve is the exit from the small intestine and the entrance to the colon. The first part of the large intestine, the **cecum** (SEE kum), has a wormlike appendage, called the **vermiform appendix** (VUR mih form ah PEN dicks) (*pl.* appendices), dangling from it. Although this organ does not seem to have any direct function related to the digestive system, it is thought to have a possible immunologic defense mechanism.

No longer called chyme, whatever has not been absorbed by the small intestines is now called **feces** (FEE sees). The feces pass from the cecum to the **ascending colon** (KOH lin), through the **transverse colon,** the **descending colon,** the **sigmoid colon** (the S-shaped part of the large intestine), and on to the **rectum** (the last straight part of the colon), where they are held until released from the body completely through the **anus** (the final sphincter in the GI tract.) The process of releasing feces from the body is called **defecation,** or a bowel movement (BM).

> ### ✖ Be Careful!
>
> *Do not confuse* -**cele,** *the suffix meaning herniation, with* **celi/o,** *a combining form for abdomen.*

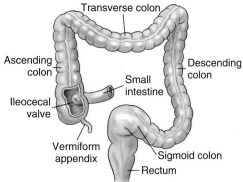

Fig. 5-4 The large intestine (colon).

> ### ✖ Be Careful!
>
> *Do not confuse* **an/o,** *the combining form for anus;* **ana-,** *the prefix meaning up or apart; and* **an-,** *the prefix meaning no, not, or without.*

## Exercise 3: The Stomach, Small Intestine, and Large Intestine

*Match the following combining forms and body parts with their terms.*

____ 1. lip/o

____ 2. plic/o

____ 3. col/o

____ 4. jejun/o

____ 5. ile/o

____ 6. rect/o

____ 7. an/o

____ 8. duoden/o

____ 9. gastr/o

____ 10. cec/o

____ 11. sigmoid/o

____ 12. lumin/o

____ 13. enter/o

____ 14. pylor/o

____ 15. proct/o

____ 16. appendic/o

A. rectum and anus
B. first part of large intestines
C. structure hanging from cecum
D. small intestines
E. tubular cavity
F. stomach
G. second part of small intestines
H. a fatty substance, fat
I. folds
J. first part of small intestines
K. muscle between stomach and first part of small intestines
L. last straight part of colon
M. large intestines
N. distal part of small intestines
O. final sphincter in GI tract
P. S-shaped part of large intestine

*Decode the terms.*

17. perirectal _____

18. intraluminal _____

19. epigastric _____

## Exercise 4: Stomach and Intestines

*Label the drawing with correct anatomic terms and combining forms where appropriate.*

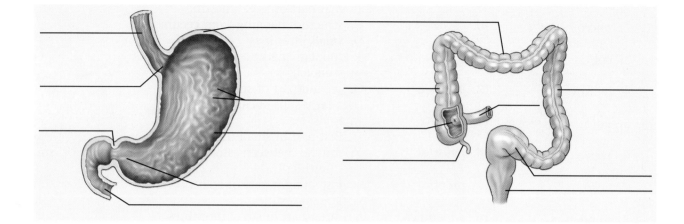

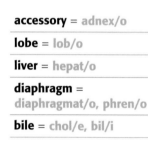

| | |
|---|---|
| **accessory** = adnex/o | |
| **lobe** = lob/o | |
| **liver** = hepat/o | |
| **diaphragm** = diaphragmat/o, phren/o | |
| **bile** = chol/e, bil/i | |
| **cholesterol** = cholesterol/o | |

### Accessory Organs (Adnexa)

The accessory organs are the gallbladder (GB), liver, and pancreas (Fig. 5-5). These organs secrete fluid into the GI tract but are not a direct part of the tube itself. Sometimes accessory structures are referred to as **adnexa** (ad NECK sah).

The two **lobes** that form the **liver** (LIH vur) virtually fill the right upper quadrant of the abdomen and extend partially into the left upper quadrant directly inferior to the **diaphragm.** The liver filters and stores blood and forms a substance called **bile,** which **emulsifies** (ee MUL sih fyez), or mechanically breaks down, fats into smaller particles so that they can be chemically digested. Bile is composed of **bilirubin** (BILL ee roo bin), the waste product formed by the normal breakdown of hemoglobin in red blood cells at the end of their life spans, and **cholesterol** (koh LESS tur all), a fatty substance found only in animal tissues. Bile is released from the liver through the right and left hepatic ducts, which join to form the **hepatic** (heh PAT ick) **duct.** The **cystic** (SISS tick) **duct** carries bile to and from the gallbladder. When the hepatic and cystic

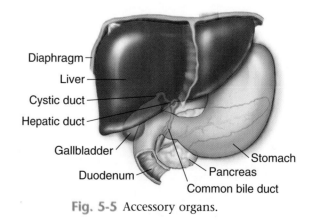

Diaphragm
Liver
Cystic duct
Hepatic duct
Gallbladder
Duodenum
Stomach
Pancreas
Common bile duct

**Fig. 5-5** Accessory organs.

ducts merge, they form the **common bile duct,** which empties into the duodenum. Collectively, all of these ducts are termed **bile vessels.** Bile is stored in the **gallbladder** (GALL blad ur), a small sac found on the underside of the right lobe of the liver. When fatty food enters the duodenum, a hormone called **cholecystokinin** (koh lee sis toh KYE nin) is secreted, causing a contraction of the gallbladder to move bile out into the cystic duct, then the common bile duct, and finally into the duodenum.

    The **pancreas** (PAN kree us) is a gland located in the upper left quadrant. It is involved in the digestion of the three types of food molecules: carbohydrates, proteins, and lipids. The pancreatic enzymes are carried through the pancreatic duct, which empties into the common bile duct. Pancreatic involvement in food digestion is an **exocrine** (ECK soh krin) function because the secretion is into a duct. Pancreatic **endocrine** (EN doh krin) functions (secretion into blood and lymph vessels) are discussed in Chapter 15.

---

**common bile duct =**
choledoch/o

---

**bile vessel** = cholangi/o

---

**gallbladder =**
cholecyst/o

---

**pancreas** = pancreat/o

---

**cholecystokinin**
  cholecyst/o =
  gallbladder
  -kinin = movement
  substance

---

**exocrine**
  exo- = outside
  -crine = to secrete

---

**endocrine**
  endo- = within
  -crine = to secrete

---

## Exercise 5: Accessory Organs

*Match the combining forms with their terms.*

| | | |
|---|---|---|
| ____ 1. pancreas | ____ 5. bile | A. lob/o |
| | | B. chol/e, bil/i |
| ____ 2. gallbladder | ____ 6. bile vessels | C. hepat/o |
| | | D. cholecyst/o |
| ____ 3. lobe | ____ 7. common bile duct | E. cholangi/o |
| | | F. choledoch/o |
| ____ 4. liver | | G. pancreat/o |

*Decode the terms.*

8. pancreatic _____

9. biliary _____

10. subhepatic _____

## Exercise 6: Accessory Organs

*Label the drawing with the correct anatomic terms and combining forms where appropriate.*

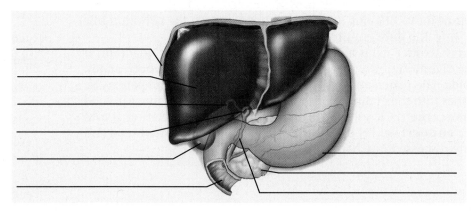

You can review the anatomy of the gastrointestinal system by clicking on **Body Spectrum Electronic Anatomy Coloring Book → Digestive.**

## *Case Study* Peter Jacobs

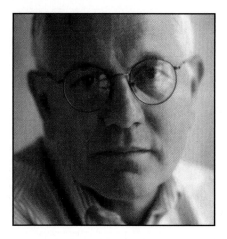

Peter Jacobs is a 62-year-old CEO of a large international company, who has come to see his physician today because he has been experiencing nausea and persistent heartburn. His physician, Dr. Wellemeyer, knows that Peter's job is stressful and has required him to travel frequently and eat a variety of unusual foods. In the past, Dr. Wellemeyer has prescribed an antacid and an antianxiety medication, which helped relieve Peter's symptoms. Today, however, Peter says that he is no longer getting relief. He has lost weight and sleep over the past 2 months.

After lab and stool tests turn out normal, Dr. Wellemeyer refers Peter to a gastroenterologist, who schedules an upper GI endoscopy, which reveals erosion and narrowing of the esophagus. He is diagnosed with Barrett esophagus, a moderate hiatal hernia, and gastritis. Peter is placed on a special antacid and is told that if his symptoms do not improve, surgery may be necessary to repair his hiatal hernia.

## Case Study   Peter Jacobs

JACOBS, PETER E - 613446 Opened by  JEROME, ALAN MD     _ ⊡ ☒

Task   Edit   View   Time Scale   Options   Help

As Of 06:15

| JACOBS, PETER E | Age: 62 | Sex: Male | Loc: WHC-SMMC |
|---|---|---|---|
| | DOB: 08/20/1950 | MRN: 613446 | FIN: 3506004 |

Reference Text Browser    Form Browser    Medication Profile

Orders   Last 48 Hours   ED   Lab   Radiology   Assessment   **Surgery**   Clinical Notes   Pt. Info   Pt. Schedule   Task List   I & O   MAR

Flowsheet:  Surgery  ▼  ...    Level:  Operative Report  ▼        ⦿ Table   ○ Group   ○ List

**Navigator**    ☒

✓  Operative Report

| PREOPERATIVE DIAGNOSIS: | Rule out GI pathology |
|---|---|
| POSTOPERATIVE DIAGNOSIS: | See "Impression" below |
| OPERATION: | Upper GI endoscopy |

Patient was brought into the endoscopy suite where continuous oximetry, blood pressure, and ECG monitoring was placed. He was given 50 mg of fentanyl before procedure. The GIF Olympus 150 video endoscope was introduced through the pharynx without difficulty. Proximal portion of the esophagus appeared normal. At approximately mid esophagus, there were noted streaks of erythema extending up into the esophagus. The squamocolumnar junction was at 33 cm where there was a smooth concentric narrowing of the esophagus. There was mild friability of this tissue and distally was a moderate hiatal hernia. The scope was advanced through this into the gastric fundus, which was visualized in both the forward and retroflexed manner. Mucosa appeared quite normal. Distally, there was marked erythema of the antrum, particularly surrounding the pylorus. Biopsy was taken for *H. pylori*. The duodenum was difficult to intubate but appeared normal. Scope was withdrawn again to the level of the lower esophageal sphincter at 36 cm. Biopsies were taken from that area and circumferentially up to approximately 32 cm. There was minimal bleeding. Patient tolerated the procedure well.

IMPRESSION:
1. Reflux esophagitis with stricture at 33 cm
2. Moderate hiatal hernia
3. Probably Barrett esophagus
4. Diffuse antral gastritis, biopsy pending

PROD  MAHAFC   23 August 2012   06:15

## Exercise 7: Operative Report

*Using the operative report above, answer the following questions. Use a dictionary as needed for this exercise.*

1. What was the route of the endoscope? _____

2. The portion of the esophagus that appeared normal was (close to/far from) the mouth. Circle one.

3. The mucosa was normal in which part of the stomach? _____

4. What are synonyms for the "lower esophageal sphincter"? _____

Choose **Hear It, Spell It** to practice spelling the anatomy and physiology terms that you have learned in this chapter. To practice pronouncing anatomy and physiology terms choose **Hear It, Say It.**

## Combining and Adjective Forms for the Anatomy of the GI System

| Meaning | Combining Form | Adjective Form |
| --- | --- | --- |
| abdomen | abdomin/o, celi/o, lapar/o | abdominal, celiac |
| accessory | adnex/o | adnexal |
| anus | an/o | anal |
| appendix | appendic/o, append/o | appendicular |
| bile | chol/e, bil/i | biliary |
| bile vessel | cholangi/o | |
| bolus | bol/o | |
| cecum | cec/o | cecal |
| cheek | bucc/o | buccal |
| cholesterol | cholesterol/o | |
| common bile duct | choledoch/o | choledochal |
| corporis, body | corpor/o | corporeal |
| duodenum | duoden/o | duodenal |
| esophagus | esophag/o | esophageal |
| fat, lipid | lip/o, lipid/o | lipid |
| feces | fec/a | fecal |
| fold, plica | plic/o | plical |
| fundus | fund/o | fundal |
| gallbladder | cholecyst/o | cholecystic |
| glucose, sugar | gluc/o | |
| gums | gingiv/o | gingival |
| ileum | ile/o | ileal |
| intestines | intestin/o | intestinal |
| jejunum | jejun/o | jejunal |
| large intestine, colon | col/o, colon/o | colonic |
| lips | cheil/o, labi/o | labial |
| liver | hepat/o | hepatic |
| lobe | lob/o | lobular |
| lower jaw | mandibul/o | mandibular |
| lumen | lumin/o | luminal |
| mouth, oral cavity | or/o, stom/o, stomat/o | oral, stomal, stomatic |
| nose | nas/o, rhin/o | nasal |
| nutrition | aliment/o | alimentary |
| palate | palat/o | palatine |
| pancreas | pancreat/o | pancreatic |
| pharynx, throat | pharyng/o | pharyngeal |
| pylorus | pylor/o | pyloric |
| rectum | rect/o | rectal |
| rectum and anus | proct/o | |
| rugae | rug/o | rugous |
| saliva | sial/o | salivary |
| salivary gland | sialaden/o | |
| sigmoid colon | sigmoid/o | sigmoidal |
| small intestine | enter/o | enteral |

## Combining and Adjective Forms for the Anatomy of the GI System—cont'd

| Meaning | Combining Form | Adjective Form |
|---------|----------------|----------------|
| starch | amyl/o | |
| stomach | gastr/o | gastric |
| teeth | dent/i, odont/o | dental |
| tongue | gloss/o, lingu/o | lingual, glossal |
| upper jaw | maxill/o | maxillary |
| uvula | uvul/o | uvular |
| villus | vill/o | villous |

## Prefixes for the Anatomy of the GI System

| Prefix | Meaning |
|--------|---------|
| endo- | within |
| exo- | outside |
| hypo- | below |
| par- | near |
| peri- | surrounding |
| sub- | under |

## Suffixes for the Anatomy of the GI System

| Suffix | Meaning |
|--------|---------|
| -al, -ar, -eal, -ic, -id, -ine, -ous | pertaining to |
| -crine | to secrete |
| -kinin | movement substance |
| -stalsis | contraction |

## PATHOLOGY

### Terms Related to Upper Gastrointestinal Complaints

| Term | Word Origin | Definition |
|------|-------------|------------|
| **dyspepsia**<br>dis PEP see ah | *dys-* abnormal, bad<br>*-pepsia* digestion condition | Feeling of epigastric discomfort that occurs shortly after eating. The discomfort may include feelings of nausea, fullness, heartburn, and/or bloating. Also called **indigestion**. |
| **eructation**<br>ee ruck TAY shun | | Release of air from the stomach through the mouth. Eructation may be caused by rapid eating or by intentionally or unintentionally swallowing air (**aerophagia**). Also called **burping** or **belching**. |
| **halitosis**<br>hal ih TOH sis | *halit/o* breath<br>*-osis* abnormal condition | Bad-smelling breath. |
| **hematemesis**<br>hee mah TEM ah sis | *hemat/o* blood<br>*-emesis* vomiting | Vomiting of blood. |
| **hiccup**<br>HICK up | | Involuntary contraction of the diaphragm, followed by a rapid closure of the glottis (which in turn causes the characteristic sound of a hiccup). Also known as **hiccough** or **singultus**. |

*Continued*

## Terms Related to Upper Gastrointestinal Complaints—cont'd

| Term | Word Origin | Definition |
|------|-------------|------------|
| **nausea**<br>NAH see ah | | Sensation that accompanies the urge to vomit but does not always lead to vomiting. The abbreviation N&V refers to nausea and vomiting. The term is derived from a Greek word meaning seasickness. |
| **pyrosis**<br>pye ROH sis | *pyr/o* fire<br>*-osis* abnormal condition | Painful burning sensation in esophagus, usually caused by reflux of stomach contents, hyperactivity, or peptic ulcer. Also known as **heartburn.** |
| **regurgitation**<br>ree gur jih TAY shun | | Return of swallowed food to the mouth. Regurgitation may, however, describe any backward flow in the body, not just that of a GI nature. |
| **vomiting**<br>VAH mih ting | | Forcible or involuntary emptying of the stomach through the mouth. The material expelled is called **vomitus** or **emesis.** |

## Terms Related to Lower Gastrointestinal Complaints

| Term | Word Origin | Definition |
|------|-------------|------------|
| **constipation**<br>kon stih PAY shun | | Infrequent, incomplete, or delayed bowel movements. **Obstipation** is intractable (difficult to manage) constipation or intestinal obstruction. |
| **diarrhea**<br>dye ah REE ah | *dia-* through, complete<br>*-rrhea* discharge, flow | Abnormal discharge of watery, semisolid stools. |
| **flatus**<br>FLAY tus | | Gas expelled through the anus. |
| **hematochezia**<br>hee mat oh KEE zee ah | *hemat/o* blood<br>*-chezia* condition of stools | Bright red, frank lower GI bleeding from the rectum that may originate in the distal colon. Passage of bloody stools. |
| **irritable bowel syndrome (IBS)** | | Diarrhea, gas, and/or constipation resulting from stress with no underlying disease. |
| **melena**<br>mah LEE nah | *melan/o* black, dark | Black, tarry stools caused by the presence of partially digested blood. |

## Exercise 8: Upper and Lower GI Complaints

*Match the GI complaints to their definitions.*

_____ 1. diarrhea      _____ 6. IBS

_____ 2. obstipation     _____ 7. constipation

_____ 3. flatus     _____ 8. nausea

_____ 4. melena     _____ 9. regurgitation

_____ 5. halitosis

A. bad breath
B. delayed defecation
C. feeling of need to vomit
D. gas passed through the anus
E. backward flow to mouth
F. black, tarry stools
G. loose, watery stools
H. extremely delayed defecation
I. diarrhea/gas/constipation resulting from stress with no underlying disease

*Match the synonyms.*

___ 10. indigestion    ___ 13. eructation    A. vomit
                                            B. hiccup
___ 11. singultus      ___ 14. emesis       C. burping
                                            D. dyspepsia
___ 12. pyrosis                             E. heartburn

*Build the terms.*

15. condition of blood in the stools _____

16. vomiting of blood _____

17. abnormal condition of digestion _____

## Terms Related to Congenital Disorders

| Term | Word Origin | Definition |
|------|-------------|------------|
| **cleft palate**<br>kleft<br>PAL it | | Failure of the palate to close during embryonic development, creating an opening in the roof of the mouth. Cleft palate often is accompanied by a cleft lip (Fig. 5-6). |
| **esophageal atresia**<br>eh soff uh JEE ul<br>ah TREE zsa | *esophag/o* esophagus<br>*-eal* pertaining to<br>*a-* without<br>*-tresia* condition of an opening | Esophagus that ends in a blind pouch and therefore lacks an opening into the stomach (Fig. 5-7). |
| **Hirschsprung disease**<br>HERSH sprung | | Congenital absence of normal nervous function in part of the colon, which results in an absence of peristaltic movement, accumulation of feces, and an enlarged colon. Also called **congenital megacolon.** |
| **pyloric stenosis**<br>pye LORE ick<br>sten OH sis | *pylor/o* pylorus<br>*-ic* pertaining to<br>*stenosis* narrowing | Condition in which the muscle between the stomach and the small intestine narrows or fails to open adequately to allow partially digested food into the duodenum. |

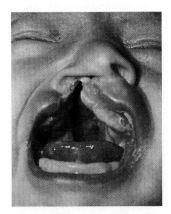

**Fig. 5-6** Cleft palate and cleft lip.

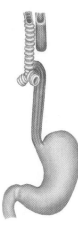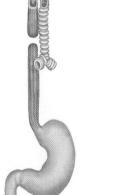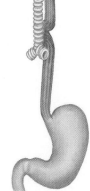

**Fig. 5-7** Esophageal atresia.

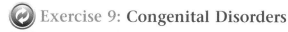

## Exercise 9: Congenital Disorders

*Fill in the blank with the correct term.*

**pyloric stenosis, cleft palate, esophageal atresia, Hirschsprung disease, congenital megacolon**

1. The term that refers to the lack of an opening in the tube that extends from the throat to the stomach is _____.

2. A congenital fissure in the roof of the mouth is called _____.

3. If the patient has a lack of normal nervous function in part of the large intestine, which results in an accumulation of feces, he or she may be diagnosed with _____.

4. Another name for the answer to question 3 is _____.

5. A narrowing of the muscle between the stomach and the duodenum is called _____.

## Terms Related to Oral Cavity Disorders

| Term | Word Origin | Definition |
|------|-------------|------------|
| **aphthous stomatitis** <br> AFF thus <br> stoh mah TYE tis | *aphth/o* ulceration <br> *-ous* pertaining to <br> *stomat/o* mouth <br> *-itis* inflammation | Recurring condition characterized by small erosions (ulcers), which appear on the mucous membranes of the mouth. Also called a **canker sore** (Fig. 5-8). |
| **cheilitis** <br> kye LYE tis | *cheil/o* lip <br> *-itis* inflammation | Inflammation of the lips. |
| **cheilosis** <br> kye LOH sis | *cheil/o* lip <br> *-osis* abnormal condition | Abnormal condition of the lips present in riboflavin (a B vitamin) deficiency. |
| **dental caries** <br> KARE ees | *dent/i* teeth <br> *-al* pertaining to | Plaque disease caused by an interaction between food and bacteria in the mouth, leading to tooth decay. Also called **cavities.** |
| **dental plaque** <br> plack | *dent/i* teeth <br> *-al* pertaining to | Film of material that coats the teeth and may lead to dental decay if not removed. |
| **gingivitis** <br> jin jih VYE tis | *gingiv/o* gums <br> *-itis* inflammation | Inflammatory disease of the gums characterized by redness, swelling, and bleeding (Fig. 5-9). |

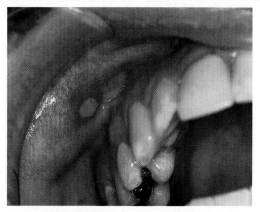

Fig. 5-8 Aphthous stomatitis.

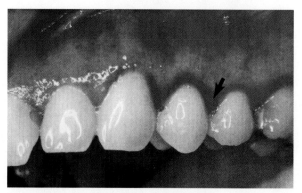

Fig. 5-9 Gingivitis.

## Terms Related to Oral Cavity Disorders—cont'd

| Term | Word Origin | Definition |
|------|-------------|------------|
| herpetic stomatitis<br>hur PET ick<br>stoh mah TYE tis | *stomat/o* mouth<br>*-itis* inflammation | Inflammation of the mouth caused by the herpes simplex virus (HSV). Also known as a **cold sore** or **fever blister**. |
| leukoplakia<br>loo koh PLAY kee ah | *leuk/o* white<br>*-plakia* condition of patches | Condition of white patches that may appear on the lips and buccal mucosa (Fig. 5-10). It usually is associated with tobacco use and may be precancerous. |
| malocclusion<br>mal oh KLOO zhun | *mal-* bad, poor<br>*-occlusion* condition of closure | Condition in which the teeth do not touch properly when the mouth is closed (abnormal bite). |
| periodontal disease<br>pair ee oh DON tul | *peri-* surrounding<br>*odont/o* tooth<br>*-al* pertaining to | Pathologic condition of the tissues surrounding the teeth. |
| pyorrhea<br>pye or REE yah | *py/o* pus<br>*-rrhea* flow, discharge | Purulent discharge from the tissue surrounding the teeth; often seen with gingivitis. |

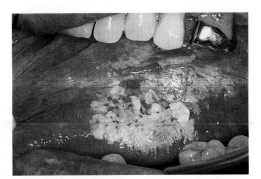

**Fig. 5-10** Leukoplakia.

## Exercise 10: Oral Cavity Disorders

*Match the oral cavity disorders to their definitions.*

_____ 1. dental caries

_____ 2. cheilosis

_____ 3. aphthous stomatitis

_____ 4. herpetic stomatitis

_____ 5. dental plaque

_____ 6. malocclusion

_____ 7. periodontal disease

A. tooth decay
B. disorder of tissue surrounding teeth
C. abnormal bite
D. canker sore
E. cold sore
F. abnormal condition of lips
G. material that coats teeth

*Build the terms.*

8. inflammation of the gums _____

9. discharge of pus _____

10. condition of white patches _____

## Terms Related to Disorders of the Esophagus

| Term | Word Origin | Definition |
|------|-------------|------------|
| **achalasia**<br>ack uh LAY zsa | *a-* without<br>*-chalasia* condition of relaxation | Impairment of esophageal peristalsis along with the lower esophageal sphincter's inability to relax. Also called **cardiospasm, esophageal aperistalsis** (a per rih STALL sis), and **megaesophagus.** |
| **dysphagia**<br>dis FAY jee ah | *dys-* difficult, bad<br>*-phagia* condition of swallowing, eating | Difficulty with swallowing that may be due to an obstruction (e.g., a tumor) or a motor disorder (e.g., a spasm). |
| **gastroesophageal reflux disease (GERD)**<br>gass troh eh sah fah JEE ul | *gastr/o* stomach<br>*esophag/o* esophagus<br>*-eal* pertaining to<br>*re-* back<br>*-flux* flow | Flowing back, or return, of the contents of the stomach to the esophagus caused by an inability of the lower esophageal sphincter (LES) to contract normally; characterized by pyrosis with or without regurgitation of stomach contents to the mouth (Fig. 5-11). Barrett esophagus is a condition caused by chronic reflux from the stomach. It is associated with an increased risk of cancer. |

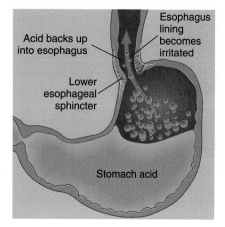

Fig. 5-11 GERD.

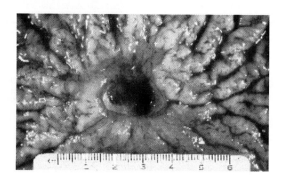

Fig. 5-12 Chronic peptic ulcer.

## Terms Related to Disorders of the Stomach

| Term | Word Origin | Definition |
|------|-------------|------------|
| **gastralgia**<br>gass TRAL zsa | *gastr/o* stomach<br>*-algia* pain | Gastric pain. Also called **gastrodynia** (gass troh DIH nee ah). |
| **gastritis**<br>gass TRY tis | *gastr/o* stomach<br>*-itis* inflammation | Acute or chronic inflammation of the stomach that may be accompanied by anorexia, nausea and vomiting, or indigestion. |
| **peptic ulcer disease (PUD)** | | An erosion of the protective mucosal lining of the stomach or duodenum (Fig. 5-12). Also called a **gastric** or **duodenal ulcer.** |

# Exercise 11: Esophageal and Stomach Disorders

*Matching. More than one answer may be correct.*

____ 1. PUD      ____ 4. achalasia

____ 2. gastralgia      ____ 5. dysphagia

____ 3. gastritis      ____ 6. GERD

A. cardiospasm
B. difficulty swallowing
C. inflammation of the stomach
D. stomach pain
E. gastrodynia
F. erosion of the gastric mucosa
G. return of the contents of the stomach to the esophagus
H. megaesophagus
I. esophageal aperistalsis

## Terms Related to Intestinal Disorders

| Term | Word Origin | Definition |
|---|---|---|
| **anal fissure** <br> A null <br> FISH ur | *an/o* anus <br> *-al* pertaining to | Cracklike lesion of the skin around the anus. |
| **anorectal abscess** <br> an oh RECK tul <br> AB sess | *an/o* anus <br> *rect/o* rectum <br> *-al* pertaining to | Circumscribed area of inflammation in the anus or rectum, containing pus. |
| **appendicitis** <br> ah pen dih SYE tis | *appendic/o* appendix <br> *-itis* inflammation | Inflammation of the vermiform appendix (Fig. 5-13). |
| **colitis** <br> koh LYE tis | *col/o* colon <br> *-itis* inflammation | Inflammation of the large intestine. |
| **Crohn disease** <br> krohn | | Inflammation of the ileum or the colon that is of idiopathic origin. Also called **regional** or **granulomatous enteritis.** |
| **diverticulitis** <br> dye vur tick yoo LYE tis | *diverticul/o* diverticulum <br> *-itis* inflammation | Inflammation occurring secondary to the occurrence of diverticulosis. |
| **diverticulosis** <br> dye vur tick yoo LOH sis | *diverticul/o* diverticulum <br> *-osis* abnormal condition | Development of diverticula, pouches in the lining of the small or large intestines (Fig. 5-14). |

*Continued*

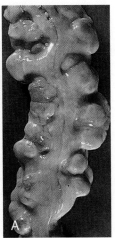

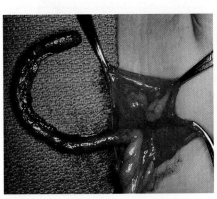

**Fig. 5-13** Appendicitis. Note the darker pink color of the appendix, indicating the inflammation.

**Fig. 5-14 A,** Diverticulosis. Diverticulosis can lead to diverticulitis **(B)** and subsequent complications.

## Terms Related to Intestinal Disorders—cont'd

| Term | Word Origin | Definition |
|------|-------------|------------|
| **fistula**<br>FIST yoo lah | | Abnormal channel between organs or from an internal organ to the surface of the body. |
| **hemorrhoid**<br>HEM uh royd | | Varicose vein in the lower rectum or anus. |
| **ileus**<br>ILL ee us | | Obstruction. **Paralytic ileus** is lack of peristaltic movement in the intestinal tract. Also called **adynamic ileus.** |
| **inflammatory bowel disease (IBD)** | | Chronic inflammation of the lining of the intestine characterized by bleeding and diarrhea. |
| **intussusception**<br>in tuh suh SEP shun | | Inward telescoping of the intestines (Fig. 5-15). |
| **mucositis**<br>myoo koh SYE tis | *mucos/o* mucus<br>*-itis* inflammation | Inflammation of the mucous membranes. Gastrointestinal mucositis may be an adverse effect of chemotherapy and can occur throughout the GI tract. |
| **peritonitis**<br>pair ih tuh NYE tis | *periton/o* peritoneum<br>*-itis* inflammation | Inflammation of the peritoneum that most commonly occurs when an inflamed appendix ruptures. |
| **polyp**<br>PAH lip | | Benign growth that may occur in the intestines. |
| **proctitis**<br>prock TYE tis | *proct/o* rectum and anus<br>*-itis* inflammation | Inflammation of the rectum and anus. Also called **rectitis.** |
| **pruritus ani**<br>proo RYE tis<br>A nye | | Common chronic condition of itching of the skin surrounding the anus. Note that pruritis is spelled with a u, not an i. |
| **ulcerative colitis**<br>UL sur uh tiv<br>koh LYE tis | *col/o* colon<br>*-itis* inflammation | Chronic inflammation of the colon and rectum manifesting with bouts of profuse watery diarrhea. |
| **volvulus**<br>VAWL vyoo lus | | Twisting of the intestine. |

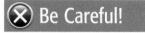 **Be Careful!**

*The correct spelling is* **pruritus,** *not pruritis.*

**Be Careful!**

*Don't confuse* **peritone/o,** *which is the membrane that lines the abdominal cavity, with* **perone/o,** *which is a combining form for the fibula and* **perine/o,** *the space between the anus and external reproductive organs.*

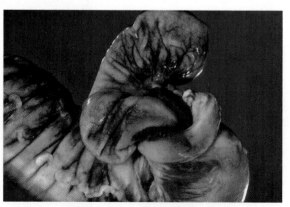

**Fig. 5-15** Intussusception.

## Exercise 12: Intestinal Disorders

*Match the intestinal disorders to their definitions.*

____ 1. polyp

____ 2. colitis

____ 3. anal fissure

____ 4. volvulus

____ 5. paralytic ileus

____ 6. fistula

____ 7. intussusception

____ 8. acute peritonitis

____ 9. pruritus ani

____ 10. ulcerative colitis

____ 11. Crohn disease

____ 12. hemorrhoids

____ 13. IBD

____ 14. diverticulitis

____ 15. anorectal abscess

____ 16. ileus

A. general term for an obstruction
B. a twisting of the intestines
C. inward telescoping of the intestines
D. idiopathic inflammation of ileum or colon
E. profuse watery diarrhea accompanies this condition
F. ruptured appendix puts a patient at risk for this
G. growth on mucous membranes
H. inflammation of pouches in GI tract
I. inflammation of the large intestine
J. itching of the skin around the anus
K. varicosities around the anus and rectum
L. cracklike lesion in the skin around the anus
M. abnormal channel that forms between organs or to the outside of the body
N. circumscribed area of purulent material in the distal end of the digestive tract
O. lack of peristaltic movement in intestines
P. erosion of intestinal lining accompanied by bleeding and diarrhea

*Build the terms:*

17. inflammation of the appendix _____

18. abnormal condition of diverticula _____

19. inflammation of the rectum and anus _____

## Terms Related to GI Accessory Organ Disorders

| Term | Word Origin | Definition |
|---|---|---|
| cholangitis<br>koh lan JYE tis | *cholangi/o* bile vessel<br>*-itis* inflammation | Inflammation of the bile vessels. |
| cholecystitis<br>koh lee sis TYE tis | *cholecyst/o* gallbladder<br>*-itis* inflammation | Inflammation of the gallbladder, either acute or chronic. May be caused by choledocholithiasis or cholelithiasis. |
| choledocholithiasis<br>koh lee doh koh lih THY ih sis | *choledoch/o* common bile duct<br>*lith/o* stones<br>*-iasis* presence of | Presence of stones in the common bile duct. |
| cholelithiasis<br>koh lee lih THY ih sis | *chol/e* gall, bile<br>*lith/o* stones<br>*-iasis* presence of | Presence of stones (**calculi**) in the gallbladder, sometimes characterized by right upper quadrant pain (**biliary colic**) with nausea and vomiting (Fig. 5-16). |

*Continued*

## Terms Related to GI Accessory Organ Disorders—cont'd

| Term | Word Origin | Definition |
|------|-------------|------------|
| **cirrhosis**<br>sur OH sis | *cirrh/o* orange-yellow<br>*-osis* abnormal condition | Chronic degenerative disease of the liver, commonly associated with alcohol abuse, chronic liver disease, and biliary tract disorders (Fig. 5-17). |
| **hepatitis**<br>heh pah TYE tis | *hepat/o* liver<br>*-itis* inflammation | Inflammation of the liver that is caused by an increasing number of viruses, alcohol, and drugs. Currently named by letter, **hepatitis A-G**, the means of viral transmission is not the same for each form. The most common forms, A to C, are discussed below. |
|    hepatitis A | *hepat/o* liver<br>*-itis* inflammation | Virus transmitted through direct contact with fecally contaminated food or water. |
|    hepatitis B | *hepat/o* liver<br>*-itis* inflammation | Virus transmitted through contaminated blood or sexual contact. |
|    hepatitis C | *hepat/o* liver<br>*-itis* inflammation | Virus transmitted through blood transfusion, percutaneous inoculation, or sharing of infected needles. |
| **jaundice**<br>JAHN diss | | Yellowing of the skin and sclerae (whites of the eyes) caused by elevated levels of bilirubin. Also called **icterus**. |
| **pancreatitis**<br>pan kree uh TYE tis | *pancreat/o* pancreas<br>*-itis* inflammation | Inflammation of the pancreas, which may be acute or chronic. |

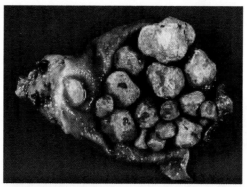

**Fig. 5-16** Cholelithiasis (stones in the gallbladder).

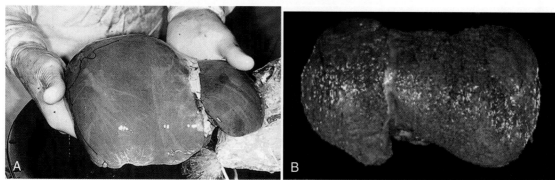

**Fig. 5-17 A,** normal liver. **B,** Cirrhosis of the liver is indicated by nodules on the surface.

Go to the Shiland Evolve site to view an **animation** of cholecystitis.

## Exercise 13: GI Accessory Organ Disorders

*Fill in the blanks using the following terms.*

**pancreatitis, hepatitis, cholangitis, choledocholithiasis, jaundice, cholelithiasis, cirrhosis, cholecystitis**

1. What is a chronic degenerative disorder of the liver, usually caused by alcohol abuse?

   _____

2. What is the term for the presence of stones in the gallbladder? _____

3. What is the term for inflammation of the bile vessels? _____

4. What is the term for the presence of stones in the common bile duct? _____

5. What is the term for an inflammation of the pancreas? _____

6. What is an inflammatory disease of the liver that is named by letter? _____

7. What is the term for an inflammation of the gallbladder? _____

8. Elevated level of bilirubin resulting in yellowing of the skin is termed _____ .

## Terms Related to Hernias

| Term | Word Origin | Definition |
|------|-------------|------------|
| **femoral hernia**<br>FEM uh rull<br>HER nee ah | *femor/o* femur<br>*-al* pertaining to | Protrusion of a loop of intestine through the femoral canal into the groin. Also called a **crural hernia.** |
| **hiatal hernia**<br>hye A tull<br>HER nee ah | *hiat/o* an opening<br>*-al* pertaining to | Protrusion of a portion of the stomach through the diaphragm. Also known as a **diaphragmatic hernia** and **diaphragmatocele** (dye uh frag MAT oh seel) (Fig. 5-18). |
| **incarcerated hernia**<br>in KAR sih ray tid<br>HER nee ah | | Loop of bowel with ends occluded (blocked) so that solids cannot pass; herniated bowel can become strangulated. Also called an **irreducible hernia.** |
| **inguinal hernia**<br>IN gwin null<br>HER nee ah | *inguin/o* groin<br>*-al* pertaining to | Protrusion of a loop of intestine into the inguinal canal. May be **indirect** (through a normal internal passage) or **direct** (through a muscle wall). |
| **strangulation** | | Constriction of a tubular structure, including intestines, leading to impedance of circulation, resulting in a lack of blood supply (ischemia) and possible tissue death. |
| **umbilical hernia**<br>um BILL ih kull<br>HER nee ah | *umbilic/o* umbilicus<br>*-al* pertaining to | Protrusion of the intestine and omentum through a weakness in the abdominal wall (Fig. 5-19). Also known as an **omphalocele** (AHM fah loh seel) |

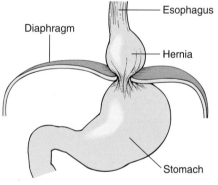

Fig. 5-18 Hiatal hernia.

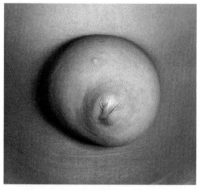

Fig. 5-19 Umbilical hernia.

## Exercise 14: Hernias

*Match the hernias to their definitions.*

____ 1. hiatal hernia      ____ 4. incarcerated hernia

____ 2. umbilical hernia     ____ 5. inguinal hernia

____ 3. strangulation      ____ 6. femoral hernia

A. diaphragmatocele
B. protrusion of part of the intestines and omentum through the abdominal wall
C. irreducible hernia
D. protrusion of intestine in the inguinal canal
E. protrusion of intestine through the femoral canal
F. constriction of a tubular structure

### Terms Related to Benign Neoplasms

| Term | Word Origin | Definition |
|---|---|---|
| **cystadenoma**<br>sist aden OH mah | *cyst/o* bladder, cyst<br>*aden/o* gland<br>*-oma* tumor, mass | Glandular tumors that are filled with cysts, these are the most common benign tumors in the pancreas. |
| **leiomyoma**<br>lye oh mye OH mah | *leiomy/o* smooth muscle<br>*-oma* tumor, mass | Smooth muscle tumor that may occur in the digestive tract. |
| **odontogenic tumor**<br>oh don toh JEN ick | *odont/o* tooth<br>*-genic* pertaining to, produced by | Benign tumors that arise around the teeth and jaw. |
| **polyps, adenomatous or hyperplastic**<br>POLL ups<br>ad eh noh MAH tuss<br>hye per PLASS tick | *aden/o* gland<br>*-oma* tumor<br>*-ous* pertaining to<br>*hyper-* excessive<br>*plas/o* formation, growth<br>*-tic* pertaining to | Adenomatous (growths that arise from glandular tissue, have potential to become malignant) or hyperplastic (generally, small growths that have no tendency to become malignant) tumors occurring throughout the digestive tract. Polyps may be sessile (flat) or pedunculated (having a stalk) (Fig. 5-20). |

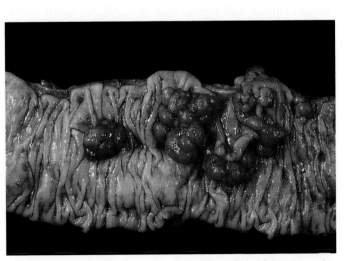

**Fig. 5-20** Multiple adenomatous polyps of the large intestine.

## Terms Related to Malignant Neoplasms

| Term | Word Origin | Definition | |
|---|---|---|---|
| adenocarcinoma<br>ad en noh kar<br>seh NOH mah | *aden/o* gland<br>*-carcinoma* cancerous tumor of epithelial origin | A malignant tumor of epithelial origin that either originates from glandular tissue or has a glandular appearance. | Adenocarcinomas occur throughout the gastrointestinal tract, but especially in the esophagus, stomach, pancreas, and colon. |
| hepatocellular carcinoma/ hepatoma<br>heh pat oh SELL you lur<br>kar seh NOH mah<br>heh puh TOH mah | *hepat/o* liver<br>*cellul/o* cell<br>*-ar* pertaining to | Malignant tumors of epithelial origin that originate in the liver cells. | Hepatocellular carcinoma (also called hepatoma) is the most common type of primary liver cancer worldwide. |
| squamous cell carcinoma<br>SKWAY muss | *squam/o* scaly<br>*-ous* pertaining to | Cancers that have a scalelike appearance. | Squamous cell carcinomas arise from the cells that cover the surfaces of the body. These occur throughout the digestive system. |

*Please note:* Metastatic carcinoma is the most common form of liver cancer. The liver is the most common site of all metastases. This is not a primary tumor, but one that has spread from another site.

## Exercise 15: Neoplasms

*Fill in the blank.*

1. What type of benign growth is described as either sessile or pedunculated? _____

2. What is the most common type of primary liver cancer? _____

3. Which type of cancer occurs throughout the GI tract, but especially in the esophagus, stomach, pancreas, and colon? _____

4. What is the term for a benign tumor that arises from around the teeth and jaw?

_____

## Age Matters

### Pediatrics

GI congential disorders are cleft palate, esophageal atresia, Hirschsprung disease, and pyloric stenosis. Although none of these are common, they do require medical intervention. Gastroenteritis and appendicitis—with their possible complications, respectively, of dehydration and peritonitis—are the most common reasons for hospital admissions of children.

### Geriatrics

An aging digestive system is more likely to develop new dysfunctional cell growths (both benign and malignant), so statistics for polyps and colorectal cancer are high for the senior age group. Other diagnoses that appear more often are GERD and dysphagia, hemorrhoids, and type 2 diabetes mellitus.

To practice spelling the pathology terms that you have learned in this chapter. click on **Hear It, Spell It.** To see how well you pronounce the pathology terms in this chapter, click on **Hear It, Say It.** To review the pathology terms in this chapter, play **Medical Millionaire.**

## DIAGNOSTIC PROCEDURES

### Terms Related to Imaging

Visualizing the internal workings of the digestive system can be achieved through a wide variety of techniques but is usually accomplished through either radiographic imaging or endoscopy, or a combination of the two. Most of the procedures below are a form of radiography, or "taking x-rays." However, because the tissues of the digestive system are soft (as opposed to bone), a radiopaque contrast medium may be necessary to outline the digestive tract. This substance may be introduced into the body through the oral or anal opening, or it may be injected. Fluoroscopy provides instant visual access to deep tissue structures.

| Term | Word Origin | Definition |
|---|---|---|
| **barium enema (BE)**<br>BAIR ee um<br>EN nuh mah | | Introduction of a barium sulfate suspension through the rectum for imaging of the lower digestive tract to detect obstructions, tumors, and other abnormalities. |
| **barium swallow (BaS)** | | Radiographic imaging done after oral ingestion of a barium sulfate suspension; used to detect abnormalities of the esophagus and stomach (Fig. 5-21). |

*Continued*

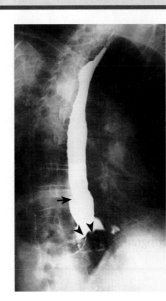

Fig. 5-21 Barium swallow.

## Terms Related to Therapeutic Interventions—cont'd

| Term | Word Origin | Definition |
|------|-------------|------------|
| colostomy<br>koh LOSS tuh mee | *col/o* colon<br>*-stomy* new opening | Surgical redirection of the bowel to a **stoma** (STOH mah), an artificial opening on the abdominal wall (Fig. 5-26). |
| enema<br>EH nih mah | | Method of introducing a solution into the rectum for therapeutic (relief of constipation) or hygienic (preparation for surgery) reasons. |
| feeding tubes | | **Enteral nutrition**—introduced through a digestive structure (Fig. 5-27). **Parenteral nutrition**—introduced through a structure outside of the alimentary canal, usually by IV. |
| gastrectomy<br>gass TRECK tuh mee | *gastr/o* stomach<br>*-ectomy* removal | Surgical removal of all or part of the stomach. |
| gastric gavage<br>gah VAHZH | | Feeding through a tube in the stomach. |
| hemorrhoidectomy<br>heh moh roy DECK tuh mee | *hemorrhoid/o* hemorrhoid<br>*-ectomy* removal | Surgical excision of hemorrhoids. |
| herniorrhaphy<br>hur nee OR rah fee | *herni/o* hernia<br>*-rrhaphy* suture | Hernia repair; suture of a hernia. |
| hyperalimentation<br>hye pur al ih men TAY shun | *hyper-* excessive<br>*aliment/o* nutrition<br>*-ation* process of | The therapeutic use of nutritional supplements that exceed recommended daily requirements. |
| laparoscopic surgery<br>lap uh roh SCAH pick | *lapar/o* abdomen<br>*-scopic* pertaining to viewing | Surgery done through several small incisions in the abdominal wall with the aid of an instrument called a **laparoscope**. A **laparoscopic cholecystectomy** is the removal of the gallbladder (see Fig. 5-25). |

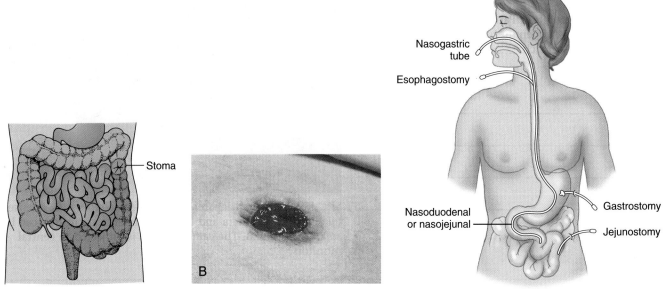

Fig. 5-26 **A,** Colostomy. **B,** Stoma.

Fig. 5-27 Common placement locations for enteral feeding tubes.

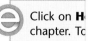

Exerc

*Match the th*

____  1. rer

____  2. su

____  3. joi

____  4. int
        rec
        pu

____  5. tyi

____  6. de

____  7. ins
        sto

____  8. art

A. anastom
B. paracent
C. laparosc
D. hemorrh
E. laparoto

*Decode the f*

16. pylorom

17. coloston

18. herniorr

19. gastrect

20. polypect

Click on **H**
chapter. To

| Terms Related to Therapeutic Interventions—cont'd | | |
|---|---|---|
| **Term** | **Word Origin** | **Definition** |
| **laparotomy**<br>lap uh RAH tuh mee | *lapar/o* abdomen<br>*-tomy* incision | Any surgical incision in the abdominal wall for the purpose of an operative approach or for exploratory purposes. |
| **ligation**<br>lye GAY shun | *ligat/o* tying<br>*-tion* the process of | Tying off of a blood vessel or duct (e.g., the cystic duct is ligated when the gallbladder is removed during a cholecystectomy). |
| **lysis of adhesions**<br>LYE sis | *lys/o* breakdown<br>*-is* noun ending | Surgical destruction of adhesions (scar tissue that binds two anatomic surfaces) (e.g., in the peritoneal cavity). |
| **nasogastric intubation**<br>nay soh GASS trick<br>in too BAY shun | *nas/o* nose<br>*gastr/o* stomach<br>*-ic* pertaining to | Placement of a tube from the nose, down the back of the throat, then into the stomach, for the purpose of enteral feeding or removing gastric contents. May be termed an NG tube. |
| **odontectomy**<br>oh don TECK tuh mee | *odont/o* teeth<br>*-ectomy* removal | Surgical excision of a tooth. |
| **paracentesis**<br>pair ah sen TEE sis | *para-* near, beside<br>*-centesis* surgical puncture | Procedure for withdrawing fluid from a body cavity, most commonly to remove fluid accumulated in the abdominal cavity. |
| **percutaneous endoscopic gastrostomy (PEG)**<br>pur kew TAY nee us<br>en doh SKOP ick<br>gass TROSS tuh mee | *per-* through<br>*cutane/o* skin<br>*-ous* pertaining to<br>*endo-* within<br>*-scopic* pertaining to viewing<br>*gastr/o* stomach<br>*-stomy* new opening | A new opening of the stomach through the skin that allows the surgeon to place a tube for the purpose of enteral feeding. |

*Continued*

Terr
Terr
poly
poll it

pylo
pye l

stom
STOH

troca
TROH

**antiemetic**
anti- = against
-emetic = pertaining
to vomiting

## PHARMACOLOGY

**anorexiants** (an nor RECK see unts): appetite suppressants designed to aid in weight control, often in an attempt to treat **morbid obesity** (an amount of body fat that threatens normal health). Examples of anorexiants are sibutramine (Meridia) and phentermine (Adipex-P).

**antacids:** a buffer (neutralizer) of hydrochloric acid in the stomach to temporarily relieve symptoms of GERD, pyrosis, and ulcers. Examples include calcium carbonate (Tums, Rolaids) and aluminum hydroxide with magnesium hydroxide (Maalox).

**antidiarrheals:** provide relief from diarrhea by reducing intestinal motility, inflammation, or loss of fluids and nutrients. Examples include loperamide (Imodium), bismuth subsalicylate (Pepto Bismol), and diphenoxylate with atropine (Lomotil).

**antiemetics:** prevent or alleviate nausea and vomiting. Examples include scopolamine (Scopace), ondansetron (Zofran), and promethazine (Phenergan).

**cathartics** (kuh THAR ticks): cause evacuation of the bowel by stimulating peristalsis, increasing the fluidity or bulk of intestinal contents, softening the feces, or lubricating the intestine. Cathartics can be classified as either mild (laxatives) or severe (purgatives). Senna (Sennacot) and mineral oil (Fleet Enema) are commonly used purgatives.

**histamine-2 receptor antagonists (H2RAs):** prevent a portion of the hydrochloric acid production in the stomach for moderate-lasting acid suppression. Examples include famotidine (Pepcid) and ranitidine (Zantac).

**laxatives:** cause mild evacuation of the bowel by increasing the bulk of the feces, softening the stool, or lubricating the intestinal wall. Examples include fiber, docusate (Colace), and bisacodyl (Dulcolax).

**proton pump inhibitors:** block production of hydrochloric acid in the stomach for long-lasting acid suppression of disorders like GERD. Examples include omeprazole (Prilosec) and pantoprazole (Protonix).

### Exercise 19: Pharmacology

*Match each disorder with the type of drug that is used to treat it.*

____ 1. nausea and vomiting     ____ 4. excessive weight gain     A. laxative
                                                                  B. antidiarrheal
____ 2. chronic GERD            ____ 5. constipation               C. proton pump inhibitor
                                                                  D. antacid
____ 3. short-term dyspepsia    ____ 6. intestinal cramping        E. antiemetic
                                        and loose, watery stools   F. anorexiant

## Abbreviations

| Abbreviation | Definition | Abbreviation | Definition |
|---|---|---|---|
| BaS | barium swallow | HBV | hepatitis B virus |
| BE | barium enema | IBD | inflammatory bowel disease |
| BM | bowel movement | IBS | irritable bowel syndrome |
| CT scan | computed tomography scan | Lap | laparoscopy, laparotomy |
| EGD | esophagogastroduodenoscopy | LES | lower esophageal sphincter |
| ERCP | endoscopic retrograde cholangiopancreatography | N&V | nausea and vomiting |
| GB | gallbladder | PEG | percutaneous endoscopic gastrostomy |
| GERD | gastroesophageal reflux disease | PTC, PTCA | percutaneous transhepatic cholangiography |
| GGT | gamma-glutamyl transferase | | |
| GI | gastrointestinal | PUD | peptic ulcer disease |
| HAV | hepatitis A virus | | |

## Exercise 20: Abbreviations

*Spell out the abbreviations used in the following examples.*

1. The 76-year-old patient complained of no BM in the last week. He had not had a/an

   _____ .

2. The patient was admitted for suspected GB disease. _____

3. The nurse recorded the patient's symptoms as N&V, without a fever.

   _____

4. Constant heartburn for Phyllis may have been a result of GERD. _____

5. Stressful situations were made even more so for Bill when his IBS flared up.

   _____

# Chapter Review

*Match the word parts to their definitions.*

## WORD PART DEFINITIONS

| Suffix | | Definition |
|--------|---|------------|
| -chezia | | 1. _____ flow, discharge |
| -emesis | | 2. _____ process of viewing |
| -pepsia | | 3. _____ condition of an opening |
| -phagia | | 4. _____ new opening |
| -rrhaphy | | 5. _____ suture, repair |
| -rrhea | | 6. _____ vomiting |
| -scopy | | 7. _____ condition of stools |
| -stalsis | | 8. _____ condition of eating, swallowing |
| -stomy | | 9. _____ contraction |
| -tresia | | 10. _____ digestion condition |

| Combining Form | | Definition |
|----------------|---|------------|
| an/o | | 11. _____ tongue |
| bucc/o | | 12. _____ gums |
| cholangi/o | | 13. _____ groin |
| cholecyst/o | | 14. _____ diaphragm |
| choledoch/o | | 15. _____ esophagus |
| col/o | | 16. _____ saliva |
| enter/o | | 17. _____ bile vessel |
| esophag/o | | 18. _____ common bile duct |
| gastr/o | | 19. _____ mouth |
| gingiv/o | | 20. _____ pus |
| inguin/o | | 21. _____ stomach |
| hepat/o | | 22. _____ rectum and anus |
| labi/o | | 23. _____ lips |
| lingu/o | | 24. _____ liver |
| lumin/o | | 25. _____ cheek |
| odont/o | | 26. _____ tooth |
| pharyng/o | | 27. _____ anus |
| phren/o | | 28. _____ gallbladder |
| proct/o | | 29. _____ throat |
| py/o | | 30. _____ lumen |
| sial/o | | 31. _____ large intestine |
| stomat/o | | 32. _____ small intestines |

# WORDSHOP

| Prefixes | Combining Forms | Suffixes |
|---|---|---|
| a- | cheil/o | -al |
| an- | chol/e | -eal |
| dys- | cholecyst/o | -ectomy |
| peri- | choledoch/o | -ia |
| pre- | col/o | -iasis |
| syn- | esophag/o | -ic |
| trans- | gastr/o | -itis |
|  | hepat/o | -pepsia |
|  | lapar/o | -phagia |
|  | lith/o | -plasty |
|  | nas/o | -rrhea |
|  | odont/o | -stomy |
|  | py/o | -tomy |
|  | stomat/o | -tresia |

*Build the following terms by combining the word parts above. Some word parts may be used more than once. Some won't be used at all. The number in parentheses indicates the number of word parts needed to build the term.*

| Definition | Term |
|---|---|
| 1. pertaining to the stomach and esophagus (3) | |
| 2. condition of no opening (2) | |
| 3. pertaining to surrounding the teeth (3) | |
| 4. pertaining to the nose and stomach (3) | |
| 5. new opening of the colon (2) | |
| 6. inflammation of the gallbladder (2) | |
| 7. new opening between the stomach and esophagus (3) | |
| 8. removal of the gallbladder (2) | |
| 9. discharge of pus (2) | |
| 10. condition of difficult/painful swallowing (2) | |
| 11. condition of bad digestion (2) | |
| 12. condition of gallstones (3) | |
| 13. condition of stones in the common bile duct (3) | |
| 14. incision of the abdomen (2) | |
| 15. surgical repair of the mouth (2) | |

Sort the terms below into their correct categories.

## TERM SORTING

| Anatomy and Physiology | Pathology | Diagnostic Procedures | Therapeutic Interventions |
|---|---|---|---|
| | | | |
| | | | |
| | | | |
| | | | |
| | | | |
| | | | |
| | | | |
| | | | |
| | | | |
| | | | |

achalasia

anastomosis

barium enema

BaS

cheilitis

cholecystectomy

cholecystography

cholecystokinin

colostomy

CT scan

cystadenoma

deglutition

dyspepsia

ERCP

esophagus

gastric gavage

GGT

halitosis

hematemesis

hematochezia

herniorrhaphy

jaundice

jejunum

laparotomy

LES

leukoplakia

ligation

lipid

manometry

mastication

oropharynx

paracentesis

PEG

peristalsis

PTCA

pyrosis

rugae

stomatoplasty

stool guaiac

total bilirubin

*Replace the highlighted words with the correct terms.*

## TRANSLATIONS

1. After having a **viewing of the large intestine,** the patient needed a **removal of a polyp.**

2. The patient was tested for **an inflammation of the liver** due to a **yellowing of the skin and sclerae.**

3. The patient's **protrusion of a loop of the intestine into the inguinal canal** was corrected with **a suture (repair) of the hernia.**

4. The patient's **impairment of esophageal peristalsis** was diagnosed through the use of a **measurement of pressure.**

5. A **fecal exam to detect hidden blood** was used to determine if the patient had bleeding in his gastrointestinal tract.

6. The patient underwent a **tying off of a blood vessel or duct** during his **surgical removal of the gallbladder.**

7. Ross underwent **surgical redirection of the bowel to a stoma** when his **inflammation of the ileum or the colon that is of idiopathic origin** became too severe.

8. Miriam took **a mild medication that causes evacuation of the bowel** when she had **infrequent, incomplete, or delayed bowel movements.**

9. The patient had **gas expelled through the anus** and **an abnormal discharge of watery, semisolid stools.**

10. Delay in treating the patient's **inflammation of the appendix** led to a nearly fatal case of **inflammation of the peritoneum.**

11. The dentist told Ava she had **inflammatory disease of the gums** and **a condition in which the teeth do not touch properly when the mouth is closed.**

12. The infant was born with a **failure of the palate to close during embryonic development.** Her twin was born with **congenital absence of normal nervous function in part of the colon.**

13. The newborn experienced **return of swallowed food to the mouth** of his formula because of **esophagus that ends in a blind pouch.**

14. **Bright red, frank lower GI bleeding from the rectum** was one of the symptoms of Frank's **varicose vein in the lower rectum.**

# *Case Study*  Mariah Hopkins

For the past 2 weeks, every time Mariah Hopkins has eaten a heavy meal, she has had upper right quadrant (RUQ) pain and occasional nausea and vomiting. The pain would last for a couple of hours and then subside. However, after a night of unremitting pain, Mariah can stand it no longer and calls her physician. He does a quick examination at his office and, suspecting cholelithiasis, sends her to the local hospital for immediate testing and admission. Elena Sanchez, one of the medical-surgical nurses on the floor that afternoon, helps Mariah get settled for her admission and notices that the patient's skin has a yellowish hue.

When the laboratory results are reported, Mariah's white blood cell count and serum

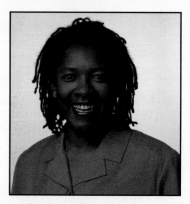

bilirubin are both well above normal limits. An oral cholecystography and sonography both indicate that she indeed has cholelithiasis. Mariah is prepped for laparoscopic surgery.

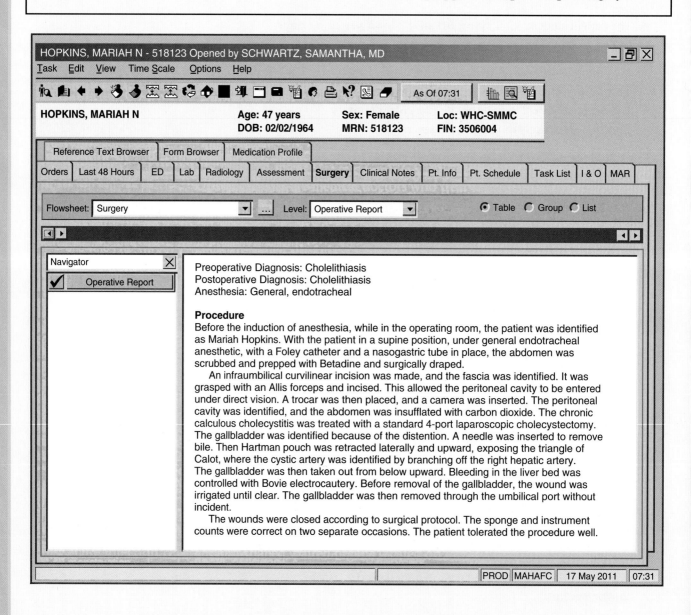

HOPKINS, MARIAH N - 518123 Opened by SCHWARTZ, SAMANTHA, MD

Task   Edit   View   Time Scale   Options   Help

| HOPKINS, MARIAH N | Age: 47 years | Sex: Female | Loc: WHC-SMMC |
| | DOB: 02/02/1964 | MRN: 518123 | FIN: 3506004 |

Reference Text Browser | Form Browser | Medication Profile

Orders | Last 48 Hours | ED | Lab | Radiology | Assessment | **Surgery** | Clinical Notes | Pt. Info | Pt. Schedule | Task List | I & O | MAR

Flowsheet: Surgery ▼ ...   Level: Operative Report ▼    ⦿ Table ○ Group ○ List

Navigator ☒

✓ Operative Report

Preoperative Diagnosis: Cholelithiasis
Postoperative Diagnosis: Cholelithiasis
Anesthesia: General, endotracheal

**Procedure**
Before the induction of anesthesia, while in the operating room, the patient was identified as Mariah Hopkins. With the patient in a supine position, under general endotracheal anesthetic, with a Foley catheter and a nasogastric tube in place, the abdomen was scrubbed and prepped with Betadine and surgically draped.

An infraumbilical curvilinear incision was made, and the fascia was identified. It was grasped with an Allis forceps and incised. This allowed the peritoneal cavity to be entered under direct vision. A trocar was then placed, and a camera was inserted. The peritoneal cavity was identified, and the abdomen was insufflated with carbon dioxide. The chronic calculous cholecystitis was treated with a standard 4-port laparoscopic cholecystectomy. The gallbladder was identified because of the distention. A needle was inserted to remove bile. Then Hartman pouch was retracted laterally and upward, exposing the triangle of Calot, where the cystic artery was identified by branching off the right hepatic artery. The gallbladder was then taken out from below upward. Bleeding in the liver bed was controlled with Bovie electrocautery. Before removal of the gallbladder, the wound was irrigated until clear. The gallbladder was then removed through the umbilical port without incident.

The wounds were closed according to surgical protocol. The sponge and instrument counts were correct on two separate occasions. The patient tolerated the procedure well.

PROD  MAHAFC   17 May 2011   07:31

## Operative Report

1. How do you know that Ms. Hopkins has gallstones? _____ .

2. Which term tells you that her gallbladder was inflamed? _____ .

3. Her gallbladder was removed through an endoscopic procedure called a/an _____ .

4. To say that the patient was in a supine position means that she was lying on her _____ .

5. To ligate a structure means to _____ .

For more interactive learning, click on:
- **Whack a Word Part** to review gastrointestinal word parts.
- **Wheel of Terminology** and **Word Shop** to practice word building.
- **Tournament of Terminology** to test your knowledge of gastrointestinal terms.
- **Terminology Triage** to practice sorting gastrointestinal terms into categories.

# 6

*What is man, when you come to think about him, but a minutely set, ingenious machine for turning, with infinite artfulness, the red wine of Shiraz into urine?*
—**Isak Dinesen**

## OBJECTIVES

- Recognize and use terms related to the anatomy and physiology of the urinary system.
- Recognize and use terms related to the pathology of the urinary system.
- Recognize and use terms related to the diagnostic procedures for the urinary system.
- Recognize and use terms related to the therapeutic interventions for the urinary system.

# Urinary System

## CHAPTER AT A GLANCE

*Use this list of key word parts and terms to assess your knowledge. Check off the ones you have mastered.*

### ANATOMY AND PHYSIOLOGY

- ☐ bladder
- ☐ hilum
- ☐ kidneys
- ☐ micturition
- ☐ nephron
- ☐ renal pelvis
- ☐ trigone
- ☐ ureters
- ☐ urethra
- ☐ urinary meatus
- ☐ urination
- ☐ voiding

### KEY WORD PARTS

#### PREFIXES
- ☐ an-
- ☐ di-
- ☐ dys-
- ☐ poly-
- ☐ re-

#### SUFFIXES
- ☐ -cele
- ☐ -dipsia
- ☐ -flux
- ☐ -graphy
- ☐ -lithotomy
- ☐ -lysis
- ☐ -pexy
- ☐ -ptosis
- ☐ -scope
- ☐ -scopy
- ☐ -tomy
- ☐ -tripsy
- ☐ -uria

#### COMBINING FORMS
- ☐ azot/o
- ☐ cyst/o
- ☐ gluc/o, glycos/o
- ☐ lith/o
- ☐ meat/o
- ☐ nephr/o
- ☐ pyel/o
- ☐ ren/o
- ☐ trigon/o
- ☐ ureter/o
- ☐ urethr/o
- ☐ urin/o, ur/o
- ☐ vesic/o

### KEY TERMS

- ☐ anuria
- ☐ catheter
- ☐ cystocele
- ☐ cystoscope
- ☐ diabetes insipidus (DI)
- ☐ diabetes mellitus (DM)
- ☐ dysuria
- ☐ glycosuria
- ☐ incontinence (urinary)
- ☐ lithotripsy
- ☐ meatotomy
- ☐ nephrolithotomy
- ☐ nephropexy
- ☐ nephroptosis
- ☐ polydipsia
- ☐ polyuria
- ☐ pyelonephritis
- ☐ retention (urinary)
- ☐ urethral stenosis
- ☐ urgency
- ☐ urinalysis
- ☐ vesicoureteral reflux
- ☐ voiding cystourethrography (VCUG)

**extracellular**
  extra = outside
  cellul/o = cell
  -ar = pertaining to

**urination**
  urin/o = urine, urinary
    system
  -ation = process of

## ⊗ Be Careful!

*-uria is a suffix that
means urinary condition;
**urea** is a chemical waste
product.*

**urology**
  ur/o = urine, urinary
    system
  -logy = study of

## ⊗ Be Careful!

*Don't confuse **ureters**
with the **urethra**.*

**kidney** = nephr/o, ren/o

**parenchymal**
  par- = near
  en- = in
  chym/o = juices
  -al = pertaining to

**ureter** = ureter/o

**bladder** = cyst/o, vesic/o

**urethra** = urethr/o

**meatus** = meat/o

**trigone** = trigon/o

**stromal tissue** = strom/o

**retroperitoneal**
  retro- = backward
  peritone/o = peritoneum
  -al = pertaining to

**cortex** = cortic/o

**medulla** = medull/o

**renal pelvis** = pyel/o

**renal calyx** = calic/o,
cali/o, calyc/o

## FUNCTIONS OF THE URINARY SYSTEM

The major function of the urinary system is to continually maintain a healthy balance of the amount and content of **extracellular fluids** within the body. Biologists use the term *homeostasis* to describe this important process. The process of metabolism changes food and liquid (with its requisite fats, carbohydrates, and proteins) into building blocks, energy sources, and waste products. To operate efficiently, the body constantly needs to monitor and rebalance the amounts of these substances in the bloodstream. The breakdown of proteins and amino acids in the liver leaves chemical wastes, such as urea, creatinine, and uric acid, in the bloodstream. These wastes are toxic nitrogenous substances that must be excreted in the urine. The act of releasing urine is called **urination, voiding,** or **micturition** (mick ter RIH shun).

Succinctly phrased by Homer William Smith in 1939, "It is no exaggeration to say that the composition of the blood is determined not by what the mouth ingests but by what the kidneys keep; they are the master chemists of our internal environment, which, so to speak, they synthesize in reverse."

## SPECIALTIES/SPECIALISTS

The medical specialist for the diagnosis, treatment, and study of urinary disorders in both sexes is called a **urologist.** Urologists also treat most disorders of the male reproductive system. The specialty is referred to as **urology.**

## ANATOMY AND PHYSIOLOGY

The urinary system is composed of two kidneys, two ureters, a urinary bladder, and a urethra (Figs. 6-1 and 6-2). The work of the urinary system is done by a specialized tissue in the **kidneys** called **parenchymal** (pair EN kuh mul) **tissue.** The kidneys function to filter the blood and eliminate waste through the passage of urine. The **ureters** (YOOR eh turs) are thin, muscular tubes that move urine in peristaltic waves from the kidneys to the bladder. The urinary **bladder** is the sac that stores the urine until it is excreted. The bladder is lined with an epithelial mucous membrane of transitional cells. Underneath, a layer termed the *lamina propria* is composed of connective tissue that holds the blood vessels and nerves. The detrusor muscle is the final coat; it normally contracts to expel urine. The **urethra** (yoo REE thrah) is the tube that conducts the urine out of the bladder. The opening of the urethra is called the **urinary meatus** (YOOR in nair ee mee ATE us). The triangular area in the bladder between the ureters' entrance and the urethral outlet is called the **trigone** (TRY gohn). The ureters, bladder, and urethra are all **stromal** (STROH mul) **tissue,** which is a supportive tissue.

### The Kidney

Because the kidneys are primarily responsible for the functioning of the urinary system, it is helpful to look at them in greater detail. Each of the two kidneys is located high in the abdominal cavity, tucked under the ribs in the back and behind the lining of the abdominal cavity **(retroperitoneal).** The normal human kidney is about the size of a fist. If a kidney were sliced open, the outer portion, the **cortex** (KORE tecks) (*pl.* cortices), and the inner portion, called the **medulla** (muh DOO lah) (*pl.* medullae), would be visible (Fig. 6-3). The **renal pelvis** and **calyces** (KAL ih seez) (*sing.* calyx) are an extension of the ureter inside of the kidney. The term **renal** means *pertaining to the kidneys.*

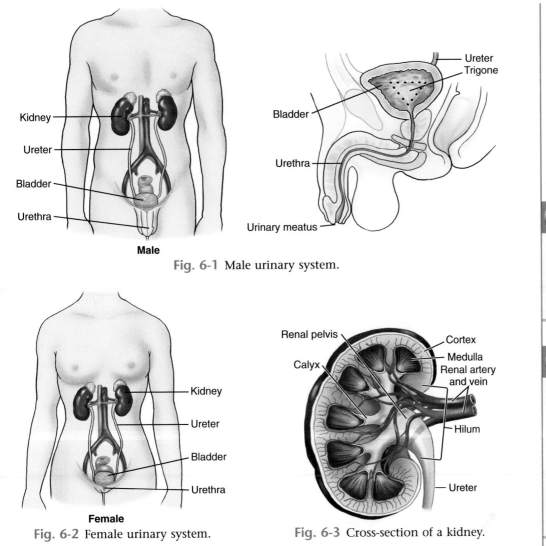

**Fig. 6-1** Male urinary system.

**Fig. 6-2** Female urinary system.

**Fig. 6-3** Cross-section of a kidney.

⊗ **Be Careful!**

Calic/o, calyc/o and cali/o are the combining forms for calyx, but calc/o is the combining form for calcium.

⊗ **Be Careful!**

It is easy to confuse the combining forms **perone/o**, which means fibula; **perine/o**, which means the space between external genitalia and the anus; and **peritone/o**, which means the abdominal lining.

hilum = hil/o

artery = arteri/o

glomerulus = glomerul/o

The **hilum** (HYE lum) (*pl.* hila) is the location on the kidney where the ureter and renal vein leave the kidney and the renal artery enters. The cortex contains tissue with millions of microscopic units called **nephrons** (NEFF rons) (Fig. 6-4). Here in the tiny nephrons, blood passes through a continuous system of urinary filtration, reabsorption, and secretion that measures, monitors, and adjusts the levels of substances in the extracellular fluid.

### The Nephron

The nephrons filter all of the blood in the body approximately every 5 minutes. The **renal afferent arteries** transport unfiltered blood to the kidneys. Once in the kidneys, the blood travels through small arteries called **arterioles** (ar TEER ree ohls) and finally into tiny balls of renal capillaries, called **glomeruli** (gloh MER yoo lye) (*sing.* glomerulus). These glomeruli cluster at the entrance to each nephron. It is here that the process of filtering the blood to form urine begins.

The nephron consists of four parts: (1) the **renal corpuscle** (KORE pus sul), which is composed of the glomerulus and its surrounding Bowman's capsule; (2) a **proximal convoluted tubule;** (3) the **nephronic loop,** also known as the loop of Henle; and (4) the **distal convoluted tubule.** As blood flows through the capillaries, water, electrolytes, glucose, and nitrogenous wastes are passed through the glomerular membrane and collected. The most common electrolytes are sodium (Na), chloride (Cl), and potassium (K). Blood cells and

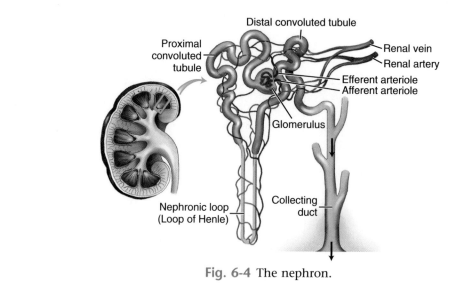

Fig. 6-4 The nephron.

**urine** = ur/o, urin/o

proteins are too large to pass through the glomerular membrane. Selective filtration and reabsorption continue along the renal tubules, with the end result of **urine** concentration and subsequent dilution occurring in the renal medulla. From there, the urine flows to the calyces and exits the kidney, flowing through the ureter into the bladder, where it is stored until it can be expelled from the body through the urethra.

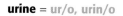 ## Exercise 1: **The Urinary System**

*Match the combining form with its term.*

____  1. opening of the urethra

____  2. tubes connecting kidneys
       and bladder

____  3. tube conducting urine out
       of the bladder

____  4. same as ren/o

____  5. sac that stores urine

____  6. area between ureters coming
       in and urethra going out in
       the sac that stores urine

____  7. urine, urinary system

____  8. renal pelvis

____  9. outer portion of the kidney

____ 10. inner portion of the kidney

____ 11. artery

____ 12. renal calyx

____ 13. location where ureter and
       renal vein leave kidney and
       renal artery enters

A. nephr/o
B. ur/o, urin/o
C. meat/o
D. urethr/o
E. cyst/o, vesic/o
F. ureter/o
G. trigon/o
H. medull/o
I. calic/o, cali/o, calyc/o
J. cortic/o
K. hil/o
L. pyel/o
M. arteri/o

*Decode the terms.*

14. transurethral _____

15. paranephric _____

16. retroperitoneal _____

17. suprarenal _____

18. perivesical _____

## Combining and Adjective Forms for the Anatomy of the Urinary System

| Meaning | Combining Form | Adjective Form |
|---|---|---|
| artery | arteri/o | arterial |
| bladder | cyst/o, vesic/o | cystic, vesical |
| calyx | calic/o, cali/o, calyc/o | caliceal, calyceal |
| cell | cellul/o | cellular |
| cortex | cortic/o | cortical |
| glomerulus | glomerul/o | glomerular |
| hilum | hil/o | hilar |
| kidney | nephr/o, ren/o | nephric, renal |
| medulla | medull/o | medullary |
| parenchyma | parenchym/o | parenchymal |
| peritoneum | peritone/o | peritoneal |
| renal pelvis | pyel/o | |
| stroma | strom/o | stromal |
| trigone | trigon/o | trigonal |
| ureter | ureter/o | ureteral |
| urethra | urethr/o | urethral |
| urinary meatus | meat/o | meatal |
| urine, urinary system | urin/o, ur/o | urinary |

## Prefixes for the Anatomy of the Urinary System

| Prefix | Meaning |
|---|---|
| extra- | outside |
| en- | in |
| par- | beside, near |
| retro- | backward |

## Suffixes for the Anatomy of the Urinary System

| Suffix | Meaning |
|---|---|
| -al, -ar, -ic | pertaining to |
| -ation, -ion | process of |

You can review the anatomy of the urinary system by clicking on **Body Spectrum Electronic Anatomy Coloring Book → Urinary Tract.** Click on **Hear It, Spell It** to practice spelling the anatomy and physiology terms you have learned in this chapter. Practice pronouncing anatomy and physiology terms by clicking on **Hear It, Say It.**

## Exercise 2: The Urinary System

*Label the urinary system drawings below with the correct anatomy and combining forms where appropriate.*

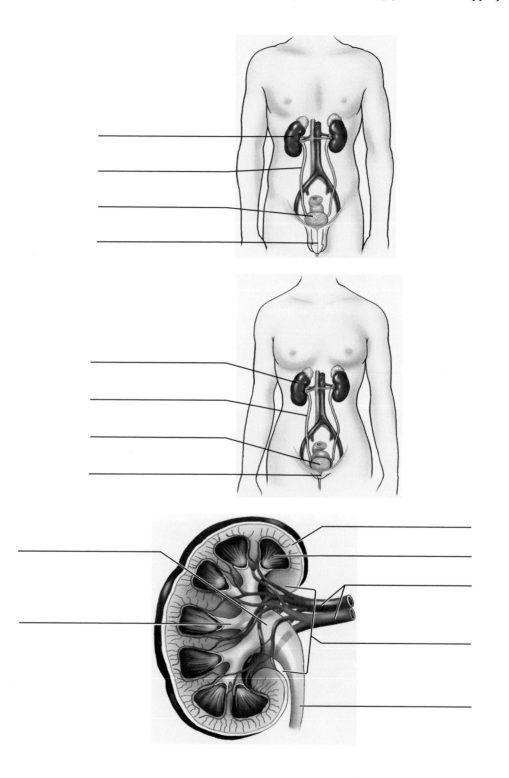

## PATHOLOGY

### Terms Related to Urinary Signs

| Term | Word Origin | Definition |
|------|-------------|------------|
| **abscess, urinary**<br>AB ses | | Cavity containing pus and surrounded by inflamed tissue in the urinary system. |
| **albuminuria**<br>al byoo mih NOOR ee ah | *albumin/o* protein<br>*-uria* urinary condition | Albumin (a protein) in the urine. Also called **proteinuria** (pro teen NOOR ee ah). |
| **azotemia**<br>a zoh TEE mee ah | *azot/o* nitrogen<br>*-emia* blood condition | Condition of excessive urea in the blood indicating nonfunctioning kidneys; also called **uremia**. |
| **azoturia**<br>a zoh TOOR ee ah | *azot/o* nitrogen<br>*-uria* urinary condition | Excessive nitrogenous compounds, including urea, in the urine. |
| **bacteriuria**<br>back tur ee YOOR ee ah | *bacteri/o* bacteria<br>*-uria* urinary condition | Bacteria in the urine. |
| **edema**<br>eh DEE mah | | Accumulation of fluid in the tissues; can result from kidney failure. |
| **glycosuria**<br>gly kohs YOOR ee ah | *glycos/o* sugar, glucose<br>*-uria* urinary condition | Sugar in the urine. |
| **hematuria**<br>hee mah TOOR ee ah | *hemat/o* blood<br>*-uria* urinary condition | Blood in the urine. |
| **hypertension**<br>hye pur TEN shun | *hyper-* excessive<br>*tens/o* stretching<br>*-ion* process of | Condition of high blood pressure. |
| **pyuria**<br>pye YOOR ee ah | *py/o* pus<br>*-uria* urinary condition | Pus in the urine. |

### Terms Related to Urinary Symptoms

| Term | Word Origin | Definition |
|------|-------------|------------|
| **anuria**<br>a NOOR ee ah | *an-* without<br>*-uria* urinary condition | Condition of no urine. |
| **diuresis**<br>dye yoor EE sis | *di-* through, complete<br>*ur/o* urine<br>*-esis* state of | Condition of increased formation and excretion of urine, of large volumes of urine. Caffeine and alcohol are diuretics (dye yoor RET icks)—that is, they increase the amount of urine produced. |
| **dysuria**<br>dis YOOR ee ah | *dys-* painful, abnormal<br>*-uria* urinary condition | Condition of painful urination. |
| **enuresis**<br>en yoor EE sis | *en-* in<br>*ur/o* urine<br>*-esis* state of | Also commonly known as "bed-wetting," enuresis can be nocturnal (at night) or diurnal (during the day). |

*Continued*

## Terms Related to Urinary Symptoms—cont'd

| Term | Word Origin | Definition |
|------|-------------|------------|
| incontinence, urinary<br>in KON tih nense | | Inability to hold urine. |
| nocturia<br>nock TOOR ee ah | *noct/i* night<br>*-uria* urinary condition | Condition of excessive urination at night. |
| oliguria<br>ah lig GYOOR ee ah | *olig/o* scanty, few<br>*-uria* urinary condition | Condition of scanty urination. |
| polydipsia<br>pah lee DIP see ah | *poly-* excessive, frequent<br>*-dipsia* condition of thirst | Condition of excessive thirst (usually accompanied by polyuria). |
| polyuria<br>pah lee YOOR ee ah | *poly-* excessive, frequent<br>*-uria* urinary condition | Condition of excessive urination. |
| retention, urinary | | Inability to release urine. |
| urgency | | Intense sensation of the need to urinate immediately. |

### Exercise 3: Urinary Signs and Symptoms

*Fill in the blank.*

1. Urinary _____ is the inability to release urine.

2. If a patient complains of an accumulation of fluid around her ankles, she may be exhibiting

    _____.

3. A patient with a renal _____ has a cavity containing pus and surrounded by inflamed tissue in the kidneys.

4. A sign of kidney failure may be excessive urea in the blood, called _____.

5. A concerned parent calls in to discuss her 4-year-old son's inability to remain dry during the night.

    This bed-wetting may be diagnosed as _____.

6. Caffeine and alcohol are substances that cause an increase in the volume of fluids excreted from the

    body, causing _____.

7. A feeling of a need to urinate immediately is called _____.

8. The elderly gentleman was seen by his physician because he was unable to control his urination. He

    was suffering from urinary _____.

*Build the terms.*

9. urinary condition of pus _____

10. condition of excessive thirst _____

11. condition of painful urination _____

*Decode the terms.*

12. glycosuria _____

13. hematuria _____

14. anuria _____

⊗ **Be Careful!**

**Py/o** *means pus, and* **pyel/o** *means renal pelvis. A dilation of the renal pelvis caused by an accumulation of pus would be pyopyelectasis.*

## Terms Related to Urinary System Disorders, Stones, and Diabetes

| Term | Word Origin | Definition |
|---|---|---|
| **diabetes insipidus (DI)**<br>dye ah BEE teez<br>in SIP ih dus | | Deficiency of antidiuretic hormone (ADH), which causes the patient to excrete large quantities of urine **(polyuria)** and exhibit excessive thirst **(polydipsia)**. |
| **diabetes mellitus (DM)**<br>dye ah BEE teez<br>meh LYE tus | | A group of metabolic disorders characterized by high glucose levels that result from inadequate amounts of insulin, resistance to insulin, or a combination of both. (See Chapter 14). |
| **nephrolithiasis**<br>neff roh lih THIGH uh sis | *nephr/o* kidney<br>*lith/o* stone<br>*-iasis* condition, presence of | Stones in the kidney. |
| **polycystic kidney disease**<br>pah lee SIS tick | *poly-* excessive, many<br>*cyst/o* sac<br>*-ic* pertaining to | Inherited disorder characterized by an enlargement of the kidneys caused by many renal cysts bilaterally that reduce functioning of renal tissue (Fig. 6-5). |
| **renal colic**<br>REE null<br>KAH lick | *ren/o* kidney<br>*-al* pertaining to | Severe pain associated with kidney stones lodged in the ureter. The term "colic" means pain. |
| **urinary tract infection (UTI)** | *urin/o* urine, urinary system | Infection anywhere in the urinary system, caused most commonly by bacteria, but also by parasites, yeast, and protozoa (*sing.* protozoon). Most frequently occurring disorder in the urinary system. |
| **urolithiasis**<br>yoo roo lih THIGH uh sis | *ur/o* urine, urinary system<br>*lith/o* stone<br>*-iasis* condition, presence of | Stones anywhere in the urinary tract, but usually in the renal pelvis or urinary bladder. Usually formed in patients with an excess of the mineral calcium. Also called **urinary calculi** (KAL kyoo lye) (Fig. 6-6). |

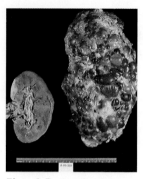

Fig. 6-5 Comparison of a polycystic kidney (*right*) with a normal kidney (*left*).

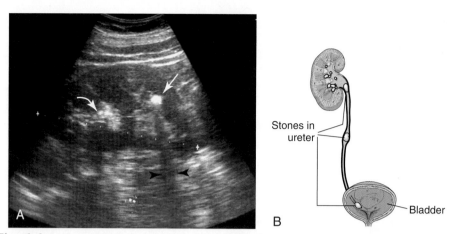

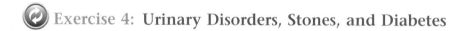

Fig. 6-6 **A,** Sonogram of stones in the renal pelvis. **B,** Locations of ureteral calculi.

## Exercise 4: Urinary Disorders, Stones, and Diabetes

*Match the disorders with their definitions.*

_____ 1. inherited congenital disorders of the kidneys

_____ 2. pain caused by a stone lodged in the ureter

_____ 3. disease caused by deficiency of insulin

_____ 4. infection anywhere in the urinary system

_____ 5. deficiency of anti-diuretic hormone

_____ 6. stones in the urinary tract

_____ 7. excessive thirst

A. urolithiasis
B. polydipsia
C. polycystic kidney disease
D. diabetes mellitus
E. urinary tract infection
F. renal colic
G. diabetes insipidus

*Build terms for the following conditions.*

8. condition of stones in the kidney _____

9. condition of stones in the ureter _____

10. condition of stones in the bladder _____

11. condition of stones in the urethra _____

## Terms Related to Kidney Disorders

| Term | Word Origin | Definition |
|------|-------------|------------|
| **glomerulonephritis (GN)**<br>gloh MUR yoo loh neh FRY tis | *glomerul/o* glomerulus<br>*nephr/o* kidney<br>*-itis* inflammation | Inflammation of the glomeruli of the kidney characterized by proteinuria, hematuria, decreased urine production, and edema. |
| **hydronephrosis**<br>hye droh neh FROH sis | *hydr/o* water<br>*nephr/o* kidney<br>*-osis* abnormal condition | Dilation of the renal pelvis and calices of one or both kidneys resulting from obstruction of the flow of urine. |
| **nephritis**<br>neh FRY tis | *nephr/o* kidney<br>*-itis* inflammation | Inflammation of the kidney; a general term that does not specify the location of the inflammation or its cause. |
| **nephropathy**<br>neh FROP ah thee | *nephr/o* kidney<br>*-pathy* disease process | Disease of the kidneys; a general term that does not specify a disorder. |
| **nephroptosis**<br>neh frop TOH sis | *nephr/o* kidney<br>*-ptosis* drooping, prolapse | Prolapse or sagging of the kidney. |
| **nephrosclerosis**<br>neh froh sklih ROH sis | *nephr/o* kidney<br>*-sclerosis* a hardening | Hardening of the arteries of the kidneys. Also known as **renal sclerosis**. |
| **nephrotic syndrome**<br>neh FRAH tick | *nephr/o* kidney<br>*-tic* pertaining to | Abnormal group of symptoms in the kidney, characterized by proteinuria, hypoalbuminemia, and edema; may occur in glomerular disease and as a complication of many systemic diseases (e.g., diabetes mellitus). Also called **nephrosis** (neh FROH sis). |
| **pyelonephritis**<br>pye uh loh neh FRY tis | *pyel/o* renal pelvis<br>*nephr/o* kidney<br>*-itis* inflammation | Infection of the renal pelvis and parenchyma of the kidney, usually the result of lower urinary tract infection. |
| **renal failure** | *ren/o* kidney<br>*-al* pertaining to | Inability of the kidneys to excrete wastes, concentrate urine, and conserve electrolytes. May be acute or chronic. |
| **acute renal failure (ARF)** | | Sudden inability of the kidneys to excrete wastes, resulting from hemorrhage, trauma, burns, toxic injury to the kidney, pyelonephritis or glomerulonephritis, or lower urinary tract obstruction. Characterized by oliguria and rapid azotemia. |
| **chronic kidney disease (CKD) (formerly chronic renal failure)** | | CKD is measured in stages of increasing severity, from 1 (mild damage with a normal glomerular filtration rate) to 5 (complete kidney failure requiring either dialysis or a renal transplant). Stage 5 is also called **end-stage renal disease (ESRD)**. |
| **renal hypertension** | *ren/o* kidney<br>*-al* pertaining to<br>*hyper-* excessive<br>*tens/o* stretching<br>*-ion* process of | High blood pressure secondary to kidney disease. |

## Terms Related to Bladder, Ureter, and Urethra Disorders

| Term | Word Origin | Definition |
|------|-------------|------------|
| **cystitis** <br> sis TYE tis | *cyst/o* urinary bladder <br> *-itis* inflammation | Inflammation of the urinary bladder. **Trigonitis** is inflammation of the trigone of the bladder. |
| **cystocele** <br> SIS toh seel | *cyst/o* urinary bladder <br> *-cele* herniation | Herniation of the urinary bladder (Fig. 6-7). |
| **ureterocele** <br> yoo REE tur oh seel | *ureter/o* urethra <br> *-cele* herniation | Prolapse of the terminal end of the ureter into the bladder. |
| **urethral stenosis** <br> yoo REE thruhl <br> sten NOH sis | *urethr/o* urethra <br> *-al* pertaining to <br> *stenosis* a narrowing | Narrowing of the urethra. Also called a **urethral stricture**. |
| **urethritis** <br> yoo ree THRY tis | *urethr/o* urethra <br> *-itis* inflammation | Inflammation of the urethra. |
| **vesicoureteral reflux** <br> ves ih koh yoo REE tur ul <br> REE flucks | *vesic/o* urinary bladder <br> *ureter/o* ureter <br> *-al* pertaining to <br> *re-* back <br> *-flux* flow | Abnormal backflow of urine from the bladder to the ureter. May be the result of an obstruction, an infection, or a congenital defect (Fig. 6-8). |

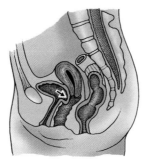

**Fig. 6-7** Cystocele. The urinary bladder is displaced downward (*arrow*), which causes bulging of the anterior vaginal wall.

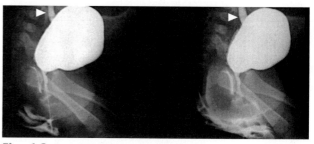

**Fig. 6-8** Serial voiding cystourethrograms in an infant girl with vesicoureteral reflux (*arrowheads*).

## Exercise 5: Kidney, Ureter, Bladder, and Urethral Disorders

*Match the kidney disorders with their definitions.*

_____ 1. inability of the kidneys to excrete wastes

_____ 2. hardening of the arteries of the kidneys

_____ 3. prolapse of the kidney

_____ 4. inflammation of the renal parenchyma and the renal pelvis

_____ 5. disease of the kidney

_____ 6. inflammation of the kidney

_____ 7. proteinuria, hypoalbuminemia, and edema characterize this syndrome

_____ 8. inflammation of the capillaries within the renal corpuscles

_____ 9. inflammation of the tube leading from the bladder to the outside of the body

_____ 10. inflammation of the bladder

_____ 11. herniation of the tube from the kidney to the bladder

_____ 12. backward flow of urine from the bladder toward the kidney

A. glomerulonephritis    E. vesicoureteral reflux    I. nephrosclerosis
B. cystitis    F. urethritis    J. nephropathy
C. nephritis    G. pyelonephritis    K. ureterocele
D. nephroptosis    H. nephrotic syndrome    L. renal failure

*Decode the terms.*

13. hydronephrosis _____

14. cystocele _____

15. nephrolithiasis _____

16. renal sclerosis _____

## Terms Related to Benign Neoplasms

| Term | Word Origin | Definition |
|------|-------------|------------|
| **renal adenoma** <br> REE nuhl <br> add ih NOH mah | *ren/o* kidney <br> *-al* pertaining to <br> *aden/o* gland <br> *-oma* tumor, mass | Small, slow-growing glandular noncancerous tumor of the kidney, usually found at autopsy. |
| **renal oncocytoma** <br> REE null <br> on koh sye TOH mah | *onc/o* tumor <br> *cyt/o* cell <br> *-oma* tumor, mass | The most common benign solid renal tumor. An adenoma composed of oncocytes, abnormal epithelial cells, that develops in the nephron of the kidney. |
| **transitional cell papilloma** <br> pap ih LOH mah | *papill/o* nipple <br> *-oma* tumor, mass | Also referred to as **bladder papilloma.** Although this type of tumor is benign when found, recurrences are occasionally malignant. |

## Terms Related to Malignant Neoplasms

| Term | Word Origin | Definition |
|------|-------------|------------|
| **nephroblastoma** <br> nef roh blass TOH mah | *nephr/o* kidney <br> *blast/o* embryonic <br> *-oma* tumor, mass | Also called **Wilms tumor**, these tumors develop from kidney cells that did not develop fully before a child's birth. These cancerous tumors of the kidney occur mainly in children (Fig. 6-9). |
| **renal cell carcinoma** <br> REE null <br> sell <br> kar sih NOH mah | *ren/o* kidney <br> *-al* pertaining to <br> *carcinoma* cancerous tumor of epithelial origin | Also referred to as **hypernephroma** or **adenocarcinoma of the kidney**, this is one of the most common cancers. Although the cause is unknown, risk factors include smoking and obesity. |
| **transitional cell carcinoma (TCC) of the bladder** <br> tran SIH shuh null <br> kar sih NOH mah | *carcinoma* cancerous tumor of epithelial origin | These malignant tumors account for approximately 90% of all bladder cancers and arise from the cells lining the bladder (Fig. 6-10). Also called **urothelial cell carcinoma**. |

# Chapter Review

Match the word parts to their definitions.

## WORD PART DEFINITIONS

| Suffix | | Definition |
|--------|---|-----------|
| -cele | 1. _____ | removal of a stone |
| -dipsia | 2. _____ | herniation |
| -esis | 3. _____ | separation, breakdown |
| -lithotomy | 4. _____ | machine to crush |
| -lysis | 5. _____ | condition of thirst |
| -pexy | 6. _____ | process of viewing |
| -ptosis | 7. _____ | suspension |
| -scopy | 8. _____ | drooping, prolapse |
| -tripter | 9. _____ | urinary condition |
| -uria | 10. _____ | state of |

| Combining Form | | Definition |
|----------------|---|-----------|
| azot/o | 11. _____ | sugar, glucose |
| albumin/o | 12. _____ | urinary bladder |
| calic/o | 13. _____ | ureter |
| cortic/o | 14. _____ | potassium |
| cyst/o | 15. _____ | night |
| glomerul/o | 16. _____ | trigone |
| glycos/o | 17. _____ | sodium |
| kal/i | 18. _____ | urine, urinary system |
| lith/o | 19. _____ | stone |
| meat/o | 20. _____ | urinary meatus |
| natr/o | 21. _____ | kidney |
| nephr/o | 22. _____ | scanty, few |
| noct/i | 23. _____ | glomerulus |
| olig/o | 24. _____ | kidney |
| pyel/o | 25. _____ | calyx |
| ren/o | 26. _____ | renal pelvis |
| trigon/o | 27. _____ | urethra |
| ureter/o | 28. _____ | urinary bladder |
| urethr/o | 29. _____ | protein |
| ur/o | 30. _____ | nitrogen |
| vesic/o | 31. _____ | cortex |

# WORDSHOP

| Prefixes | Combining Forms | Suffixes |
|---|---|---|
| a- | azot/o | -al |
| an- | cyst/o | -cele |
| dys- | glomerul/o | -dipsia |
| per- | glycos/o | -emia |
| peri- | hemat/o | -graphy |
| poly- | lith/o | -iasis |
| pre- | nephr/o | -itis |
|  | pyel/o | -lysis |
|  | py/o | -oma |
|  | tom/o | -scope |
|  | ureter/o | -scopy |
|  | urethr/o | -tomy |
|  | ur/o | -tripsy |
|  | vesicul/o | -uria |

*Build the following terms by combining the above word parts. Some word parts may be used more than once. Some may not be used at all. The number in parenthesis is the number of word parts needed to build the term.*

| Definition | Term |
|---|---|
| 1. pertaining to surrounding the bladder (3) | |
| 2. process of recording a section of kidney (3) | |
| 3. instrument to visually examine the kidney (2) | |
| 4. herniation of a ureter (2) | |
| 5. condition of painful/difficult urination (2) | |
| 6. condition of blood in the urine (2) | |
| 7. inflammation of the glomerulus in the kidney (3) | |
| 8. condition of stones in the urinary tract (3) | |
| 9. condition of no urination (2) | |
| 10. process of crushing stones (2) | |
| 11. condition of urea in the blood (2) | |
| 12. freeing from adhesions in the urethra (2) | |
| 13. condition of excessive urination (2) | |
| 14. inflammation of the renal pelvis of the kidney (3) | |
| 15. condition of excessive thirst (2) | |

Sort the terms below into the correct categories.

## TERM SORTING

| Anatomy and Physiology | Pathology | Diagnostic Procedures | Therapeutic Interventions |
|---|---|---|---|
| | | | |
| | | | |
| | | | |
| | | | |
| | | | |
| | | | |
| | | | |
| | | | |
| | | | |
| | | | |

| | | | |
|---|---|---|---|
| albuminuria | hemodialysis | nephropexy | urea |
| BUN | hilum | nephroptosis | urethra |
| CAPD | IVU | nephrostomy | urethral stenosis |
| cortex | KUB | nephrotomography | urethrolysis |
| cystoscopy | lithotripsy | pyuria | urinalysis |
| cystourethroscopy | medulla | renal adenoma | urinary meatus |
| DM | meatotomy | renal colic | urinometer |
| enuresis | micturition | renal dialysis | UTI |
| GFR | nephritis | renal medulla | VCUG |
| glomeruli | nephrolithotomy | trigone | vesicotomy |

*Replace the highlighted words with the correct terms.*

## TRANSLATIONS

1. Emily was admitted with **accumulation of fluid in the tissues** and **condition of high blood pressure.**

2. Dr. Garcia ordered a **blood test that measures the amount of nitrogenous waste** and a **test of kidney function that measures the rate at which nitrogenous waste is removed from the blood.**

3. Moumoud was admitted for **severe pain associated with kidney stones lodged in the ureter** and **stones anywhere in the urinary tract.**

4. Mr. Samuels was treated for his **stones in the kidney** with **process of crushing stones to prevent or clear an obstruction in the urinary system.**

5. Once **an infection anywhere in the urinary system** was ruled out, Rebecca was evaluated for ongoing **bed-wetting.**

6. A/an **instrument for visual examination of the inside of the bladder** was used to locate the site of a **herniation of the urinary bladder.**

7. Mr. Alton's acute renal failure was diagnosed after examination findings that included **condition of scanty urination** and **condition of excessive urea in the blood.**

8. The patient's **prolapse or sagging of the kidney** was surgically corrected with a suspension or **fixation of the kidney.**

9. A **sectional radiographic exam of the kidneys** was performed to diagnose Mr. Woo's **adenoma composed of oncocytes.**

10. Mary's DM was diagnosed after she presented with **condition of excessive urination** and **condition of excessive thirst.**

11. Kevin Allen was afraid he had **a group of metabolic disorders characterized by high glucose levels** but was instead diagnosed with **deficiency of ADH.**

12. The patient showed symptoms of **infection of the renal pelvis and parenchyma of the kidney.**

13. Dr. Simons told Marqueta that she had **high blood pressure secondary to kidney disease** due to **inability of the kidneys to excrete wastes.**

14. After several years of **process of diffusing blood across a semipermeable membrane**, Johnna underwent **a surgical transfer of a complete kidney from a donor.**

# *Case Study* Brian Coulter

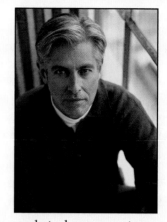

**B**rian Coulter has been experiencing sharp pain in his back, which has radiated to his lower left quadant for the past few days. Now, Friday night, it seems worse than it has ever been, so he drives to his local emergency department hoping for some relief.

After consulting with the resident on call, Brian is immediately sent for imaging and lab studies. The imaging order calls for an x-ray of the abdomen, a renal ultrasound, and a spiral CT scan to rule out a suspected urinary calculus. The CBC result is normal, but the urinalysis reveals a finding of blood in the urine and an abnormally low pH.

Brian's CT scan shows a left distal ureteral stone and hydronephrosis. His physician tells him that he needs to have a ureteroscopic stone extraction. A cystoscopy is scheduled for the next morning.

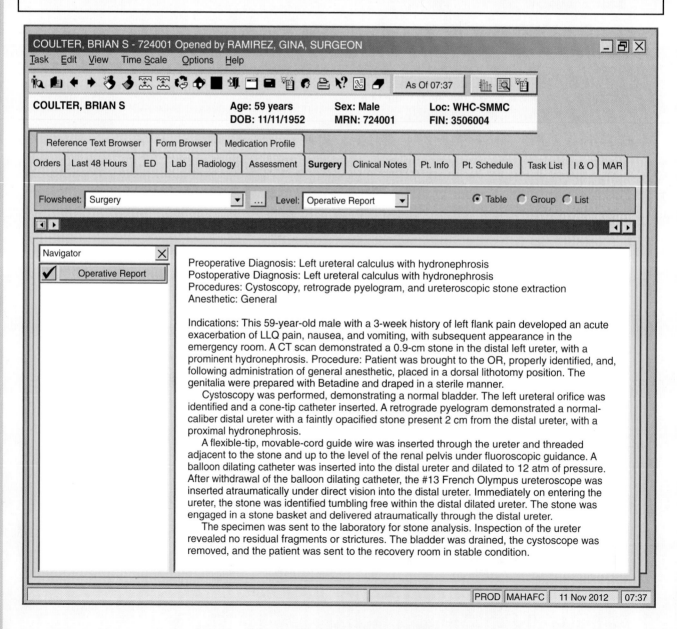

COULTER, BRIAN S - 724001 Opened by RAMIREZ, GINA, SURGEON

Task   Edit   View   Time Scale   Options   Help

As Of 07:37

**COULTER, BRIAN S**

| | Age: 59 years | Sex: Male | Loc: WHC-SMMC |
| | DOB: 11/11/1952 | MRN: 724001 | FIN: 3506004 |

Reference Text Browser | Form Browser | Medication Profile

Orders | Last 48 Hours | ED | Lab | Radiology | Assessment | **Surgery** | Clinical Notes | Pt. Info | Pt. Schedule | Task List | I & O | MAR

Flowsheet: Surgery          Level: Operative Report          ○ Table ○ Group ○ List

Navigator
✓ Operative Report

Preoperative Diagnosis: Left ureteral calculus with hydronephrosis
Postoperative Diagnosis: Left ureteral calculus with hydronephrosis
Procedures: Cystoscopy, retrograde pyelogram, and ureteroscopic stone extraction
Anesthetic: General

Indications: This 59-year-old male with a 3-week history of left flank pain developed an acute exacerbation of LLQ pain, nausea, and vomiting, with subsequent appearance in the emergency room. A CT scan demonstrated a 0.9-cm stone in the distal left ureter, with a prominent hydronephrosis. Procedure: Patient was brought to the OR, properly identified, and, following administration of general anesthetic, placed in a dorsal lithotomy position. The genitalia were prepared with Betadine and draped in a sterile manner.
    Cystoscopy was performed, demonstrating a normal bladder. The left ureteral orifice was identified and a cone-tip catheter inserted. A retrograde pyelogram demonstrated a normal-caliber distal ureter with a faintly opacified stone present 2 cm from the distal ureter, with a proximal hydronephrosis.
    A flexible-tip, movable-cord guide wire was inserted through the ureter and threaded adjacent to the stone and up to the level of the renal pelvis under fluoroscopic guidance. A balloon dilating catheter was inserted into the distal ureter and dilated to 12 atm of pressure. After withdrawal of the balloon dilating catheter, the #13 French Olympus ureteroscope was inserted atraumatically under direct vision into the distal ureter. Immediately on entering the ureter, the stone was identified tumbling free within the distal dilated ureter. The stone was engaged in a stone basket and delivered atraumatically through the distal ureter.
    The specimen was sent to the laboratory for stone analysis. Inspection of the ureter revealed no residual fragments or strictures. The bladder was drained, the cystoscope was removed, and the patient was sent to the recovery room in stable condition.

PROD | MAHAFC | 11 Nov 2012 | 07:37

### Operative Report

*Answer the questions using the operative report on p. 236.*

1. What is a left ureteral calculus? _____

2. How do we know that there was no abnormal narrowing of the ureter? _____

3. What term describes the sudden onset of symptoms? _____

4. Did the ureteral calculus cause an obstruction? _____

   How do you know? _____

5. What were all the instruments and/or procedures that were used to visualize the problem?

   _____

6. What term indicates that no further injury was caused by the surgery? _____

For more interactive learning, go to the Shiland Evolve site and click on:
• **Whack a Word Part** to review urinary word parts.
• **Wheel of Terminology** and **Word Shop** to practice word building.
• **Tournament of Terminology** to test your knowledge of urinary terms.
• **Terminology Triage** to pratice sorting urinary terms into categories.

# 7

*Recognizing and preventing men's health problems is not just a man's issue. Because of its import on wives, mothers, daughters, and sisters, men's health is truly a family issue.*
**—Congressman Bill Richardson**

## OBJECTIVES

- Recognize and use terms related to the anatomy and physiology of the male reproductive system.
- Recognize and use terms related to the pathology of the male reproductive system.
- Recognize and use terms related to the diagnostic procedures for the male reproductive system.
- Recognize and use terms related to the therapeutic interventions for the male reproductive system.

# Male Reproductive System

## CHAPTER AT A GLANCE

*Use this list of word parts and key terms to assess your knowledge. Check off the ones you've mastered.*

### ANATOMY AND PHYSIOLOGY

- ☐ coitus
- ☐ conception
- ☐ copulation
- ☐ ductus deferens
- ☐ epididymis
- ☐ foreskin
- ☐ gametes
- ☐ genitalia
- ☐ glans penis
- ☐ gonads
- ☐ penis
- ☐ prepuce
- ☐ prostate
- ☐ scrotum
- ☐ semen
- ☐ seminal vesicle
- ☐ seminiferous tubules
- ☐ spermatic cord
- ☐ spermatogenesis
- ☐ spermatozoon
- ☐ testis
- ☐ testosterone
- ☐ urethra

### KEY WORD PARTS

**PREFIXES**
- ☐ a-, an-
- ☐ circum-
- ☐ crypt-
- ☐ hyper-
- ☐ hypo-
- ☐ non-
- ☐ trans-

**SUFFIXES**
- ☐ -cision
- ☐ -ectomy
- ☐ -genesis
- ☐ -graphy
- ☐ -itis
- ☐ -spadias
- ☐ -stomy

**COMBINING FORMS**
- ☐ balan/o
- ☐ epididym/o
- ☐ olig/o
- ☐ orchid/o, orchi/o, orch/o
- ☐ pen/i
- ☐ phall/o
- ☐ plethysm/o
- ☐ preputi/o
- ☐ prostat/o
- ☐ scrot/o
- ☐ semin/i
- ☐ sperm/o, spermat/o
- ☐ test/o
- ☐ urethr/o
- ☐ vas/o
- ☐ vesicul/o

### KEY TERMS

- ☐ anorchism
- ☐ azoospermia
- ☐ balanitis
- ☐ benign prostatic hyperplasia (BPH)
- ☐ circumcision
- ☐ cryptorchidism
- ☐ epididymitis
- ☐ erectile dysfunction (ED)
- ☐ human papillomavirus (HPV)
- ☐ hypospadias
- ☐ nongonococcal urethritis (NGU)
- ☐ oligospermia
- ☐ phimosis
- ☐ plethysmography
- ☐ prostatectomy
- ☐ prostate-specific antigen (PSA)
- ☐ testitis
- ☐ transurethral resection of the prostate (TURP)
- ☐ vasectomy
- ☐ vasovasostomy
- ☐ vesiculitis

## FUNCTIONS OF THE MALE REPRODUCTIVE SYSTEM

The function of the male reproductive system is to reproduce. In the process of providing half of the genetic material (in the form of spermatozoa) necessary to form a new person—and then successfully storing, transporting, and delivering this material to fertilize the female counterpart, the ovum—the species survives.

## SPECIALTIES/SPECIALISTS

**Andrology** is the study of the male reproductive system, especially in reference to fertility issues. **Urologists** treat male urinary and reproductive disorders.

## ANATOMY AND PHYSIOLOGY

Both male and female anatomy can be divided into two parts: **parenchymal** (puh REN kih mul), or **primary tissue,** which produces sex cells for reproduction; and **stromal** (STROH mul), or **secondary tissue,** which includes all of the glands nerves, ducts, and other tissues that serve a supportive function in producing, maintaining, and transmitting these sex cells. Together these types of reproductive tissue, in either sex, are called **genitalia** (jen ih TAIL ee ah). The parenchymal organs that produce the sex cells in both sexes are called **gonads** (GOH nads). The sex cells themselves are called **gametes** (GAM eets).

In the male, the gonads are the **testes** (TESS teez) (*sing.* testis) or **testicles** (TESS tick kuls), paired organs that produce the gametes called **spermatozoa** (spur mat ah ZOH ah) (*sing.* spermatozoon). The testes are suspended in a sac called the **scrotum** (SKROH tum) (*pl.* scrota) outside the body's trunk (Fig. 7-1).

At **puberty** (PYOO bur tee), the stage of life in which males and females become functionally capable of sexual reproduction, the interstitial cells in the testicles begin to produce **testosterone** (tess TOSS tur rohn), a sex hormone responsible for the growth and development of male sex characteristics. The spermatozoa are formed in a series of tightly coiled tiny tubes in each testis called the **seminiferous tubules** (sem ih NIFF ur us TOO byools). The formation of sperm is called **spermatogenesis** (spur mat toh JEN ih sis). The serous membrane that surrounds the front and sides of the testicle is called the **tunica vaginalis testis** (TOON ih kah vaj ih NAL is TESS tis). From the seminiferous tubules, the formed spermatozoa travel to the **epididymis** (eh pih DID ih mis) (*pl.* epididymides), where they are stored.

When the seminal fluid is about to be ejected from the urethra (**ejaculation),** the spermatozoa travel through the left and right **vas deferens** (vas DEH fur ens), also called the **ductus deferens** (DUCK tus DEH fur ens), from the epididymides, around the bladder. The **spermatic cord** is an enclosed sheath that includes the vas deferens, along with arteries, veins, and nerves.

To survive and thrive, the sperm are nourished by fluid from a series of glands. The **seminal vesicles** (SEM ih nul VESS ih kuls), **Cowper's** (or **bulbourethral** [bul boh yoo REE thrul]) **glands,** and the **prostate** (PROS tate) **gland** provide fluid either to nourish or to aid in motility and lubrication. The sperm and the fluid together make up a substance called **semen** (SEE men). The **ejaculatory duct** (ee JACK yoo lah tore ee) begins where the seminal vesicles join the vas deferens, and this "tube" joins the urethra. Once the sperm reach the **urethra,** they travel out through the shaft, or body, of the **penis** (PEE nuss), which is composed of three columns of highly vascular erectile tissue. There are two columns of **corpora cavernosa** (KORE poor ah kav ur NOH suh) and one of **corpus spongiosum** (KORE puss spun jee OH sum) that fill with blood through the dorsal veins during sexual arousal. During ejaculation, the sperm exit through the enlarged tip of the penis, the **glans penis.** At birth, the glans

---

**andrology**
   andr/o = male
   -logy = the study of

**parenchymal**
   par- = near
   en- = in
   chym/o = juice
   -al = pertaining to

**stromal tissue** = strom/o

**gonad** = gonad/o

**testis, testicle** = test/o, testicul/o, orchi/o, orchid/o, orch/o

**spermatozoon** = sperm/o, spermat/o

**scrotum** = scrot/o

**testosterone**
   test/o = testis
   ster/o = steroid
   -one = substance that forms

**seminiferous**
   semin/i = semen
   -ferous = pertaining to carrying

**spermatogenesis**
   spermat/o = spermatozoon
   -genesis = production

**epididymis** = epididym/o

**vas deferens, ductus deferens** = vas/o

**seminal vesicle** = vesicul/o

**prostate** = prostat/o

**semen** = semin/i

**urethra** = urethr/o

**penis** = pen/i, phall/o

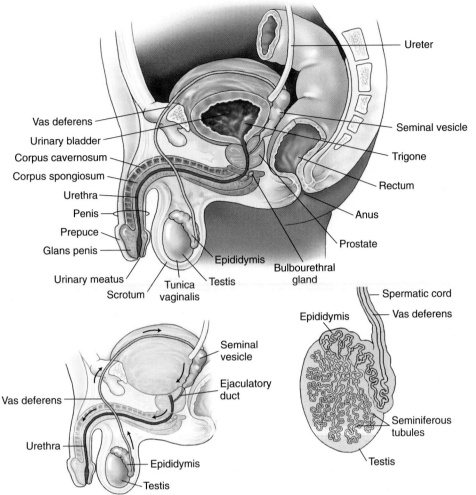

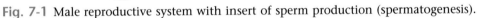

**Fig. 7-1** Male reproductive system with insert of sperm production (spermatogenesis).

⊗ **Be Careful!**

*Don't confuse **vesic/o**, which means the urinary bladder, and **vesicul/o**, which means the seminal vesicle.*

⊗ **Be Careful!**

*Don't confuse **phall/o**, which means penis, and **phalang/o**, which is a bone in the finger or toe.*

⊗ **Be Careful!**

*Don't confuse **urethr/o**, which means urethra, and **ureter/o**, which means the ureter.*

penis is surrounded by a fold of skin called the **prepuce** (PREE pyoos), or **foreskin.** The removal of this skin is termed **circumcision** (sur kum SIH zhun).

When ejaculation occurs during sexual intercourse (**coitus** [KOH ih tus] or **copulation** [kop yoo LAY shun]), the sperm then race toward the female sex cell, or ovum. If a specific sperm penetrates and unites with the ovum, **conception** takes place, and formation of an embryo begins.

**glans penis = balan/o**

**prepuce, foreskin = preputi/o**

🔄 Exercise 1: **Anatomy of the Male Reproductive System**

*Match the word parts with their meanings.*

____ 1. penis

____ 2. prostate

____ 3. seminal vesicle

____ 4. scrotum

____ 5. prepuce

____ 6. semen

____ 7. urethra

____ 8. glans penis

____ 9. ductus deferens

____ 10. spermatozoon

____ 11. epididymis

____ 12. testis

A. vesicul/o
B. preputi/o
C. orchid/o
D. phall/o
E. epididym/o
F. spermat/o

G. scrot/o
H. vas/o
I. semin/i
J. urethr/o
K. prostat/o
L. balan/o

# Chapter 7

*Decode the terms.*

13. unitesticular _____

14. preputial _____

15. vesicular _____

16. periprostatic _____

17. intrascrotal _____

You can review the anatomy of the male reproductive system by clicking on **Body Spectrum Electronic Anatomy Coloring Book** → **Reproductive** → **Male.** Click on **Hear It, Spell It** to practice spelling the anatomy and physiology terms you have learned in this chapter. To practice pronouncing male reproductive anatomy and physiology terms, click on **Hear It, Say It.**

## Exercise 2: Anatomy of the Male Reproductive System

*Label the drawing with the correct anatomic terms and combining forms where appropriate.*

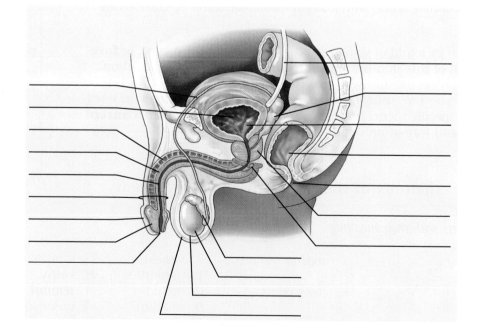

## Combining and Adjective Forms for the Anatomy of the Male Reproductive System

| Meaning | Combining Form | Adjective Form |
|---|---|---|
| epididymis | epididym/o | epididymal |
| glans penis | balan/o | balanic |
| gonad | gonad/o | gonadal |
| juices | chym/o | chymal |
| male | andr/o | |
| penis | pen/i, phall/o | penile, phallic |
| prepuce, foreskin | preputi/o | preputial |
| prostate | prostat/o | prostatic |
| scrotum | scrot/o | scrotal |
| semen | semin/i | seminal |
| seminal vesicle | vesicul/o | vesicular |
| spermatozoon | sperm/o, spermat/o | spermatic |
| steroid | ster/o | steroidal |
| stroma | strom/o | stromal |
| testis, testicle | test/o, testicul/o, orchid/o, orch/o | testicular |
| urethra | urethr/o | urethral |
| vas deferens, ductus deferens | vas/o | vasal, ductal |

## Prefixes for the Anatomy of the Male Reproductive System

| Prefix | Meaning |
|---|---|
| en- | in |
| par- | near |

## Suffixes for the Anatomy of the Male Reproductive System

| Suffix | Meaning |
|---|---|
| -al, -ous, -ar, -ile, -atic, -ic | pertaining to |
| -ferous | pertaining to carrying |
| -genesis | production |
| -logy | the study of |
| -one | substance that forms |

## PATHOLOGY

### Terms Related to Congenital Disorders

| Term | Word Origin | Definition |
|---|---|---|
| **anorchism**<br>AN or kih zum | *an-* without<br>*orch/o* testis<br>*-ism* condition | Condition of being born without a testicle. May also be an acquired condition due to trauma or disease. |
| **chordee**<br>KORE dee | *chord/o* cord | Congenital defect resulting in a downward (ventral) curvature of the penis due to a fibrous band (cord) of tissue along the corpus spongiosum. Often associated with hypospadias (Fig. 7-2). |
| **cryptorchidism**<br>kript OR kid iz um | *crypt-* hidden<br>*orchid/o* testis<br>*-ism* condition | Condition in which the testicles fail to descend into the scrotum before birth. Also called **cryptorchism** (Fig. 7-3). |
| **epispadias**<br>eh pee SPAY dee ahs | *epi-* above<br>*-spadias* a rent or tear | Urethral opening on the dorsum (top) of the penis rather than on the tip. Also called **hyperspadias**. |
| **hypospadias**<br>hye poh SPAY dee ahs | *hypo-* below<br>*-spadias* a rent or tear | Urethral opening on the ventral surface (underside) of the penis instead of on the tip (Fig. 7-4). May be acquired as a result of the disease process. |
| **phimosis**<br>fih MOH sis | | Congenital condition of tightening of the prepuce around the glans penis so that the foreskin cannot be retracted. |

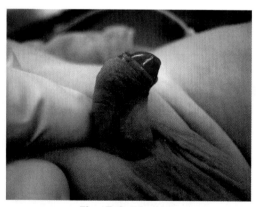

Fig. 7-2 Chordee.

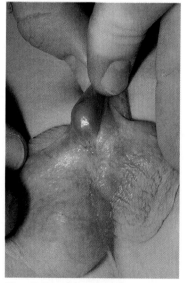

Fig. 7-3 Cryptorchidism in left testicle of a neonate.

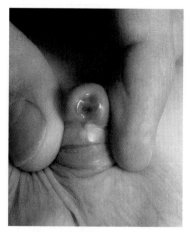

Fig. 7-4 Hypospadias.

## Terms Related to Other Male Reproductive Disorders

| Term | Word Origin | Definition |
|------|-------------|------------|
| **aspermia**<br>a SPUR mee ah | *a-* without<br>*sperm/o* sperm<br>*-ia* condition | Condition in which no spermatozoa are present, nor any semen formed or ejaculated. |
| **azoospermia**<br>a zoh uh SPUR mee ah | *a-* without<br>*zo/o* animal<br>*sperm/o* sperm<br>*-ia* condition | Condition of no living sperm in the semen. This may be a desired condition, as when it follows a vasectomy. |
| **balanitis**<br>bal en EYE tis | *balan/o* glans penis<br>*-itis* inflammation | Inflammation of the glans penis. |
| **benign prostatic hyperplasia (BPH)**<br>beh NYNE<br>pros TAT ick<br>hye pur PLAY zsa | *prostat/o* prostate<br>*-ic* pertaining to<br>*hyper-* excessive<br>*-plasia* formation | Abnormal enlargement of the prostate gland surrounding the urethra, leading to difficulty with urination (Fig. 7-5). Also known as **benign prostatic hypertrophy.** |
| **epididymitis**<br>ep ih did ih MYE tis | *epididym/o* epididymis<br>*-itis* inflammation | Inflammation of the epididymis, usually as a result of an ascending infection through the genitourinary tract. |
| **erectile dysfunction (ED)** | | Inability to achieve or sustain a penile erection for sexual intercourse. Also known as **impotence** (IM poh tense). |
| **gynecomastia**<br>gye neh koh MASS tee ah | *gynec/o* female<br>*mast/o* breast<br>*-ia* condition | Enlargement of either unilateral or bilateral breast tissue in the male. The *gynec/o* is a reference to the appearance of the breast, not to a female (Fig. 7-6). |
| **hydrocele**<br>HYE droh seel | *hydr/o* water, fluid<br>*-cele* herniation, protrusion | Accumulation of fluid in the tunica vaginalis testis (Fig. 7-7). |
| **oligospermia**<br>oh lih goh SPUR mee ah | *olig/o* scanty<br>*sperm/o* sperm<br>*-ia* condition | Condition of temporary or permanent deficiency of sperm in the seminal fluid; related to azoospermia. |
| **orchitis**<br>or KYE tis | *orch/o* testis<br>*-itis* inflammation | Inflammation of one or both of the testicles; may or may not be associated with the mumps virus. Also known as **testitis** (tess TYE tis). |

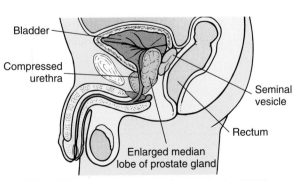

Fig. 7-5 Benign prostatic hyperplasia (BPH).

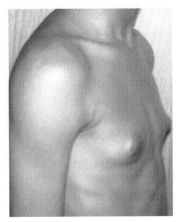

Fig. 7-6 Gynecomastia.

## Terms Related to Other Male Reproductive Disorders–cont'd

| Term | Word Origin | Definition |
|---|---|---|
| priapism<br>PRY ah piz um | | An abnormally prolonged erection. |
| prostatitis<br>pros tah TYE tis | *prostat/o* prostate<br>*-itis* inflammation | Inflammation of the prostate gland. |
| testicular torsion<br>tes TICK kyoo lur | *testicul/o* testicle<br>*-ar* pertaining to | Twisting of a testicle on its spermatic cord, usually caused by trauma. May lead to ischemia of the testicle. |
| varicocele<br>VAIR ih koh seel | *varic/o* varices<br>*-cele* herniation, protrusion | Abnormal dilation of the veins of the spermatic cord; can lead to infertility (Fig. 7-8). |
| vesiculitis<br>veh sick yoo LYE tis | *vesicul/o* seminal vesicle<br>*-itis* inflammation | Inflammation of a seminal vesicle, usually associated with prostatitis. |

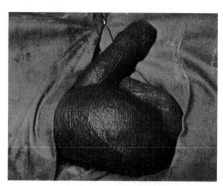

Fig. 7-7 Hydrocele.

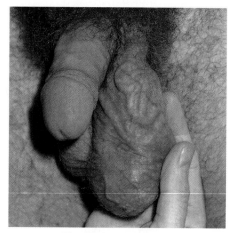

Fig. 7-8 Varicocele.

## Exercise 3: Male Reproductive Disorders

*Match the male reproductive disorders with their definitions.*

\_\_\_\_ 1. tightening of foreskin

\_\_\_\_ 2. opening of urethra on underside of penis

\_\_\_\_ 3. twisting of testicle on spermatic cord

\_\_\_\_ 4. inability to achieve or sustain a penile erection

\_\_\_\_ 5. accumulation of fluid in tunica vaginalis testis

\_\_\_\_ 6. opening of urethra on dorsum of penis

\_\_\_\_ 7. enlargement of breast tissue in a male

\_\_\_\_ 8. abnormal dilation of veins of the spermatic cord

A. hypospadias
B. varicocele
C. gynecomastia
D. epispadias
E. testicular torsion
F. erectile dysfunction
G. phimosis
H. hydrocele

*Build the terms.*

9. inflammation of the glans penis _____

10. condition of no living sperm (in the semen) _____

11. inflammation of the prostate _____

12. excessive formation, pertaining to the prostate (2 words) _____

*Decode the terms.*

13. orchitis _____

14. oligospermia _____

15. vesiculitis _____

To see an animation of testicular torsion, click on **Animations.**

## Terms Related to Sexually Transmitted Infections (STIs)

The pathogens that cause STIs are various, but what they have in common is that all are most efficiently transmitted by sexual contact. The other term for STIs is venereal disease, abbreviated VD.

| Term | Word Origin | Definition |
|---|---|---|
| **gonorrhea**<br>gon uh REE ah | *gon/o* seed<br>*-rrhea* flow, discharge | Disease caused by the gram-negative diplococcus *Neisseria gonorrhoeae* bacterium (Gc), which manifests itself as inflammation of the urethra, prostate, rectum, or pharynx. The cervix and fallopian tubes may also be involved in females, although they may appear to be **asymptomatic**, meaning without symptoms (Fig. 7-9). |
| **herpes genitalis (herpes simplex virus, HSV-2)**<br>HER peez<br>jen ih TAL is | | Form of the herpesvirus transmitted through sexual contact, causing recurring painful vesicular eruptions (Fig. 7-10). |
| **human papillomavirus (HPV)**<br>pap ih LOH mah | | Virus that causes common warts of the hands and feet and lesions of the mucous membranes of the oral, anal, and genital cavities. A genital wart is referred to as a **condyloma** (kon dih LOH mah) (*pl.* condylomata). |
| **nongonococcal urethritis (NGU)**<br>non gon uh KOCK ul<br>yoor ih THRY tis | *urethr/o* urethra<br>*-itis* inflammation | Inflammation of the urethra caused by *Chlamydia trachomatis, Mycoplasma genitalium,* or *Ureaplasma urealyticum.* |
| **syphilis**<br>SIFF ill is | | Multistage STI caused by the spirochete *Treponema pallidum* bacterium. A highly infectious **chancre** (SHAN kur), a painless, red pustule, appears in the first stage, usually on the genitals. |

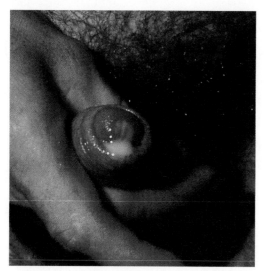

Fig. 7-9 Gonorrhea in a male patient.

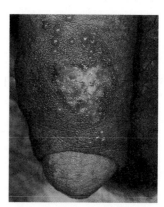

Fig. 7-10 Genital herpes.

## Exercise 4: Sexually Transmitted Infections

*Fill in the blanks with one of the following terms.*

**condylomata, asymptomatic, human papillomavirus, chancres, herpes simplex virus-2, nongonococcal urethritis, syphilis, gonorrhea**

1. HPV causes genital warts that are referred to as _____.

2. Which STI has multiple stages? _____

3. Inflammation of the urethra not caused by the gonorrhea bacterium is called _____.

4. An STI caused by gram-negative bacteria is called _____.

5. Syphilitic lesions that are painless ulcers are called _____.

6. When a patient has no symptoms, he is considered to be _____.

7. Genital warts are caused by the _____.

8. A viral infection that results in painful, recurring vesicular eruptions is called _____.

| Terms Related to Benign Neoplasms | | |
|---|---|---|
| **Term** | **Word Origin** | **Definition** |
| Leydig and Sertoli cell tumors <br> LAY dig <br> sur TOH lee | | These testicular tumors arise from the stromal tissue of the testes that produce hormones. They are usually benign. |

## Terms Related to Malignant Neoplasms

| Term | Word Origin | Definition |
|---|---|---|
| adenocarcinoma of the prostate<br>ad eh noh<br>kar sih NOH mah | *aden/o* gland<br>*-carcinoma* cancer of epithelial origin | Prostate cancer is diagnosed in one of every six men. With early detection, however, this cancer is treatable (Fig. 7-11). |
| seminoma<br>seh mih NOH mah | *semin/i* semen<br>*-oma* tumor, mass | This malignancy is one type of germ cell tumor (GCT) that develops from the cells that form sperm (Fig. 7-12). |
| nonseminoma<br>non seh mih NOH mah | *non-* not<br>*semin/i* semen<br>*-oma* tumor, mass | Nonseminoma is the second type of GCT. It accounts for the majority of testicular cancer cases and occurs in younger men, usually between the ages of 15 and 35. |
| teratoma, malignant<br>tair uh TOH mah | *terat/o* deformity<br>*-oma* tumor, mass | This tumor is a type of nonseminoma that is usually benign in children. Because these tumors are created from germ cells, they have half of the necessary genetic information to form an individual. A synonym is the term **dermoid cyst**. |

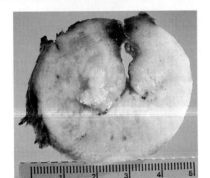

Fig. 7-11 Adenocarcinoma of the prostate.

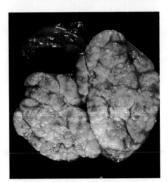

Fig. 7-12 Seminoma of the testicle.

## Exercise 5: Neoplasms

*Match the neoplasms with their definitions.*

____ 1. nonseminoma

____ 2. teratoma

____ 3. seminoma

____ 4. adenocarcinoma of the prostate

____ 5. Leydig and Sertoli cell tumors

A. benign tumors that arise from testicular stromal tissue
B. prostate cancer
C. majority of germ cell tumors
D. germ cell tumor developing from cells that form sperm
E. synonym is dermoid cyst

*Build the terms.*

6. tumor of semen _____

7. glandular cancerous tumor of epithelial origin _____

Click on **Hear It, Spell It** to practice spelling the pathology terms you have learned. To see how well you can pronounce the pathology terms in this chapter, click on **Hear It, Say It**. To review the pathology terms you've learned in this chapter, play **Medical Millionaire**.

## Age Matters

**Pediatrics**

Aside from the congenital disorders that a male child may be born with, very few male reproductive system disorders are specific to childhood. Seminoma, a cancer of the testicles, is one of the few cancers that afflicts youth. Fortunately, early detection makes this cancer almost 100% curable.

**Geriatrics**

Senior men have some very significant disorders. Disorders of the prostate gland are common and are usually accompanied by difficulty with urination because of the location of the prostate around the urethra. Usually benign, this also has a malignant form, and prostate cancer is the second greatest cause of cancer deaths. Erectile disorders, now treatable with a variety of different medications on the market, have also emerged as a significant "reason for visit" to the family physician.

## DIAGNOSTIC PROCEDURES

### Terms Related to Diagnostic Procedures

| Term | Word Origin | Definition |
|---|---|---|
| digital rectal examination (DRE) | *digit/o* digit (finger or toe) <br> *-al* pertaining to <br> *rect/o* rectum <br> *-al* pertaining to | Insertion of a gloved finger into the rectum to palpate the prostate (Fig. 7-13). |
| epididymo-vesiculography <br> eh pih did ih moh veh sih kuh LAH grah fee | *epididym/o* epididymis <br> *vesicul/o* seminal vesicle <br> *-graphy* process of recording | Imaging of the epididymis and seminal vesicle using a contrast medium. |
| fluorescent treponemal antibody absorption test (FTA-ABS) <br> floor ES unt <br> trep uh NEE mul | | Definitive test for diagnosing syphilis (Fig. 7-14). |
| Gram stain | | A laboratory method of staining microorganisms as a means of identifying them as either gram-negative or gram-positive. Gonorrhea, a gram-negative bacteria, is diagnosed using Gram stain (Fig. 7-15). |
| plethysmography, penile <br> pleth iz MAH grah fee | *plethysm/o* volume <br> *-graphy* process of recording | The measurement of changes in volume of organs or body parts. |
| prostate-specific antigen (PSA) <br> AN tih jen | | Blood test for prostatic hypertrophy. Very high levels may indicate prostate cancer. Above 2.6 ng/mL is considered elevated. |
| sonography, transrectal | *son/o* sound <br> *-graphy* process of recording | Use of high-frequency sound waves to examine the prostate for abnormalities (Fig. 7-16). |

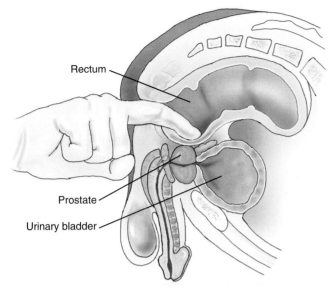

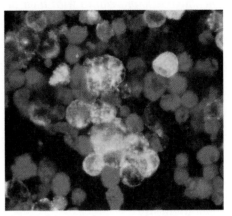

Fig. 7-13 Digital rectal examination (DRE).

Fig. 7-14 Fluorescent treponemal antibody absorption test (FTA-ABS).

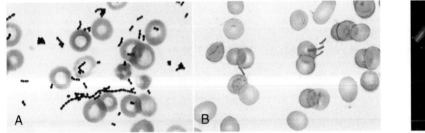

Fig. 7-15 Gram stain. **A,** Red blood cells and gram-positive cocci. **B,** RBs with gram-negative bacilli.

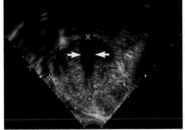

Fig. 7-16 Transrectal ultrasound scan of the prostate, showing BPH.

## Terms Related to Diagnostic Procedures—cont'd

| Term | Word Origin | Definition |
|---|---|---|
| sperm analysis | | Count and analysis of the number and health of the spermatozoa as a test for male fertility. Also called **sperm count** or **semen analysis.** |
| testicular self-examination (TSE) | *testicul/o* testicle<br>*-ar* pertaining to | Examination of the testicles by the patient. |
| Venereal Disease Research Laboratory (VDRL) test | | Test used to screen for syphilis. |

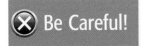 **Be Careful!**      *Don't confuse* **proct/o**, *which means rectum and anus, and* **prostat/o**, *which means prostate.*

## Exercise 6: Diagnostic Procedures

*Match the diagnostic procedures with their definitions.*

____ 1. DRE

____ 2. FTA-ABS

____ 3. Gram stain

____ 4. PSA

____ 5. sperm analysis

____ 6. sonography

____ 7. VDRL

A. imaging with high-frequency sound waves
B. test used to screen for syphilis
C. test of male fertility
D. blood test for prostatic hypertrophy
E. insertion of a gloved finger to palpate the prostate
F. definitive test for diagnosing syphilis
G. test used to diagnose gonorrhea

*Decode the terms.*

8. plethysmography _____

9. epididymovesiculography _____

## THERAPEUTIC INTERVENTIONS

### Terms Related to Therapeutic Interventions

| Term | Word Origin | Definition |
|------|-------------|------------|
| ablation<br>ah BLAY shun | | Removal of tissue by surgery, chemical destruction, cryoprobe, electrocautery, or radiofrequency energy. |
| castration<br>kas TRAY shun | | Removal of both gonads in the male or the female. |
| circumcision<br>sur kum SIH zhun | *circum-* around<br>*-cision* process of cutting | Surgical procedure in which the prepuce of the penis (or that of the clitoris of the female) is excised. |
| orchidectomy<br>or kih DECK tuh mee | *orchid/o* testis<br>*-ectomy* removal | Removal of one or both testicles. |
| orchiopexy<br>or kee oh PECK see | *orchi/o* testis<br>*-pexy* fixation | Surgical procedure to mobilize an undescended testicle, attaching it to the scrotum. |
| prostatectomy<br>pros tuh TECK tuh mee | *prostat/o* prostate<br>*-ectomy* removal | Removal of the prostate gland. If termed a **radical prostatectomy,** the seminal vesicles and area of vas ampullae of the vas deferens are also removed. |
| transurethral resection of the prostate (TUR, TURP)<br>trans yoo REE thrul | *trans-* through<br>*urethr/o* urethra<br>*-al* pertaining to | Removal of the prostate in sections through a urethral approach (Fig. 7-17). This procedure is the most common type of prostatectomy. |
| sterilization | | Process of rendering a male or female unable to conceive a child while retaining gonads. |
| transurethral incision of the prostate (TUIP)<br>trans yoo REE thruhl | *trans-* through<br>*urethr/o* urethra<br>*-al* pertaining to | Form of prostate surgery involving tiny incisions of the prostate. The prostate is not removed. |

## Terms Related to Therapeutic Interventions—cont'd

| Term | Word Origin | Definition |
|------|-------------|------------|
| **vasectomy**<br>vas SECK tuh mee | *vas/o* vas deferens<br>*-ectomy* removal | Incision, ligation, and cauterization of both of the vas deferens for the purpose of male sterilization (Fig. 7-18). |
| **vasovasostomy**<br>vas zoh vuh SOS tuh mee | *vas/o* vas deferens<br>*-stomy* new opening | Anastomosis of the ends of the vas deferens as a means of reconnecting them to reverse the sterilization procedure. |

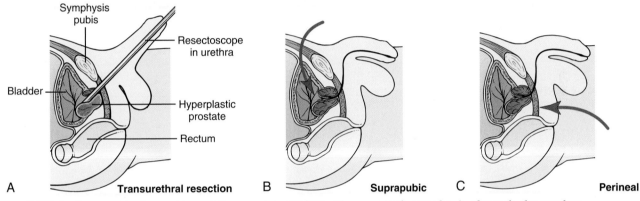

Symphysis pubis

Resectoscope in urethra

Bladder

Hyperplastic prostate

Rectum

A        **Transurethral resection**        B        **Suprapubic**        C        **Perineal**

Fig. 7-17 **A,** Transurethral resection of the prostate (TURP). The approach may be **A,** through the urethra (transurethral), **B,** above the public bone (suprapubic), or **C,** through the perineum (perineal).

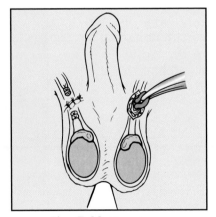

Fig. 7-18 Vasectomy.

## Exercise 7: Therapeutic Interventions

*Match the therapeutic interventions with their definitions.*

_____ 1. removal of both gonads

_____ 2. destruction of tissue

_____ 3. removal of prepuce

_____ 4. removal of testicle

_____ 5. fixation of a testicle

_____ 6. rendering barren

_____ 7. ligation of ductus deferens

A. orchidectomy
B. ablation
C. circumcision
D. sterilization
E. vasectomy
F. castration
G. orchiopexy

*Decode the terms.*

8. vasovasostomy _____

9. transurethral _____

10. prostatectomy _____

## Case Study  Tyson Bernard

Tyson, a 64-year-old real estate broker from Chicago, is visiting his urologist, Dr. Worth, for a prostate exam. Tyson had undergone a PSA test and biopsy 6 months previously, both of which were normal, but his problems with urination have been getting worse, and Dr. Worth decides to perform another PSA test and biopsy.

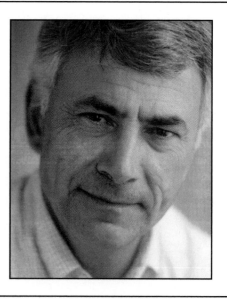

## Case Study    Tyson Bernard

BERNARD, TYSON Q. - 732723 Opened by PEREZ, RAECHAL, MD    _ 🗗 X

Task    Edit    View    Time Scale    Options    Help

🏃📖 ← → 🔥 🥄 🔀 🔀 🔄 ⬆ ■ 📲 🖵 🖴 📑 🕐 🖨 ❓ 🖳 ✒    As Of 11:04    📊 🔍 📋

| BERNARD, TYSON Q. | Age: 64 years<br>DOB: 05/05/1948 | Sex: Male<br>MRN: 732723 | Loc: WHC-SMMC<br>FIN: 3506004 |
|---|---|---|---|

| Reference Text Browser | Form Browser | Medication Profile |

Orders | Last 48 Hours | ED | Lab | Radiology | Assessments | **Surgery** | Clinical Notes | Pt. Info | Pt. Schedule | Task List | I & O | MAR

Flowsheet: Surgery ▼ ...    Level: Operative Report ▼    ● Table  ○ Group  ○ List

◄ ►                                                                                ◄ ►

| Navigator            X |
| ✓   Operative Report |

| Preoperative diagnosis: | Elevated prostate-specific antigen |
| Surgical procedure: | Transrectal ultrasound of prostate |

A 64-year-old male with PSA of 21.8. He had normal biopsy results 6 months ago. The PSA continues to rise incrementally and the patient comes in now for repeat prostate ultrasound with biopsy.

Patient was placed in the left lateral decubitus position. A lubricated ultrasound probe passed per rectum without difficulty. Multiple images of the prostate were obtained, transverse and sagittal axes. Seminal vesicles were nondilated. Prostate capsule intact. There were prostatic calcifications especially toward the base of the gland. At this point, the needle biopsy device was positioned, and under ultrasound guidance, five biopsies were obtained from the right side and five biopsies from the left. Prostate volume measured 71 mL. Patient tolerated the procedure well and was returned to the recovery room in good condition.

PROD | MAHAFC | 03 April 2012 | 11:04

## Exercise 8: Operative Report

1. What was the route of the approach for the ultrasound? _____

2. What is the significance of an elevated PSA? _____

3. The report says that the "seminal vesicles were nondilated." What is the function of the seminal

   vesicles? _____

## PHARMACOLOGY

**alpha-adrenergic inhibitors:** block alpha-1 adrenergic receptors to relax smooth muscle in prostate to improve urinary flow. Examples include tamsulosin (Flomax) and terazosin (Hytrin).

**alternative medicine:** saw palmetto (Serenoa repens), which has been shown to be as effective as finasteride (Propecia) for treatment of symptoms of BPH.

andr/o = male

**androgen hormone inhibitors:** block the conversion of testosterone to the more potent hormone 5-alpha-dihydrotestosterone (DHT) to suppress growth of and even shrink the enlarged prostate. Examples include finasteride (Proscar) and dutasteride (Avodart).

**antibiotics:** treat bacterial infection. Penicillin G, tetracycline, and doxycycline all can be used to treat syphilis.

anti- = against

**antifungals:** treat fungal infection. Butenafine (Lotrimin) and terbinafine (Lamisil) can be used topically for jock-itch.

**antiimpotence agents:** used to alleviate erectile dysfunction. Sildenafil (Viagra), tadalafil (Cialis), and vardenafil (Levitra) are the oral agents currently available. Alprostadil (Caverject) is injected directly into the corpus cavernosum of the penis.

**antivirals:** treat viral infections. Acyclovir (Zovirax) is used to treat genital herpes virus.

## Exercise 9: **Pharmacology**

*Match the pharmacology terms with their definitions.*

_____ 1. class of drug used to treat bacterial infection

_____ 2. class of drug used to treat viral infections

_____ 3. class of drug used to treat erectile dysfunction

_____ 4. an example of a drug used to treat BPH

_____ 5. class of drug used to improve urine flow in patients with BPH

A. antivirals
B. antiimpotence agents
C. alpha-adrenergic inhibitors
D. antibiotics
E. finasteride

Click on **Hear It, Spell It** to practice spelling the diagnostic and therapeutic terms you have learned in this chapter. To practice pronouncing these terms correctly, click on **Hear It, Say It.**

## Abbreviations

| Abbreviation | Definition | Abbreviation | Definition |
|---|---|---|---|
| BPH | benign prostatic hyperplasia/ hypertrophy | PSA | prostate-specific antigen |
| | | STI | sexually transmitted infection |
| Bx | biopsy | TSE | testicular self-examination |
| DRE | digital rectal exam | TUIP | transurethral incision of the prostate |
| FTA-ABS | fluorescent treponemal antibody test | TUR | transurethral resection (of the prostate) |
| Gc | gonococcus | | |
| GCT | germ cell tumor | TURP | transurethral resection of the prostate |
| HPV | human papillomavirus | | |
| HSV-2 | herpes simplex virus-2, herpes genitalis | VD | venereal disease |
| | | VDRL | Venereal Disease Research Laboratory test (for syphilis) |
| NGU | nongonococcal urethritis | | |

## Exercise 10: **Abbreviations**

1. The patient had a TURP to relieve his _____ (answer with another abbreviation).

2. Someone who has a Gc infection has a/an _____ (answer with another abbreviation).

3. A patient tested with VDRL may be suspected of having _____.

4. What is a DRE, and for what is it used? _____

5. If condylomata are present, the patient may have _____.

6. What is the GU system? _____

**⊗ Be Careful!**   *Don't confuse the gastrointestinal* **(GI)** *system with the genitourinary* **(GU)** *system.*

# Chapter Review

Match the word parts to their definitions.

## WORD PART DEFINITIONS

| Prefix/Suffix | | Definition |
|---|---|---|
| a- | 1. _____ | below |
| -cele | 2. _____ | excessive |
| circum- | 3. _____ | tumor, mass |
| -cision | 4. _____ | through |
| crypt- | 5. _____ | inflammation |
| -ectomy | 6. _____ | around |
| -genesis | 7. _____ | process of recording |
| -graphy | 8. _____ | herniation, protrusion |
| hyper- | 9. _____ | without |
| hypo- | 10. _____ | hidden |
| -itis | 11. _____ | removal |
| -oma | 12. _____ | production |
| -plasia | 13. _____ | process of cutting |
| -spadias | 14. _____ | a rent or tear |
| trans- | 15. _____ | formation |

| Combining Form | | Definition |
|---|---|---|
| andr/o | 16. _____ | male |
| balan/o | 17. _____ | semen |
| epididym/o | 18. _____ | glans penis |
| hydr/o | 19. _____ | spermatozoon |
| olig/o | 20. _____ | epididymis |
| orchid/o | 21. _____ | testis |
| pen/i | 22. _____ | foreskin |
| phall/o | 23. _____ | seminal vesicle |
| plethysm/o | 24. _____ | penis |
| preputi/o | 25. _____ | scrotum |
| prostat/o | 26. _____ | vas deferens |
| scrot/o | 27. _____ | scanty |
| semin/i | 28. _____ | prostate |
| sperm/o | 29. _____ | volume |
| vas/o | 30. _____ | water, fluid |
| vesicul/o | 31. _____ | animal |
| zo/o | 32. _____ | penis |

# WORDSHOP

| Prefixes | Combining Forms | Suffixes |
|----------|-----------------|----------|
| a- | andr/o | -cision |
| an- | balan/o | -ectomy |
| circum- | epididym/o | -genesis |
| crypt- | olig/o | -ia |
| dys- | orchid/o | -ism |
| e- | orchi/o | -itis |
| post- | orch/o | -logy |
| pre- | prostat/o | -pexy |
| syn- | spermat/o | -plasty |
| | sperm/o | -stomy |
| | vas/o | -tomy |
| | vesicul/o | |
| | zo/o | |

Build the following terms by combining the above word parts. Some word parts may be used more than once. Some won't be used at all. The number in parenthesis is the number of word parts needed to build the terms.

| Definition | Term |
|------------|------|
| 1. condition of scanty sperm (3) | |
| 2. inflammation of a seminal vesicle (2) | |
| 3. fixation of a testicle (2) | |
| 4. surgical repair of the glans penis (2) | |
| 5. removal of the prostate (2) | |
| 6. inflammation of the glans penis (2) | |
| 7. the study of the male reproductive system (2) | |
| 8. production of sperm (2) | |
| 9. condition of no animals (life) in the sperm (4) | |
| 10. process of cutting around (2) | |
| 11. condition of a "hidden" testicle (3) | |
| 12. inflammation of the vessels that store sperm (2) | |
| 13. removal of the epididymis (2) | |
| 14. condition of no testicle (3) | |
| 15. removal of a testicle (2) | |

*Sort the terms below into the correct categories.*

## TERM SORTING

| Anatomy and Physiology | Pathology | Diagnostic Procedures | Therapeutic Interventions |
|---|---|---|---|
|  |  |  |  |
|  |  |  |  |
|  |  |  |  |
|  |  |  |  |
|  |  |  |  |
|  |  |  |  |
|  |  |  |  |
|  |  |  |  |
|  |  |  |  |
|  |  |  |  |
|  |  |  |  |

ablation                epididymovesiculography        orchiopexy          sterilization

anorchism               gametes                        plethysmography     TSE

castration              genitalia                      prepuce             TUIP

circumcision            glans penis                    prostatectomy       TURP

corpora cavernosa       gonorrhea                      semen               tunica vaginalis

ductus deferens         Gram stain                     seminoma            vasectomy

epididymis              oligospermia                   sperm analysis

epididymitis            orchidectomy                   spermatogenesis

*Raplace the highlighted words with the correct term.*

## TRANSLATIONS

1. A **count and analysis of the number and health of spermatozoa** revealed a **condition of temporary or permanent deficiency of sperm in the seminal fluid** that caused the couple's infertility.

2. Mr. Steinman's **abnormal enlargement of the prostate gland** was treated with a **form of prostate surgery involving tiny incision of the prostate.**

3. Sam's painful testicular swelling was diagnosed as **an inflammation of the epididymis.**

4. The physician suggested a **surgical procedure in which the prepuce of the penis is excised** to treat the patient's **congenital condition of tightening of the prepuce around the glans penis.**

5. Dr. Adams explained that **the painless, red, highly infectious pustule** was the first stage of **a multistage STI caused by the** spirochete *Treponema pallidum* bacterium.

6. The physician ordered **a laboratory method of staining microorganisms as a means of identifying them as gram-negative or gram-positive** to diagnose the patient's disease caused by the gram-negative diplococcus *Neisseria gonorrhoeae* bacterium.

7. When Ken remarried, he decided to have his **incision, ligation, and cauterization of both of the vas deferens** reversed and was scheduled for a/an **anatomosis of the ends of the vas deferens as a means of reconnecting them.**

8. Hunter underwent a **removal of one or both testicles** to treat his **condition in which the testicles fail to descend into the scrotum before birth.**

9. As part of a work-up for **the inability to achieve or sustain a penile erection for sexual intercourse,** the patient underwent **the measurement of changes in volume of organs or body parts.**

10. The patient was treated for the **genital warts** that accompanied his **form of the herpesvirus transmitted through sexual contact, causing painful eruptions.**

11. Harold was diagnosed with a/an **germ cell tumor that develops from the cells that form sperm.**

12. **The healthcare specialist who treats male urinary and reproductive disorders** treated Mr. Mason's **abnormal dilation of the veins of the spermatic cord.**

13. Tanner was embarrassed about his **enlargement of breast tissue in the male.**

14. Robert's **condition of no living sperm in the semen, following a vasectomy** was the result of **the process of rendering a male unable to to conceive a child while retaining gonads.**

## *Case Study* Sam Trudell

Sam Trudell, a 67-year-old retired postman, has come to see Adam Duncan, a physician assistant (PA) in a large urologist practice. Mr. Trudell has been suffering from a decreased ability to urinate and suspects he has another urinary tract infection (UTI), the second in as many months. Adam tells Mr. Trudell that he suspects an enlarged prostate is causing his problem.

Adam explains that standard blood and urine laboratory tests are necessary, along with a digital rectal examination (DRE) and a prostate-specific antigen (PSA) test. Diagnostic imaging will probably include an intravenous urogram (IVU) or a renal ultrasound. Mr. Trudell is not overjoyed about the DRE, but is anxious to get some relief.

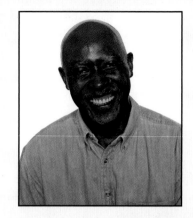

Mr. Trudell's test results come back positive for benign prostatic hyperplasia (BPH) and Sam's urologist tells him he will need to have surgery.

---

TRUDELL, SAMUEL H. - 453768 Opened by JAMES, ZACHARY MD    — 🗗 ☒

Task   Edit   View   Time Scale   Options   Help

As Of 16:24

| **TRUDELL, SAMUEL H.** | **Age: 67 years** | **Sex: Male** | **Loc: WHC-SMMC** |
| | **DOB: 10/17/1945** | **MRN: 453768** | **FIN: 3506004** |

Reference Text Browser | Form Browser | Medication Profile

Orders | Last 48 Hours | ED | Lab | Radiology | Assessments | **Surgery** | Clinical Notes | Pt. Info | Pt. Schedule | Task List | I & O | MAR

Flowsheet: Surgery ▼ ...   Level: Operative Report ▼      ⦿ Table  ○ Group  ○ List

**Navigator** ☒

✓ Operative Report

Preoperative Diagnosis: benign prostatic hyperplasia, urinary retention
Postoperative Diagnosis: benign prostatic hyperplasia, urinary retention

   History of Present Illness: Patient is a 67-year-old African American male with past medical history of hiatal hernia with gastritis, BPH, and UTI with a history of urinary retention. Patient denies dysuria, incontinence, hematuria, urgency, and urinary frequency. Urinary retention has been managed with a Foley catheter after a bout of UTI on past admission.

   Operation: TURP
   Anesthesia: Spinal
   Procedure: The patient was brought to the operating room, was properly identified, and, following adequate administration of spinal anesthetic, was placed in the dorsal lithotomy position, and the genitalia prepared with Betadine and draped in the sterile manner.

   A #26 French scope was used to inspect the urethra and bladder. Bilobar hypertrophy of the prostate was easily identified.

   A transurethral resection of the prostate was carried out in the usual fashion. Chips of prostatic tissue were evacuated from the bladder with a Toomey syringe. Hemostasis was achieved with a Bovie. On final inspection, the urethra was free of obstruction, and both the external sphincter and the ureteral orifices were intact. A Foley catheter was attached for drainage, and the patient was sent to the recovery room in satisfactory condition.

PROD | MAHAFC | 01 August 2012 | 16:24

### Operative Report

1. The patient's past medical history included BPH. Describe this condition.

   _____

   _____

2. Define what the patient does *not* complain of:

   A. dysuria_____

   B. incontinence _____

   C. urgency _____

   D. urinary frequency _____

   E. hematuria _____

3. How many lobes of the prostate were enlarged? _____

4. What does the abbreviation TURP mean? _____

5. If this patient had had periprostatic lesions, where would they have been?

   _____

---

For more interactive learning, go to the Shiland Evolve site, and click on:
- **Whack a Word Part** to review male reproductive word parts.
- **Wheel of Terminology** and **Word Shop** to practice word building.
- **Tournament of Terminology** to test your knowledge of male reproductive terms.
- **Terminology Triage** to practice sorting male reproductive terms into categories.

# 8

*A woman's health is her capital.*
**—Harriet Beecher Stowe**

## OBJECTIVES

- Recognize and use terms related to the anatomy and physiology of the female reproductive system.
- Recognize and use terms related to the pathology of the female reproductive system.
- Recognize and use terms related to the diagnostic procedures for the female reproductive system.
- Recognize and use terms related to the therapeutic interventions for the female reproductive system.

# Female Reproductive System

## CHAPTER AT A GLANCE

Use this list of key word parts and terms to assess your knowledge. Check off the ones you have mastered.

### ANATOMY AND PHYSIOLOGY

- [ ] amnion
- [ ] areola
- [ ] Bartholin glands
- [ ] breast
- [ ] cervix
- [ ] chorion
- [ ] clitoris
- [ ] corpus luteum
- [ ] endometrium
- [ ] estrogen
- [ ] fallopian tubes
- [ ] fetus
- [ ] fimbriae
- [ ] gestation
- [ ] hCG
- [ ] hymen
- [ ] labia majora
- [ ] labia minora
- [ ] mammary papilla
- [ ] menarche
- [ ] menopause
- [ ] menstruation
- [ ] mons pubis
- [ ] myometrium
- [ ] ovary
- [ ] ovulation
- [ ] ovum
- [ ] parturition
- [ ] perimetrium
- [ ] perineum
- [ ] placenta
- [ ] progesterone
- [ ] puerperium
- [ ] rectouterine pouch
- [ ] uterus
- [ ] vagina
- [ ] vulva
- [ ] zygote

## KEY WORD PARTS

### PREFIXES

- [ ] an-
- [ ] dys-
- [ ] multi-
- [ ] nulli-
- [ ] poly-
- [ ] pre-

### SUFFIXES

- [ ] -centesis
- [ ] -graphy
- [ ] -gravida
- [ ] -lysis
- [ ] -para
- [ ] -pexy
- [ ] -plasia
- [ ] -ptosis
- [ ] -rrhagia
- [ ] -rrhea
- [ ] -scopy
- [ ] -tocia
- [ ] -tomy

### COMBINING FORMS

- [ ] amni/o
- [ ] cervic/o
- [ ] chori/o
- [ ] colp/o
- [ ] culd/o
- [ ] endometri/o
- [ ] episi/o
- [ ] hyster/o
- [ ] mamm/o
- [ ] mast/o
- [ ] men/o
- [ ] metr/o, metri/o
- [ ] nat/o
- [ ] olig/o
- [ ] oophor/o
- [ ] part/o
- [ ] puerper/o
- [ ] salping/o
- [ ] thel/e
- [ ] vagin/o
- [ ] vulv/o

## KEY TERMS

- ☐ AFP test
- ☐ amenorrhea
- ☐ amniocentesis
- ☐ anovulation
- ☐ antenatal
- ☐ cervical dysplasia
- ☐ cervicitis
- ☐ cesarean section (CS)
- ☐ choriocarcinoma
- ☐ colposcopy
- ☐ culdocentesis

- ☐ dysmenorrhea
- ☐ ectopic pregnancy
- ☐ endometriosis
- ☐ episiotomy
- ☐ erythroblastosis fetalis
- ☐ hysteropexy
- ☐ hysteroptosis
- ☐ hysterosalpingography
- ☐ leiomyoma
- ☐ mammography
- ☐ mastopexy

- ☐ meconium
- ☐ menorrhagia
- ☐ metrorrhagia
- ☐ multigravida
- ☐ nullipara
- ☐ oligohydramnios
- ☐ oophorectomy
- ☐ polycystic ovary
  syndrome (PCOS)
- ☐ postpartum
- ☐ preeclampsia

- ☐ puerperal
- ☐ salpingitis
- ☐ salpingolysis
- ☐ theleplasty
- ☐ tubal ligation
- ☐ uterine artery
  embolization (UAE)
- ☐ vulvovaginitis

---

**female** = gynec/o

**ovum** = o/o, ov/o, ov/i, ovul/o

**gynecologist**
  gynec/o = female
  -logist = one who
  specializes in the study of

### ⊗ Be Careful!

*The term **germ** comes from the Latin word for sprout or fetus, here referring to its reproductive nature; however, it can also mean a type of microorganism that can cause disease.*

**menarche**
  men/o = menstruation
  -arche = beginning

**menopause**
  men/o = menstruation
  -pause = stop, cease

## FUNCTIONS OF THE FEMALE REPRODUCTIVE SYSTEM

The role of the female reproductive system is to keep one's genetic material in the world's gene pool. Through sexual reproduction, the 23 pairs of chromosomes of the **female** must join with 23 pairs of chromosomes from a male to create new life. To do this, the system must produce the hormones necessary to provide a hospitable environment for the **ovum** (OH vum) (*pl.* **ova**), the female gamete, to connect with the spermatozoon, the male gamete, for fertilization to occur. Once an egg is fertilized, it is nurtured throughout its growth process until the delivery of the neonate (newborn).

## SPECIALTIES/SPECIALISTS

**Obstetricians** are medical doctors who treat women during pregnancy, deliver infants, and follow women through the postpartum period. Many obstetricians are also trained as **gynecologists,** medical doctors who monitor health and treat diseases of the female reproductive system. The medical specialties for these fields are called **obstetrics** and **gynecology,** respectively.

  **Midwives** are healthcare providers, usually nurses, who assist women through labor and delivery.

  **Doulas** care for a pregnant mother through labor and delivery and/or after delivery provide care for the mother and baby.

## ANATOMY AND PHYSIOLOGY

### Internal Anatomy

Because the primary function of the female reproductive system is to create new life through the successful fertilization of an ovum, discussion of this system begins with this very important germ cell.

### Ova and Ovaries

From **menarche** (meh NAR kee), the first menstrual period, to **menopause** (MEN oh poz), the cessation of menstruation, mature ova are produced by the female gonads, the **ovaries** (OH vuh reez) (Fig. 8-1). The ovaries are small, almond-shaped, paired organs located on either side of the uterus in the female pelvic cavity. They are attached to the uterus by the ovarian ligaments and lie close to the opening of the **fallopian** (fuh LOH pee un) **tubes**, the ducts that

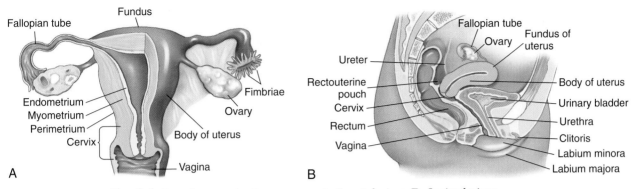

Fig. 8-1 Female reproductive organs, **A,** Frontal view. **B,** Sagittal view.

convey the ova from the ovaries to the uterus. Approximately every 28 days, in response to hormonal stimulation, the ovaries alternate releasing one ovum. This egg matures in one of the **follicles** (FALL ih kuls), which are tiny secretory sacs within an ovary. The **pituitary** (pih TOO ih tair ee) **gland**, an endocrine gland located in the cranial cavity, secretes two hormones that influence the activity of the ovaries. **Follicle-stimulating hormone (FSH)** causes the ovarian follicles to begin to mature and secrete estrogen. Because of the increase of estrogen in the bloodstream, **luteinizing** (LOO tin eye zing) **hormone (LH)** is released by the anterior lobe of the pituitary gland. LH then stimulates the follicle to mature and release its ovum **(ovulation)** and aids in the development of the **corpus luteum** (KORE pus LOO tee um). The corpus luteum is then responsible for secreting **estrogen** (ES troh jen) and **progesterone** (proh JES teh roan), hormones responsible for female secondary sex characteristics and the cyclical maintenance of the uterus for pregnancy.

If two eggs are released and fertilized, the resulting twins will be termed **fraternal,** because they will be no more or less alike in appearance than brothers (or sisters) occurring in sequential pregnancies. If, however, one of the fertilized eggs divides and forms two infants, these are **identical** twins, who share the same appearance and genetic material.

### Fallopian Tubes

Once the mature ovum has been released, it is drawn into the **fimbriae** (FIM bree ee) (*sing.* fimbria), the feathery ends of the fallopian tube (see Fig. 8-1). These tubes, about the width of a pencil, and about as long (10 to 12 cm), transport the ovum to the uterus. The fallopian tubes (also called *oviducts* or *uterine tubes*) and the ovaries make up what is called the **uterine adnexa** (YOO tuh rin add NECKS ah), or accessory organs of the uterus.

### Uterus

Once the ovum has traversed the fallopian tube, it is secreted into the uterus, or womb, a pear-shaped organ that is designed to nurture a developing embryo/ fetus (see Fig. 8-1). The uterus is composed of three layers: the outer layer, called the **perimetrium** (pair ih MEE tree um), or serosa; the **myometrium** (mye oh MEE tree um), or muscle layer; and the **endometrium** (en doh MEE tree um), the lining of the uterus. As a whole, it can be divided into several areas. The body or **corpus** (which means *body* in Latin) is the large central area; the **fundus** (FUN dus) is the raised area at the top of the uterus between the outlets for the fallopian tubes; and the **cervix** (SUR vicks) is the narrowed lower area, often referred to as the neck of the uterus.

### Rectouterine Pouch

An area associated with the female reproductive system that does not play a direct role in its function, the **rectouterine pouch** (reck toh YOO tur in), is

---

**menstruation** = men/o, menstru/o

**ovary** = oophor/o, ovari/o

**uterus** = hyster/o, metri/o, metr/o, uter/o

**fallopian tube** = salping/o, -salpinx

**ovulation**
  ovul/o = egg
  -ation = process of

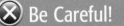

## Be Careful!

*Do not confuse* **ureter/o**, *which means the ureter, with* **uter/o**, *which means uterus.*

---

**perimetrium** = perimetri/o

**myometrium** = myometri/o

**endometrium** = endometri/o

**fundus** = fund/o

**cervix** = cervic/o

**rectouterine pouch** = culd/o

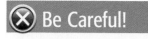 **Be Careful!**

*Don't confuse* **culd/o**, *which means the rectouterine pouch, with* **colp/o**, *which means vagina.*

**vagina** = colp/o, vagin/o

also called **Douglas' cul-de-sac,** a space in the pelvic cavity between the uterus and the rectum.

### Vagina

If the ovum does not become fertilized by a spermatozoon, the corpus luteum stops producing estrogen and progesterone, and the lining of the uterus is shed through the muscular, tubelike vagina by the process of **menstruation (menses).** The vagina extends from the uterine cervix to the vulva (the external genitalia).

## Exercise 1: Combining Forms for Internal Female Genitalia

*Match the following. There may be more than one answer per question. Answers may be used more than once.*

____ 1. culd/o      ____ 5. colp/o      ____ 9. ovari/o

____ 2. oophor/o    ____ 6. ov/o       ____ 10. uter/o

____ 3. metr/o      ____ 7. salping/o  ____ 11. vagin/o

____ 4. hyster/o    ____ 8. cervic/o   ____ 12. men/o

A. uterus
B. vagina
C. fallopian tube
D. cervix
E. rectouterine pouch
F. ovary
G. female germ cell
H. menstruation, menses

*Decode the terms.*

13. supracervical _____

14. intrauterine _____

15. premenstrual _____

16. transvaginal _____

## Exercise 2: Internal Female Anatomy

*Label the drawings below with the correct anatomy and combining forms where appropriate.*

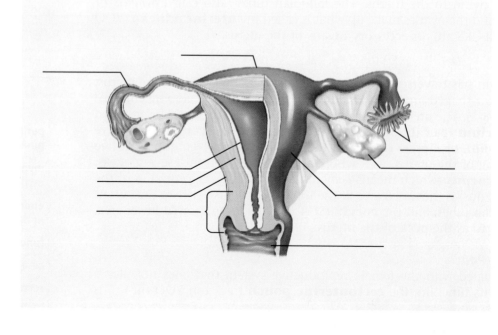

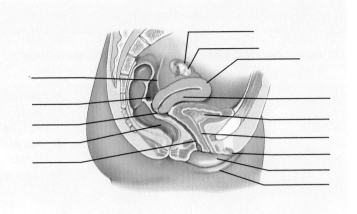

⊗ Be Careful!

*The combining form* **cervic/o** *has two meanings: the neck and the cervix (the neck of the uterus).*

## External Genitalia

The external female genitalia collectively are called the **vulva** (VUL vah) (Fig. 8-2). The vulva consists of the vaginal opening, or **orifice** (ORE ih fis); the membrane covering the opening, or **hymen** (HYE men); the two folds of skin surrounding the opening, or **labia majora** (LAY bee ah muh JOR ah) (the larger folds) and **labia minora** (LAY bee ah min NOR uh) (the smaller folds); the **clitoris** (KLIT uh ris), which is sensitive, erectile tissue; and the **perineum** (pair ih NEE um), the area between the opening of the vagina and the anus. The paired glands in the vulva that secrete a mucous lubricant for the vagina are the **Bartholin** (BAR toh lin) **glands.** The **mons pubis** (mons PYOO bis) is a fatty cushion of tissue over the pubic bone.

| | |
|---|---|
| **vulva** = vulv/o, episi/o | |
| **hymen** = hymen/o | |
| **labia** = labi/o | |
| **clitoris** = clitorid/o | |
| **perineum** = perine/o | |
| **Bartholin gland** = bartholin/o | |

## The Breast

The **breasts,** or mammary glands, function to secrete milk. The breast tissue is composed of glandular **milk**-producing, fatty, and fibrous tissue. The **nipple** of the breast is the **mammary papilla** (MAM uh ree puh PILL ah) (*pl.* **papillae**), and the darker colored skin surrounding the nipple is the **areola** (ah REE oh lah) (*pl.* **areolae**) (Fig. 8-3).

| | |
|---|---|
| **breast** = mamm/o, mast/o | |
| **milk** = lact/o, galact/o | |
| **nipple** = papill/o, thel/e | |

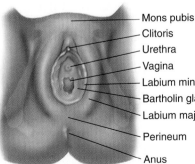

Mons pubis
Clitoris
Urethra
Vagina
Labium minora
Bartholin gland
Labium majora
Perineum
Anus

**Fig. 8-2** Female external genitalia

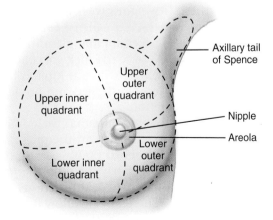

Axillary tail of Spence

Upper outer quadrant

Upper inner quadrant

Nipple

Areola

Lower outer quadrant

Lower inner quadrant

**Fig. 8-3** Breast quadrants.

## Exercise 3: External Female Genitalia and the Breast

*Match the following combining forms with their meanings. There may be more than one answer.*

____ 1. vulva

____ 2. nipple

____ 3. hymen

____ 4. milk

____ 5. labia

____ 6. breast

____ 7. perineum

____ 8. Bartholin glands

____ 9. clitoris

A. galact/o
B. episi/o
C. bartholin/o
D. papill/o
E. mamm/o
F. thel/e
G. hymen/o

H. perine/o
I. lact/o
J. vulv/o
K. mast/o
L. labi/o
M. clitorid/o

*Decode the terms.*

10. interlabial _____

11. intramammary _____

You can review the anatomy of the female reproductive system by clicking on **Body Spectrum Electronic Anatomy Coloring Book → Reproductive → Female.**

## Pregnancy And Delivery

**pregnancy** = gravid/o, -gravida, -cyesis

**Pregnancy** begins with the fertilization of an ovum by a spermatozoon, often in the fallopian tube, as the ovum travels toward the uterus. Conception is usually the result of sexual intercourse (also termed *copulation* or *coitus*). However, other methods of conception are possible if the couple has difficulty conceiving. These methods are discussed in the section on therapeutic interventions and may include artificial insemination and in vitro fertilization.

The fertilized egg, or **zygote** (ZYE gote), divides as it moves through the fallopian tube to the uterus, where it becomes implanted. From the third to the eighth week of life, it is called an **embryo** (EM bree oh). From the ninth through the thirty-eighth week of life (a normal length for **gestation** [jes TAY shun], or pregnancy), it is called a **fetus** (FEE tus). During implantation, the zygote functions as an endocrine gland by secreting **human chorionic gonadotropin (hCG)** (kore ee AH nick goh nad doh TROH pin). The function of the hormone is to prevent the corpus luteum from deteriorating, which allows the continued production of estrogen and progesterone to support the pregnancy and prevent menstruation.

**fetus** = fet/o

At the same time that the embryo is developing, extraembryonic membranes are forming to sustain the pregnancy: Two of these, the **amnion** (AM nee on) and the **chorion** (KORE ee on), form the inner and outer sacs that contain the embryo (Fig. 8-4). The fluid that forms inside the amnion is the **amniotic** (am nee AH tick) **fluid.** It functions to cushion the embryo, protect it against temperature changes, and allow it to move. The **placenta** (plah SEN tah) is a highly vascular structure that acts as a physical communication between the mother

**amnion** = amni/o, amnion/o, -amnios

**chorion** = chori/o, chorion/o

**placenta** = placent/o

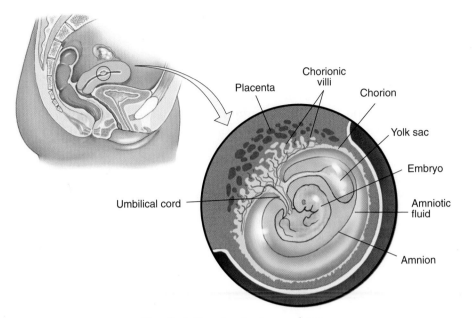

Fig. 8-4 The developing embryo.

and the embryo. The **umbilical** (um BILL ih kul) **cord** is the tissue that connects the embryo to the placenta (and hence to the mother). When the baby is delivered, the umbilical cord is cut, and the baby is then dependent on his/her own body for all physiologic processes. The remaining "scar" is the **umbilicus** (um BILL il kus), or navel. The delivery of an infant is termed **parturition** (par tur RIH shun).

A woman who is pregnant for the first time is a **primigravida.** If she has two or more pregnancies, she is referred to as a **multigravida.** If she has never been pregnant, she is a **nulligravida.**

A woman who has delivered her first baby is referred to as a **primipara.** If she delivers more than one baby, she is a **multipara.** A woman who has never delivered a child is referred to as a **nullipara.**

The abbreviation GPA is used in obstetric notation to indicate the *number of pregnancies* (G for gravida), *the number of deliveries* of a live or stillborn infant at more than 20 weeks of gestation (P for para), and *the number of miscarriages/ abortions* that occur before 20 weeks of gestation (A for abortion). A woman described as G4P3A1 has had 4 pregnancies, 3 deliveries, and 1 abortion.

The terms **antenatal** and **prenatal** both mean "pertaining to before birth," and **postnatal** means "Pertaining to after birth." **Antepartum** means "before delivery," and **postpartum** means "after delivery." The **puerperium** is the approximate 6-week time period after childbirth.

Babies born before 37 weeks are referred to as *premature infants*. Those weighing less than 2500 g (5 lb, 8 oz) are referred to as *low–birth-weight infants*.

Each pregnancy is divided into three equal trimesters of 3 months each. The first trimester is week 1-14, the second trimester is week 15-28, and the third trimester is week 29 to the day of delivery.

---

**umbilicus** = omphal/o, umbilic/o

---

**parturition** = part/o, -para, -partum, -tocia

---

**birth, born** = nat/o

---

**primigravida**
  primi- = first
  -gravida = pregnancy

---

**multigravida**
  multi- = many
  -gravida = pregnancy

---

**nulligravida**
  nulli- = none
  -gravida = pregnancy

---

**primipara**
  primi- = first
  -para = delivery

---

**multipara**
  multi- = many
  -para = delivery

---

**nullipara**
  nulli- = none
  -para = delivery

---

**puerper/o** = childbirth

## ⊘ Exercise 4: Pregnancy

*Match the word parts with their correct meanings. There may be more than one answer.*

____ 1. pregnancy

____ 2. navel

____ 3. labor, delivery

____ 4. organ of
communication
between mother
and baby

____ 5. inner sac that
encircles the
embryo

____ 6. outer sac that
encircles the
embryo

____ 7. fetus

____ 8. birth

A. -tocia
B. omphal/o
C. gravid/o
D. amni/o
E. umbilic/o
F. chori/o
G. nat/o
H. -para

I. -cyesis
J. chorion/o
K. -gravida
L. fet/o
M. placent/o

*Decode the terms.*

9. antenatal  _____

10. periumbilical  _____

## ⊘ Exercise 5: Pregnancy

*Label the drawing with the correct anatomic terms and combining forms where appropriate.*

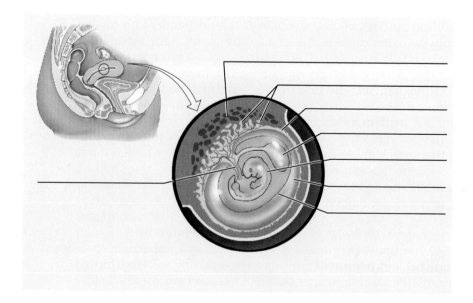

⊖   Choose **Hear It, Spell It** to practice spelling the anatomy and physiology terms you have learned in this chapter. To
practice pronouncing anatomy and physiology terms choose **Hear It, Say It.**

The following word part tables can be used as a reference and a review of the anatomy and physiology word parts you've learned for the female reproductive system.

## Combining and Adjective Forms for the Anatomy and Physiology of the Female Reproductive System

| Meaning | Combining Form | Adjective Form |
|---|---|---|
| amnion | amni/o, amnion/o | amniotic |
| Bartholin gland | bartholin/o | |
| birth, born | nat/o | natal |
| breast | mamm/o, mast/o | mammary |
| cervix | cervic/o | cervical |
| chorion | chori/o, chorion/o | chorionic |
| clitoris | clitorid/o | |
| endometrium | endometri/o | endometrial |
| fallopian tube | salping/o, fallopi/o | salpingeal, fallopian |
| female | gynec/o | |
| fetus | fet/o | fetal |
| fundus | fund/o | fundal |
| hymen | hymen/o | hymenal |
| labia | labi/o | labial |
| menstruation, menses | men/o | menstrual |
| milk | lact/o, galact/o | lactic, galactic |
| myometrium | myometri/o | myometrial |
| nipple | papill/o, thel/e | papillary, thelial |
| ovary | oophor/o, ovari/o | ovarian |
| ovum, egg | ov/o, ov/i, ovul/o, o/o | |
| parturition, delivery | part/o | |
| perimetrium | perimetri/o | perimetrial |
| perineum | perine/o | perineal |
| placenta | placent/o | placental |
| pregnancy | gravid/o | |
| puerperium | puerper/o | |
| rectouterine pouch | culd/o | |
| umbilicus, navel | omphal/o, umbilic/o | umbilical, omphalic |
| uterus | hyster/o, metri/o, metr/o, uter/o | uterine |
| vagina | colp/o, vagin/o | vaginal |
| vulva | vulv/o, episi/o | vulvar |

## Prefixes for the Anatomy and Physiology of the Female Reproductive System

| Prefix | Meaning |
|--------|---------|
| endo- | within |
| multi- | many |
| neo- | new |
| nulli- | none |
| peri- | surrounding |
| primi- | first |

## Suffixes for the Anatomy and Physiology of the Female Reproductive System

| Suffix | Meaning |
|--------|---------|
| -arche | beginning |
| -ation | process of |
| -gravida, -cyesis | pregnancy, gestation |
| -ic, -al, -ine | pertaining to |
| -ician, -logist | one who specializes in the study of |
| -para, -partum, -tocia | delivery, parturition |
| -pause | stop, cease |
| -salpinx | fallopian tube |
| -um | structure |

# PATHOLOGY

## Terms Related to Disorders of the Ovaries

| Term | Word Origin | Definition |
|------|-------------|------------|
| **anovulation**<br>an ah vyoo LAY shun | *an-* without<br>*ovul/o* ovum<br>*-ation* process of | Failure of the ovary to release an ovum. |
| **oophoritis**<br>oh off oh RYE tis | *oophor/o* ovary<br>*-itis* inflammation | Inflammation of an ovary. |
| **polycystic ovary syndrome (PCOS)**<br>pall ee SIS tick | *poly-* many<br>*cyst/o* sac, cyst<br>*-ic* pertaining to | Bilateral presence of numerous cysts, caused by a hormonal abnormality leading to the secretion of androgens. Can cause acne, facial hair, and infertility. |

## Terms Related to Disorders of the Fallopian Tubes

| Term | Word Origin | Definition |
|------|-------------|------------|
| adhesions, fallopian tubes<br>add HEE zhuns | | Scar tissue that binds surfaces together; a sequela of pelvic inflammatory disease (PID), in which, as a result of the inflammation, the tubes heal closed, causing infertility. |
| hematosalpinx<br>hee mah toh SAL pinks | *hemat/o* blood<br>*-salpinx* fallopian tube | Condition of blood in a fallopian tube. |
| hydrosalpinx<br>hye droh SAL pinks | *hydr/o* fluid, water<br>*-salpinx* fallopian tube | Condition of fluid in a fallopian tube. |
| pyosalpinx<br>pye oh SAL pinks | *py/o* pus<br>*-salpinx* fallopian tube | Condition of pus in a fallopian tube. |
| salpingitis<br>sal pin JYE tis | *salping/o* fallopian tube<br>*-itis* inflammation | Inflammation of a fallopian tube. |

To view an animation of PID, click on **Animations.**

## Exercise 6: Ovarian and Fallopian Tube Disorders

*Fill in the blanks with the terms provided.*

**polycystic ovary syndrome, adhesions, hematosalpinx, salpingitis, hydrosalpinx, pyosalpinx**

1. condition of pus in the fallopian tubes _____

2. scar tissue that binds surfaces together _____

3. inflammation of the fallopian tubes _____

4. condition of fluid in the fallopian tubes _____

5. condition of multiple cysts on both ovaries leading to acne, facial hair, and infertility

_____

*Decode the terms.*

6. oophoritis _____

7. anovulation _____

8. hematosalpinx _____

## Terms Related to Disorders of the Uterus

| Term | Word Origin | Definition |
|------|-------------|------------|
| endometritis<br>en doh mee TRY tis | *endometri/o* endometrium<br>*-itis* inflammation | Inflammation of the inner layer of the uterus, the endometrium. |
| endometriosis<br>en doh mee tree OH sis | *endometri/o* endometrium<br>*-osis* abnormal condition | Condition in which the tissue that makes up the lining of the uterus, the endometrium, is found ectopically (outside the uterus); causes are unknown (Fig. 8-5). |
| hysteroptosis<br>hiss tur op TOH sis | *hyster/o* uterus<br>*-ptosis* drooping, sagging | Falling or sliding of the uterus from its normal location in the body. Also called **uterine prolapse** (Fig. 8-6). |
| retroflexion of uterus<br>reh troh FLECK shun | *retro-* backward<br>*flex/o* bend<br>*-ion* process | Condition in which the body of the uterus is bent backward, forming an angle with the cervix. |

## Terms Related to Disorders of the Cervix

| Term | Word Origin | Definition |
|------|-------------|------------|
| cervicitis<br>sur vih SYE tis | *cervic/o* cervix<br>*-itis* inflammation | Inflammation of the cervix. |
| leukorrhea<br>loo kuh REE ah | *leuk/o* white<br>*-rrhea* discharge, flow | Whitish discharge usually resulting from an inflammation of the cervix. |

## Exercise 7: Disorders of the Uterus and Cervix

*Fill in the blanks with the terms provided.*

**leukorrhea, endometriosis, retroflexion of uterus**

1. white cervical discharge _____

2. uterus bent toward spine _____

3. condition of ectopic endometrial tissue _____

*Decode the terms.*

4. endometritis _____

5. hysteroptosis _____

6. cervicitis _____

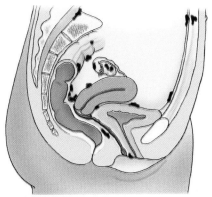

Fig. 8-5 Black spots indicate common sites of endometriosis.

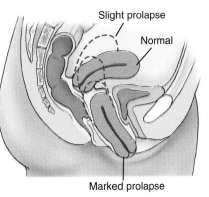

Fig. 8-6 Prolapse of uterus.

## Terms Related to Disorders of the Vagina and Vulva

| Term | Word Origin | Definition |
|------|-------------|------------|
| **vaginal prolapse**<br>PRO laps | *pro-* forward<br>*-lapse* fall | Downward displacement of the vagina. Also called colpoptosis (kohl pop TOH sis). |
| **vaginitis**<br>vaj ih NYE tis | *vagin/o* vagina<br>*-itis* inflammation | Inflammation of the vagina. |
| **vulvitis**<br>vul VYE tis | *vulv/o* vulva<br>*-itis* inflammation | Inflammation of the external female genitalia. |
| **vulvodynia**<br>vul voh DIN ee ah | *vulv/o* vulva<br>*-dynia* pain | Idiopathic syndrome of nonspecific complaints of pain of the vulva. |
| **vulvovaginitis**<br>vul voh vaj ih NYE tis | *vulv/o* vulva<br>*vagin/o* vagina<br>*-itis* inflammation | Inflammation of the vulva and the vagina. |

## Terms Related to Disorders of the Breast

| Term | Word Origin | Definition |
|------|-------------|------------|
| **galactorrhea**<br>gah lack toh REE ah | *galact/o* milk<br>*-rrhea* flow, discharge | An abnormal discharge of milk from the breasts. |
| **mastitis**<br>mass TYE tis | *mast/o* breast<br>*-itis* inflammation | Inflammation of the breast. |
| **mastoptosis**<br>mass top TOH sis | *mast/o* breast<br>*-ptosis* drooping, sagging | Downward displacement of the breasts. |
| **thelitis**<br>thee LYE tis | *thel/e* nipple<br>*-itis* inflammation | Inflammation of the nipples; also referred to as **acromastitis** (ack kroh mass TYE tis), meaning an inflammation of the extremities of the breast. |

## Exercise 8: Disorders of the Vagina, Vulva, and Breasts

*Fill in the blanks with the terms provided.*

**vulvitis, thelitis, mastitis, vulvodynia, vaginal prolapse, vulvovaginitis**

1. also known as colpoptosis _____

2. inflammation of the external female genitalia _____

3. pain of external female genitalia _____

4. also known as acromastitis _____

5. inflammation of the breast _____

6. inflammation of female external genitalia and vagina _____

*Decode the terms.*

7. galactorrhea _____

8. mastoptosis _____

9. vaginitis _____

## Terms Related to Menstrual Disorders

| Term | Word Origin | Definition |
|---|---|---|
| **amenorrhea**<br>ah men uh REE ah | *a-* without<br>*men/o* menses<br>*-rrhea* discharge | Lack of menstrual flow. This is a normal, expected condition before puberty, after menopause, and during pregnancy. |
| **dysfunctional uterine bleeding (DUB)** | | Abnormal uterine bleeding not caused by a tumor, inflammation, or pregnancy. **PMB** stands for postmenopausal bleeding. |
| **dysmenorrhea**<br>diss men uh REE ah | *dys-* painful<br>*men/o* menses<br>*-rrhea* discharge | Painful menstrual flow, cramps. |
| **menometrorrhagia**<br>men oh meh troh RAH zsa | *men/o* menses<br>*metr/o* uterus<br>*-rrhagia* bursting forth | Excessive menstrual flow and uterine bleeding other than that caused by menstruation. |
| **menorrhagia**<br>men or RAH zsa | *men/o* menses<br>*-rrhagia* bursting forth | Abnormally heavy or prolonged menstrual period. May be an indication of fibroids. |
| **metrorrhagia**<br>meh troh RAH zsa | *metr/o* uterus<br>*-rrhagia* bursting forth | Uterine bleeding other than that caused by menstruation. May be caused by uterine lesions. |
| **oligomenorrhea**<br>oh lig oh men oh REE ah | *olig/o* scanty, few<br>*men/o* menses<br>*-rrhea* discharge | Abnormally light or infrequent menstrual flow; **menorrhea** refers to the normal discharge of blood and tissue from the uterus. |

## Terms Related to Menstrual Disorders—cont'd

| Term | Word Origin | Definition |
|------|-------------|------------|
| polymenorrhea<br>pol ee men or REE ah | *poly-* many<br>*men/o* menses<br>*-rrhea* discharge | Abnormally frequent menstrual flow. |
| premenstrual dysphoric<br>disorder (PMDD) | *pre-* before<br>*menstru/o* menses<br>*-al* pertaining to<br>*dys-* abnormal<br>*phor/o* carry, bear<br>*-ic* pertaining to | Mood disorder that includes depression, irritability, fatigue, changes in appetite or sleep, and difficulty in concentrating; occurs 1 to 2 weeks before the onset of the menstrual flow. |
| premenstrual<br>syndrome (PMS) | *pre-* before<br>*menstru/o* menses<br>*-al* pertaining to<br>*syn-* together<br>*-drome* run | Poorly understood group of symptoms that occur in some women on a cyclical basis: Breast pain, irritability, fluid retention, headache, and lack of coordination are some of the symptoms. |

Exercise 9: **Menstrual Disorders**

*Fill in the blanks with the terms provided.*

**premenstrual syndrome, menometrorrhagia, dysfunctional uterine bleeding, menorrhagia, premenstrual dysphoric disorder**

1. What is the term for an excessively heavy menstrual period? _____

2. What is the term for bleeding from the uterus that is not a result of menstruation?

   _____

3. What is the term for the group of symptoms that occurs on a cyclical basis that include irritability,

   retention of fluid, and lack of coordination? _____

4. What is the term for excessive menstrual and dysfunctional bleeding? _____

5. What mood disorder occurs before menstruation and includes depression, appetite loss, and sleep

   disorders? _____

6. What is the term for uterine bleeding not caused by a tumor, inflammation, or pregnancy?

   _____

*Decode the terms.*

7. dysmenorrhea _____

8. amenorrhea _____

9. polymenorrhea _____

10. oligomenorrhea _____

## Infertility

Couples who are infertile are unable to produce offspring. The causes of infertility in the female may be endometriosis, ovulation problems, poor egg quality, polycystic ovarian syndrome, or female tube blockages. In the male, the problem may be lack of sperm production or viability, or male tube blockages. His partner may even be allergic to his sperm. Treatments are dependent on the variety of causal factors and are discussed in the **Therapeutic Interventions** and **Pharmacology** sections.

### Terms Related to Pregnancy Disorders

| Term | Word Origin | Definition |
|---|---|---|
| abruptio placentae<br>ah BRUP she oh<br>plah SEN tee | | Premature separation of the placenta from the uterine wall; may result in a severe hemorrhage that can threaten both infant and maternal lives. Also called **ablatio placentae** (ah BLAY she oh) (Fig. 8-7). |
| agalactia<br>a gah LACK tee ah | *a-* without<br>*galact/o* milk<br>*-ia* condition | Condition of mother's inability to produce milk. |
| cephalopelvic disproportion<br>seh fah loh PELL vick | *cephal/o* head<br>*pelv/i* pelvis<br>*-ic* pertaining to | Condition in which the infant's head is larger than the pelvic outlet it must pass through, thereby inhibiting normal labor and birth. It is one of the indications for a cesarean section. |
| eclampsia<br>eh KLAMP see ah | | Extremely serious form of hypertension secondary to pregnancy. Patients are at risk for coma, convulsions, and death. |
| ectopic pregnancy<br>eck TAH pick | *ec-* out<br>*top/o* place<br>*-ic* pertaining to | Implantation of the embryo in any location but the uterus (Fig. 8-8). |
| erythroblastosis fetalis<br>eh RITH roh blas toh sis<br>feh TAL is | *erythr/o* red (blood cell)<br>*blast/o* immature<br>*-osis* abnormal condition | Condition in which the mother is Rh negative and her fetus is Rh positive, causing the mother to form antibodies to the Rh-positive factor. Subsequent Rh-positive pregnancies will be in jeopardy because the mother's anti-Rh antibodies will cross the placenta and destroy fetal blood cells (Fig. 8-9). |
| miscarriage/abortion | | Termination of a pregnancy before the fetus is viable. If spontaneous, it may be termed a **miscarriage** or a **spontaneous abortion**. If induced, it can be referred to as a **therapeutic abortion**. |
| oligohydramnios<br>oh lih goh hye DRAM nee ohs | *olig/o* scanty<br>*hydr/o* water, fluid<br>*-amnios* amnion | Condition of low or missing amniotic fluid. |
| placenta previa<br>plah SEN tah PREE vee ah | *previa* in front of | Placenta that is malpositioned in the uterus, so that it covers the opening of the cervix. |

## Terms Related to Pregnancy Disorders—cont'd

| Term | Word Origin | Definition |
|---|---|---|
| **polyhydramnios**<br>pah lee hye DRAM nee ohs | *poly-* excessive<br>*hydr/o* water, fluid<br>*-amnios* amnion | Condition of excessive amniotic fluid. |
| **preeclampsia**<br>pree eh KLAMP see ah | *pre-* before | Abnormal condition of pregnancy with unknown cause, marked by hypertension, edema, and proteinuria. Also called **toxemia of pregnancy**. |

## Terms Related to Neonatal Disorders

| Term | Word Origin | Definition |
|---|---|---|
| **meconium staining**<br>meh KOH nee um | | Refers to fetal defecation while in utero and indicates fetal distress. Meconium is the first feces of the newborn. |
| **nuchal cord**<br>NOO kul | *nuch/o* neck<br>*-al* pertaining to | Abnormal but common occurrence of the umbilical cord wrapped around the neck of the neonate. |

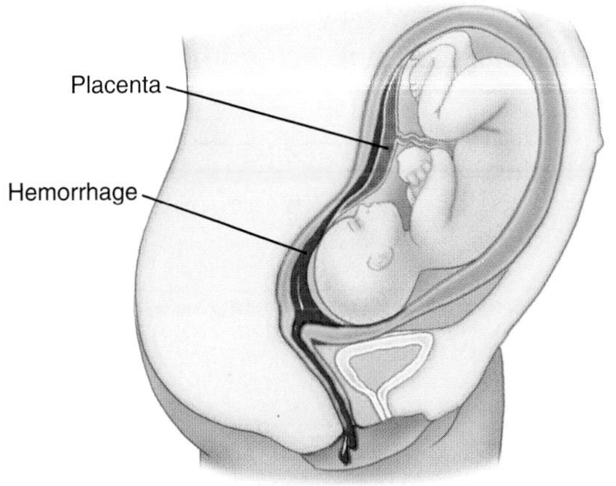

Fig. 8-7 Abruptio placentae.

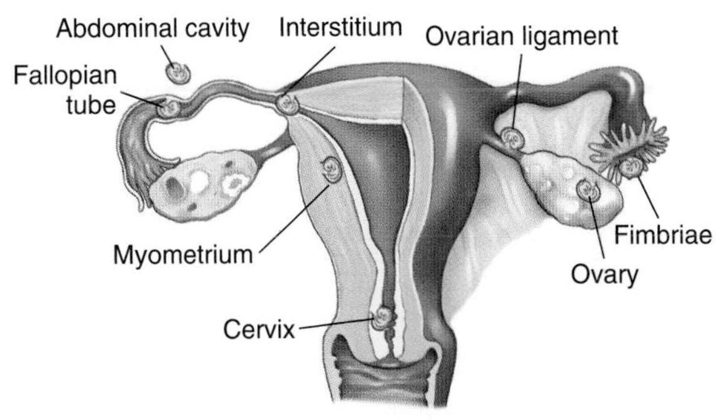

Fig. 8-8 Sites of ectopic pregnancy.

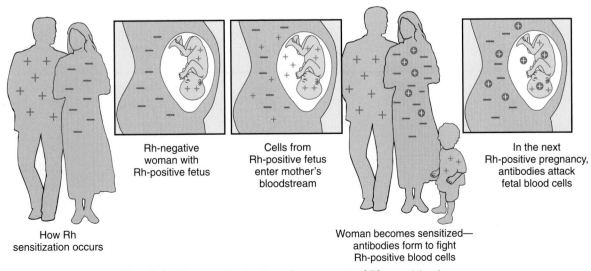

Fig. 8-9 Diagram illustrating the concept of Rh sensitization.

## Exercise 10: Disorders of Pregnancy and the Newborn

*Fill in the blanks with the terms provided.*

**ectopic pregnancy, nuchal cord, abortion, eclampsia, placenta previa, meconium, erythroblastosis fetalis, preeclampsia, abruptio placentae, cephalopelvic disproportion**

1. What are the first feces of the newborn called? _____

2. What is the term for the cord wrapped around the neck of the neonate?

   _____

3. What is the term for a placenta that separates prematurely from the wall of the uterus?

   _____

4. What is the term for a baby's head being larger than the pelvic outlet?

   _____

5. What is the term for a pregnancy that takes place anywhere but in the uterus?

   _____

6. What is the term for the termination of a pregnancy, intentionally or not, before the fetus is viable?

   _____

7. What is the term for a complication of pregnancy characterized by protein in the mother's urine,

   hypertension, and swelling? _____

8. What is the term for a placenta that is attached to the opening of the cervix?

   _____

9. What is the term for a severe form of toxemia that may result in convulsions, coma, and death?

   _____

10. Incompatibility between Rh factors of mother and baby that leads to destruction of red blood

    cells in the fetus is called _____

*Build the terms.*

11. condition of no milk _____

12. excessive amniotic fluid _____

13. scanty amniotic fluid _____

## Terms Related to Benign Neoplasms

| Term | Word Origin | Definition |
|------|-------------|------------|
| cervical intraepithelial neoplasia (CIN)<br>SUR vih kull<br>intruh ehp ih THEE lee ahl<br>nee oh PLAY zha | *cervic/o* cervix<br>*-al* pertaining to<br>*neo-* new<br>*-plasia* formation, development | Also termed "cervical dysplasia," this abnormal cell growth may or may not develop into cancer. It is reported in grades I, II, and III, with I being the mildest and III the most severe. |
| endometrial hyperplasia<br>en doh MEE tree uhl<br>hye pur PLAY zha | *endometri/o* endometrium<br>*-al* pertaining to<br>*hyper-* excessive<br>*-plasia* formation, development | An excessive development of cells in the lining of the uterus; this condition is benign but can become malignant. |
| fibroadenoma of the breast<br>fye broh add eh NOH mah | *fibr/o* fiber<br>*aden/o* gland<br>*-oma* tumor, mass | Noncancerous breast tumors composed of fibrous and glandular tissue (Fig. 8-10). |
| fibrocystic changes of the breast | *fibr/o* fiber<br>*cyst/o* sac, cyst<br>*-ic* pertaining to | Formerly called fibrocystic disease, this benign condition affects the glandular and stromal tissue. The changes may take a variety of forms with typical symptoms of cysts, lumpiness, and/or pain. |
| leiomyoma of the uterus<br><br>lye oh mye OH mah | *leiomy/o* smooth muscle<br>*-oma* tumor, mass | Also termed **fibroids**, these smooth muscle tumors of the uterus are usually nonpainful growths, which may be removed surgically (Fig. 8-11). |

*Continued*

To view an animation of an ovarian cyst, click on **Animations.**

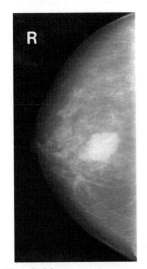
**Fig. 8-10** Fibroadenoma in the right (R) breast.

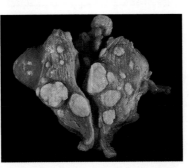
**Fig. 8-11** Leiomyoma of the uterus.

## Terms Related to Benign Neoplasms—cont'd

| Term | Word Origin | Definition |
|------|-------------|------------|
| **mature teratoma of the ovary**<br>tare ih TOH mah | *terat/o* deformity<br>*-oma* tumor, mass | Also termed "dermoid cysts," these usually noncancerous ovarian growths arise from germ cells. |
| **ovarian cyst** | *ovari/o* ovary<br>*-an* pertaining to | Benign, fluid-filled sac. Can be either a follicular cyst, which occurs when a follicle does not rupture at ovulation, or a cyst of the corpus luteum, caused when it does not continue its transformation (Fig. 8-12). |

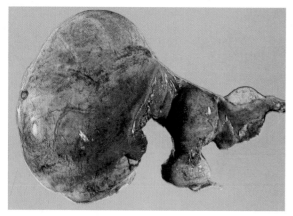
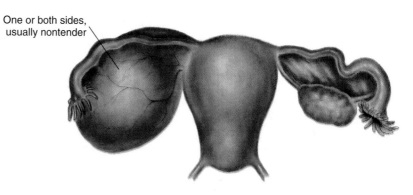

One or both sides, usually nontender

Fig. 8-12 Ovarian cyst.

## Terms Related to Malignant Neoplasms

| Term | Word Origin | Definition |
|------|-------------|------------|
| **choriocarcinoma**<br>kore ee oh kar sih NOH mah | *chori/o* chorion<br>*-carcinoma* cancer of epithelial origin | A malignant tumor arising from the chorionic membrane surrounding the fetus. |
| **endometrial adenocarcinoma**<br>en doh MEE tree uhl<br>add eh noh kar sih NOH mah | *endometri/o* endometrium<br>*-al* pertaining to<br>*aden/o* gland<br>*-carcinoma* cancer of epithelial origin | By far the most common cancer of the uterus, this type develops from the cells that line the uterus. |
| **epithelial ovarian cancer (EOC)**<br>epp ih THEE lee uhl | *epitheli/o* epithelium<br>*-al* pertaining to<br>*ovari/o* ovary<br>*-an* pertaining to | An inherited mutation of the *BRCA1* or *BRCA2* gene is linked to the risk of this malignancy and breast cancer. |
| **infiltrating ductal carcinoma (IDC)** | *duct/o* carry<br>*-al* pertaining to<br>*-carcinoma* cancer of epithelial origin | The most common type of breast cancer, infiltrating ductal carcinoma arises from the cells that line the milk ducts. |

## Terms Related to Malignant Neoplasms—cont'd

| Term | Word Origin | Definition |
| --- | --- | --- |
| leiomyosarcoma<br>lye oh mye oh sar KOH mah | *leiomy/o* smooth muscle<br>*-sarcoma* cancerous tumor of connective tissue | A rare type of cancer of the smooth muscle of the uterus. |
| lobular carcinoma<br>LAH byoo lure<br>kar sih NOH mah | *lobul/o* small lobe<br>*-ar* pertaining to<br>*-carcinoma* cancer of epithelial origin | About 15% of breast cancers are lobular carcinomas. These tumors begin in the glandular tissue of the breast at the ends of the milk ducts (Fig. 8-13). |
| Paget disease of the breast<br>PAJ ett | | A rare form of cancer, this malignancy of the nipple can occur in men and women. |
| squamous cell carcinoma of the cervix<br>SKWAY muss | *squam/o* scaly<br>*-ous* pertaining to<br>*-carcinoma* cancer of epithelial origin | The most common type of cervical cancer. Thought to be caused by the human papilloma virus (HPV), it is also one of the most curable cancers if detected in its early stage. |

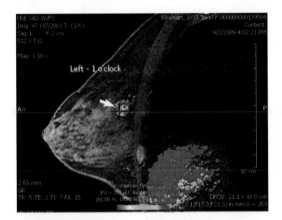

**Fig. 8-13** MRI breast image using contrast and demonstrating lobular carcinoma in the left breast (*arrow*).

## Exercise 11: Neoplasms

*Match the benign neoplasms with their definitions.*

____ 1. ovarian cyst

____ 2. endometrial hyperplasia

____ 3. CIN

____ 4. fibroadenoma of breast

____ 5. mature teratoma of ovary

____ 6. fibrocystic changes of breast

____ 7. leiomyoma of uterus

A. fibroid
B. dermoid cyst
C. benign breast tumors of fibrous and glandular tissue
D. cervical dysplasia
E. benign, fluid-filled sac
F. excessive cell development in lining of uterus
G. benign breast condition with symptoms of cysts, lumpiness, and/or pain

*Match the malignant neoplasms with their definitions.*

____ 8. endometrial adenocarcinoma

____ 9. lobular carcinoma

____ 10. Paget disease of the breast

____ 11. infiltrating ductal carcinoma

____ 12. EOC

____ 13. squamous cell carcinoma of the cervix

____ 14. leiomyosarcoma of the uterus

A. most common cancer of the uterus
B. rare smooth muscle tumor of uterus
C. breast cancer arising from ends of milk ducts
D. most common type of cervical cancer
E. inherited mutation linked to this form of ovarian cancer
F. most common type of breast cancer arising from cells that line milk ducts
G. malignancy of nipple

## *Case Study* Olivia Carter

Olivia Carter is a 19-year-old female who works full time at a fast food restaurant and attends the community college part time. Lately, she has been experiencing pelvic pain and heavy menstrual bleeding. She tells her gynecologist that she had a severe pelvic infection when she was 16 years old, but that it was treated with antibiotics and she has not had any other problems until just recently. She reports being on oral birth control pills since she delivered her son. Her last period, she states, was "different"; it lasted 10 days, and she had very heavy bleeding with lots of clots. Her cramping was so bad that she had to miss a day of work and her classes that evening.

The gynecologist orders blood tests and performs a Pap smear, among other tests. He suspects complications of PID.

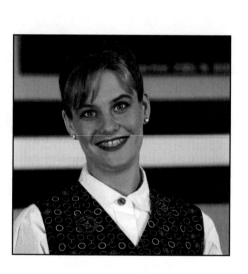

## Case Study  Olivia Carter

CARTER, OLIVIA M. - 599333 Opened by MACHARIA, LOUIS MD    _ □ X

Task   Edit   View   Time Scale   Options   Help

| CARTER, OLIVIA M. | Age: 19 years DOB: 05/27/1993 | Sex: Female MRN: 599333 | Loc: WHC-SMMC FIN: 3506004 |

Reference Text Browser | Form Browser | Medication Profile

Orders | Last 48 Hours | ED | Lab | Radiology | **Assessments** | Surgery | Clinical Notes | Pt. Info | Pt. Schedule | Task List | I & O | MAR

Flowsheet: Assessments   ▼ ...    Level: Progress Note   ▼      ⦿ Table  ○ Group  ○ List

**Navigator**   X

✓ | Progress Note

This 19-year-old female states that her last menstrual period ended approximately 2 weeks ago. She reports she had heavy vaginal bleeding with passage of clots and crampy lower abdominal pain, and she felt weak. She is on OCPs.

Gravida 1 para 1, history of normal vaginal delivery approximately 1 year ago. History of PID before pregnancy and recurrent dysmenorrhea.

There is a minimum amount of blood in the vaginal vault. No tissue noted. Cervix is normal in appearance. The os is closed. The fundus of the uterus is not well appreciated. Serum pregnancy test was negative. WBC was 11,300 with normal Hgb and Hct.

Vaginal bleeding, possibly involving past pelvic inflammatory disease.

PROD  MAHAFC    25 May 2012    13:02

---

### Exercise 12: Progress Note

*Using the progress note above, answer the following questions.*

1. What does gravida 1 para 1 mean? _____

2. What is the meaning of the abbreviation for the disorder she had before pregnancy?

_____

3. How do you know that she experienced painful menstrual periods? _____

4. What type of pregnancy test is a "serum pregnancy test"?

_____

Click on **Hear It, Spell It** to practice spelling the pathology terms you have learned in this chapter. To see how well you pronounce the pathology terms in this chapter, click on **Hear It, Say It.** To review the pathology terms in this chapter play **Medical Millionaire.**

## *Age Matters*

### Pediatrics

A review of the most recent national statistics for all diagnoses for hospital inpatients for newborns and children under the age of 17 revealed some surprises. For neonates (28 days old and younger), diagnoses that included complications of delivery were common. Meconium staining and cord entanglement were high on the list. However, for fertile females between the ages of 1 and 17, the delivery of a single liveborn is second only to hypovolemia for all diagnoses. (Pneumonia and asthma follow close behind.) Still within the top 50 diagnoses are a large number of complications of delivery.

### Geriatrics

Later in life, senior women are seen most often for neoplasms of the breast, uterus, cervix, and ovaries. Breast cancer alone will be diagnosed in one in eight women in their lifetime in this country.

## DIAGNOSTIC PROCEDURES

### Terms Related to Imaging

| Term | Word Origin | Definition |
|---|---|---|
| cervicography<br>sur vih KAH gruh fee | *cervic/o* cervix<br>*-graphy* process of recording | Photographic procedure in which a specially designed 35-mm camera is used to image the entire cervix to produce a slide called a **cervigram.** It is used to detect early cervical intraepithelial neoplasia (CIN) or invasive cervical cancer. Can be combined with **colposcopy** or can be done independently. |
| hysterosalpingography (HSG)<br>his tur oh sal pin GAH gruh fee | *hyster/o* uterus<br>*salping/o* fallopian tube<br>*-graphy* process of recording | X-ray procedure in which contrast medium is used to image the uterus and fallopian tubes (Fig. 8-14). |
| mammography<br>mam MOG gruh fee | *mamm/o* breast<br>*-graphy* process of recording | Imaging technique for the early detection of breast cancer. The record produced is called a **mammogram** (see Fig. 8-10). |
| pelvimetry<br>pell VIH meh tree | *pelv/i* pelvis<br>*-metry* process of measurement | Measurement of the birth canal. Types of pelvimetry include clinical and x-ray, although x-ray pelvimetry is not commonly done. |
| sonography | *son/o* sound<br>*-graphy* process of recording | Use of high-frequency sound waves to image the pelvic area (**pelvic sonography**) and the uterus (**sonohysterography**). **Transvaginal sonography** of the pelvic cavity is obtained through the use of a probe introduced into the vagina (Fig. 8-15). |

> **⊗ Be Careful!**     *Don't confuse the suffix -**metry**, which means the process of measurement, with **metr/o**, the combining form for the uterus.*

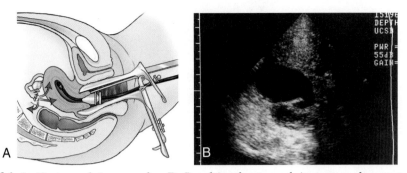

**Fig. 8-14 A,** Hysterosalpingography. **B,** Resulting hysterosalpingogram demonstrating coronal image of a very dilated fallopian tube. When swollen with fluid, the tube bends and curls.

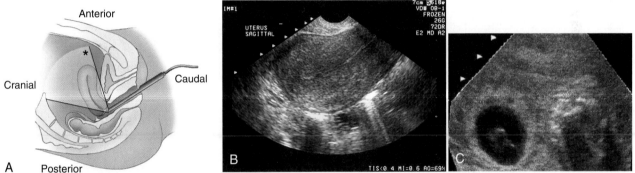

**Fig. 8-15 A,** Transvaginal sonography. **B,** Transvaginal sagittal view of the uterus. **C,** Uterus with fibroids *(right)* and fetus *(left)*.

## Terms Related to Endoscopies

| Term | Word Origin | Definition |
|---|---|---|
| **colposcopy**<br>kohl PAH skuh pee | *colp/o* vagina<br>*-scopy* process of viewing | Endoscopic procedure used for a cervical/vaginal biopsy. The instrument used is called a **colposcope** (Fig. 8-16). |
| **culdoscopy**<br>kull DAH skuh pee | *culd/o* cul-de-sac<br>*-scopy* process of viewing | Endoscopic procedure used for biopsy of Douglas cul-de-sac. The instrument used is called a **culdoscope**. |
| **hysteroscopy**<br>hiss tuh RAH skuh pee | *hyster/o* uterus<br>*-scopy* process of viewing | Endoscopic procedure used for a myomectomy (fibroid removal) or polypectomy (polyp removal). The instrument used is called a **hysteroscope**. |
| **laparoscopy**<br>lap uh RAH skuh pee | *lapar/o* abdomen<br>*-scopy* process of viewing | Endoscopic procedure for removing lesions (lysis) or performing a hysterectomy or an ovarian biopsy. The instrument used is called a **laparoscope**. |

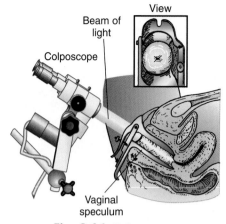

Fig. 8-16 Colposcopy.

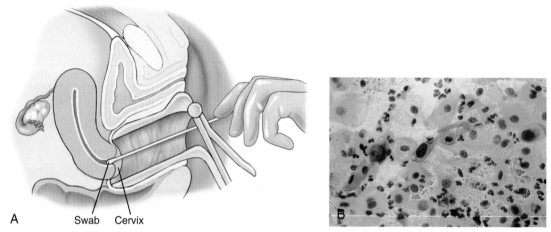

Fig. 8-17 **A,** Obtaining a Pap smear. **B,** Malignant cells have enlarged hyperchromatic nuclei in contrast to the small nuclei of normal cells.

## Terms Related to Laboratory Tests

| Term | Word Origin | Definition |
|---|---|---|
| culdocentesis<br>kull doh sen TEE sis | *culd/o* cul-de-sac<br>*-centesis* surgical puncture | Removal of fluid and cells from the rectouterine pouch to detect dysplasia. |
| hormone levels | | Laboratory measurements of the presence and extent of specific hormones in specimens of blood, urine, or body tissues. Information is useful in evaluating a range of conditions from pregnancy to menopause. |
| Pap smear | | Exfoliative cytology procedure useful for the detection of vaginal and cervical cancer (Fig 8-17). |

Exercise 13: **Female Reproductive Imaging Techniques, Endoscopies, and Laboratory Tests**

*Fill in the blanks with the terms provided.*

**cervicography, pelvimetry, hysterosalpingography, sonohysterography, hysteroscopy, laparoscopy, hormone levels, Pap smear**

1. process of imaging the uterus and fallopian tubes _____

2. measurement of the birth canal _____

3. photographic recording of the cervix _____

4. endoscopic procedure for fibroid/polyp removal _____

5. high-frequency sound waves used to image the uterus _____

6. endoscopic procedure for removing lesions _____

7. lab test to detect a range of conditions from pregnancy to menopause _____

8. removal of cells from the cervix to detect abnormal cells _____

*Decode the terms.*

9. culdocentesis _____

10. mammography _____

11. culdoscopy _____

12. colposcopy _____

| Signs of Pregnancy | | |
| --- | --- | --- |
| Presumptive | Probable | Positive |
| amenorrhea | Goodell's sign (softening of cervix) | Fetal heart tones (FHT) heard |
| chloasma (hyperpigmentation of face, "mask of pregnancy") | Hegar's sign (softening of lower segment of uterus) | Fetal movement felt by examiner |
| nausea and vomiting (N&V) | Ballottement of fetus (palpation to detect floating object) | Fetus observed on ultrasound |
| fatigue | Positive pregnancy test | |
| quickening | Chadwick's sign (vaginal hyperemia) | |

## Terms Related to Prenatal Diagnosis

| Term | Word Origin | Definition |
|------|-------------|------------|
| **alpha fetoprotein (AFP) test** <br> al fah fee toh PROH teen | | Maternal serum (blood) alpha fetoprotein test performed between 14 and 19 weeks of gestation; may indicate a variety of conditions, such as neural tube defects (spina bifida is the most common finding) and multiple gestation. |
| **amniocentesis** <br> am nee oh sen TEE sis | *amni/o* amnion <br> *-centesis* surgical puncture | Removal and analysis of a sample of the amniotic fluid with the use of a guided needle through the abdomen of the mother into the amniotic sac to diagnose fetal abnormalities (Fig. 8-18). |
| **chorionic villus sampling (CVS)** <br> kore ee AH nick VILL us | *chorion/o* chorion <br> *-ic* pertaining to | Removal of a small piece of the chorionic villi that develop on the surface of the chorion, either transvaginally or through a small incision in the abdomen, to test for chromosomal abnormalities. |
| **contraction stress test (CST)** | | Test to predict fetal outcome and risk of intrauterine asphyxia by measuring fetal heart rate throughout a minimum of three contractions within a 10-minute period. Also called a **stress test** or **oxytocin challenge test**. |
| **nonstress test (NST)** | | The fetus is monitored for a normal, expected acceleration of the fetal heart rate. A reactive nonstress test should be followed by a CST and possible ultrasound studies. |
| **pregnancy test** | | Test available in two forms: a standard over-the-counter pregnancy test, which examines urine for the presence of hCG; and a serum (blood) pregnancy test performed in a physician's office or laboratory to get a quantitative hCG. A "triple-screen" is a blood test for hCG, AFP, and uE3 (unconjugated estradiol). |

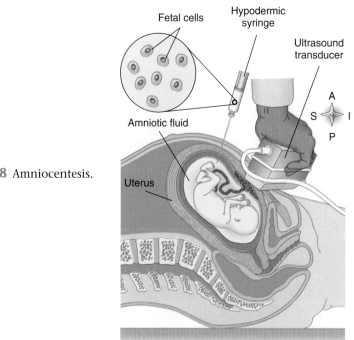

**Fig. 8-18** Amniocentesis.

## Terms Related to Postnatal Diagnosis

| Term | Word Origin | Definition |
|------|-------------|------------|
| Apgar score | | Rates the physical health of the infant with a set of criteria 1 minute and 5 minutes after birth. |
| congenital hypothyroidism<br>kon JEN ih tuhl<br>hye poh THIGH royd iz um | *hypo-* below<br>*thyroid/o* thyroid<br>*-ism* condition | Test for deficient thyroid hormones. Undiscovered and untreated, this condition can lead to retarded growth and brain development. If caught at birth, oral doses of the missing thyroid hormone will allow normal development. |
| phenylketonuria (PKU)<br>fee null kee tone YOOR ee ah | | Test for deficiency of enzyme phenylalanine hydroxylase, which is responsible for converting phenylalanine, found in certain foods, into tyrosine. Failure to treat this condition will lead to brain damage and mental retardation. |

 Exercise 14: Prenatal and Postnatal Diagnosis

*Fill in the blanks with the terms provided.*

**alpha fetoprotein, human chorionic gonadotropin, Apgar score, nonstress test, chorionic villus sampling, contraction stress test, congenital hypothyroidism**

1.  What hormone does a pregnancy test look for? _____

2.  What is the name of the test done 1 and 5 minutes after birth that scores the physical health of the

    neonate? _____

3.  What is a measurement of fetal heart rate through contractions? _____

4.  What test determines fetal health by measuring the heart rate? _____

5.  What test of maternal blood between 14 and 19 weeks indicates neural tube defects and/or multiple

    gestation? _____

6.  What is a condition of deficient thyroid hormones that is present at birth? _____

7.  What test of a sample from the outer covering of the fetus determines chromosomal abnormalities?

    _____

*Build the term.*

8.  removal of amniotic fluid for diagnostic testing _____

## THERAPEUTIC INTERVENTIONS

### Terms Related to Nonpregnancy Procedures

| Term | Word Origin | Definition |
| --- | --- | --- |
| cervicectomy<br>sur vih SECK tuh mee | *cervic/o* cervix<br>*-ectomy* removal | Resection (removal) of the uterine cervix. |
| clitoridectomy<br>klit er oh DECK toh mee | *clitorid/o* clitoris<br>*-ectomy* removal | Removal of the clitoris. Referred to as "female circumcision" in some cultures. |
| colpopexy<br>KOHL poh peck see | *colp/o* vagina<br>*-pexy* fixation, suspension | Fixation of the vagina to an adjacent structure to hold it in place. |
| colpoplasty<br>KOHL poh plas tee | *colp/o* vagina<br>*-plasty* surgical repair | Surgical repair of the vagina. |
| culdoplasty<br>KULL doh plas tee | *culd/o* cul-de-sac<br>*-plasty* surgical repair | Surgical repair of the cul-de-sac. |
| dilation and curettage (D & C)<br>dye LAY shun<br>kyoor ih TAHZH | | Procedure involving widening (dilation) of the cervix until a curette, a sharp scraping tool, can be inserted to remove the lining of the uterus (curettage). Used to treat and diagnose conditions such as heavy menstrual bleeding, or to empty the uterus of the products of conception. |
| hymenotomy<br>hye meh NAH tuh mee | *hymen/o* hymen<br>*-tomy* incision | Incision of the hymen to enlarge the vaginal opening. |
| hysterectomy<br>hiss tur RECK tuh mee | *hyster/o* uterus<br>*-ectomy* removal | Resection (removal) of the uterus; may be partial, pan- (all), or include other organs as well (e.g., total abdominal hysterectomy with a bilateral salpingo-oophorectomy [TAH-BSO]). The surgical approach is usually stated: whether it is laparoscopic, vaginal, or abdominal. |
| hysteropexy<br>HISS tur roh peck see | *hyster/o* uterus<br>*-pexy* fixation, suspension | Suspension and fixation of a prolapsed uterus. |
| loop electrocautery excision procedure (LEEP)<br>ee leck troh KAH tur ee | *electr/o* electricity<br>*cauter/i* burning<br>*-y* process of | A procedure done to remove abnormal cells in cervical dysplasia. |
| lumpectomy<br>lum PECK tuh mee | *-ectomy* removal | Removal of a tumor from the breast. |
| mammoplasty<br>MAM oh plas tee | *mamm/o* breast<br>*-plasty* surgical repair | Surgical or cosmetic repair of the breast. Options may include augmentation, to increase the size of the breasts, or reduction, to reduce the size of the breasts. |
| mastectomy<br>mass TECK tuh mee | *mast/o* breast<br>*-ectomy* removal | Removal of the breast; may be unilateral or bilateral. |

## Terms Related to Nonpregnancy Procedures—cont'd

| Term | Word Origin | Definition |
|---|---|---|
| mastopexy<br>MASS toh peck see | *mast/o* breast<br>*-pexy* fixation, suspension | Reconstructive procedure to lift and fixate the breasts. |
| oophorectomy<br>oo ah fore ECK tuh mee | *oophor/o* ovary<br>*-ectomy* cut out | Resection of an ovary; may be unilateral or bilateral. |
| oophorocystectomy<br>oo off oh roh sis TECK<br>tuh mee | *oophor/o* ovary<br>*cyst/o* sac, cyst<br>*-ectomy* cut out | Removal of an ovarian cyst (Fig 8-19). |
| pelvic exenteration<br>eck sen tuh RAY shun | | Removal of the contents of the pelvic cavity. Pelvic exenteration is usually done in response to widespread cancer to remove the uterus, fallopian tubes, ovaries, bladder, vagina, rectum, and lymph nodes (Fig. 8-20). |
| salpingectomy<br>sal pin JECK tuh mee | *salping/o* fallopian tube<br>*-ectomy* cut out | Resection of a fallopian tube; may be unilateral or bilateral. |
| salpingolysis<br>sal ping GALL ih sis | *salping/o* fallopian tube<br>*-lysis* freeing from adhesions; destruction | Removal of the adhesions in a fallopian tube to reestablish patency, with the goal of fertility. |
| theleplasty<br>THEE leh plas tee | *thel/e* nipple<br>*-plasty* surgical repair | Surgical and/or cosmetic repair of the nipple. |
| uterine artery<br>  embolization (UAE)<br>em boh lye ZAY shun | | Injection of particles to block a uterine artery supplying blood to a fibroid with resultant death of fibroid tissue. |

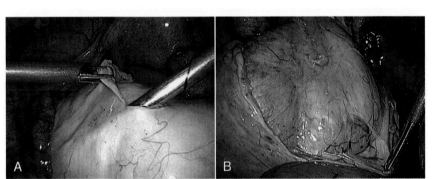
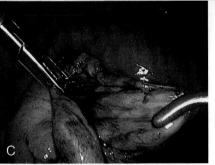

Fig. 8-19 Oophorocystectomy.

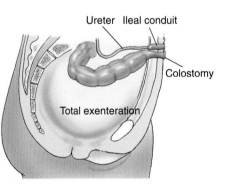

Fig. 8-20 Total pelvic exenteration.

## Exercise 15: Therapeutic Interventions Not Related to Pregnancy

*Fill in the blanks with the terms provided.*

**lumpectomy, dilation and curettage, salpingolysis, colpoplasty, hysteropexy, pelvic exenteration, uterine artery embolization, mastopexy, bilateral oophorectomy, TAH-BSO**

1. What surgical procedure suspends the uterus? _____

2. What surgical procedure removes adhesions from the fallopian tubes? _____

3. What surgical procedure resects both ovaries? _____

4. What surgical procedure resects the entire uterus, fallopian tubes, and ovaries through an incision in the abdomen? _____

5. What is removal of a tumor from the breast called? _____

6. What is the term for the removal of the contents of the pelvic cavity? _____

7. What procedure treats fibroids without surgically removing them? _____

8. What is the term for a procedure that widens the cervix to remove the lining of the uterus?

   _____

9. What is surgical repair of the vagina called? _____

10. What is the term for the lifting and fixation of sagging breasts? _____

*Decode the terms.*

11. clitoridectomy _____

12. culdoplasty _____

13. hymenotomy _____

*Build the terms.*

14. removal of an ovarian cyst _____

15. surgical repair of the nipple _____

## Terms Related to Pregnancy and Delivery Procedures

| Term | Word Origin | Definition |
| --- | --- | --- |
| cephalic version<br>seh FAL ick | *cephal/o* head<br>*-ic* pertaining to<br>*version* process of turning | Process of turning the fetus so that the head is at the cervical outlet for a vaginal delivery. |
| cerclage<br>sur KLAHZH | | Suturing the cervix closed to prevent a spontaneous abortion in a woman with an incompetent cervix. The suture is removed when the pregnancy is at full term to allow the delivery to proceed normally (Fig. 8-21). |
| cesarean section<br>(C-section, CS)<br>seh SARE ree un | | Delivery of an infant through a surgical abdominal incision (Fig. 8-22). |
| episiotomy<br>eh pee zee AH tuh mee | *episi/o* vulva<br>*-tomy* incision | Incision to widen the vaginal orifice to prevent tearing of the tissue of the vulva during delivery (Fig. 8-23). |
| oxytocia<br>ock see TOH sha | *oxy-* rapid<br>*-tocia* labor, delivery | Rapid birth. **Dystocia** is a difficult labor. **Eutocia** is a normal, "good" delivery. |
| vaginal birth after<br>C-section (VBAC)<br>VAJ ih nul | *vagin/o* vagina<br>*-al* pertaining to | Delivery of subsequent babies vaginally after a C-section. In the past, women were told "once a C-section, always a C-section." Currently, this is being changed by recent developments in technique. |
| vaginal delivery | *vagin/o* vagina<br>*-al* pertaining to | (Usually) cephalic presentation (head first) through the vagina. Feet or buttock presentation is a **breech** delivery. |

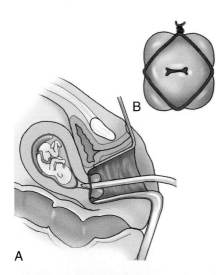

Fig. 8-21 **A,** Cerclage correction of premature dilation of the cervix. **B,** Cross-sectional view of closed cervix.

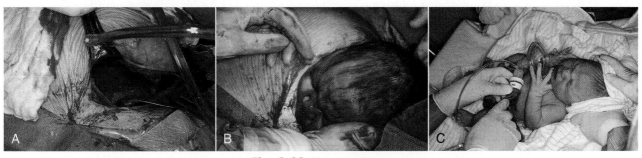

Fig. 8-22 Cesarean birth.

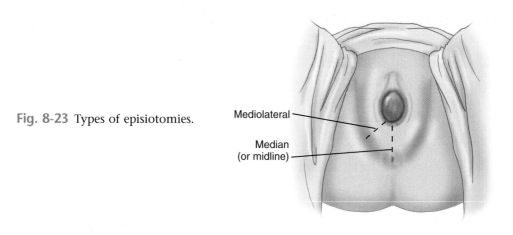

Fig. 8-23 Types of episiotomies.

## Terms Related to Infertility Procedures

| Term | Word Origin | Definition |
|------|-------------|------------|
| **artificial insemination (AI)** | *in-* in<br>*semin/i* semen<br>*-ation* process of | Introduction of semen into the vagina by mechanical or instrumental means. |
| **gamete intrafallopian transfer (GIFT)**<br>GAM eet<br>in trah fah LOH pee un | *intra-* within<br>*fallopi/o* fallopian tube<br>*-an* pertaining to | Laboratory mixing and injection of the ova and sperm into the fallopian tubes so that fertilization occurs naturally within the body. |
| **intracytoplasmic sperm injection (ICSI)**<br>in trah sye toh PLAZ mick | *intra-* within<br>*cyt/o* cell<br>*plasm/o* formation<br>*-ic* pertaining to | Injection of one sperm into the ovum and subsequent transplantation of the resulting zygote into the uterus (Fig. 8-24). |
| **in vitro fertilization (IVF)**<br>in VEE tro | *in* in<br>*vitro* life | Procedure that allows the mother's ova to be fertilized outside the body and then implanted in the uterus of the biologic mother or a surrogate to carry to term. |
| **zygote intrafallopian transfer (ZIFT)**<br>ZYE gote<br>in trah fuh LOH pee un | *intra-* within<br>*fallopi/o* fallopian tube<br>*-an* pertaining to | Mixing of the ova and sperm in the laboratory, with fertilization confirmed before the zygotes are returned to the fallopian tubes. |

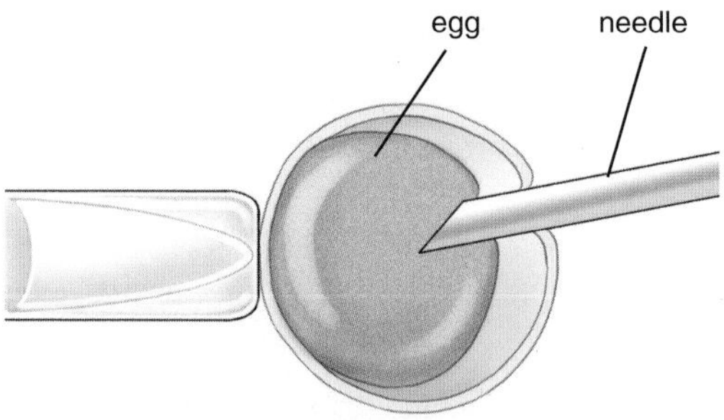

Fig. 8-24 Intracytoplasmic sperm injection (ICSI).

## Terms Related to Sterilization

| Term | Word Origin | Definition |
|---|---|---|
| **salpingosalpingostomy** <br> sal pin goh sal pin GOS tuh mee | *salping/o* fallopian tube <br> *salping/o* fallopian tube <br> *-stomy* new opening | The rejoining of previously cut fallopian tubes to re-establish patency. A reversal of a tubal ligation. |
| **sterilization** | | Surgical procedure rendering a person unable to produce children; for women, may involve hysterectomy, bilateral oophorectomy, or tubal ligation. |
| **tubal ligation** <br> TOO bul <br> lye GAY shun | *tub/o* tube <br> *-al* pertaining to <br> *ligat/o* tying <br> *-ion* process of | Sterilization procedure in which the fallopian tubes are cut, ligated (tied), and cauterized to prevent released ova from being fertilized by spermatozoa (Fig. 8-25). |

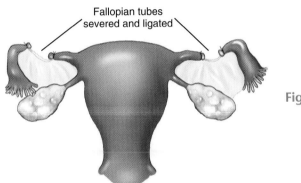

Fallopian tubes severed and ligated

**Fig. 8-25** Tubal ligation.

## Exercise 16: Interventions Related to Procreation and Contraception

*Fill in the blanks with the terms provided.*

**C-section, VBAC, tubal ligation, cerclage, cephalic version, sterilization, eutocia**

1. The fallopian tubes are cut, tied, and cauterized in which procedure? _____

2. A patient who has a baby vaginally after having a cesarean section may have what abbreviation on

    her chart? _____

3. What is the term for a normal, good delivery? _____

4. What is the procedure to turn the infant if its head is not down? _____

5. What is the term for a delivery via an incision? _____

6. A bilateral oophorectomy would effectively cause _____.

7. A procedure to keep an incompetent cervix closed until the due date is called _____.

*Match the abbreviations with the type of fertilization technique.*

____  8. IVF

____  9. ZIFT

____  10. AI

____  11. GIFT

____  12. ICSI

A. ova fertilized outside of the body, then implanted in the uterus of biologic mother or surrogate

B. semen introduced in vagina by means other than sexual intercourse

C. ova and sperm mixed outside of the body; confirmed zygotes are implanted in fallopian tubes

D. ova and sperm injected in oviducts; fertilization occurs within the body

E. ovum injected with one sperm; confirmed zygote is implanted in uterus

*Decode the terms.*

13. episiotomy _____

14. oxytocia _____

15. salpingosalpingostomy _____

## *Case Study*  Hortencia Garcia

Hortencia is a 27-year-old massage therapist. She has two children and is pregnant with the third. She does not want to get pregnant again, so she is here to discuss family planning for after delivery, which will occur in about 2 weeks. Various options, including IUD, OCPs, injections, and implants are reviewed, as are the more permanent forms, such as tubal ligation or vasectomy. Her gynecologist recommends that she consider the tubal ligation because this can be done in the hospital right after she delivers her baby. She agrees that this is the best option for her, and she successfully undergoes the procedure after her son is born.

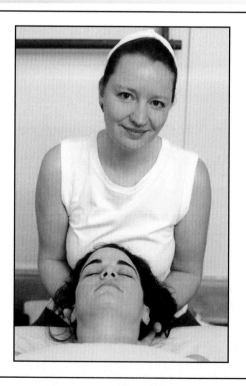

*Case Study*  *Hortencia Garcia*

GARCIA, HORTENCIA T. - 538437 Opened by Chung, Patrick MD          _ ⊡ ☒

Task   Edit   View   Time Scale   Options   Help

As Of 11:27

**GARCIA, HORTENCIA T.**     Age: 27 years        Sex: Female       Loc: WHC-SMMC
                            DOB: 04/04/1985      MRN: 538437        FIN: 3506004

| Reference Text Browser | Form Browser | Medication Profile |
|---|---|---|

| Orders | Last 48 Hours | ED | Lab | Radiology | Assessments | **Surgery** | Clinical Notes | Pt. Info | Pt. Schedule | Task List | I & O | MAR |

Flowsheet: Surgery        Level: Operative Report          ⦿ Table  ○ Group  ○ List

**Navigator**     ☒
✓  Operative Report

Diagnosis:        Desired sterilization, multiparity
Surgery:          Laparoscopic tubal ligation

This 27-year-old multigravida female desired tubal sterilization. The patient was taken to the operating room, where, under adequate general anesthetic, the abdomen and perineum were prepped and draped in a sterile fashion. The bladder was drained. An infraumbilical incision was made, and the Veress needle was used for institution of pneumoperitoneum. A 10-mm and a 5-mm port were placed. Both tubes were electrocoagulated and divided under direct vision. After hemostasis was ensured, the wounds were closed with 2-0 Vicryl and 4-0 Vicryl subcuticular. Skin incisions were infiltrated with Marcaine. The patient went to the recovery room in stable condition.

PROD | MAHAFC | 13 July 2012 | 11:27

## Exercise 17: Operative Report

*Using the operative report above, answer the following questions.*

1. What does this diagnosis mean, "Desired sterilization, multiparity"? (Define sterilization and

   multiparity.) _____

2. The patient is also described as being "multigravida." What is the difference between multiparous and

   multigravida? _____

3. What approach is used for the procedure? _____

4. What does the term "ligation" mean? _____

5. Where was the incision made? _____

Click on **Hear It, Spell It** to practice spelling the diagnostic and therapeutic terms you have learned in this chapter. To practice pronouncing these terms, click on **Hear It, Say It.**

## PHARMACOLOGY

### Contraceptive Management

**abortifacient** (ah bore tih FAY shee ent): medication that terminates pregnancy. Mifepristone (Mifeprex) and dinoprostone (Prostin E2) may be used as abortifacients.

**abstinence:** total avoidance of sexual intercourse as a contraceptive option.

**barrier methods:** see *diaphragm* and *cervical cap.*

**birth control patch:** timed-release contraceptive worn on the skin that delivers hormones transdermally.

**cervical cap:** small rubber cup that fits over the cervix to prevent sperm from entering.

**contraceptive sponge:** intravaginal barrier with a spermicidal additive.

**diaphragm:** soft, rubber hemisphere that fits over the cervix, which can be lined with a spermicidal lubricant prior to insertion.

**emergency contraception pill (ECP):** medication that can prevent pregnancy after unprotected vaginal intercourse; does not affect existing pregnancies or cause abortions. Plan B is a popular brand-name available ECP that is now available OTC behind the counter. Commonly called the "day-after pill".

**female condom:** soft, flexible sheath that fits within the vagina and prevents sperm from entering the vagina.

**hormone implant:** timed-release medication placed under the skin of the upper arm, providing long-term protection. The Norplant system is an example.

**hormone injection:** contraceptive hormones such as Depo-Provera that may be given every few months to provide reliable pregnancy prevention.

**intrauterine device (IUD):** small, flexible device inserted into the uterus that prevents implantation of a zygote (Fig. 8-26).

**male condom:** soft, flexible sheath that covers the penis and prevents sperm from entering the vagina. If may also be coated with a spermicide.

**oral contraceptive pill (OCP) or birth control pill (BCP):** pill containing estrogen and/or progesterone that is taken daily to fool the body into thinking it is pregnant, so that ovulation is suppressed.

**procreative and contraceptive management:** term for a variety of medications and techniques that describe the options available for women's reproductive health.

**cervix** = cervic/o

**intrauterine**
intra- = within
uter/o = uterus

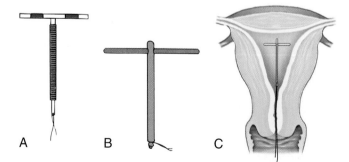

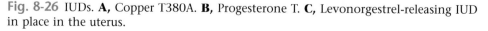
**Fig. 8-26** IUDs. **A,** Copper T380A. **B,** Progesterone T. **C,** Levonorgestrel-releasing IUD in place in the uterus.

**rhythm method:** a natural family planning method that involves charting the menstrual cycle to recognize fertile and infertile periods.
**spermicides:** foam or gel applied as directed prior to intercourse to kill sperm.

sperm/o = **sperm**
-cide = to kill

## Exercise 18: Contraceptive Options

*Fill in the blanks with the terms provided.*

**abstinence, rhythm method, abortifacient, OCP, spermicides, IUDs, condoms, ECP, barrier methods**

1. A contraceptive oral medication that works by suppressing ovulation is _____

2. Diaphragms and cervical caps are examples of what type of contraceptive method? _____

   _____

3. Soft, flexible sheaths that prevent sperm from entering the vagina are called _____

   _____.

4. Small flexible devices that fit within the uterus are called _____

   _____.

5. A medication intended to terminate a pregnancy is a/an _____.

6. A natural family planning method that has participants chart the woman's menstrual cycle

   to determine fertile and infertile periods is _____.

7. The only 100% effective contraceptive method is _____.

8. Foams and gels that kill sperm are called _____.

9. An emergency contraceptive measure that prevents pregnancy but does not affect an existing

   pregnancy is called a/an _____.

## Fertility Drugs

All of the following fertility drugs support or trigger ovulation and may be referred to as *ovulation stimulants:*

**bromocriptine (Parlodel):** oral medication typically used with in vitro fertilization to reduce prolactin levels, which suppresses ovulation.
**clomiphene (Clomid, Serophene):** oral medication that stimulates the pituitary gland to produce the hormones that trigger ovulation.
**gonadotropin-releasing hormone (GRH) agonist (Lupron):** agent injected or inhaled nasally to prevent premature release of eggs.
**human chorionic gonadotropin (hCG) (Novarel):** hormone given intramuscularly to trigger ovulation and typically given with another hormone that will stimulate the release of developed eggs.

**human menopausal gonadotropins (hMG) (Repronex):** dual gonadotropins that both stimulate the production of egg follicles and cause the eggs to be released once they are developed. These are given by intramuscular or subcutaneous injection.

**lutropin alfa (Luveris):** a gonadotropin that stimulates the production of egg follicles.

**urofollitropin (Fertinex):** hormone given subcutaneously that mimics follicle-stimulating hormone (FSH) to directly stimulate the ovaries to produce egg follicles.

### Drugs to Manage Delivery

**⊗ Be Careful!**

*Do not confuse*
**oxytocin**, *a labor-inducing drug, with*
**oxytocia**, *which means rapid birth.*

**oxytocic:** medication given to induce labor by mimicking the body's natural release of the oxytocin hormone or to manage postpartum uterine hemorrhage. Oxytocin (Pitocin) is the most commonly used agent to induce labor. Other available oxytocic agents are methylergonovine (Methergine) and ergonovine (Ergotrate).

**tocolytic:** medication given to slow down or stop preterm labor by inhibiting uterine contractions. Also referred to as a uterine relaxant. Ritodrine (Yutopar) is the only FDA-approved tocolytic, but terbutaline (Brethine) is commonly used for this purpose.

### Hormone Replacements

**hormone replacement therapy (HRT), and estrogen replacement therapy (ERT):** the healthcare replacement of estrogen alone (ERT) or with progesterone (HRT) perimenopausally in several forms (tablet, transdermal patch, injection, or vaginal suppository) to relieve symptoms of menopause and protect against osteoporosis.

**phytoestrogens:** an alternative source of estrogen replacement that occurs through the ingestion of certain plants like soy beans. Phytoestrogens act similarly to human estrogens in the body.

### ⟳ Exercise 19: Fertility, Delivery, and Hormone Replacement Drugs

*Underline the correct answer in parentheses.*

1. Bromocriptine, clomiphene, and hMG all are used to *(increase, decrease)* fertility.
2. Use of drugs to replace hormones that are missing as a result of menopause is called *(hormone replacement therapy, contraceptive management)*.
3. A natural source of estrogen is in *(carbohydrates, soy beans)*.
4. Oxytocin is used to *(inhibit, induce)* labor.
5. Medications given to slow down or stop labor are called *(tocolytics, phytoestrogens)*.

## Abbreviations

| Abbreviation | Definition |
|---|---|
| AFP | alpha fetoprotein test |
| AI | artificial insemination |
| CIN | cervical intraepithelial neoplasia |
| CS | cesarean section |
| CST | contraction stress test |
| CVS | chorionic villus sampling |
| Cx | cervix |
| D & C | dilation and curettage |
| DUB | dysfunctional uterine bleeding |
| ECP | emergency contraceptive pill |
| EDD | estimated delivery date |
| EOC | epithelial ovarian cancer |
| ERT | estrogen replacement therapy |
| FHR | fetal heart rate |
| FSH | follicle-stimulating hormone |
| GIFT | gamete intrafallopian transfer |
| GPA | gravida, para, abortion |
| hCG | human chorionic gonadotropin |
| hMG | human menopausal gonadotropin |
| HRT | hormone replacement therapy |
| HSG | hysterosalpingography |
| ICSI | intracytoplasmic sperm injection |
| IDC | infiltrating ductal carcinoma |

| Abbreviation | Definition |
|---|---|
| IUD | intrauterine device |
| IVF | in vitro fertilization |
| LEEP | loop electrocautery excision procedure |
| LH | luteinizing hormone |
| LMP | last menstrual period |
| LN | luteinizing hormone |
| NST | nonstress test |
| OB | obstetrics |
| OCP | oral contraceptive pill |
| PCOS | polycystic ovary syndrome |
| PID | pelvic inflammatory disease |
| PKU | phenylketonuria |
| PMB | postmenopausal bleeding |
| PMDD | premenstrual dysphoric disorder |
| PMS | premenstrual syndrome |
| Rh | Rhesus factor |
| TAH-BSO | total abdominal hysterectomy with a bilateral salpingo-oophorectomy |
| UAE | uterine artery embolization |
| VBAC | vaginal birth after cesarean section |
| ZIFT | zygote intrafallopian transfer |

## Exercise 20: Abbreviations

*Matching.*

____ 1. baby is due

____ 2. pregnancy hormone

____ 3. multiple cysts on ovaries

____ 4. birth control medication

____ 5. bleeding after menopause

____ 6. removal of uterine lining

____ 7. test for cervical/vaginal cancer

____ 8. removal of uterus, oviducts, and ovaries

A. TAH-BSO
B. OCP
C. Pap smear
D. hCG
E. D & C
F. PCOS
G. PMB
H. EDD

# Chapter Review

*Match the word parts to their definitions.*

## WORD PARTS

| Prefix/Suffix | Definition | |
|---|---|---|
| -gravida | 1. _____ | new |
| multi- | 2. _____ | first |
| neo- | 3. _____ | pregnancy |
| nulli- | 4. _____ | delivery |
| -para | 5. _____ | fallopian tube |
| primi- | 6. _____ | many |
| -ptosis | 7. _____ | none |
| -rrhea | 8. _____ | drooping, sagging |
| -salpinx | 9. _____ | discharge, flow |
| -tocia | 10. _____ | condition of labor, delivery |

| Combining Form | Definition | |
|---|---|---|
| amni/o | 11. _____ | cervix |
| cervic/o | 12. _____ | pregnancy |
| chori/o | 13. _____ | milk |
| colp/o | 14. _____ | breast |
| culd/o | 15. _____ | birth |
| episi/o | 16. _____ | nipple |
| gravid/o | 17. _____ | breast |
| gynec/o | 18. _____ | amnion |
| hyster/o | 19. _____ | nipple |
| lact/o | 20. _____ | female |
| mamm/o | 21. _____ | ovum, egg |
| mast/o | 22. _____ | scanty, few |
| men/o | 23. _____ | uterus |
| metr/o | 24. _____ | menstruation |
| nat/o | 25. _____ | delivery |
| o/o | 26. _____ | chorion |
| olig/o | 27. _____ | vagina |
| oophor/o | 28. _____ | uterus |
| papill/o | 29. _____ | rectourine pouch |
| part/o | 30. _____ | fallopian tube |
| salping/o | 31. _____ | ovary |
| thel/e | 32. _____ | vulva |

## WORDSHOP

| Prefixes | Combining Forms | Suffixes |
|----------|-----------------|----------|
| a- | colp/o | -ectomy |
| an- | episi/o | -graphy |
| dys- | galact/o | -gravida |
| eu- | gynec/o | -ia |
| multi- | hyster/o | -lysis |
| nulli- | mamm/o | -para |
| poly- | mast/o | -partum |
| post- | men/o | -pexy |
| pre- | metr/o | -plasty |
|  | oophor/o | -rrhea |
|  | py/o | -salpinx |
|  | salping/o | -tocia |
|  | thel/e | -tomy |

Build the following terms by combining the above word parts. Some word parts may be used more than once. Some may not be used at all. The number in parentheses indicates how many word parts are needed to build the term.

| Definition | Term |
|------------|------|
| 1. no menstrual flow (3) | |
| 2. process of recording the uterus and fallopian tube (3) | |
| 3. frequent menstrual flow (3) | |
| 4. no pregnancies (2) | |
| 5. after delivery (2) | |
| 6. many (more than one) deliveries (2) | |
| 7. painful menstrual flow (3) | |
| 8. removal of the uterus (2) | |
| 9. freeing from adhesions in a fallopian tube (2) | |
| 10. fixation of the breast (2) | |
| 11. pus in a fallopian tube (2) | |
| 12. condition of no milk (3) | |
| 13. incision of the perineum (2) | |
| 14. process of healthy, normal delivery, labor (2) | |
| 15. surgical repair of the nipple (2) | |

*Sort the terms below into the correct categories.*

## TERM SORTING

| Anatomy and Physiology | Pathology | Diagnostic Procedures | Therapeutic Interventions |
|---|---|---|---|
| | | | |
| | | | |
| | | | |
| | | | |
| | | | |
| | | | |
| | | | |
| | | | |
| | | | |
| | | | |

| | | | |
|---|---|---|---|
| AFP | CST | hysteroptosis | Pap smear |
| amniocentesis | culdocentesis | LEEP | parturition |
| anovulation | CVS | leiomyoma | pelvimetry |
| Apgar | D&C | tubal ligation | PKU |
| areola | eclampsia | vulvodynia | polyhydramnios |
| cerclage | endometrium | mastopexy | progesterone |
| cervicectomy | fimbriae | menopause | puerperium |
| cervix | gestation | menorrhagia | pyosalpinx |
| colpopexy | hCG | oophorectomy | salpingolysis |
| colposcopy | hematosalpinx | oophoritis | theleplasty |

*Replace the highlighted words with the correct terms.*

## TRANSLATIONS

1. Ms. Costello made an appointment with her **medical doctor who monitors health and treat diseases of the female reproductive system** to discuss her **painful menstrual flow.**

2. Anna Walker's **medical doctor who treats women during pregnancy, delivery, and during the postpartum period** scheduled her for a **removal and analysis of a sample of amniotic fluid.**

3. The **newborn** was born with a/an **umbilical cord around his neck.**

4. Maria Olmos had a **white discharge** that was a symptom of **inflammation of the cervix.**

5. Ms. Robinson was treated for **closure of the uterine tubes** with **destruction of adhesions within the fallopian tubes.**

6. After her third **implantation of the embryo in any location but the uterus**, the patient requested a **sterilization procedure in which the fallopian tubes are cut, ligated, and cauterized.**

7. The 42-year-old **woman who is pregnant for the first time** was sent for a **stimulation of the fetus to monitor for a normal, expected acceleration of the fetal heart rate.**

8. Ms. Graf had a **removal of the breast** to treat her **breast cancer that arises from the cells that line the milk ducts.**

9. Because of an abnormal **exfoliative cytology procedure used for the detection of vaginal and cervical cancer**, the patient was scheduled for a/an **endoscopic procedure used for a cervical/vaginal biopsy.**

10. After delivering a baby two weeks ago, the patient was seen to treat **inflammation of the breast** and **inflammation of the nipples.**

11. The doctor ordered a/an **x-ray procedure in which contrast medium is used to image the uterus and fallopian tubes** to image the patient's **inflammation of the fallopian tubes.**

12. Janice had a **resection of the uterus** to treat her **rare cancer of the smooth muscle of the uterus.**

13. Maria experienced **rapid birth**, and her obstetrician did not have time to do an **incision to widen the vaginal orifice.**

14. Because of a/an **condition in which the infant's head is larger than the mother's pelvic outlet**, Suzanne had to have a **delivery of an infant through a surgical abdominal incision.**

# *Case Study*    *Suzanne Banfield*

After several years of trying, Suzanne Banfield and her husband are finally expecting their first baby. Suzanne is ecstatic, and she immediately begins to read everything she can get her hands on to make sure that she does what she can to ensure her delivery is normal and her baby is healthy. She had already been doing yoga and had swum regularly, and after consulting with her obstetrician to make sure that it was okay, she continues with those activities. She eats healthfully and doesn't smoke or drink. Her monthly check-ups go well. The baby develops as she should, and Suzanne feels quite well. She is certain that the birth will be uneventful and that she can deliver vaginally.

However, at her examination in the 34th week of her pregnancy, her obstetrician suspects the fetus may be in trouble. He orders a nonstress test and intravaginal sonography, both of which indicate low amniotic fluid volume and a distressed fetus. A cesarian section is immediately

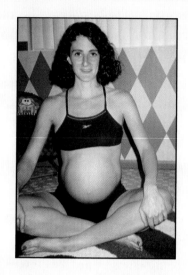

scheduled. Suzanne is nervous and worried about her baby, but everything goes well, and within an hour she is holding her new daughter, Thea.

---

BARFIELD, SUZANNE W. - 600001 Opened by MACHARIA, LOUIS, MD

Task    Edit    View    Time Scale    Options    Help

**BANFIELD, SUZANNE W.**

| | | | |
|---|---|---|---|
| | Age: 36 years | Sex: Female | Loc: WHC-SMMC |
| | DOB: 08/09/1976 | MRN: 600001 | FIN: 3506004 |

Reference Text Browser | Form Browser | Medication Profile

Orders | Last 48 Hours | ED | Lab | Radiology | Assessments | **Surgery** | Clinical Notes | Pt. Info | Pt. Schedule | Task List | I & O | MAR

Flowsheet: Surgery ▼ ...    Level: Operative Report ▼    ⊙ Table  ○ Group  ○ List

Navigator ✕
✓ Operative Report

Preoperative Diagnosis: Pregnancy at 34 weeks, poor nonstress test, oligohydramnios
Postoperative Diagnosis: Pregnancy at 34 weeks, poor nonstress test, oligohydramnios
Procedure: Low transverse cervical cesarean section
Estimated Blood Loss: 300 ml
Anesthesia: Epidural anesthesia
Description of Procedure: Routine preparation and draping of the abdomen. Abdominal cavity was opened with a Pfannenstiel skin incision. Bladder flap of peritoneum was incised and bluntly stripped downward over the lower uterine segment.

A transverse incision was made in the lower uterine segment, and a normal, viable female neonate weighing 6 lb 1 oz was delivered with meconium-stained amniotic fluid. Her Apgars were 5 and 9. Cord blood was obtained. Placenta was removed complete with membranes.

Edge of uterine incision was then closed with two layers of a continuous #1 chromic catgut, with the second layer placed in a running type of Lembert suture. All bleeding was controlled. Bladder flap of peritoneum was replaced.

Sponge and pack counts were correct before and after the abdomen was closed. Routine closure of the abdomen. Staples were used for the skin.

Immediate postoperative condition of mother and baby was good. Amniotic fluid was noted to be meconium stained.

PROD | MAHAFC | 09 Aug 2012 | 06:29

**⟳ Operative Report**

1. An infant born at 34 weeks of gestation would be considered what type of infant?

   _____

2. What is meconium? _____

3. What is a nuchal cord? _____

4. What does an Apgar score measure? _____

5. The nonstress test probably was done because there was concern about _____

   _____

C

*Use*

AN

☐ a
☐ a
☐ a
☐ a
☐ a
☐ a
☐ B

KE

PRI

☐ a
☐ a
☐ c
☐ iı
☐ p
☐ p
☐ t

For more interactive learning, go to Evolve and click on:
- **Whack a Word** Part to review female reproductive word parts.
- **Wheel of Terminology** and **Word Shop** to practice word building.
- **Tournament of Terminology** to test your knowledge of female reproductive terms.
- **Terminology Triage** to practice sorting female reproductive terms into categories.

KE

☐ /
☐ a
☐ a
☐ a
☐ a
☐ b
☐ b

## PATHOLOGY

**Dyscrasia** (dis KRAY zsa), a term that means a bad (dys-) mixture (-crasia), is used more specifically to describe diseases of the blood or bone marrow. Many disorders of the blood have to do with too many or too few of certain types of blood cells. **Anemia** is a decrease in red blood cells, hemoglobin, and/or hematocrit. Many others have to do with abnormalities of cell morphology or shape.

### Terms Related to Deficiency Anemias

| Term | Word Origin | Definition |
| --- | --- | --- |
| acute posthemorrhagic anemia<br>post heh moh RAJ ick ah NEE mee uh | *post-* after<br>*hem/o* blood<br>*-rrhagic* pertaining to bursting forth<br>*an-* no, not<br>*-emia* blood condition | RBC deficiency caused by blood loss. |
| B$_{12}$ deficiency | | Insufficient blood levels of cobalamin, also called vitamin B$_{12}$, which is essential for red blood cell maturation. Condition may be caused by inadequate dietary intake, as in some extreme vegetarian diets, or it may result from absence of **intrinsic factor,** a substance in the GI system essential to vitamin B$_{12}$ absorption. |
| chronic blood loss | | Long-term internal bleeding. May cause anemia. |
| folate deficiency<br>FOH late | | Anemia as a result of a lack of folate from dietary, drug-induced, congenital, or other causes. |
| hypovolemia<br>hye poh voh LEE me ah | *hypo-* deficient<br>*vol/o* volume<br>*-emia* blood condition | Deficient volume of circulating blood. |
| sideropenia<br>sih dur roh PEE nee ah | *sider/o* iron<br>*-penia* deficiency | Condition of having reduced numbers of RBCs because of chronic blood loss, inadequate iron intake, or unspecified causes. A type of **iron deficiency anemia.** |
| pernicious anemia<br>pur NIH shush | *an-* no, not<br>*-emia* blood condition | Progressive anemia that results from a lack of intrinsic factor essential for the absorption of vitamin B$_{12}$. |

### Terms Related to Aplastic and Hemolytic Anemias

| Term | Word Origin | Definition |
| --- | --- | --- |
| aplastic anemia<br>a PLAS tick | *a-* no, not<br>*plast/o* formation<br>*-ic* pertaining to<br>*an-* no, not<br>*-emia* blood condition | Suppression of bone marrow function leading to a reduction in RBC production. Although causes of this often fatal type of anemia may be hepatitis, radiation, or cytotoxic agents, most causes are idiopathic. Also called **hypoplastic anemia.** |
| hemolytic anemia<br>hee moh LIH tick | *hem/o* blood<br>*-lytic* pertaining to destruction | A group of anemias caused by destruction of red blood cells. |

## Terms Related to Aplastic and Hemolytic Anemias—cont'd

| Term | Word Origin | Definition |
|---|---|---|
| **autoimmune acquired hemolytic anemia**<br>hee moh LIT ick | *auto-* self<br>*immune* safety, protection<br>*hem/o* blood<br>*-lytic* pertaining to destruction<br>*an-* no, not<br>*-emia* blood condition | Anemia caused by the body's destruction of its own RBCs by serum antibodies. |
| **nonautoimmune acquired hemolytic anemia** | *non-* not<br>*hem/o* blood<br>*-lytic* pertaining to destruction<br>*an-* no, not<br>*-emia* blood condition | Anemia that may be drug induced or may be caused by an infectious disease, in which the RBCs are destroyed. |
| **sickle cell anemia** | *an-* no, not<br>*-emia* blood condition | Inherited anemia characterized by crescent-shaped RBCs. This abnormality in morphology causes RBCs to block small-diameter capillaries, thereby decreasing the oxygen supply to the cells (Fig. 9-9). A **sickle cell crisis** is an acute, painful exacerbation of sickle-cell anemia. |
| **thalassemia**<br>thal ah SEE mee ah | *thalass/o* sea<br>*-emia* blood condition | Group of inherited disorders of people of Mediterranean, African, and Southeast Asian descent, in which the anemia is the result of a decrease in the synthesis of hemoglobin, resulting in decreased production and increased destruction of RBCs. |
| **pancytopenia**<br>pan sye toh PEE nee ah | *pan-* all<br>*cyt/o* cell<br>*-penia* deficiency | Deficiency of all blood cells caused by dysfunctional stem cells (Fig. 9-10). |

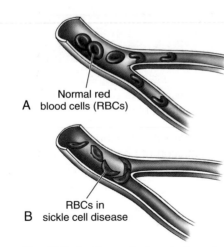

Fig. 9-9 **A,** Normal, donut-shaped red blood cells bend to fit through capillaries. **B,** Sickled red blood cells cannot bend and therefore block the flow of blood through the vessel.

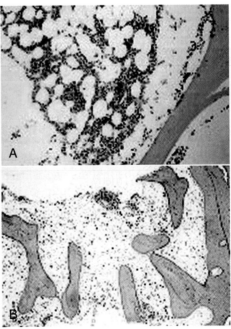

Fig. 9-10 **A,** Normal cellularity.
**B,** Hypocellularity in pancytopenia.

# Chapter Review

Match the word parts to their definitions.

## WORD PARTS

| Suffix | | Definition |
|--------|---|------------|
| -cyte | 1. _____ | cell |
| -cytosis | 2. _____ | producing |
| -edema | 3. _____ | abnormal increase in cells |
| -emia | 4. _____ | protein substance |
| -gen | 5. _____ | formation |
| -globin | 6. _____ | swelling |
| -penia | 7. _____ | attraction condition |
| -philia | 8. _____ | deficiency |
| -poiesis | 9. _____ | iron substance |
| -siderin | 10. _____ | blood condition |

| Combining Form | | Definition |
|----------------|---|------------|
| axill/o | 11. _____ | blood |
| cyt/o | 12. _____ | rosy-colored |
| eosin/o | 13. _____ | groin |
| erythr/o | 14. _____ | nucleus |
| granul/o | 15. _____ | lymph vessel |
| hemat/o | 16. _____ | bone marrow |
| inguin/o | 17. _____ | spleen |
| leuk/o | 18. _____ | fever, fire |
| lymphaden/o | 19. _____ | red |
| lymphangi/o | 20. _____ | clotting, clot |
| lymph/o | 21. _____ | lymph gland (node) |
| morph/o | 22. _____ | cell |
| myel/o | 23. _____ | neutral |
| neutr/o | 24. _____ | armpit |
| nucle/o | 25. _____ | white |
| plasm/o | 26. _____ | serum |
| pyr/o | 27. _____ | little grain |
| ser/o | 28. _____ | plasma |
| splen/o | 29. _____ | thymus |
| thromb/o | 30. _____ | lymph |
| thym/o | 31. _____ | shape |
| tonsill/o | 32. _____ | tonsil |

# WORDSHOP

| Prefixes | Combining Forms | Suffixes |
|---|---|---|
| an- | adenoid/o | -cytosis |
| dys- | cyt/o | -ectomy |
| hyper- | erythr/o | -edema |
| hypo- | hem/o | -graphy |
| pan- | leuk/o | -ia |
| par- | lymphaden/o | -ic |
| | lymphangi/o | -in |
| | lymph/o | -ism |
| | phag/o | -itis |
| | sider/o | -lysis |
| | splen/o | -penia |
| | thromb/o | -stasis |

Build the following terms by combining the above word parts. Some word parts may be used more than once. Some may not be used at all. The number in parentheses is the number of word parts needed to correctly build the term.

| Definition | Term |
|---|---|
| 1. deficiency of all cells (3) | |
| 2. abnormal increase of white blood cells (2) | |
| 3. inflammation of a lymph gland/node (2) | |
| 4. deficiency of clotting cells (3) | |
| 5. process of recording a lymph gland (2) | |
| 6. abnormal increase of red blood cells (2) | |
| 7. removal of the adenoids (2) | |
| 8. swelling (due to) lymph (fluid) (2) | |
| 9. stopping/controlling bleeding (2) | |
| 10. break down of blood (2) | |
| 11. blood iron substance (3) | |
| 12. iron deficiency anemia (2) | |
| 13. process of recording a lymph vessel (2) | |
| 14. condition of excessive spleen (3) | |
| 15. removal of the spleen (2) | |

Sort the terms below into the correct categories.

## TERM SORTING

| Anatomy and Physiology | Pathology | Diagnostic Procedures | Therapeutic Interventions |
|---|---|---|---|
| | | | |
| | | | |
| | | | |
| | | | |
| | | | |
| | | | |
| | | | |
| | | | |
| | | | |
| | | | |

| | | | |
|---|---|---|---|
| adenoidectomy | CMP | hemoglobin | plasma |
| agglutination | coagulation | hemostasis | plateletpheresis |
| anaphylaxis | diff count | hemostatics | Schilling test |
| antibody | dyscrasia | hypovolemia | septicemia |
| antiretrovirals | edema | leukocytosis | sideropenia |
| apheresis | ELISA | lymphangiography | splenectomy |
| blood transfusion | eosinophil | lymphangitis | thalassemia |
| BMP | Hct | MCHC | thrombocyte |
| BMT | hematinic | mononucleosis | thymus |
| CBC | hematopoiesis | monospot | vaccine |

*Replace the highlighted words with the correct terms.*

## TRANSLATIONS

1. On physical examination, Ms. Cooper's physician observed **an enlarged spleen** and she was scheduled for a **removal of the spleen.**

2. Laboratory findings indicated **deficiency of all blood cells** and Mrs. Hamilton was diagnosed with **suppression of bone marrow function leading to a reduction in RBC production.**

3. Laboratory testing revealed that Marc Douglas had an **abnormal increase in WBCs** and **blood samples submitted to propagate microorganisms that may be present** was positive for staphylococci.

4. Tyra was stung by a bee and suffered **an extreme form of allergic response.**

5. The patient underwent a **transplantation of bone marrow to stimulate production of normal blood cells** to treat his **rapidly progressive form of leukemia that develops from immature bone marrow stem cells.**

6. Mr. Washington was admitted with **an acute, painful exacerbation of sickle-cell anemia** that was complicated by **an increased function of the spleen that results in hemolysis.**

7. **Removal of thrombocytes from a donor** was used to treat Mrs. Alverez' **deficiency of platelets that causes an inability of the blood to clot.**

8. The patient was diagnosed with **RBC deficiency caused by blood loss** and needed **an intravenous transfer of blood from a donor to a recipient.**

9. Tommy was seen for cervical **disease of the lymph nodes** and was diagnosed with **an increase in the number of mononuclear cells.**

10. The physician suspected that Alex had **a deficiency of one of the factors necessary for the coagulation of blood** and ordered **a test of blood plasma to detect coagulation defects of the intrinsic system.**

11. Dr. Martinez thought Amanda had **progressive anemia that results from a lack of intrinsic factor** ordered a **nuclear medicine test used to diagnose B$_{12}$ deficiency.**

12. Francis had **a bleeding disorder characterized by hemorrhage into the tissues** and was diagnosed with **a systemic infection with pathologic microbes in the blood.**

13. Greta's doctor ordered blood tests to see if she had **an abnormal decrease in WBCs** or **an abnormal decrease in neutrophils due to disease process.**

14 The patient was diagnosed with **a group of inherited bleeding disorders characterized by a deficiency of one of the factors necessary for the coagulation of blood.**

## Case Study   Ozzie Samuelson

Ozzie Samuelson is a 42-year-old African American with a history of sickle-cell disease. Diagnosed as a child, he has been treated for the disease and its complications numerous times at the hospital. On this day, Ozzie is admitted for a probable sickle-cell crisis accompanied by acute bronchitis.

Sickle-cell anemia causes RBCs to become sickle shaped, which causes them to block up small blood vessels and stop the flow of blood. Pain is the main symptom, but respiratory infections are common, and severe anemia sometimes occurs, necessitating blood transfusions.

Ozzie is exhausted by this most recent, painful sickle-cell crisis episode, which this time has been accompanied by bronchitis. Sickle-cell crisis is an acute exacerbation of sickle-cell anemia.

Ozzie's blood work reveals the low hematocrit and the high WBC that accompany a sickle-cell crisis. Ozzie is given intravenous pain medication, along with antibiotics for his bronchitis. Luckily, the RBC is not low enough to necessitate a blood transfusion.

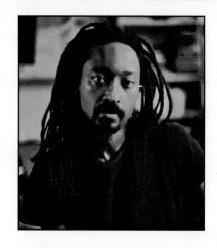

SAMUELSON, OZZIE P. - 499483 Opened by WATERFIELD, WENDY

Task   Edit   View   Time Scale   Options   Help

| SAMUELSON, OZZIE P. | Age: 42 years | Sex: Male | Loc: WHC-SMMC |
| | DOB: 01/27/1969 | MRN: 499483 | FIN: 3506004 |

As Of 12:52

Reference Text Browser | Form Browser | Medication Profile

Orders | Last 48 Hours | ED | Lab | Radiology | Assessments | Surgery | **Clinical Notes** | Pt. Info | Pt. Schedule | Task List | I & O | MAR

Flowsheet: Clinical Notes    Level: Clinical Notes    ○ Table ○ Group ○ List

Navigator

✓   Clinical Notes

Principal Diagnosis: Sickle-Cell Crisis
Surgical Procedure: None
History of Present Illness: The patient was admitted via the emergency room, with a chief complaint of pain all over his body since the night before.
    The patient, a 42-year-old African American male with a history of sickle-cell anemia, stated that he started having pain all over his body, especially at the back of the legs. He also notes having chills, but denies sweats.
Medical History: The patient has a medical history of sickle-cell anemia and pneumonia in 2004.
Surgical History: Surgical history includes a total hip replacement and an appendectomy.
Allergies: The patient has no history of allergies.
Medications: Motrin and Darvon.
Occupation: The patient is unemployed, on disability. The patient is a nonsmoker and a nondrinker.
Family History: The patient's family history reveals mother and father with sickle-cell trait; otherwise unremarkable.
Review of Systems: Unremarkable except for global body pain.
Physical Examination: Temperature was 98.1 degrees, blood pressure was 155/90, heart rate of 75, respiratory rate of 23.
Consultations: The consultations included Dr. Smith for sickle-cell disease.
Pertinent Laboratory Studies: Reticulocyte count of 13.8; white blood cell count of 12.9; hemoglobin and hematocrit of 12.0 and 29.4, respectively; albumin of 2.1.
Hospital Course: The patient was admitted and progressed steadily with intravenous analgesic support until discharge, when the patient was deemed stable.
Condition on Discharge: Stable.
Discharge Instructions: The patient is to limit activity and should follow up with Dr. Rohr in his office in 1 week.
Medications on Discharge: Biaxin, Suprax, Trental, folic acid, Toradol, and vitamin E.

PROD | MAHAFC | 11 Nov 2011 | 12:52

## Clinical Notes

1. What statement in the discharge summary indicates that the patient was in sickle-cell crisis?

_____

2. What medications were used to treat the patient's symptoms?

_____

3. The patient's past healthcare history mentions a resection of his _____ .

For more interactive learning, go to the Shiland Evolve site and click on:
- **Whack a Word Part** to review blood, lymph, and immune word parts.
- **Wheel of Terminology** and **Word Shop** to practice word building.
- **Tournament of Terminology** to test your knowledge of blood, lymph, and immune terms.
- **Terminology Triage** to practice sorting blood, lymph, and immune terms, into categories.

# 10

*A good exercise for the heart is bending down and helping someone to get up.*
**—Proverb**

## OBJECTIVES

- Recognize and use terms related to the anatomy and physiology of the cardiovascular system.
- Recognize and use terms related to the pathology of the cardiovascular system.
- Recognize and use terms related to the diagnostic procedures for the cardiovascular system.
- Recognize and use terms related to the therapeutic interventions for the cardiovascular system.

# Cardiovascular System

## CHAPTER AT A GLANCE

*Use this list of key word parts and terms to assess your knowledge. Check off the ones you have mastered.*

### ANATOMY AND PHYSIOLOGY

- [ ] aorta
- [ ] aortic semilunar valve
- [ ] arteriole
- [ ] artery
- [ ] atrioventricular bundle
- [ ] atrium
- [ ] AV node
- [ ] capillary
- [ ] coronary arteries
- [ ] diastole
- [ ] ejection fraction
- [ ] endocardium
- [ ] inferior vena cava
- [ ] mitral valve (MV)
- [ ] myocardium
- [ ] normal sinus rhythm (NSR)
- [ ] pericardium
- [ ] pulmonary semilunar valve
- [ ] Purkinje fibers
- [ ] SA node
- [ ] septum
- [ ] superior vena cava
- [ ] systole
- [ ] tricuspid valve (TV)
- [ ] vein
- [ ] ventricle
- [ ] venule

### KEY WORD PARTS

#### PREFIXES

- [ ] a-
- [ ] brady-
- [ ] echo-
- [ ] electro-
- [ ] end-
- [ ] hyper-
- [ ] per-
- [ ] tachy-
- [ ] trans-

#### SUFFIXES

- [ ] -cardia
- [ ] -centesis
- [ ] -ectomy
- [ ] -graphy
- [ ] -itis
- [ ] -megaly
- [ ] -osis
- [ ] -pathy
- [ ] -plasty
- [ ] -sclerosis
- [ ] -tension
- [ ] -therapy

#### COMBINING FORMS

- [ ] angi/o
- [ ] arteri/o
- [ ] ather/o
- [ ] atri/o
- [ ] cardi/o
- [ ] coron/o
- [ ] cyan/o
- [ ] endocardi/o
- [ ] lumin/o
- [ ] myocardi/o
- [ ] pericardi/o
- [ ] phleb/o
- [ ] scler/o
- [ ] sept/o
- [ ] thromb/o
- [ ] valvul/o
- [ ] ventricul/o

### KEY TERMS

- [ ] aneurysm
- [ ] angina pectoris
- [ ] angioplasty
- [ ] arrhythmia
- [ ] atrial septal defect
- [ ] arteriosclerosis
- [ ] atherectomy
- [ ] bradycardia
- [ ] CABG
- [ ] cardiac catheterization
- [ ] cardiomegaly
- [ ] cardiomyopathy
- [ ] coronary artery disease (CAD)
- [ ] cyanosis
- [ ] diaphoresis
- [ ] echocardiography (ECHO)
- [ ] electrocardiography
- [ ] endarterectomy
- [ ] heart failure (HF)
- [ ] hypertension (HTN)
- [ ] myocardial infarction (MI)
- [ ] palpitations
- [ ] pericardiocentesis
- [ ] phlebectomy
- [ ] PTCA
- [ ] sclerotherapy
- [ ] tachycardia
- [ ] thrombophlebitis
- [ ] valvuloplasty

## FUNCTIONS OF THE CARDIOVASCULAR SYSTEM

The primary function of the **cardiovascular** (kar dee oh VAS kyoo lur) **system** (CV), also called the **circulatory system,** is to provide transportation of oxygen, nutrients, water, body salts, hormones, and other substances to every cell in the body. It also acts to carry waste products, such as carbon dioxide ($CO_2$), away from the cells, eventually to be excreted. The **heart** functions as a pump; the blood **vessels** act as "pipes"; and the blood is the transportation medium. If the system does not function properly, causing oxygen or the other critical substances to be withheld from the cells, dysfunction results, and the cells (and the person) may be injured or die.

## SPECIALISTS/SPECIALTIES

**Cardiology** is the diagnosis, treatment, and prevention of disorders of the heart. The specialist in this field is called a **cardiologist.**

## ANATOMY AND PHYSIOLOGY

### Pulmonary and Systemic Circulation

To accomplish its task of pumping substances to and from the cells of the body, the heart is in the center of two overlapping cycles of circulation: **pulmonary** and **systemic.**

#### Pulmonary Circulation

In short, pulmonary circulation goes from the heart to the lungs and then back to the heart. Pulmonary circulation begins with the right side of the heart, sending blood to the lungs to absorb oxygen ($O_2$) and release carbon dioxide ($CO_2$). Note in Fig. 10-1 that the vessels that carry blood to the lungs from the heart are blue to show the blood as being **deoxygenated** (dee OCK sih juh nay tid), or oxygen deficient. Once the oxygen is absorbed, the blood is considered **oxygenated,** or oxygen rich. Note in Fig. 10-1 that the vessels traveling away from the lungs are red to show oxygenation. The blood then progresses back to the left side of the heart, where it is pumped out to begin its route through the systemic circulatory system.

#### Systemic Circulation

The systemic circulation carries blood from the heart to the cells of the body, where nutrient and waste exchange takes place; the wastes, such as $CO_2$, are carried back to the heart on the return trip. This blood is then pumped out of the right side of the heart to the lungs to dispose of its $CO_2$, absorb $O_2$, and repeat the cycle. In systemic circulation, the blood traveling away from the heart first passes through the largest artery in the body called the **aorta** (a ORE tuh). From the aorta, the vessels branch into conducting **arteries** (AR tur reez), then into smaller **arterioles** (ar TEER ee olez), and finally to the **capillaries** (CAP ih lair eez). Arteries are blood vessels that carry blood *away* from the heart (Fig. 10-2, *A*). Note in Fig. 10-3 that the color has changed from the red of oxygenated blood to a purple color at the capillaries. This is the site of exchange between the cells' fluids and the plasma of the circulatory system. Oxygen and other substances are supplied, and carbon dioxide collected, along with a number of other wastes. Once the blood begins its journey back to the heart, it first goes through **venules** (VEEN yools), then **veins** (vayns), and finally into one of the two largest veins, either the **superior** or the **inferior vena cava** (VEE nuh

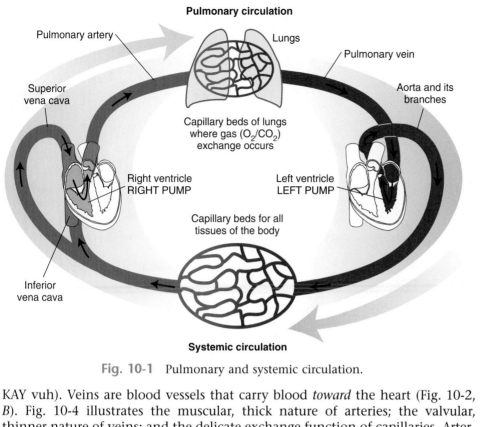

**Pulmonary circulation**

Pulmonary artery

Lungs

Pulmonary vein

Superior
vena cava

Aorta and its
branches

Capillary beds of lungs
where gas (O$_2$/CO$_2$)
exchange occurs

Right ventricle
RIGHT PUMP

Left ventricle
LEFT PUMP

Capillary beds for all
tissues of the body

Inferior
vena cava

**Systemic circulation**

Fig. 10-1  Pulmonary and systemic circulation.

KAY vuh). Veins are blood vessels that carry blood *toward* the heart (Fig. 10-2, *B*). Fig. 10-4 illustrates the muscular, thick nature of arteries; the valvular, thinner nature of veins; and the delicate exchange function of capillaries. Arteries are generally thicker than veins, because they must withstand the force of the heart's pumping action. Veins do not have the thick muscle coat of the arteries to propel the blood on its journey through the circulatory system but instead rely on one-way valves that prevent the backflow of blood. In addition, skeletal muscle contraction provides pumping action. The capillaries' diameters are so tiny that only one blood cell at a time can pass through them.

## Exercise 1: Pulmonary and Systemic Circulation

*Match the following combining forms with their meanings. More than one answer may be correct.*

____ 1. vein

____ 2. artery

____ 3. heart

____ 4. venule

____ 5. capillary

____ 6. lung

____ 7. aorta

____ 8. arteriole

____ 9. vessel

A. vas/o
B. pulmon/o
C. angi/o
D. phleb/o
E. arteri/o
F. ven/o

G. cardi/o
H. capillar/o
I. vascul/o
J. arteriol/o
K. aort/o
L. venul/o

*Decode the terms.*

10. endovascular _____

11. intravenous _____

12. pericardial _____

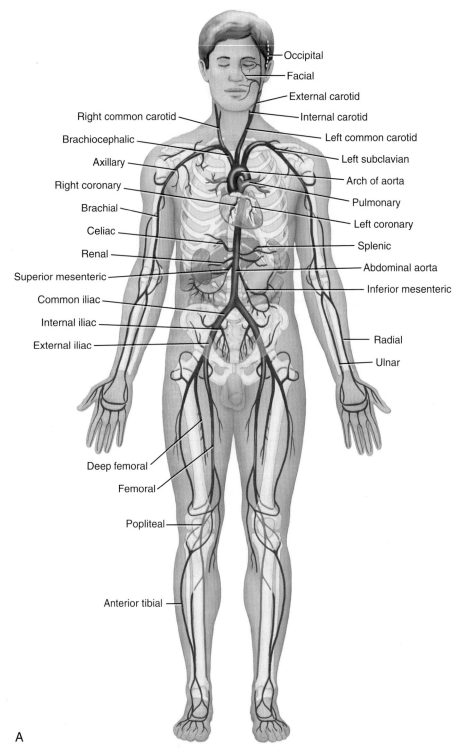

Fig. 10-2  **A,** Principal arteries of the body.

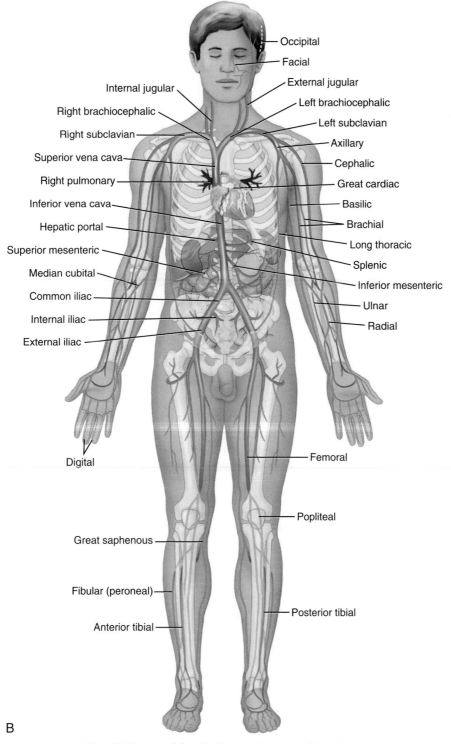

Fig. 10-2, cont'd    **B,** Principal veins of the body.

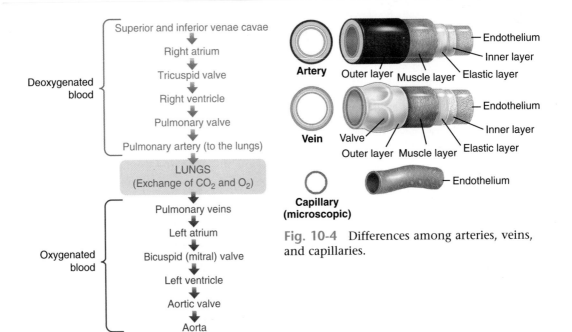

Fig. 10-3   Oxygenated/deoxygenated status.

**Fig. 10-4**   Differences among arteries, veins, and capillaries.

## Anatomy of the Heart

apex = apic/o

precordium
    pre- = before
    cordi/o = heart
    -um = structure

atrium = atri/o

ventricle = ventricul/o

septum = sept/o

valve = valvul/o

endocardium = endocardi/o

myocardium = myocardi/o

visceral = viscer/o

parietal = pariet/o

pericardium = pericardi/o

epicardium
    epi- = above, on top of
    cardi/o = heart
    -um = structure

The human heart is about the size of a fist. It is located in the mediastinum of the thoracic cavity, slightly left of the midline. Its pointed tip, the **apex,** rests just above the diaphragm. The area of the chest wall anterior to the heart and lower thorax is referred to as the **precordium** (pree KORE dee um). The heart muscle has its own dedicated system of blood supply, the **coronary** (KORE ih nair ee) **arteries** (Fig. 10-5, *A*). The two main coronary arteries are called the left and right coronary arteries (LCA, RCA). They supply a constant, uninterrupted blood flow to the heart. The areas of the heart wall that they feed are designated as *inferior, lateral, anterior,* and *posterior.*

The heart has four chambers (Fig. 10-5, *B*). The upper chambers are called **atria** (A tree uh) (*sing.* atrium). The lower chambers are called **ventricles** (VEN trih kuls). Between the atria and ventricles, and between the ventricles and vessels, are valves that allow blood to flow through in one direction. Those values are opened and closed with the assistance of the papillary muscles and their connecting cords, the chordae tendinae. The tissue walls between the chambers are called **septa** (SEP tuh) (*sing.* septum). The heart wall is constructed of three layers. The **endocardium** (en doh KAR dee um) is the thin tissue that acts as a lining of each of the chambers and **valves.** The **myocardium** (mye oh KAR dee um) is the cardiac muscle surrounding each of these chambers. The **pericardium** (pare ee KAR dee um) is the double-folded layer of connective tissue that surrounds the heart. The inner surface of this double fold is called the **visceral** (VIS uh rul) **pericardium,** and the outer membrane, closest to the body wall, is the **parietal** (puh RYE uh tul) **pericardium.** Another name for the visceral pericardium is the **epicardium** (eh pee KAR dee um) because it is the structure on top of the heart.

    **⊗ Be Careful!**   *Do not confuse* **aort/o,** *meaning aorta;* **atri/o,** *meaning atrium;* **arteri/o,** *meaning artery; and* **arteriol/o,** *meaning arteriole.*

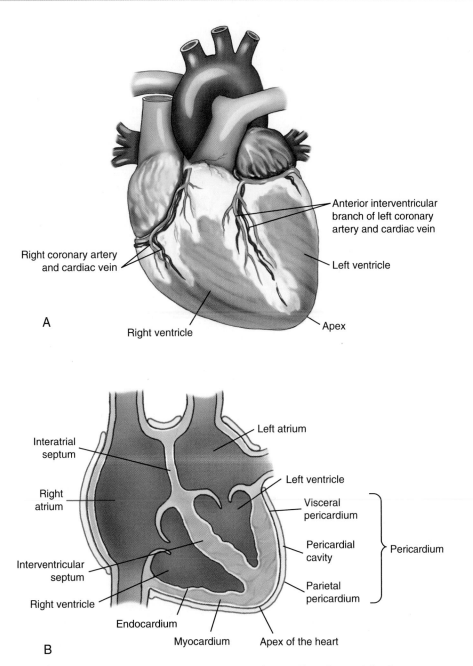

Anterior interventricular branch of left coronary artery and cardiac vein

Right coronary artery and cardiac vein

Left ventricle

Apex

Right ventricle

A

Left atrium

Interatrial septum

Right atrium

Left ventricle

Visceral pericardium

Pericardial cavity

Pericardium

Interventricular septum

Right ventricle

Parietal pericardium

Endocardium

Myocardium

Apex of the heart

B

Fig. 10-5  **A,** The heart and great vessels. **B,** Chambers of the heart.

## Exercise 2: Anatomy of the Heart

*Match the combining form with the correct body part.*

_____ 1. sept/o

_____ 2. valvul/o

_____ 3. atri/o

_____ 4. ventricul/o

_____ 5. aort/o

_____ 6. cardi/o, cordi/o, coron/o

_____ 7. apic/o

_____ 8. endocardi/o

_____ 9. myocardi/o

_____ 10. pericardi/o

_____ 11. pulmon/o

_____ 12. arteri/o

A. upper chamber of the heart
B. lower chamber of the heart
C. heart
D. largest artery
E. inner lining of chambers of heart
F. outer sac surrounding the heart
G. lung
H. muscle layer of the heart
I. valve
J. vessel that carries blood away from the heart
K. wall between chambers
L. the pointed extremity of a conical structure

*Build the terms.*

13. pertaining to between the ventricles _____

14. pertaining to surrounding the tip (of the heart) _____

15. pertaining to before the heart _____

16. pertaining to through the heart muscle _____

## Exercise 3: Anatomy of the Heart

*Label the drawing of the heart below with correct anatomic terms and combining forms where appropriate.*

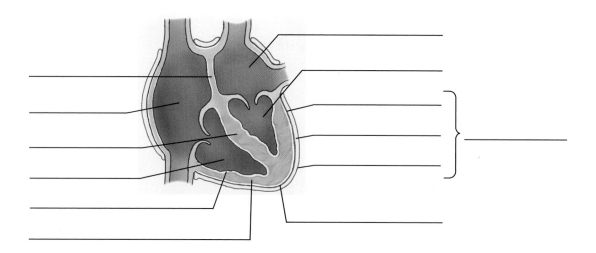

## Blood Flow Through the Heart

Using Fig. 10-6 as a guide, follow the route of the blood through the heart. The pictures and words in this diagram are shaded red and blue to represent oxygenated and deoxygenated blood. Blood is squeezed from the **right atrium** (RA) to the **right ventricle** (RV) through the **tricuspid** (try KUSS pid) **valve** (TV). Valves are considered to be competent if they open and close properly, letting through or holding back an expected amount of blood. Once in the right ventricle, the blood is squeezed out through the **pulmonary semilunar valve** through the short, wide **pulmonary trunk** and into the **pulmonary arteries** (PA), which carry blood to the lungs and are the only arteries that carry deoxygenated blood. In the capillaries of the lungs, the $CO_2$ is passed out of the blood and $O_2$ is taken in. The now-oxygenated blood continues its journey back to the left side of the heart through the **pulmonary veins.** These are the only veins that carry oxygenated blood. The blood then enters the heart through the **left atrium** (LA) and has to pass the **mitral** (MYE trul) **valve** (MV), also termed the **bicuspid valve,** to enter the **left ventricle** (LV). When the left ventricle contracts, the blood is finally pushed out through the **aortic semilunar valve** into the **aorta** and begins yet another cycle through the body.

The amount of blood expelled from the left ventricle compared with the total volume of blood filling the ventricle is referred to as the stroke volume and is a measure of the **ejection fraction** of cardiac output. Typically around 65%, this amount is reduced in certain types of heart disease.

If a woman's heart rate is 80 beats per minute (bpm), then that means her heart contracts almost 5000 times per hour and more than 100,000 beats per day, every day, for a lifetime. Truly an amazing amount of work is accomplished by an individual's body without a bit of conscious thought!

**ejection**
e- = out
ject/o = throwing
-ion = process of

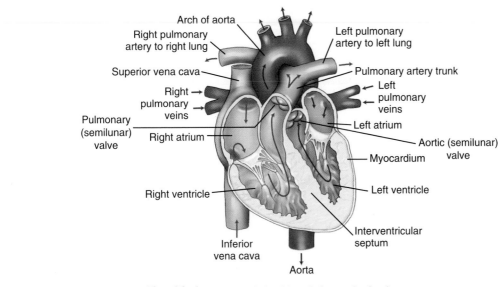

**Fig. 10-6**  Route of the blood through the heart.

---

## ⊘ Exercise 4:   Blood Flow Through the Heart

*Fill in the correct answer.*

1. _____ are the only arteries that carry deoxygenated blood.

2. The _____ valve is between the right atrium and right ventricle.

3. The _____ valve is between the left atrium and left ventricle.

4. _____ valves open and close properly.

5. The amount of blood expelled from the left ventricle compared with total heart volume is a measure

   of the _____.

**contraction**
  con- = together
  tract/o = pull
  -ion = process of

## The Cardiac Cycle

Systemic and pulmonary circulations occur as a result of a series of coordinated, rhythmic pulsations, called **contractions** and **relaxations,** of the heart muscle. The normal *rate* of these pulsations in humans is 60 to 100 beats per minute (BPM) and is noted as a patient's **heart rate.** Fig. 10-7 illustrates various pulse points, places where heart rate can be measured in the body. **Blood pressure (BP)** is the resulting *force* of blood against the arteries. The contractive phase is **systole** (SIS toh lee), and the relaxation phase is **diastole** (dye AS toh lee). Blood pressure is recorded in millimeters of mercury (Hg) as a fraction representing the systolic pressure over the diastolic pressure. Optimum blood pressure is a systolic reading less than 120 and a diastolic reading less than 80. This is written as 120/80. Normal blood pressure is represented by a range. See the table below for blood pressure guidelines.

| Blood Pressure Guidelines | | | |
|---|---|---|---|
| | Systolic | | Diastolic |
| Normal | Under 120 | and | Under 80 |
| Prehypertension | 120-139 | or | 80-89 |
| Stage 1 hypertension | 140-159 | or | 90-99 |
| Stage 2 hypertension | over 160 | or | over 100 |

*Modified from U.S. Department of Health and Human Services.*

**sinoatrial**
  sin/o = sinus
  atri/o = atrium
  -al = pertaining to

**atrioventricular**
  atri/o = atrium
  ventricul/o = ventricle
  -ar = pertaining to

**arrhythmia**
  a- = without
  rhythm/o = rhythm
  -ia = condition

The cues for the timing of the heartbeat come from the electrical pathways in the muscle tissue of the heart (Fig. 10-8). The heartbeat begins in the right atrium in the tissue referred to as the **sinoatrial** (sin oh A tree ul) **(SA) node,** also called the natural pacemaker of the heart. The initial electrical signal causes the atria to undergo electrical changes that signal contraction. This electrical signal is sent to the **atrioventricular** (a tree oh ven TRICK yoo lur) **(AV) node,** which is located at the base of the right atrium proximal to the interatrial septum. From the AV node, the signal travels next to the **bundle of His** (also called the **atrioventricular bundle).** This bundle, a band of specialized cardiac muscle fibers, is in the interatrial septum, and its right and left bundle branches transmit the impulse to the **Purkinje** (poor KIN jee) **fibers** in the right and left ventricles. Once the Purkinje fibers receive stimulation, they cause the ventricles to undergo electrical changes that signal contraction to force blood out to the pulmonary arteries and the aorta. If the electrical activity is normal, it is referred to as a **normal sinus rhythm (NSR)** or **heart rate.** Any deviation of this electronic signaling may lead to an **arrhythmia** (ah RITH mee ah), an abnormal heart rhythm that compromises an individual's cardiovascular functioning by pumping too much or too little blood during that segment of the cardiac cycle.

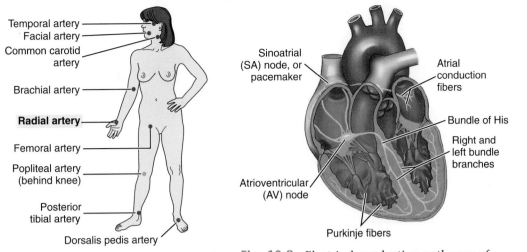

Fig. 10-7 Pulse points. The radial artery is the most commonly used pulse point.

Fig. 10-8 Electrical conduction pathways of the heart.

---

Choose **Hear It, Spell It** to practice spelling the anatomy and physiology terms you have learned in this chapter. To practice pronouncing anatomy and physiology terms choose **Hear It, Say It.** You can review the anatomy of the cardiovascular system by clicking on **Body Spectrum Electronic Anatomy Coloring Book → Circulatory.**

---

*Case Study* William Woodward

William is a 58-year-old coach of a baseball double A farm team. He travels a lot, eats out almost every day, is very stressed, and gets very little exercise. His family history consists of a mother with high blood pressure and high cholesterol, a father and grandfather with coronary artery disease and high blood pressure, and a grandmother who had a stroke at the age of 72.

William's past medical history includes high blood pressure, high cholesterol and triglycerides, and, most recently, fatigue and dizzy spells, which finally force him to visit his cardiologist, who orders a left carotid endarterectomy. After the procedure, an arteriogram shows that the endarterectomy was successful.

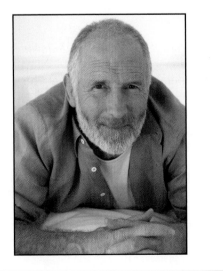

## *Case Study*   William Woodward

WOODWARD, WILLIAM W - 52243                                        ⊟ ⊡ ☒

Task   Edit   View   Time Scale   Options   Help

| WOODWARD, WILLIAM W | Age: 58 years | Sex: Male | Loc: VVH |
|---|---|---|---|
| | DOB: 06/06/1952 | MRN: 52243 | FIN: 884401 |

| Reference Text Browser | Form Browser | Medication Profile |
|---|---|---|

| Orders | Last 48 Hours | ED | Lab | **Radiology** | Assessments | Surgery | Clinical Notes | Pt. Info | Pt. Schedule | Task List | I & O | MAR |

Flowsheet: Radiology ▼ ... Level: Radiology ▼        ⦿ Table  ○ Group  ○ List

**Navigator** ☒
✓ Radiology

**Intraoperative Left Carotid Arteriogram**

A single intraoperative left carotid arteriogram is submitted. The catheter tip is located within the distal common carotid artery. The injection has opacified a widely patent endarterectomy site. The former stenosis located at the origin of the right internal carotid artery has been completely reduced. The left internal carotid artery is widely patent into the intracranial circulation. The external carotid artery is also widely patent.

Impression: Intraoperative arteriogram demonstrating a widely patent left carotid endarterectomy site.

PROD  MAHAFC   07 Aug 2010   12:37

## Exercise 5: Imaging Report

*Fill in the correct answer in the following questions using the report provided above.*

1. "Intraoperative" tells you that the procedure was done _____ the operation.

2. The carotid arteries are located in the _____ and supply blood to the _____.

3. An "endarterectomy" site would refer to an area _____ an artery.

4. The term "stenosis" in the report refers to a _____ of the artery.

## Combining and Adjective Forms for the Anatomy and Physiology of the Cardiovascular System

| Meaning | Combining Form | Adjective Form |
|---|---|---|
| aorta | aort/o | aortic |
| apex | apic/o | apical |
| arteriole | arteriol/o | |
| artery | arteri/o | arterial |
| atrium | atri/o | atrial |
| carbon dioxide | capn/o | |
| endocardium | endocardi/o | endocardial |
| epicardium | epicardi/o | epicardial |
| heart | cardi/o, coron/o, cordi/o | cardiac, coronary, cordial |
| lung | pulmon/o, pneum/o, pneumat/o | pulmonary, pneumatic |
| myocardium | myocardi/o | myocardial |
| oxygen | ox/i, ox/o | |
| pericardium | pericardi/o | pericardial |
| pull | tract/o | |
| rhythm | rhythm/o | rhythmic |
| septum, wall | sept/o | septal |
| sinus | sin/o | |
| system | system/o | systemic |
| valve | valvul/o | valvular |
| vein | ven/o, phleb/o | venous |
| ventricle | ventricul/o | ventricular |
| venule | venul/o | |
| vessel | vascul/o, angi/o, vas/o | vascular |
| viscera | viscer/o | visceral |
| wall | pariet/o | parietal |

## Prefixes for Anatomy and Physiology of the Cardiovascular System

| Prefix | Meaning |
|---|---|
| a- | without |
| con- | together |
| e- | out |
| pre- | before |

## Suffixes for Anatomy and Physiology of the Cardiovascular System

| Suffix | Meaning |
|---|---|
| -ar, -ary, -ic, -al | pertaining to |
| -ia | condition |
| -ion | process of |
| -logy | study of |
| -um | structure |

# PATHOLOGY

## Terms Related to Cardiac Signs and Symptoms

| Term | Word Origin | Definition |
|---|---|---|
| **bradycardia**<br>brad dee KAR dee ah | *brady-* slow<br>*-cardia* heart condition | Slow heartbeat, with ventricular contractions less than 60 bpm (Fig. 10-9, *B*). |
| **bruit**<br>BROO ee | | Abnormal sound heard when an artery is auscultated. Usually a blowing or swishing sound, higher pitched than a murmur. |
| **cardiodynia**<br>kar dee oh DIN ee uh | *cardi/o* heart<br>*-dynia* pain | Heart pain that may be described as atypical or ischemic. **Atypical pain** is a stabbing or burning pain that is variable in location and intensity and unrelated to exertion. **Ischemic pain** is a pressing, squeezing, or weightlike cardiac pain caused by decreased blood supply that usually lasts only minutes. **Precordial pain** is pain in the area over the heart. Also called **cardialgia.** |
| **cardiomegaly**<br>kar dee oh MEG uh lee | *cardi/o* heart<br>*-megaly* enlargement | Enlargement of the heart. |
| **claudication**<br>klah dih KAY shun | | Cramplike pains in the calves caused by poor circulation in the leg muscles. |
| **cyanosis**<br>sye uh NOH sis | *cyan/o* blue<br>*-osis* abnormal condition | A bluish or grayish discoloration of skin, nail beds, and/or lips caused by a lack of oxygen in the blood. |
| **diaphoresis**<br>dye uh foh REE sis | | Profuse secretion of sweat. |
| **dyspnea; dyspnea on exertion (DOE)**<br>DISP nee uh | *dys-* difficult<br>*-pnea* breathing | Difficult and/or painful breathing; if DOE, it is experienced when effort is expended. |
| **edema**<br>eh DEE muh | | Abnormal accumulation of fluid in interstitial spaces of tissues. |
| **emesis**<br>EM uh sis | *emesis* to vomit | Forcible or involuntary emptying of the stomach through the mouth. |
| **ischemia** | *isch/o* to hold back<br>*-emia* blood condition | Lack of blood in a body part due to a blockage or functional constriction. |

## Terms Related to Cardiac Signs and Symptoms—cont'd

| Term | Word Origin | Definition |
|------|-------------|------------|
| **murmur** | | Abnormal heart sound heard during systole, diastole, or both, which may be described as a gentle blowing, fluttering, or humming sound. |
| **nausea** <br> NAH zsa | | Sensation that accompanies the urge to vomit, but does not always lead to vomiting. |
| **pallor** <br> PAL ur | | Paleness of skin and/or mucous membranes. On darker pigmented skin, it may be noted on the inner surfaces of the lower eyelids or the nail beds. |
| **palpitations** <br> pal pih TAY shuns | | Pounding or racing of the heart, such that the patient is aware of his/her heartbeat. |
| **pulmonary congestion** | *pulmon/o* lung <br> *-ary* pertaining to | Excessive amount of blood in the pulmonary vessels. Usually associated with heart failure. |
| **shortness of breath (SOB)** | | Breathlessness, air hunger. |
| **syncope** <br> SING kuh pee | | Fainting, loss of consciousness. |
| **tachycardia** <br> tack ee KAR dee ah | *tachy-* rapid <br> *-cardia* heart condition | Rapid heartbeat, more than 100 bpm (Fig. 10-9, *C*). |
| **thrill** | | Fine vibration felt by the examiner on palpation. |
| **venous distention** | *ven/o* vein <br> *-ous* pertaining to | Enlarged or swollen veins. |

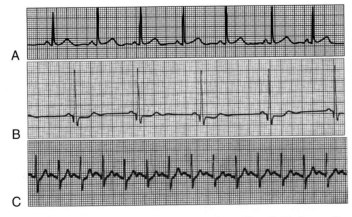

Fig. 10-9  ECGs. **A,** Normal. **B,** Bradycardia. **C,** Tachycardia.

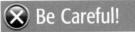 Be Careful!

*Do not confuse* **palpation,** *which means examination by touch,* **palpebration,** *which means blinking, and* **palpitation,** *which means a pounding or racing of the heart.*

## Exercise 6: Cardiac Signs and Symptoms

*Matching.*

____ 1. claudication

____ 2. syncope

____ 3. diaphoresis

____ 4. bruit

____ 5. murmur

____ 6. thrill

____ 7. emesis

____ 8. ischemia

____ 9. nausea

____ 10. pallor

____ 11. palpitations

____ 12. dyspnea

____ 13. cyanosis

____ 14. SOB

A. fainting
B. paleness of skin
C. air hunger
D. fine vibration felt on palpation
E. difficult breathing
F. abnormal sound heard upon auscultation of an artery
G. cramplike pains in legs
H. abnormal heart sound
I. blue color due to lack of oxygen
J. urge to vomit
K. vomiting
L. decreased blood supply
M. profuse sweating
N. pounding of the heart

*Decode the terms.*

15. bradycardia _____

16. tachycardia _____

17. cardiomegaly _____

## Terms Related to Congenital Disorders of the Heart

| Term | Word Origin | Definition |
|------|-------------|------------|
| **coarctation of the aorta** <br> koh ark TAY shun | | Congenital cardiac anomaly characterized by a localized narrowing of the aorta. **Coarctation** is another term for a narrowing (Fig. 10-10). |
| **patent ductus arteriosus (PDA)** <br> PAY tent <br> DUCK tus <br> ar teer ee OH sis | | Abnormal opening between the pulmonary artery and the aorta caused by failure of the fetal ductus arteriosus to close after birth, most often in premature infants. **Patent** means *open.* **Occluded** means *closed.* |
| **septal defect** <br> SEP tul | *sept/o* septum, wall <br> *-al* pertaining to | Any congenital abnormality of the walls between the heart chambers. **Atrial septal defect** (ASD) is a hole in the wall between the upper chambers of the heart. **Ventricular septal defect** (VSD) is a hole in the wall between the lower two chambers of the heart. |
| **tetralogy of Fallot** <br> teh TROL uh jee <br> fah LOH | *tetra-* four <br> *-logy* study of | Congenital cardiac anomaly that consists of four defects: pulmonic stenosis; ventricular septal defect; malposition of the aorta, so that it arises from the septal defect or the right ventricle; and right ventricular hypertrophy. |

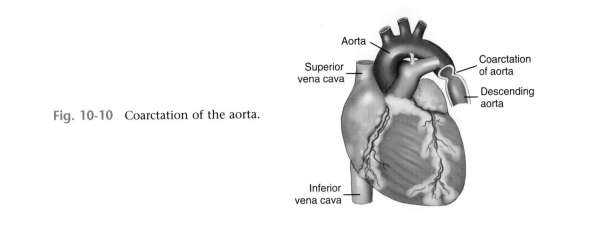

**Fig. 10-10** Coarctation of the aorta.

## Exercise 7: Congenital Disorders

*Match the congenital disorders with their definitions.*

___ 1. patent ductus arteriosus

___ 2. septal defect

___ 3. coarctation of the aorta

___ 4. tetralogy of Fallot

A. cardiac anomaly of four defects
B. narrowing of the largest artery of the body
C. abnormal opening between the pulmonary artery and the aorta
D. hole in the wall between the upper or lower chambers of the heart

## Terms Related to Valvular Heart Disease

The following valvular heart diseases (VHDs) present as incompetent or insufficient valvular function as a result of **stenosis** (narrowing), **regurgitation** (backflow), or **prolapse** (drooping). The causes are either congenital or acquired.

| Term | Word Origin | Definition |
|---|---|---|
| **aortic stenosis (AS)**<br>a OR tick<br>sten OH sis | *aort/o* aorta<br>*-ic* pertaining to<br>*stenosis* narrowing | Narrowing of the aortic valve, which may be acquired or congenital (Fig. 10-11). |
| **mitral regurgitation (MR)**<br>MYE trul<br>ree gur jih TAY shun | | Backflow of blood from the left ventricle into the left atrium in systole across a diseased valve. It may be the result of congenital valve abnormalities, rheumatic fever, or mitral valve prolapse (MVP). |
| **mitral stenosis (MS)**<br>MYE trul<br>sten OH sis | *stenosis* narrowing | Narrowing of the valve between the left atrium and left ventricle caused by adhesions on the leaflets of the valve, usually the result of recurrent episodes of rheumatic endocarditis. Left atrial hypertrophy develops and may be followed by right-sided heart failure and pulmonary edema (cor pulmonale) (see Fig. 10-11). |
| **mitral valve prolapse (MVP)**<br>MYE trul<br>valv<br>PRO laps | *pro-* forward<br>*-lapse* fall | Protrusion of one or both cusps of the mitral valve back into the left atrium during ventricular systole (Fig. 10-12). |

*Continued*

## Terms Related to Valvular Heart Disease—cont'd

| Term | Word Origin | Definition |
|------|-------------|------------|
| **orthopnea**<br>or THOP nee uh | *orth/o* straight, upright<br>*-pnea* breathing | Condition in which a person must sit or stand to breathe comfortably. |
| **tricuspid stenosis (TS)**<br>try KUSS pid<br>sten OH sis | *stenosis* narrowing | Relatively uncommon narrowing of the tricuspid valve associated with lesions of other valves caused by rheumatic fever. Symptoms include jugular vein distention and pulmonary congestion (see Fig. 10-11). |
| **valvulitis**<br>val vyoo LYE tis | *valvul/o* valve<br>*-itis* inflammation | Inflammatory condition of a valve, especially a cardiac valve, caused most commonly by rheumatic fever and less frequently by bacterial endocarditis or syphilis. Results are stenoses and obstructed blood flow. |

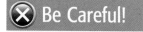 Be Careful!

*Do not confuse* **stenosis,** *which means a narrowing, with* **sclerosis,** *which means a hardening.*

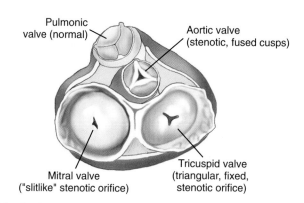

Fig. 10-11   Valvular heart disease: disorders of the aortic, mitral, and tricuspid valves.

Fig. 10-12   Mitral valve prolapse.

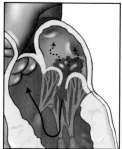

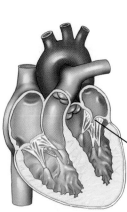

# Exercise 8: Valvular Heart Disorders

*Matching.*

____ 1. stenosis

____ 2. regurgitation

____ 3. prolapse

____ 4. orthopnea

____ 5. valvulitis

A. breathing in an upright position
B. drooping, falling forward
C. narrowing
D. backflow
E. inflammation of a valve

## Terms Related to Cardiac Dysrhythmias (Arrhythmias)

A dysrhythmia is an abnormal heartbeat (dys- means "abnormal," rhythm/o means "rhythm," and -ia means "condition"). Remember that a normal heart rate is referred to as a "normal sinus rhythm (NSR)."

| Term | Word Origin | Definition |
|---|---|---|
| arrhythmia<br>ah RITH mee ah | *a-* without<br>*rhythm/o* rhythm<br>*-ia* condition | Abnormal variation from the normal heartbeat rhythm. Also called **dysrhythmia.** |
| atrioventricular block<br>a tree oh ven TRICK yoo lur | *atri/o* atrium<br>*ventricul/o* ventricle<br>*-ar* pertaining to | Partial or complete heart block that is the result of a lack of electrical communication between the atria and the ventricles. Also termed "heart block." |
| bundle branch block (BBB) | | Incomplete electrical conduction in the bundle branches, either left or right. |
| ectopic beats<br>eck TOP ick | *ec-* out of<br>*top/o* place<br>*-ic* pertaining to | Heartbeats that occur outside of a normal rhythm. |
| atrial | *atri/o* atrium<br>*-al* pertaining to | Atrial ectopic beats (AEB) are irregular contractions of the atria. Also termed premature atrial contractions (PAC). |
| ventricular | *ventricul/o* ventricle<br>*-ar* pertaining to | Ventricular ectopic beats (VEB) are irregular contractions of the ventricles. Also called premature ventricular contractions (PVC). Are not always considered pathologic. |
| fibrillation<br>fibrill LAY shun | | Extremely rapid and irregular contractions (300-600/min) occurring with or without an underlying cardiovascular disorder, such as coronary artery disease. |
| atrial | *atri/o* atrium<br>*-al* pertaining to | Atrial fibrillation (AF) is the most common type of cardiac arrhythmia. |
| ventricular | *ventricul/o* ventricle<br>*-ar* pertaining to | Rapid, irregular ventricular contractions; may be fatal unless reversed. |
| flutter | | Extremely rapid but regular heartbeat (250-350).<br>**Atrial flutter** is a rapid, regular atrial rhythm. |

*Continued*

## Terms Related to Cardiac Dysrhythmias (Arrhythmias)—cont'd

| Term | Word Origin | Definition |
|------|-------------|------------|
| sick sinus syndrome (SSS) | | Any abnormality of the sinus node that may include the necessity of an implantable pacemaker. |
| ventricular tachycardia<br>ven TRICK yoo lur<br>tack ee KAR dee ah | *ventricul/o* ventricle<br>*-ar* pertaining to<br>*tachy-* rapid<br>*-cardia* heart condition | Condition of ventricular contractions >100 bpm. |

## Exercise 9: Cardiac Dysrhythmias

*Fill in the blank.*

1. Another general term for an arrhythmia is a/n _____.

2. Extremely rapid and irregular contractions are _____.

3. An extremely rapid but regular heartbeat is _____.

4. The general term for a lack of electrical communication is heart _____.

5. Any abnormality of the sinus node is termed _____.

6. Another term for premature ventricular contractions is _____.

7. The term for ventricular contractions over 100 beats per minute is _____.

## Terms Related to Other Disorders of Coronary Circulation

| Term | Word Origin | Definition |
|------|-------------|------------|
| angina pectoris<br>an JYE nuh<br>PECK tore us | *pector/o* chest<br>*-is* structure | Paroxysmal chest pain that is often accompanied by shortness of breath and a sensation of impending doom (Fig. 10-13). |
| coronary artery disease (CAD)<br>KORE uh nare ee | *coron/o* heart, crown<br>*-ary* pertaining to | Accumulation and hardening of plaque in the coronary arteries that eventually can deprive the heart muscle of oxygen, leading to **angina (heart pain)**. |
| myocardial infarction (MI)<br>mye oh KAR dee ul<br>in FARCK shun | *myocardi/o* heart muscle<br>*-al* pertaining to | Cardiac tissue death that occurs when the coronary arteries are occluded (blocked) by an **atheroma** (ath uh ROH mah), a mass of fat or lipids on the wall of an artery, or a blood clot caused by an atheroma, and thus are unable to carry enough oxygenated blood to the heart muscle. Depending on the area affected, the patient may die if enough of the heart muscle is destroyed (Fig. 10-14). Also called a **heart attack.** |

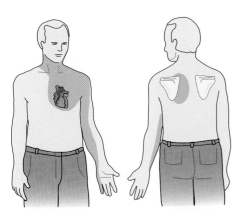

Fig. 10-13 Common sites of pain in angina pectoris.

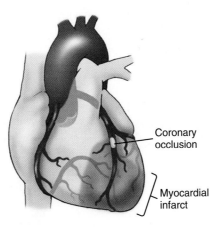

Coronary occlusion

Myocardial infarct

Fig. 10-14 Myocardial infarction.

⊗ **Be Careful!**

**Infarction** *refers to tissue death. An* **infraction** *refers to a breaking, as in an incomplete bone fracture.*

## Inflammation and Heart Disease

Research has uncovered a link between higher levels of a protein present in the blood when blood vessels are inflamed and cardiovascular disease risk. Elevated C-reactive protein (CRP) levels are associated with a dramatically increased risk for heart attack and stroke, independent of an individual's cholesterol levels, obesity, smoking history, or blood pressure. Although the research indicates that diagnosis and treatment of the inflammation may reduce one's risk of heart disease, the American Heart Association continues to recommend that individuals stop smoking, eat a healthy diet, exercise, maintain a healthy blood pressure, and manage diabetes if present for optimal cardiovascular health.

## Terms Related to Other Cardiac Conditions

| Term | Word Origin | Definition |
|---|---|---|
| **cardiac tamponade** <br> tam pon ADE | | Compression of the heart caused by fluid in the pericardial sac. |
| **cardiomyopathy** <br> kar dee oh mye AH puh thee | *cardiomy/o* myocardium <br> *-pathy* disease | Progressive disorder of the ventricles of the heart. |
| **endocarditis** <br> en doh kar DYE tis | *endocardi/o* endocardium <br> *-itis* inflammation | Inflammation of the endocardium and heart valves, characterized by lesions and caused by a number of different microbes (Fig. 10-15). |
| **heart failure (HF)** | | Inability of the heart muscle to pump blood efficiently, so that it becomes overloaded. The heart enlarges with unpumped blood, and the lungs fill with fluid. Previously referred to as **congestive heart failure** (CHF). |
| **pericarditis** <br> pair ee kar DYE tis | *pericardi/o* pericardium <br> *-itis* inflammation | Inflammation of the sac surrounding the heart, with the possibility of **pericardial effusion** (the escape of blood into the pericardium). |

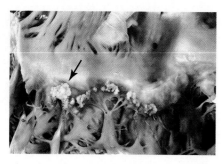

**Fig. 10-15**  Acute bacterial endocarditis. The valve is covered with large irregular vegetations (arrow).

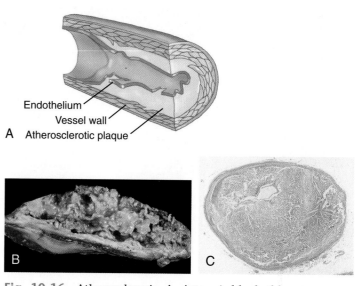

Endothelium
Vessel wall
A   Atherosclerotic plaque

B

C

**Fig. 10-16**  Atherosclerosis. **A,** Artery is blocked by an atheroma. **B,** Fatty deposits on wall of artery. **C,** Image of the resultant narrowed coronary artery.

## Exercise 10: Other Disorders of Coronary Circulation and Cardiac Conditions

*Fill in the blank.*

1. The medical term for a heart attack is a/an (2 words) _____.

2. The inability for the heart muscle to pump blood efficiently is (2 words)

   _____.

3. A compression of the heart caused by fluid in the pericardial sac is (2 words)

   _____.

4. Paroxysmal chest pain accompanied by shortness of breath is (2 words)

   _____.

5. An accumulation and hardening of plaque in the coronary arteries is (3 words)

   _____, abbreviated CAD.

*Build the terms.*

6. inflammation of the pericardium _____

7. inflammation of the endocardium _____

8. disease of the heart muscle _____

## Terms Related to Vascular Disorders

| Term | Word Origin | Definition |
|------|-------------|------------|
| **aneurysm**<br>AN yoo rizz um | | Localized dilation of an artery caused by a congenital or acquired weakness in the wall of the vessel. The acquired causes may be arteriosclerosis, trauma, infection, and/or inflammation. |
| **arteriosclerosis**<br>ar teer ee oh sklah ROH sis | *arteri/o* artery<br>*-sclerosis* abnormal condition of hardening | Disease in which the arterial walls become thickened and lose their elasticity, without the presence of atheromas. |
| **atherosclerosis**<br>ath uh roh sklah ROH sis | *ather/o* fat, plaque<br>*-sclerosis* abnormal condition of hardening | Form of arteriosclerosis in which medium and large arteries have atheromas, which can reduce or obstruct blood flow. Patients with peripheral atherosclerosis complain of intermittent claudication (Fig 10-16). |
| **esophageal varices**<br>eh sof uh JEE ul VARE ih seez | *esophag/o* esophagus<br>*-eal* pertaining to<br>*varic/o* dilated vein | Varicose veins that appear at the lower end of the esophagus as a result of portal hypertension; they are superficial and may cause ulceration and bleeding. |
| **hemorrhoid**<br>HEM uh royd | | Varicose condition of the external or internal rectal veins that causes painful swellings at the anus. |
| **hypertension (HTN)**<br>hye pur TEN shun | *hyper-* excessive<br>*tens/o* stretching<br>*-ion* process of | Condition of high or elevated blood pressure, also known as **arterial hypertension**; occurs in two forms—**primary (or essential) hypertension,** which has no identifiable cause; and **secondary hypertension,** which occurs in response to another disorder. **Malignant hypertension** is very high blood pressure that results in organ damage. |
| **hypotension**<br>hye poh TEN shun | *hypo-* below, deficient<br>*tens/o* stretching<br>*-ion* process of | Condition of below normal blood pressure. **Orthostatic hypotension** occurs when a patient experiences an episode of low blood pressure upon rising to a standing position. |
| **peripheral arterial occlusion**<br>puh RIFF uh rul<br>ar TEER ree ul<br>oh KLOO zhun | *arteri/o* artery<br>*-al* pertaining to<br>*occlus/o* blockage<br>*-ion* process of | Blockage of blood flow to the extremities. Acute or chronic conditions may be present, but patients with both types of conditions are likely to have underlying atherosclerosis. Occlusion means blockage. |
| **peripheral vascular disease (PVD)**<br>puh RIFF uh rul<br>VAS kyoo lur | *vascul/o* vessel<br>*-ar* pertaining to | Any vascular disorder limited to the extremities; may affect not only the arteries and veins but also the lymphatics. |
| **Raynaud disease**<br>ray NODE | | **Idiopathic** disease—that is, of unknown cause—of the peripheral vascular system that causes intermittent cyanosis/erythema of the distal ends of the fingers and toes, sometimes accompanied by numbness; occurs almost exclusively in young women. Presentation is bilateral. **Raynaud phenomenon** is secondary to rheumatoid arthritis, scleroderma, or trauma. Presentation is unilateral. |

*Continued*

## Terms Related to Vascular Disorders—cont'd

| Term | Word Origin | Definition |
|---|---|---|
| **thrombophlebitis**<br>throm boh fluh BYE tis | *thromb/o* clotting, clot<br>*phleb/o* vein<br>*-itis* inflammation | Inflammation of either deep veins (**deep vein thrombosis,** or **DVT**) or superficial veins (**superficial vein thrombosis,** or **SVT**), with the formation of one or more blood clots (Fig. 10-17). |
| **varicose veins**<br>VARE ih kose | *varic/o* varices<br>*-ose* pertaining to | Elongated, dilated superficial veins (varices) with incompetent valves that permit reverse blood flow. These veins may appear in various parts of the anatomy, but the term varicose vein(s) has been reserved for those in the lower extremities. |
| **vasculitis**<br>vas kyoo LYE tis | *vascul/o* vessel<br>*-itis* inflammation | Inflammation of the blood vessels. Also called **angiitis**. |

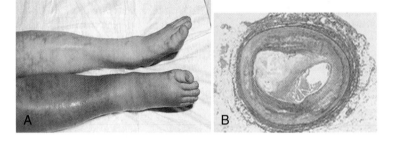

**Fig. 10-17　A,** Deep vein thrombophlebitis (DVT). **B,** Large embolus derived from a lower extremity DVT and now located in a pulmonary artery branch.

## Exercise 11: Vascular Disorders

*Fill in the blanks with one of the following terms.*

**essential, primary, secondary, varicose veins, claudication, hemorrhoids, esophageal varices, aneurysm, peripheral artery occlusion, Raynaud disease**

1. A localized dilation of an artery caused by a weakness in the vessel wall is a/an

   _____.

2. Cramplike pain in the calves caused by poor circulation is called _____.

3. If hypertension is idiopathic, it is called _____ or _____ hypertension.

4. _____ hypertension is due to another disorder.

5. Swollen, twisted veins in the region of the anus are called _____.

6. Varicose veins of the lower end of the tube from the throat to the stomach are called

   _____.

7. A blockage of blood flow to the extremities is called _____.

8. An idiopathic disease of the peripheral vascular system is called _____.

9. Elongated superficial dilated veins are called _____.

*Decode the terms.*

10. vasculitis _____

11. hypotension _____

12. hypertension _____

13. thrombophlebitis _____

## Terms Related to Benign Neoplasms

| Term | Word Origin | Definition |
|------|-------------|------------|
| **atrial myxoma**<br>A tree uhl<br>mick SOH mah | *atri/o* atrium<br>*-al* pertaining to<br>*myx/o* mucus<br>*-oma* tumor, mass | Benign growth usually occurring on the interatrial septum (Fig. 10-18). |
| **hemangioma**<br>heh man jee OH mah | *hemangi/o* blood vessel<br>*-oma* tumor, mass | Noncancerous tumor of the blood vessels. May be congenital ("stork bite") or may develop later in life. |

## Terms Related to Malignant Neoplasms

| Term | Word Origin | Definition |
|------|-------------|------------|
| **cardiac myxosarcoma**<br>mick soh sar KOH mah | *myx/o* mucus<br>*-sarcoma* connective tissue cancer | Rare cancer of the heart usually originating in the left atrium (Fig. 10-19). |
| **hemangiosarcoma**<br>hee man jee oh sar KOH mah | *hemangi/o* blood vessel<br>*-sarcoma* connective tissue cancer | Rare cancer of the cells that line the blood vessels. |

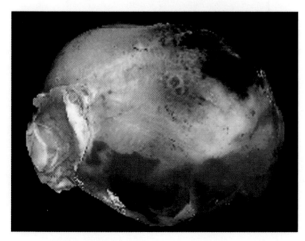

Fig. 10-18  Left atrial myxoma.

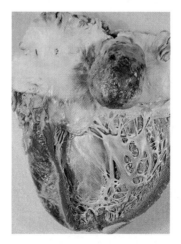

Fig. 10-19  Myxosarcoma of the heart.

## Exercise 12: Neoplasms

*Fill in the blank.*

1. What is a benign tumor of the blood vessels? _____.

2. What is a rare malignant tumor of the heart? _____.

3. What is a benign tumor that originates in the atria of the heart? _____.

4. What is a rare malignant tumor of the lining of the blood vessels? _____.

## Age Matters

### Pediatrics

Most children's cardiovascular disorders are of a congenital nature. Patent ductus arteriosus, tetralogy of Fallot, septal defects, and coarctation of the aorta are the most common. If a child is born with a healthy heart, it is unlikely that problems will occur with this system during childhood.

### Geriatrics

Seniors exhibit a variety of heart disorders. Hypertension, coronary artery disease, myocardial infarctions, arrhythmias, and peripheral vascular disease are seen frequently as diagnoses on patient charts. Contributing factors that exacerbate cardiovascular disorders are obesity, smoking, and lack of exercise.

## Case Study    Helen Podrasky

Helen has been looking forward to Thanksgiving for months because her scattered family is coming to her house for the holiday. As she rolls out the dough for her pumpkin pie, she notices that her heart is beating a little faster but attributes it to nerves. As the family gathers around the dinner table, she starts to feel warm and light-headed, and she can feel her heart racing, although she has no chest pain. Her daughter calls the ambulance, and she is taken to the hospital. She is placed on a monitor; an IV for fluids is started and blood work is ordered. A chest x-ray reveals an enlarged heart, but no CHF is noted. She was admitted to the hospital for further workup and observation.

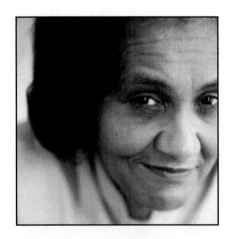

## Case Study    Helen Podrasky

```
PODRASKY, HELEN P - 612347 Opened by ADAMS, JOHANNA MD        _ ⊟ ✕
Task   Edit   View   Time Scale   Options   Help
```

```
🛉 📑 ← → 🔥 🔥 🔀 🔀 🔄 ⬆ ■ 📑 📄 📁 📁 🔗 ❓ 🖼 📄    As Of 15:09      📊 🔍 📄
```

| PODRASKY, HELEN P | Age: 63 years | Sex: Female | Loc: WHC-SMMC |
|---|---|---|---|
|  | DOB: 03/02/1949 | MRN: 612347 | FIN: 3506004 |

| Reference Text Browser | Form Browser | Medication Profile |
|---|---|---|

| Orders | Last 48 Hours | ED | Lab | Radiology | Assessments | Surgery | **Clinical Notes** | Pt. Info | Pt. Schedule | Task List | I & O | MAR |

Flowsheet: Clinical Notes ▼ ...   Level: Progress Note ▼      ⦿ Table ○ Group ○ List

| Navigator | ✕ |
|---|---|
| ✓ | Progress Note |

Patient is status post coronary bypass grafting approximately 1 year ago. Today, she developed a rapid pulse of approximately 145, no chest pain, and no SOB, but indicated she felt weak as a result.

| PAST MEDICAL HISTORY: | As above |
|---|---|
| MEDICATIONS: | verapamil, digoxin, Coumadin, iron |

PHYSICAL EXAM:

| Vital signs: | BP 150/66, pulse 136 and irregular, temp. 97.2º F |
|---|---|
| Chest: | Clear |
| Heart: | Rhythm is irregular |
| Abdomen: | Soft and nontender |
| LABORATORY FINDINGS: | ECG showed atrial flutter 125-145. Chest x-ray showed cardiomegaly. Patient given 5 mg verapamil and converted to sinus rhythm at a rate of 85 almost immediately. Patient will be admitted to Cardiology Services at the hospital. |
| DIAGNOSIS: | Atrial flutter, converted. Cardiomegaly. |

| PROD | MAHAFC | 07 May 2012 | 15:09 |

## ⟳ Exercise 13: Progress Note

*Using the report above, answer the following questions by underlining the correct answer:*

1. Which vessels in the cardiovascular system were operated on 1 year ago? *(heart vessels/veins/intracranial vessels)*.

2. "Sinus rhythm" refers to *(irregular heartbeat/normal heartbeat)*.

3. "Flutter" is an example of a/n *(arrhythmia/valve disorder/occlusion)*.

4. "Atrial" refers to *(the pericardium/the upper chambers of the heart/the lower chambers of the heart)*.

5. "Cardiomegaly" means that the heart is *(inflamed/prolapsed/enlarged)*.

6. An "ECG" is a/n *(electroencephalogram/electrocardiogram/electromyogram)*.

Click on **Hear It, Spell It** to practice spelling the pathology terms you have learned in this chapter. To see how well you pronounce the pathology terms in this chapter, click on **Hear it, Say It.** To review pathology terms play **Medical Millionaire.**

## Heart Disease in Women

Heart disease is not just a man's disease. In fact 1 in 4 women in the U.S. will die from heart disease. Heart disease is the number one killer of women in the United States, killing more women every year than men. The Office of Research on Women's Health at the National Institutes of Health is charged with understanding how biologic and physiologic differences between the sexes affect health. As a result of this research, hormonal fluctuations are now believed to account for the variations in the results of a number of diagnostic tests and the optimal time for certain types of treatments. Visit www.womenshealth.gov to view the latest results of studies that examine the differences gender makes in cardiovascular and other diseases.

## DIAGNOSTIC PROCEDURES

### Terms Related to General Diagnostic Procedures

| Term | Word Origin | Definition |
|---|---|---|
| blood pressure (BP) | | A measure of the systolic over the diastolic pressure. The instrument used is a **sphygmomanometer.** |
| auscultation and percussion (A&P)<br>oss kull TAY shun<br>pur KUH shun | | Listening to internal sounds in the body, usually with a **stethoscope,** or by tapping (percussing). |

### Terms Related to Imaging

| Term | Word Origin | Definition |
|---|---|---|
| angiocardiography<br>an jee oh kar dee AH gruh fee | *angi/o* vessel<br>*cardi/o* heart<br>*-graphy* process of recording | Injection of a radiopaque substance during cardiac catheterization for the purpose of imaging the heart and related structures (Fig. 10-20). |
| cardiac catheterization<br>KAR dee ack<br>kath ih tur ih ZAY shun | *cardi/o* heart<br>*-ac* pertaining to | Threading of a catheter (thin tube) into the heart under fluoroscopic guidance to collect diagnostic information about structures in the heart, coronary arteries, and great vessels; also used to aid in treatment of CAD, congenital abnormalities, and heart failure (Fig. 10-21). |
| digital subtraction angiography (DSA)<br>an jee AH gruh fee | *sub-* under<br>*tract/o* pulling<br>*-ion* process of<br>*angi/o* vessel<br>*-graphy* process of recording | Digital imaging process wherein contrast images are used to "subtract" the noncontrast image of surrounding structures, leaving only a clear image of blood vessels (Fig. 10-22). |

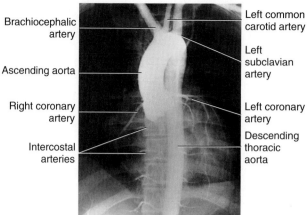

Brachiocephalic artery

Ascending aorta

Right coronary artery

Intercostal arteries

Left common carotid artery

Left subclavian artery

Left coronary artery

Descending thoracic aorta

**Fig. 10-20** Angiocardiography. Aorta and right and left coronary arteries are shown.

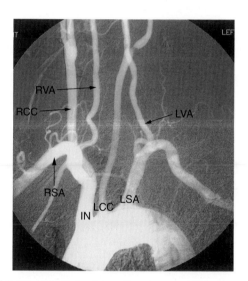

RVA

RCC

LVA

RSA

LCC   LSA

IN

**Fig. 10-22** Digital subtraction image of the aorta.

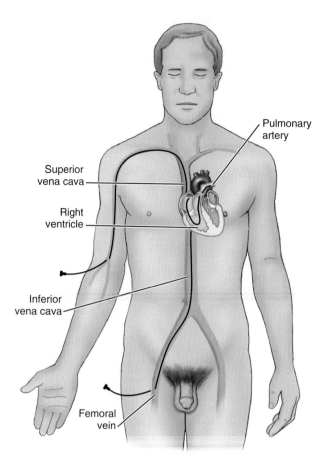

Pulmonary artery

Superior vena cava

Right ventricle

Inferior vena cava

Femoral vein

**Fig. 10-21** Right-sided heart catheterization. The catheter is inserted into the femoral or brachial vein and advanced through the inferior vena cava through the superior vena cava, right atrium, and right ventricle and into the pulmonary artery.

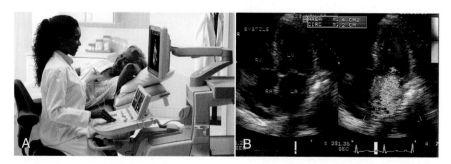

**Fig. 10-23** **A,** person undergoing echocardiography. **B,** Color Doppler image of the heart.

## Terms Related to Imaging—cont'd

| Term | Word Origin | Definition |
|------|-------------|------------|
| echocardiography (ECHO)<br>eck oh kar dee AH gruh fee | *echo-* sound<br>*cardi/o* heart<br>*-graphy* process of recording | Use of ultrasonic waves directed through the heart to study the structure and motion of the heart (Fig. 10-23). **Transesophageal echocardiography (TEE)** images the heart through a transducer introduced into the esophagus. |
| electrocardiography (ECG, EKG)<br>ee leck troh kar dee AH gruf ee | *electr/o* electricity<br>*cardi/o* heart<br>*-graphy* process of recording | Recording of electrical impulses of the heart as wave deflections of a needle on an instrument called an electrocardiograph. The record, or recording, is called an **electrocardiogram.** |
| exercise stress test (EST) | | Imaging of the heart during exercise on a treadmill; may include the use of radioactive substance. |
| fluoroscopy | *fluor/o* to flow<br>*-scopy* process of viewing | Special kind of x-ray procedure that allows visualization of structures in real time directly on a monitor screen. |
| Holter monitor<br>HOLE tur | | Portable electrocardiograph that is worn to record the reaction of the heart to daily activities (Fig. 10-24). |
| magnetic resonance imaging (MRI) | | Computerized imaging that uses radiofrequency pulses in a magnetic field to detect areas of myocardial infarction, stenoses, and areas of blood flow. |
| MUGA scan<br>MOO guh | | **Mu**ltiple-**g**ated **a**cquisition scan is a noninvasive method of imaging a beating heart by tagging RBCs with a radioactive substance. A gamma camera captures the outline of the chambers of the heart as the blood passes through them. |
| myocardial perfusion imaging<br>mye oh KAR dee ul pur FYOO zhun | *myocardi/o* myocardium<br>*-al* pertaining to<br>*per-* through<br>*-fusion* process of pouring | Use of radionuclide to diagnose CAD, valvular or congenital heart disease, and cardiomyopathy. |
| phlebography<br>fleh BAH gruh fee | *phleb/o* vein<br>*-graphy* process of recording | X-ray imaging of a vein after the introduction of a contrast dye. |
| positron emission tomography (PET)<br>POZ ih tron ee MIH shun toh MAH gruh fee | *e-* out<br>*-mission* sending<br>*tom/o* slice<br>*-graphy* process of recording | Computerized nuclear medicine procedure that uses inhaled or injected radioactive substances to help identify how much a patient will benefit from revascularization procedures. |
| radiography | *radi/o* rays<br>*-graphy* process of recording | Posteroanterior and lateral chest x-rays may be used to evaluate the size and shape of the heart. |
| Swan-Ganz catheter<br>swann ganz | | Long, thin cardiac catheter with a tiny balloon at the tip that is fed into the femoral artery near the groin and extended up to the left ventricle. This instrument then is used to determine left ventricular function by measuring pulmonary capillary wedge pressure. |

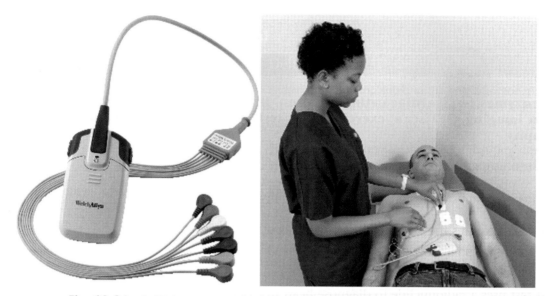

Fig. 10-24  **A,** Holter monitor. **B,** Placement of the leads on the chest.

## Terms Related to Laboratory Tests

| Term | Word Origin | Definition |
|---|---|---|
| **cardiac enzymes test** | | Blood test that measures the amount of cardiac enzymes characteristically released during a myocardial infarction; determines the amount of lactate dehydrogenase (LDH) and creatine phosphokinase (CK or CPK) in the blood. |
| **lipid profile** | | Blood test to measure the lipids (cholesterol and triglycerides) in the circulating blood (see a sample lipid profile in the box below). |
| **phlebotomy**<br>fleh BAH tuh mee | *phleb/o* vein<br>*-tomy* incision | The opening of a vein to withdraw a blood sample. Also called **venipuncture.** |

## Sample Lipid Profile

| Test | Your results | Date | Normal Range |
|---|---|---|---|
| Total Cholesterol | 171 | 11/02/2011 | Under 200 |
| HDL ("good cholesterol") | 55 | 11/02/2011 | Over 40 |
| Triglycerides | 84 | 11/02/2011 | Under 150 |
| LDL ("bad cholesterol") | 99 | 11/02/2011 | Under 100 |
| TSH (Thyroid) | 2.470 | 11/03/2011 | 0.35-5.50 |
| Blood Count | Normal | | |
| Vitamin D | 30.8 | | 32-100 |

# Chapter Review

*Match the word parts to their definitions.*

## WORD PARTS

| Prefix/Suffix | | Definition |
|---|---|---|
| brady- | | 1. _____ heart condition |
| -cardia | | 2. _____ four |
| echo- | | 3. _____ disease |
| -graphy | | 4. _____ slow |
| -megaly | | 5. _____ abnormal condition of hardening |
| -pathy | | 6. _____ sound |
| -sclerosis | | 7. _____ rapid |
| tachy- | | 8. _____ process of recording |
| tetra- | | 9. _____ structure |
| -um | | 10. _____ enlargement |

| Combining Form | | Definition |
|---|---|---|
| angi/o | | 11. _____ artery |
| aort/o | | 12. _____ heart |
| arteri/o | | 13. _____ lung |
| ather/o | | 14. _____ vessel |
| atri/o | | 15. _____ lumen |
| cardi/o | | 16. _____ endocardium |
| coron/o | | 17. _____ vessel |
| corpor/o | | 18. _____ wall |
| cyan/o | | 19. _____ myocardium |
| endocardi/o | | 20. _____ vein |
| epicardi/o | | 21. _____ blood vessel |
| hemangi/o | | 22. _____ aorta |
| isch/o | | 23. _____ body |
| lumin/o | | 24. _____ heart |
| myocardi/o | | 25. _____ fat, plaque |
| pariet/o | | 26. _____ epicardium |
| pericardi/o | | 27. _____ clotting, clot |
| phleb/o | | 28. _____ atrium |
| pulmon/o | | 29. _____ wall, septum |
| sept/o | | 30. _____ to hold back |
| thromb/o | | 31. _____ blue |
| vascul/o | | 32. _____ pericardium |

# WORDSHOP

| Prefixes | Combining Forms | Suffixes |
|----------|-----------------|----------|
| brady- | angi/o | -al |
| dys- | arteri/o | -ar |
| echo- | ather/o | -ary |
| extra- | cardi/o | -cardia |
| tachy- | corpor/o | -dynia |
| trans- | myocardi/o | -eal |
| | pericardi/o | -ectomy |
| | phleb/o | -graphy |
| | pulmon/o | -ia |
| | rhythm/o | -itis |
| | thromb/o | -plasty |
| | | -sclerosis |
| | | -tomy |

Build the following terms by combining the above word parts. Some word parts may be used more than once. Some may not be used at all. The number in parentheses is the number of word parts needed to build the term.

| Definition | Term |
|------------|------|
| 1. inflammation of the sac surrounding the heart (2) | |
| 2. inflammation of a vein with a clot (3) | |
| 3. condition of a rapid heart (beat) (2) | |
| 4. process of recording the heart using sound (3) | |
| 5. process of recording a vessel (2) | |
| 6. surgical repair of a vessel (2) | |
| 7. condition of abnormal rhythm (3) | |
| 8. abnormal condition of hardening of the arteries (2) | |
| 9. heart pain (2) | |
| 10. removal of fatty plaque (2) | |
| 11. pertaining to the heart and lungs (3) | |
| 12. removal of a vein (2) | |
| 13. pertaining to the outside of the body (3) | |
| 14. pertaining to through the heart muscle (3) | |
| 15. process of recording a vein (2) | |

Sort the terms into the correct categories.

## TERM SORTING

| Anatomy and Physiology | Pathology | Diagnostic Procedures | Therapeutic Interventions |
|---|---|---|---|
| | | | |
| | | | |
| | | | |
| | | | |
| | | | |
| | | | |
| | | | |
| | | | |
| | | | |
| | | | |

| | | | |
|---|---|---|---|
| aneurysm | CABG | EST | phlebography |
| angiocardiography | CAD | EVLT | phlebotomy |
| aorta | capillary | fluoroscopy | PTCA |
| arrhythmia | claudication | hemangiosarcoma | Purkinje fibers |
| atrium | commissurotomy | HTN | septum |
| auscultation | diastole | lipid profile | SOB |
| BP | ECC | LVAD | systole |
| bradycardia | ECG | MIDCAB | thromboendarterectomy |
| bruit | endocarditis | MUGA scan | valvuloplasty |
| bundle of His | endocardium | pericardiocentesis | ventricle |

*Replace the highlighted words with the correct terms.*

## TRANSLATIONS

1. Monique LaPlante was born with **an abnormal opening between the pulmonary artery and the aorta** that was originally detected by her pediatrician, who noted the presence of a **continuous abnormal heart sound heard during systole, diastole, or both.**

2. The child's **congenital cardiac anomaly that consists of four defects** was noted on **use of ultrasonic waves directed through the heart to study the structure and motion of the heart.**

3. Mrs. Williams had **an excessive amount of blood in the pulmonary vessels** and was diagnosed with **the inability of the heart muscle to pump blood efficiently.**

4. The 72-year-old man had an advanced case of **accumulation and hardening of plaque in the coronary arteries.** He had a history of cigarette smoking and **heart pain.**

5. The patient underwent **an x-ray imaging of a vein after the introduction of a contrast dye** to diagnose **his inflammation and formation of clots of either deep veins or superficial veins.**

6. Mr. Singh was admitted with **profuse secretion of sweat** and **rapid heartbeat.**

7. **A blood test that measures the amount of cardiac enzymes characteristically released during an MI** and **a recording of electrical impulses of the heart** was performed on the patient.

8. **Thermal destruction of veins using laser fibers within a vein** was used to treat Maria Lope's **elongated, dilated superficial veins.**

9. The patient was diagnosed with **paroxysmal chest pain** and was prescribed **drugs that relax blood vessels and reduce myocardial oxygen consumption.**

10. The cardiologist ordered **an aspiration of fluid from the pericardium** to treat Hugo's **compression of the heart caused by fluid in the pericardial sac.**

11. **A small, battery-operated device that helps the heart beat in a regular rhythm** was implanted in Mrs. Dawson's left chest to treat her **abnormality of the sinus node.**

12. Because Mr. Lin was unable to tolerate **a surgical procedure in which a catheter is threaded into the coronary artery,** his cardiologist ordered **a procedure in which a series of holes in made in the heart tissue using a laser.**

13. Malcolm's **narrowing of the tricuspid valve caused by rheumatic fever** was treated with **a repair of a stenosed heart valve with the use of a balloon-tipped catheter.**

14 Because the patient's **progressive disorder of the ventricles of the heart** had worsened she was put on **a mechanical pump device that assists a patient's weakened heart.**

## Case Study   Cheryl Miller

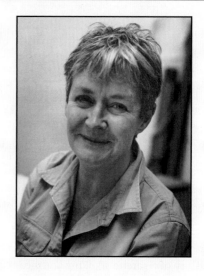

Cheryl Miller has been shopping all day and is tired. She stops for a quick burger and fries at the food court and then heads out of the mall. As Cheryl walks toward her car, she begins to experience symptoms of sweating, nausea, and extreme pain and pressure in her chest.

Cheryl is admitted through the ED. During her admission, she has an ECG and echocardiogram, a lipid profile, and a cardiac catheterization. The results indicate extensive coronary artery disease, an inferolateral wall myocardial infarction, hypercholesterolemia, and hypertension. When surgery is recommended, she is surprised and frightened. She had not thought of herself as someone who could have serious heart disease. She is scheduled for a coronary artery bypass graft.

Four weeks after being discharged, Cheryl has recovered from her coronary artery bypass. She makes her first return visit to the mall, this time to buy a new pair of walking shoes and a comfortable set of sweats. She has given her husband a list for the supermarket. It includes lots of her favorite fruits, vegetables, and low-fat alternatives for the high-cholesterol foods she had been eating. When she looks back at how poorly she had taken care of herself, Cheryl can't help but be excited about looking forward to a happy, healthier lifestyle.

 **Discharge Summary**

*Using the report on p. 403, answer the following questions.*

1. Define the symptoms presented by Ms. Miller.

   A. dyspnea _____

   B. diaphoresis _____

   C. hypertension _____

2. Where was the chest pain perceived? _____

3. How do you know that Ms. Miller did not lack oxygen in her extremities?

4. What was the name of the ultrasound procedure performed to assess her cardiac function?

   _____

5. What procedure was done to treat her CAD? _____

6. Which structures were evaluated by tapping and listening?

   _____

MILLER, CHERYL Y - 644497 Opened by TRUSKOWSKI, ABIGAIL MD     _ 🗗 ☒

Task   Edit   View   Time Scale   Options   Help

As Of 17:16

**MILLER, CHERYL Y**

| | | | |
|---|---|---|---|
| | Age: 54 years | Sex: Female | Loc: WHC-SMMC |
| | DOB: 10/10/1957 | MRN: 644497 | FIN: 3506004 |

Reference Text Browser | Form Browser | Medication Profile

Orders | Last 48 Hours | ED | Lab | Radiology | Assessments | Surgery | **Clinical Notes** | Pt. Info | Pt. Schedule | Task List | I & O | MAR

Flowsheet: Clinical Notes     ...     Level: Discharge Summary     ● Table  ○ Group  ○ List

---

Navigator     ☒

✔ Discharge Summary

**Principal Diagnosis:** Inferolateral myocardial infarction
**Secondary Diagnoses:** Coronary artery disease; hypertension
**Procedure:** Coronary artery bypass graft
**History of Present Illness:** The patient, a 45-year-old Caucasian female, has a history of substernal chest pain, nausea, dyspnea, and diaphoresis for 1½ hours before being seen in the ED.
**Medical History:** Significant for hypertension.
**Social History:** Positive for social alcohol use, and patient has smoked 1 pack per day for the past 30 years.
**Medications:** The patient is not currently taking any medication.
**Physical Examination:** On physical examination, the patient's vital signs showed a blood pressure of 165/105, a pulse rate of 88, and a temperature of 98.6 degrees. The patient was a well-developed, well-nourished, Caucasian female in mild distress. The patient's head, eyes, ears, nose, and throat were unremarkable. The neck was supple, with no jugular venous distension. Heart showed regular rhythm. The lungs were clear to auscultation and percussion. The abdominal examination was soft and nontender. Extremities had no cyanosis, clubbing, or edema. The neurologic examination was nonfocal.
**Laboratory Studies:** White blood cell count 19, hematocrit 39.9, platelets 385. Differential included 89 neutrophils, 2 bands, 5 lymphocytes, and 1 mono. Sodium 142, potassium 4.3, BUN 11, creatinine 1.0, glucose 229, calcium 7.8, magnesium 1.9, phosphorus 8.4, CPK 375. Urinalysis revealed no abnormal findings. ECG revealed normal sinus rhythm at 85 bpm.
**Hospital Course:** The patient was admitted and started on intravenous nitroglycerin, heparin, aspirin, and Lopressor. Cardiac catheterization demonstrated 94% occlusion of the RCA. Echocardiogram showed an ejection fraction of 29%.
   Patient underwent the bypass without incident and has progressed at a moderate pace through postoperative physical rehabilitation. At the time of discharge, she was ambulating well and demonstrated a good understanding of necessary lifestyle changes to maintain her health. Medications on Discharge: Ascriptin, 325 mg po daily; atenolol, 50 mg daily; clodripogel 75 mg daily; pravastatin 40 mg daily.

| | | | |
|---|---|---|---|
| | PROD | MAHAFC | 10 Nov 2011 | 17:16 |

---

For more interactive learning, click on:
• **Whack a Word Part** to review cardiovascular word parts.
• **Wheel of Terminology** and **Word Shop** to practice word building.
• **Tournament of Terminology** to test your knowledge of cardiovascular terms.
• **Terminology Triage** to practice sorting cardiovascular terms in categories.

# 11

*Roses are red, Violets are blue, Without your lungs, Your blood would be too.*
*—Susan Ott*

## OBJECTIVES

- Recognize and use terms related to the anatomy and physiology of the respiratory system.
- Recognize and use terms related to the pathology of the respiratory system.
- Recognize and use terms related to the diagnostic procedures for the respiratory system.
- Recognize and use terms related to the therapeutic interventions for the respiratory system.

# Respiratory System

## CHAPTER AT A GLANCE

*Use this list of key word parts and terms to assess your knowledge. Check off the ones you have mastered.*

### ANATOMY AND PHYSIOLOGY

- ☐ alveolus
- ☐ auscultation and percussion (A&P)
- ☐ bronchiole
- ☐ bronchus
- ☐ diaphragm
- ☐ epiglottis
- ☐ eustachian tube
- ☐ exhalation/expiration
- ☐ inhalation/inspiration
- ☐ laryngopharynx
- ☐ larynx
- ☐ mediastinum
- ☐ nasopharynx
- ☐ olfaction
- ☐ oropharynx
- ☐ paranasal sinuses
- ☐ pharynx
- ☐ pleura
- ☐ respiration
- ☐ sinus
- ☐ tonsils, palatine
- ☐ tonsils, pharyngeal
- ☐ trachea

### KEY WORD PARTS

**PREFIX**
- ☐ a-
- ☐ brady-
- ☐ dys-
- ☐ eu-
- ☐ ex-
- ☐ hyper-
- ☐ in-
- ☐ para-
- ☐ re-
- ☐ tachy-

**SUFFIX**
- ☐ -dynia
- ☐ -ectasis
- ☐ -metry
- ☐ -pnea
- ☐ -ptysis
- ☐ -rrhea
- ☐ -thorax

**COMBINING FORMS**
- ☐ adenoid/o
- ☐ alveol/o
- ☐ bronch/o
- ☐ bronchiol/o
- ☐ coni/o
- ☐ cyan/o
- ☐ laryng/o
- ☐ lob/o
- ☐ myc/o
- ☐ nas/o
- ☐ orth/o
- ☐ ox/o, ox/i
- ☐ pharyng/o
- ☐ phon/o
- ☐ pleur/o
- ☐ pneum/o, pneumon/o
- ☐ pulmon/o
- ☐ rhin/o
- ☐ salping/o
- ☐ sept/o
- ☐ sin/o, sinus/o
- ☐ spir/o
- ☐ thorac/o
- ☐ tonsill/o
- ☐ trache/o

### KEY TERMS

- ☐ asthma
- ☐ atelectasis
- ☐ bronchitis
- ☐ bronchoscopy
- ☐ chronic obstructive pulmonary disease (COPD)
- ☐ cyanosis
- ☐ dyspnea
- ☐ emphysema
- ☐ eupnea
- ☐ hemoptysis
- ☐ hypercapnia
- ☐ laryngitis
- ☐ lobectomy
- ☐ orthopnea
- ☐ oximetry
- ☐ pharyngitis
- ☐ pleurisy
- ☐ pneumoconiosis
- ☐ pneumonia
- ☐ rhinomycosis
- ☐ rhinorrhea
- ☐ septoplasty
- ☐ sinusitis
- ☐ spirometry
- ☐ sputum
- ☐ thoracodynia
- ☐ tonsillectomy
- ☐ tracheostomy
- ☐ tracheotomy
- ☐ tuberculosis (TB)

## FUNCTIONS OF THE RESPIRATORY SYSTEM

The respiratory system handles the following functions for the body:
- Delivering oxygen ($O_2$) to the blood for transport to cells in the body.
- Excreting the waste product of cellular respiration, carbon dioxide ($CO_2$).
- Filtering, cleansing, warming, and humidifying air taken into the lungs.
- Helping to regulate blood pH.
- Helping the production of sound for speech and singing.
- Providing the tissue that receives the stimulus for the sense of smell, olfaction.

Analyzing the name for this system gives a clue as to its first two functions. The word **respiratory** (RES pur uh tore ee) comes from the combining form spir/o, which means *to breathe*. As a matter of fact, to breathe in is to **inspire,** and to breathe out is to **expire.** When one dies, one breathes out and no longer breathes in again—hence the expression that the patient has "expired." **Inhalation** (in hull LAY shun) and **exhalation** (ex hull LAY shun) are alternative terms for **inspiration** and **expiration.**

The next two functions—filtering air and regulating blood pH—take place during breathing. The function of producing sound for speech and singing is accomplished by the interaction of air and the structures of the voice box, the larynx, and the hollow cavities, the sinuses, connected to the nasal passages.

Although the sense of smell, **olfaction** (ohl FACK shun), is not strictly a function of respiration, it is accomplished by the tissue in the nasal cavity, which receives the stimulus for smell and routes it to the brain through the nervous system.

## SPECIALTIES/SPECIALISTS

**Pulmonology** is the diagnosis, treatment, and prevention of disorders of the respiratory tract. The specialist in this field is called a **pulmonologist.**

## ANATOMY AND PHYSIOLOGY

The respiratory system is anatomically divided into the upper respiratory tract—the nose, pharynx, and larynx—and the lower respiratory tract—the trachea, bronchial tree, and lungs (Fig. 11-1). Physiologically, it is divided into conduction passageways and gas exchange surfaces.

There are two forms of respiration: **external respiration** and **internal respiration.** External respiration is the process of exchanging $O_2$ and $CO_2$ between the external environment and the lungs. Internal respiration is the exchange of gases between the lungs and the blood.

### Upper Respiratory Tract

The upper respiratory system encompasses the area from the nose to the larynx (Fig. 11-2). Air can enter the body through the mouth, but for the most part, it enters the body through the two **nares** (NAIR eez) (nostrils) of the **nose** that are separated by a partition called the **nasal septum** (NAY zul SEP tum). The hairs in the nose serve to filter out large particulate matter, and the mucous membrane and **cilia** (SEE lee uh) (small hairs) of the respiratory tract provide a further means of keeping air clean, warm, and moist as it travels to the lungs. The cilia continually move in a wavelike motion to push mucus and debris out of the respiratory tract. The air then travels up and backward, where it is filtered, warmed, and humidified by the environment in the upper portion of the nasal cavity. Fig. 11-3 illustrates the route of air into the body. The receptors for

---

**respiratory**
re- = again
spir/o = to breathe
-atory = pertaining to

**inspiration**
in- = in
spir/o = to breathe
-ation = process of

**expiration**
ex- = out
(s)pir/o = to breathe
-ation = process of

**inhalation**
in- = in
hal/o = to breathe
-ation = process of

**exhalation**
ex- = out
hal/o = to breathe
-ation = process of

**air** = pneum/o, aer/o

**pulmonologist**
pulmon/o = lung
-logist = one who specializes in the study of

**oxygen ($O_2$)** = ox/i, ox/o

**carbon dioxide ($CO_2$)** = capn/o

**nose** = nas/o, rhin/o

**septum**
sept/o = wall
-um = structure

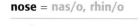
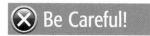 Be Careful!

*The plural of* **sinus** *is not* sini, *but* **sinuses**.

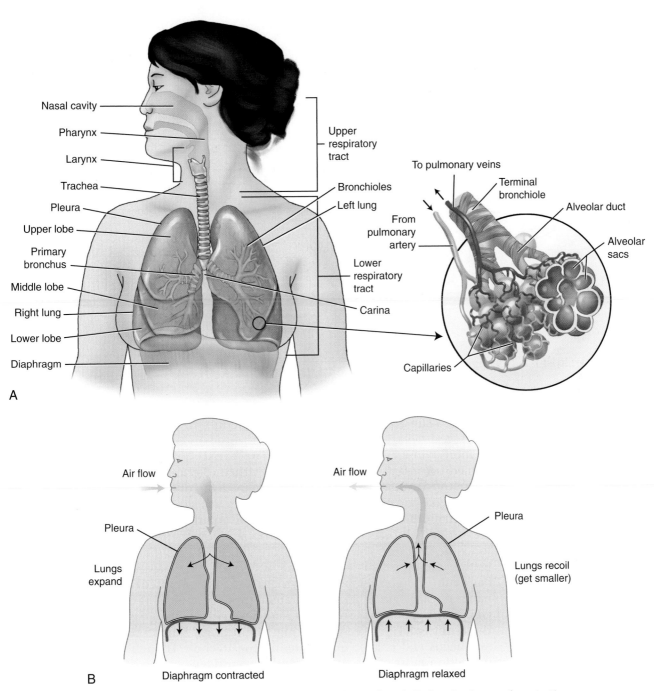

Fig. 11-1 **A,** The respiratory system showing a bronchial tree *(inset).* **B,** Inspiration and expiration.

olfaction are located in the nasal cavity. The nasal cavity is connected to the **paranasal sinuses** (pair uh NAY zul SYE nus suhs), named for their proximity to the nose.

These sinuses, divided into the frontal, maxillary, sphenoid, and ethmoid cavities, acquire their names from the bones in which they are located. The function of sinus cavities in the skull is to warm and filter the air taken in and to assist in the production of sound. They are lined with a mucous membrane that drains into the nasal cavity and can be the site of painful inflammation.

Air continues to travel past into the **nasopharynx** (NAY zoh fair inks), which is the part of the throat **(pharynx)** behind the nasal cavity. The **eustachian** (yoo STAY shun) **tubes** from the ears connect with the throat at this point to equalize pressure between the ears and the throat. This is the site of lymphatic tissue, the **pharyngeal tonsils** (fur IN jee ul TAHN suls), which are

| **paranasal** |
|---|
| para- = near |
| nas/o = nose |
| -al = pertaining to |
| **sinus** = sinus/o, sin/o |
| **mucus** = muc/o |
| **nasopharynx** |
| nas/o = nose |
| pharyng/o = throat, pharynx |
| **pharynx** = pharyng/o |
| **eustachian tube** = salping/o |

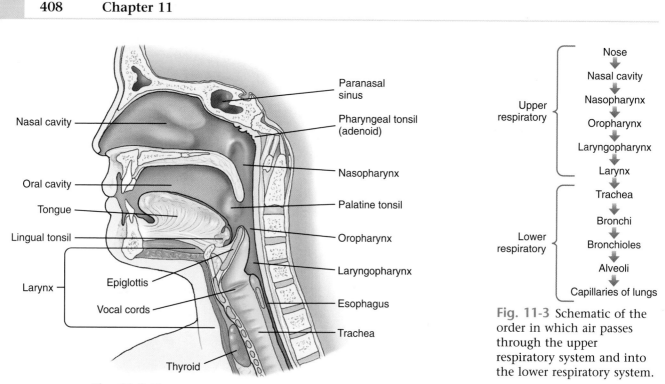

Fig. 11-2 The upper respiratory system.

**Fig. 11-3** Schematic of the order in which air passes through the upper respiratory system and into the lower respiratory system.

**adenoids** = adenoid/o

**oropharynx**
or/o = mouth
pharyng/o = throat, pharynx

**tonsils** = tonsill/o

**laryngopharynx**
laryng/o = larynx
pharyng/o = pharynx

**epiglottis** = epiglott/o

**trachea, windpipe** = trache/o

**mediastinum** = mediastin/o

**chest** = thorac/o, steth/o, pector/o

**bronchus** = bronch/o, bronchi/o

**bronchiole** = bronchiol/o

**alveolus** = alveol/o

also termed the **adenoids** (AD uh noyds). These pharyngeal tonsils help to protect against pathogens. The next structure, the **oropharynx** (or oh FAIR inks), is the part of the throat posterior to the oral cavity and also the location of more lymphatic tissue, the **palatine tonsils** (PAL ah tyne TAHN suls), so named because they are continuous with the roof of the mouth (the palate). These tonsils, just like the adenoids, are made up of protective lymphatic tissue. The lingual tonsil, located on the posterior aspect of the tongue, also serves a protective function. The oropharynx is also part of the digestive system; food and air pass through it. Below the oropharynx is the part of the throat referred to as the **laryngopharynx** (luh ring goh FAIR inks) because of its proximity to the adjoining structure, the **larynx** (LAIR inks), or voice box. As air passes back out through the opening of the larynx, the **vocal cords**, which are paired bands of cartilaginous tissue, vibrate to produce speech. The **epiglottis** (eh pee GLOT is) is a flap of cartilage at the opening to the larynx that closes access to the **trachea** (TRAY kee uh) during swallowing so that food is routed into the esophagus and is kept from entering the trachea. Though this is an effective protection most of the time, it can be overridden accidentally if the individual tries to talk and eat at the same time. When this happens, food can be pulled into the trachea, with possible serious consequences.

## Lower Respiratory Tract

The lower respiratory tract begins with the **trachea** (or windpipe), which extends from the larynx into the chest cavity. The trachea lies within the space between the lungs called the **mediastinum** (mee dee uh STY num). Air travels into the lungs as the trachea bifurcates (branches) at the **carina** (kuh RIH nuh), where the right and left airways called bronchi (BRONG kee) (*sing.* bronchus) divide into smaller branches called **bronchioles** (BRONG kee ohls). These bronchioles end in microscopic ducts capped by air sacs called **alveoli** (al VEE oh lye) (*sing.* alveolus). Each alveolus is in contact with a blood capillary to provide a means of exchange of gases. It is at this point that $O_2$ is diffused across cell membranes into the blood cells, and $CO_2$ is diffused out to be expired. Each alveolus is coated with a substance called **surfactant** (sur FACK tunt) that keeps it from collapsing.

Each **lung** is composed of sections called **lobes.** The right lung is made up of three sections, whereas the left has only two. The abbreviations for the lobes of the lungs are RUL (right upper lobe), RML (right middle lobe), RLL (right lower lobe), LUL (left upper lobe), and LLL (left lower lobe).

Each lung is also enclosed by a double-folded, serous membrane called the **pleura** (PLOOR uh) (*pl.* pleurae). The side of the membrane that coats the lungs is the **visceral pleura** (VIH sur ul PLOOR ah); the side that lines the inner surface of the rib cage is the **parietal pleura** (puh RYE uh tul PLOOR ah). The two sides of the pleural membrane contain fluid that facilitates the expansion and contraction of the lungs with each breath.

The muscles responsible for normal, quiet respiration are the **diaphragm** (DYE uh fram), the large dome-shaped muscle between the thoracic and abdominal cavities, and the **intercostal** (in tur KOS tul) **muscles**, which are located between the ribs. On inspiration, the diaphragm is pulled down as it contracts and the intercostal muscles expand, pulling air into the lungs (see Fig. 11-1, *B*).

**lung** = pneumon/o, pulmon/o, pneum/o

**lobe** = lob/o, lobul/o

**pleura** = pleur/o

**viscera** = viscer/o

**wall** = pariet/o

**diaphragm** = diaphragm/o, diaphragmat/o, phren/o

**intercostal**
  inter- = between
  cost/o = rib
  -al = pertaining to

| ⊗ **Be Careful!** | ⊗ **Be Careful!** | ⊗ **Be Careful!** |
|---|---|---|
| *Salping/o means both eustachian tubes and fallopian tubes.* | *Don't confuse the combining form **ox/i**, which means oxygen, with the prefix **oxy-**, which means rapid.* | *Don't confuse **bronchi/o**, which means the bronchial tubes, with **brachi/o**, which means the arm.* |

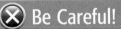 Exercise 1: **Anatomy and Physiology of the Respiratory System**

*Match the respiratory structure with its combining form or prefix. More than one letter may be correct.*

____ 1. pleura

____ 2. lobe

____ 3. tonsil

____ 4. mucus

____ 5. diaphragm

____ 6. windpipe

____ 7. adenoids

____ 8. eustachian tube

____ 9. bronchiole

____ 10. rib

____ 11. breathe

____ 12. throat

____ 13. alveolus

____ 14. lung

____ 15. sinus

____ 16. bronchus

____ 17. voice box

____ 18. mouth

____ 19. nose

____ 20. mediastinum

____ 21. in

____ 22. air

____ 23. out

____ 24. epiglottis

____ 25. wall

____ 26. carbon dioxide

____ 27. oxygen

A. ox/o
B. bronch/o, bronchi/o
C. salping/o
D. pneum/o, pneumon/o
E. phren/o
F. hal/o, spir/o
G. pharyng/o
H. adenoid/o
I. sept/o
J. rhin/o
K. pneum/o, aer/o
L. pulmon/o
M. capn/o
N. lob/o, lobul/o
O. diaphragm/o, diaphragmat/o
P. nas/o
Q. trache/o
R. alveol/o

S. tonsill/o
T. pleur/o
U. sin/o, sinus/o
V. muc/o
W. epiglott/o
X. laryng/o
Y. in-
Z. bronchiol/o
AA. cost/o
BB. mediastin/o
CC. ex-
DD. or/o

*Decode the terms.*

28. intercostal _____

29. inspiratory _____

30. paranasal _____

31. endotracheal _____

---

You can review the anatomy of the respiratory system by clicking on **Body Spectrum Electronic Anatomy Coloring Book → Respiratory.** Choose **Hear It, Spell It** to practice spelling the anatomy and physiology terms you have learned in this chapter. To practice pronouncing anatomy and physiology terms, choose **Hear It, Say It.**

---

## Exercise 2: Respiratory System

*Label the drawing below with the correct anatomic terms and combining forms where appropriate.*

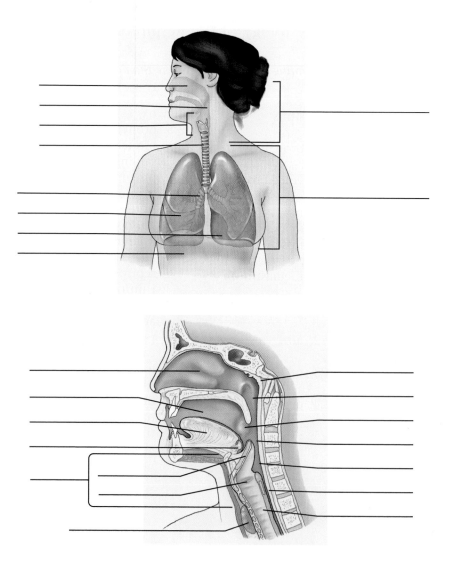

## Combining and Adjective Forms for the Anatomy and Physiology of the Respiratory System

| Meaning | Combining Form | Adjective Form |
|---------|----------------|----------------|
| adenoid | adenoid/o | adenoidal |
| air | pneum/o, aer/o | pneumatic |
| alveolus | alveol/o | alveolar |
| bronchiole | bronchiol/o | bronchiolar |
| bronchus | bronch/o, bronchi/o | bronchial |
| carbon dioxide | capn/o | |
| chest | steth/o, thorac/o, pector/o | thoracic, pectoral |
| diaphragm | diaphragm/o, diaphragmat/o, phren/o | diaphragmatic |
| eustachian tube | salping/o | salpingeal |
| larynx (voicebox) | laryng/o | laryngeal |
| lobe | lob/o, lobul/o | lobular, lobar |
| lung | pulmon/o, pneumon/o, pneum/o | pulmonary, pneumatic |
| mediastinum | mediastin/o | mediastinal |
| mouth | or/o, stomat/o | oral |
| mucus | muc/o | mucous |
| nose | nas/o, rhin/o | nasal, rhinal |
| oxygen | ox/i, ox/o | |
| pharynx (throat) | pharyng/o | pharyngeal |
| pleura | pleur/o | pleural |
| rib | cost/o | costal |
| septum, wall | sept/o | septal |
| sinus | sinus/o, sin/o | |
| to breathe | spir/o, hal/o | |
| tonsil | tonsill/o | tonsillar |
| trachea (windpipe) | trache/o | tracheal |
| viscera | viscer/o | visceral |
| wall | pariet/o | parietal |

## Prefixes for Anatomy and Physiology of the Respiratory System

| Prefix | Meaning |
|--------|---------|
| ex- | out |
| in- | in |
| inter- | between |
| para- | near |
| re- | again |

## Suffixes for Anatomy of the Respiratory System

| Suffix | Meaning |
|---|---|
| -atory, -al | pertaining to |
| -ation | process of |
| -logist | one who specializes in the study of |
| -um | structure |

## PATHOLOGY

### Terms Related to Respiratory Symptoms

| Term | Word Origin | Definition |
|---|---|---|
| **aphonia**<br>ah FOH nee ah | *a-* without<br>*phon/o* sound<br>*-ia* condition | Loss of ability to produce sounds. **Dysphonia** is difficulty making sounds. |
| **Cheyne-Stokes respiration**<br>chayne stokes | | Deep, rapid breathing followed by a period of apnea. |
| **clubbing**<br>KLUH bing | | Abnormal enlargement of the distal phalanges as a result of diminished $O_2$ in the blood (Fig. 11-4). |
| **cyanosis**<br>sye uh NOH sis | *cyan/o* blue<br>*-osis* abnormal condition | Lack of oxygen in blood seen as bluish or grayish discoloration of the skin, nailbeds, and/or lips. |
| **dyspnea**<br>DISP nee ah | *dys-* difficult<br>*-pnea* breathing | Difficult, and/or painful breathing. **Eupnea** is good, normal breathing (Eu- means healthy, normal). |
| **apnea**<br>AP nee ah | *a-* without<br>*-pnea* breathing | Abnormal, periodic cessation of breathing. |
| **bradypnea**<br>brad IP nee ah | *brady-* slow<br>*-pnea* breathing | Abnormally slow breathing. |
| **hyperpnea**<br>hye PURP nee ah | *hyper-* excessive<br>*-pnea* breathing | Excessively deep breathing. **Hypopnea** is extremely shallow breathing. |
| **orthopnea**<br>or THOP nee ah | *orth/o* straight<br>*-pnea* breathing | Condition of difficult breathing unless in an upright position. |
| **tachypnea**<br>tack ip NEE ah | *tachy-* fast<br>*-pnea* breathing | Rapid, shallow breathing. |
| **epistaxis**<br>ep ih STACK sis | | Nosebleed. Also called **rhinorrhagia.** |
| **hemoptysis**<br>heh MOP tih sis | *hem/o* blood<br>*-ptysis* spitting | Coughing up blood or blood-stained sputum. |
| **hypercapnia**<br>hye pur KAP nee ah | *hyper-* excessive<br>*capn/o* carbon dioxide<br>*-ia* condition | Condition of excessive $CO_2$ in the blood. |

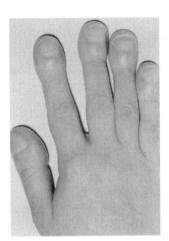

**Fig. 11-4** Clubbing.

## Terms Related to Respiratory Symptoms—cont'd

| Term | Word Origin | Definition |
|---|---|---|
| **hyperventilation**<br>hye pur ven tih LAY shun | *hyper-* excessive | Abnormally increased breathing. |
| **hypoxemia**<br>hye pock SEE mee ah | *hypo-* deficient<br>*ox/o* oxygen<br>*-emia* blood condition | Condition of deficient $O_2$ in the blood. **Hypoxia** is the condition of deficient oxygen in the tissues. |
| **pleurodynia**<br>ploor oh DIN ee ah | *pleur/o* pleura<br>*-dynia* pain | Pain in the chest caused by inflammation of the intercostal muscles. |
| **pyrexia**<br>pye RECK see ah | *pyr/o* fire<br>*-exia* condition | Fever. |
| **rhinorrhea**<br>rye noh REE ah | *rhin/o* nose<br>*-rrhea* discharge | Discharge from the nose. |
| **shortness of breath (SOB)** | | Breathlessness; air hunger. |
| **sputum**<br>SPYOO tum | | Mucus coughed up from the lungs and expectorated through the mouth. If abnormal, may be described as to its amount, color, or odor. |
| **thoracodynia**<br>thor uh koh DIN ee ah | *thorac/o* chest<br>*-dynia* pain | Chest pain. |

## Terms Related to Abnormal Chest Sounds

| Term | Word Origin | Definition |
|------|-------------|------------|
| friction sounds | | Sounds made by dry surfaces rubbing together. |
| hiccup<br>HICK up | | Sound produced by the involuntary contraction of the diaphragm, followed by rapid closure of the glottis. Also called **hiccough, singultus**. |
| rales<br>rayls | | Also called **crackles**, an abnormal lung sound heard on auscultation, characterized by discontinuous bubbling noises. |
| rhonchi<br>RONG kye | | Abnormal rumbling sound heard on auscultation, caused by airways blocked by secretions or muscle contractions. |
| stridor<br>STRY dur | | High-pitched inspiratory sound from the larynx; a sign of upper airway obstruction. |
| tympany, chest<br>TIM puh nee | *tympan/o* drum | Low-pitched resonant sound from the chest. |
| wheezing<br>WHEE zeeng | | Whistling sound made during breathing. |

## Exercise 3: Symptoms of Respiratory Disease and Abnormal Chest Sounds

*Fill in the blank.*

1. Ms. Sims visits her physician's office complaining of orthopnea. She has _____.

2. A person who has a bout of epistaxis has _____.

3. Singultus is another name for _____.

4. Rapid, shallow breathing is called _____.

5. When Samuel Wrightson had laryngitis, he experienced aphonia. He could not _____.

6. A temporary lack of breathing is called _____.

7. What is the term that means blue color of the skin due to lack of oxygen?

   _____.

8. Another name for rales is _____.

9. Pain caused by inflamed intercostal muscles and their points of attachment to the diaphragm is

   referred to as _____.

10. A whistling sound made during inhalation is called _____.

11. The distal phalanges are abnormally enlarged in which symptom of advanced chronic pulmonary

    disease? _____.

*Build the terms.*

12. nose discharge _____

13. chest pain _____

14. spitting blood _____

15. good breathing _____

16. excessive (deep) breathing _____

## Terms Related to Disorders of the Upper Respiratory Tract

| Term | Word Origin | Definition |
|------|-------------|------------|
| coryza<br>koh RYE zah | | The common cold. |
| croup<br>croop | | Acute viral infection of early childhood, marked by stridor caused by spasms of the larynx, trachea, and bronchi. |
| deviated septum<br>DEE vee a tid<br>SEP tum | *sept/o* wall, septum<br>*-um* structure | Deflection of the nasal septum that may obstruct the nasal passages, resulting in infection, sinusitis, shortness of breath, headache, or recurring epistaxis. |
| epiglottitis<br>eh pee glah TYE tis | *epiglott/o* epiglottis<br>*-itis* inflammation | Inflammation of the epiglottis (Fig. 11-5). |
| laryngitis<br>lair in JYE tis | *laryng/o* voice box (larynx)<br>*-itis* inflammation | Inflammation of the voice box. |
| obstructive sleep apnea (OSA)<br>APP nee ah | *a-* without<br>*-pnea* breathing | A temporary lack of breathing that occurs during sleep when the posterior pharynx relaxes and covers the trachea. |
| pharyngitis<br>fair in JYE tis | *pharyng/o* throat (pharynx)<br>*-itis* inflammation | Inflammation or infection of the pharynx, usually causing symptoms of a sore throat. |
| polyps, nasal and vocal cord<br>PAWL ups | | Small, tumorlike growth that projects from a mucous membrane surface, including the inside of the nose, the paranasal sinuses, and the vocal cords (Fig. 11-6). |
| rhinitis<br>rye NYE tis | *rhin/o* nose<br>*-itis* inflammation | Inflammation of the mucous membrane of the nose. |
| rhinomycosis<br>rye noh mye KOH sis | *rhin/o* nose<br>*myc/o* fungus<br>*-osis* abnormal condition | Abnormal condition of fungus in the nose. |
| rhinosalpingitis<br>rye noh sal pin JYE tis | *rhin/o* nose<br>*salping/o* eustachian tube<br>*-itis* inflammation | Inflammation of the mucous membranes of the nose and eustachian tubes. |
| sinusitis<br>sye nuh SYE tis | *sinus/o* sinus<br>*-itis* inflammation | Inflammation of one or more of the paranasal sinuses. |

*Continued*

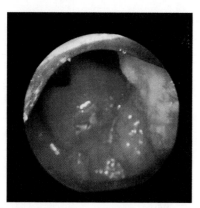

Fig. 11-5 Epiglottitis. The epiglottis is red and swollen.

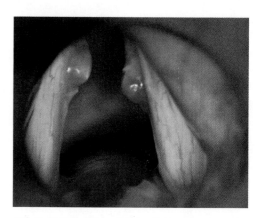

Fig. 11-6 Polypoid nodules of the vocal cords.

## Terms Related to Disorders of the Upper Respiratory Tract—cont'd

| Term | Word Origin | Definition |
|------|-------------|------------|
| **tracheomalacia**<br>tray kee oh mah LAY see ah | *trache/o* windpipe (trachea)<br>*-malacia* softening | Softening of the tissues of the trachea. |
| **tracheostenosis**<br>tray kee oh sten OH sis | *trache/o* windpipe (trachea)<br>*-stenosis* narrowing | Narrowing of the windpipe. |
| **upper respiratory infection (URI)** | | Inflammation and/or infection of structures of the upper respiratory tract. |

## Terms Related to Disorders of the Lower Respiratory Tract

| Term | Word Origin | Definition |
|------|-------------|------------|
| **acute respiratory failure (ARF)** | | A sudden inability of the respiratory system to provide oxygen and/or remove $CO_2$ from the blood. |
| **asthma**<br>AZ muh | | Respiratory disorder characterized by recurring episodes of **paroxysmal** (sudden, episodic) dyspnea. Patients exhibit coughing, wheezing, and shortness of breath. If the attack becomes continuous (termed **status asthmaticus**), it may be fatal (Fig. 11-7). |
| **atelectasis**<br>at ih LECK tuh sis | *a-* not<br>*tel/o* complete<br>*-ectasis* dilation | Collapse of lung tissue or an entire lung. |
| **bronchiectasis**<br>brong kee ECK tuh sis | *bronchi/o* bronchus<br>*-ectasis* dilation | Chronic dilation of the bronchi. Symptoms include dyspnea, expectoration of foul-smelling sputum, and coughing. |
| **bronchiolitis**<br>brong kee oh LYE tis | *bronchiol/o* bronchiole<br>*-itis* inflammation | Viral inflammation of the bronchioles; more common in children younger than 18 months. |
| **bronchitis**<br>brong KYE tis | *bronchi/o* bronchus<br>*-itis* inflammation | Inflammation of the bronchi. May be acute or chronic. |

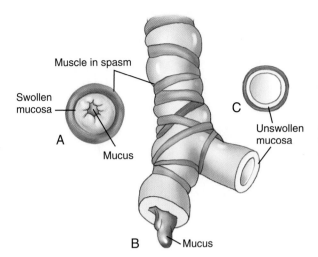

**Fig. 11-7** Factors causing expiratory obstruction in asthma. **A,** Cross section of a bronchiole occluded by muscle spasm, swollen mucosa, and mucus. **B,** Longitudinal section of an obstructed bronchiole. **C,** Cross-section of a clear bronchiole.

## Terms Related to Disorders of the Lower Respiratory Tract—cont'd

| Term | Word Origin | Definition |
|------|-------------|------------|
| **bronchospasm** <br> brong koh SPAZZ um | *bronch/o* bronchus <br> *-spasm* sudden, involuntary contraction | A sudden involuntary contraction of the bronchi, as in an asthma attack. |
| **chronic obstructive pulmonary disease (COPD)** | *pulmon/o* lung <br> *-ary* pertaining to | Respiratory disorder characterized by a progressive and irreversible diminishment in inspiratory and expiratory capacity of the lungs. Patient experiences **dyspnea on exertion (DOE),** difficulty inhaling or exhaling, and a chronic cough. |
| **cystic fibrosis (CF)** <br> SIS tick <br> fye BROH sis | | Inherited disorder of the exocrine glands resulting in abnormal, thick secretions of mucus that cause COPD. |
| **diphtheria** <br> diff THEER ee ah | | Bacterial respiratory infection characterized by a sore throat, fever, and headache. |
| **emphysema** <br> em fah SEE mah | | Abnormal condition of the pulmonary system characterized by distention and destructive changes of the alveoli. The most common cause is tobacco smoking, but exposure to environmental particulate matter may also cause the disease. |
| **flail chest** | | A condition in which multiple rib fractures cause instability in part of the chest wall and in which the lung under the injured area contracts on inspiration and bulges out on expiration (Fig. 11-8). |

*Continued*

Fig. 11-8 Flail chest. **A,** Fractured rib sections are unattached to the rest of the chest wall. **B,** On inspiration, the flail segment of ribs is sucked inward, causing the lung to shift inward. **C,** On expiration, the flail segment of ribs bellows outward, causing the lung to shift outward. Air moves back and forth between the lungs instead of through the upper airway.

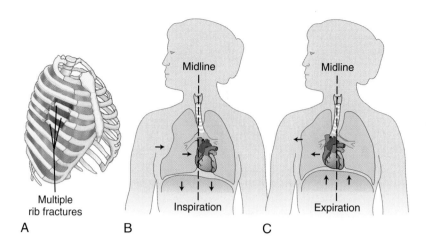

Multiple rib fractures

A          B          C

Midline          Midline

Inspiration          Expiration

## Terms Related to Disorders of the Lower Respiratory Tract—cont'd

| Term | Word Origin | Definition |
|---|---|---|
| **hemothorax**<br>hee moh THOR acks | *hem/o* blood<br>*-thorax* chest (pleural cavity) | Blood in the pleural cavity (Fig. 11-9). |
| **influenza**<br>in floo EN zah | | Also known as the **flu**. Acute infectious disease of the respiratory tract caused by a virus. **Avian (bird) flu** is caused by type A influenza virus. **Swine flu** is caused by H1N1 virus. |
| **pertussis**<br>pur TUSS is | | Bacterial infection of the respiratory tract with a characteristic high-pitched "whoop." Also called **whooping cough**. |
| **pleural effusion**<br>PLOOR ul<br>eh FYOO zhun | *pleur/o* pleura<br>*-al* pertaining to | Abnormal accumulation of fluid in the intrapleural space. |
| **pleurisy**<br>PLOOR ih see | *pleur/o* pleura | Inflammation of the parietal pleura of the lungs. May be caused by cancer, pneumonia, or tuberculosis. |
| **pneumoconiosis**<br>noo moh koh nee OH sis | *pneum/o* lung<br>*coni/o* dust<br>*-osis* abnormal condition | Loss of lung capacity caused by an accumulation of dust in the lungs. Types may include **asbestosis** (abnormal condition of asbestos in the lungs), **silicosis** (sil ih KOH sis) (abnormal accumulation of glass dust in the lungs), and **anthracosis** (abnormal accumulation of coal dust in the lungs—also known as **black lung disease** or **coal workers' pneumoconiosis [CWP]**) (Fig. 11-10). |
| **pneumonia**<br>noo MOH nya | *pneumon/o* lung<br>*-ia* condition | Inflammation of the lungs caused by a variety of pathogens. If infectious, it is termed pneumonia; if noninfectious, **pneumonitis**. The name(s) of the lobes are used to describe the extent of the disease (e.g., **RML pneumonia** is pneumonia of the right middle lobe). If both lungs are affected, it is termed **double pneumonia**. |

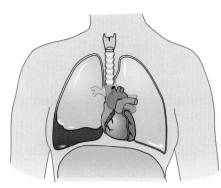

Fig. 11-9 Hemothorax. Blood below the left lung causes the lung to collapse.

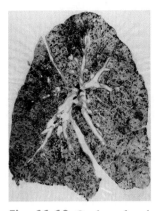

Fig. 11-10 Coal workers' pneumoconiosis. The lungs show increased black pigmentation.

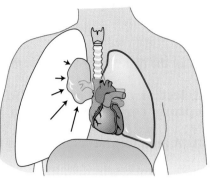

Fig. 11-11 Pneumothorax. The lung collapses as air gathers in the pleural space.

## Terms Related to Disorders of the Lower Respiratory Tract—cont'd

| Term | Word Origin | Definition |
|------|-------------|------------|
| **pneumothorax**<br>noo moh THOR acks | *pneum/o* air<br>*-thorax* chest (pleural cavity) | Air or gas in the pleural space causing the lung to collapse (Fig. 11-11). |
| **pulmonary abscess**<br>PULL mun nair ee<br>AB ses | *pulmon/o* lung<br>*-ary* pertaining to | Localized accumulation of pus in the lung. |
| **pulmonary edema**<br>PULL mun nair ee<br>eh DEE mah | *pulmon/o* lung<br>*-ary* pertaining to | Accumulation of fluid in the lung tissue. Often present in congestive heart failure, it is caused by the inability of the heart to pump blood. |
| **pyothorax**<br>pye oh THOR acks | *py/o* pus<br>*-thorax* chest (pleural cavity) | Pus in the pleural cavity. Also called **empyema**. |
| **respiratory syncytial virus (RSV)**<br>RES pur uh tore ee<br>sin SISH uhl<br>VYE rus | | Acute respiratory disorder usually occurring in the lower respiratory tract in children and the upper respiratory tract in adults. Most common cause of bronchiolitis and pneumonia in infants and highly contagious in young children. |
| **severe acute respiratory syndrome (SARS)** | *syn-* together, with<br>*-drome* to run | Viral respiratory disorder caused by a coronavirus. Usually results in pneumonia. |
| **tuberculosis (TB)**<br>too bur kyoo LOH sis | | Chronic infectious disorder caused by an acid-fast bacillus, *Mycobacterium tuberculosis*. Transmission is normally by inhalation or ingestion of infected droplets. **Multidrug-resistant tuberculosis (MDR TB)** is fatal in 80% of cases. |

To view animations of asthma and pneumonia, click on **Animations.**

## ⟳ Exercise 4: Disorders of the Upper and Lower Respiratory Tract

*Fill in the blank with one of the following terms:*

**atelectasis, vocal polyps, URI, asthma, cystic fibrosis, pleurisy, croup, pertussis, deviated septum, coryza, emphysema, pneumoconiosis, flail chest, pulmonary abscess**

1. A term for the common cold is _____.

2. An inflammation and/or infection of the structures of the upper respiratory tract is

    _____.

3. A deflection of the nasal wall that may result in nosebleeds, shortness of breath, infection, and/or

    headaches is _____.

4. Growths that occur on the mucous membranes of the larynx are referred to as

    _____.

5. An inflammation of the parietal pleura is _____.

6. An acute, infectious viral disease of the respiratory tract is _____.

7. The term for collapse of a lung is _____

8. A chronic pulmonary disease marked by distention of the alveoli is

    _____.

9. A respiratory disorder characterized by episodes of paroxysmal dyspnea is

    _____.

10. Localized accumulation of pus in the lung is _____.

11. Loss of lung capacity caused by dust in the lung is _____.

12. An inherited disorder of the exocrine glands that causes COPD is _____.

13. Patients with chest trauma who experience breathing in which the lung contracts on inspiration and

    expands on expiration have _____.

14. This is also called whooping cough. _____

*Decode the terms.*

15. pneumonia _____.

16. pneumothorax _____.

17. pyothorax _____.

*Build the terms.*

18. blood in the pleural cavity _____

19. inflammation of the bronchi _____

20. spasm of the bronchi _____

Because organs are composed of tissues and tissues are constructed from a variety of cell types, cancer of an organ can occur in a number of different varieties, depending on which types of cells mutate. Fig. 11-12 shows the three main categories of lung cancer along with the types of cells from which they originate.

## Terms Related to Benign Neoplasms

| Term | Word Origin | Definition |
|------|-------------|------------|
| hamartoma, pulmonary<br>ham ar TOH mah | *hamart/o* defect<br>*-oma* tumor, mass | A benign tumor of limited abnormal tissue formed in the respiratory tract. Also called a **chondroadenoma**. |
| mucous gland adenoma<br>ad ih NOH mah | *muc/o* mucus<br>*-ous* pertaining to<br>*aden/o* gland<br>*-oma* tumor, mass | A benign tumor of the mucous glands of the respiratory system. |
| papilloma<br>pap ih LOH mah | *papill/o* nipple<br>*-oma* tumor, mass | A benign tumor of epithelial origin named for its nipplelike appearance. |

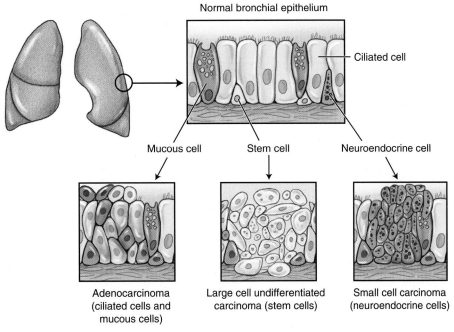

Fig. 11-12 Types of lung cancer.

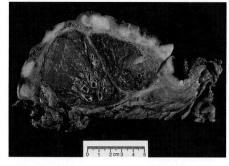

Fig. 11-13 Mesothelioma.

## Terms Related to Malignant Neoplasms

| Term | Word Origin | Definition |
|------|-------------|------------|
| mesothelioma<br>mee soh thee lee OH ma | *-oma* tumor, mass | A rare malignancy of the pleura or other protective tissues that cover the internal organs of the body. Often caused by exposure to asbestos (Fig. 11-13). |
| non–small cell lung cancer (NSCLC) | | Most prevalent type of lung cancer. |
| adenocarcinoma<br>ad ih noh kar sih NOH mah | *aden/o* gland<br>*-carcinoma* cancer of epithelial origin | NSCLC derived from the mucus-secreting glands in the lungs. |
| large cell carcinoma | *carcinoma* cancer of epithelial origin | NSCLC originating in the lining of the smaller bronchi. |
| squamous cell carcinoma<br>SKWAY muss | *squam/o* scaly<br>*-ous* pertaining to<br>*carcinoma* cancer of epithelial origin | NSCLC originating in the squamous epithelium of the larger bronchi. |
| small cell lung cancer (carcinoma) (SCLC) | *carcinoma* cancer of epithelial origin | Second most common type of lung cancer. Associated with smoking. Derived from neuroendocrine cells in the bronchi. Also called **oat cell carcinoma**. |

## Exercise 5: Neoplasms

*Fill in the blank.*

1. Hamartomas, adenomas, and papillomas are examples of _____ lung tumors.

2. Another name for a hamartoma is a/n _____.

3. Squamous cell carcinoma is an example of a _____.

4. Another name for small cell carcinoma is _____.

*Age Matters*

### Pediatrics

Respiratory disorders account for three of the top ten reasons for hospitalization among children and adolescents. These top three include pneumonia, asthma, and acute bronchitis—all disorders of the lower respiratory system. Five of the top 10 diagnoses for newborns are also respiratory problems or infections.

### Geriatrics

Although pneumonia is one of the most common diagnoses for elderly patients, pulmonary edema, chronic obstructive pulmonary disease, respiratory failure, and cancer have become the other most common disorders.

Click on **Hear It, Spell It** to practice spelling the pathology terms you have learned in this chapter. To see how well you pronounce the pathology terms in this chapter, click on **Hear It, Say It.** To review the pathology terms in this chapter, play **Medical Millionaire.**

## *Case Study*   Josiah Montgomery

Josiah is a 39-year-old truck driver who drives a rig from Seattle to Portland several times a week. A few days ago, he started to feel feverish. He figures he just has a touch of the flu, as several of his workers have had the flu over the past couple of weeks. He feels tired and chilled occasionally, but the frequency increases, and he begins to have back and side pains. As he completes his Friday delivery to Portland, he has a buddy take him to the ED. He has a high fever and an elevated pulse. Urinalysis, blood test, and chest x-ray are performed, which reveal a collapsed area in his lung and a UTI.

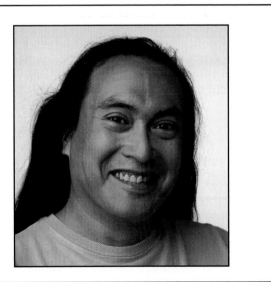

*Case Study* **Josiah Montgomery**

---

MONTGOMERY, JOSIAH N - 707418 Opened by OLNACK, PAUL MD     ▭ ⧉ ☒

Task   Edit   View   Time Scale   Options   Help

🖎 🗏 ◄ ► 🥄 🥄 🖾 🖾 🖙 ⬆ ■ 🕮 ▭ 🖫 🕮 🕮 🖨 📧 🖳 ◢    As Of 11:20    🏛 🔍 🕮

| **MONTGOMERY, JOSIAH N** | **Age: 39 years** | **Sex: Male** | **Loc: WHC-SMMC** |
|---|---|---|---|
| | DOB: 04/23/1972 | MRN: 707418 | FIN: 3506004 |

| Reference Text Browser | Form Browser | Medication Profile |
|---|---|---|

| Orders | Last 48 Hours | **ED** | Lab | Radiology | Assessments | Surgery | Clinical Notes | Pt. Info | Pt. Schedule | Task List | I & O | MAR |

Flowsheet: ED ▼ ...    Level: ED Note ▼      ● Table  ○ Group  ○ List

◄ ►                                       ◄ ►

| Navigator      ☒ |
|---|
| ✔   ED Note |

Patient comes to the emergency room complaining of fever off and on since 7 days ago. He states he has also had some chills and urinary urgency. Denies sore throat, nausea, vomiting, diarrhea, and cough. Also states has been having some low back pain and headache occasionally with fever.

| | |
|---|---|
| PMH: | HTN |
| MEDICATION: | None |
| ALLERGIES: | Penicillin |
| SH: | Nonsmoker, married |
| PHYSICAL EXAM: | |
| Vitals: | Temp 103.6, pulse 96, respirations 20, BP 168/88 |
| Lungs: | Clear to auscultation, no wheezes or crackles |
| Heart: | Regular rate and rhythm |
| Abdomen: | Nondistended, positive bowel sounds, nontender |
| LABORATORY FINDINGS: | Chest x-ray shows left lower lobe atelectasis, urinalysis shows findings compatible with urinary tract infection. |
| DIAGNOSIS: | Left lower lobe atelectasis |
| PLAN: | Patient will be treated with Cipro for his left lower lobe atelectasis and urinary tract infection symptoms. |

                          PROD | MAHAFC | 12 Dec 2011 | 11:20

---

🔄 Exercise 6: **Emergency Room Note**

---

*Using the emergency room note above, answer the following questions.*

1. What phrase in the emergency room note tells you that the patient's chest is free of fluid or exudates?

   _____

2. What term tells you that the patient has not exhibited a whistling sound made during breathing?

   _____

3. What term tells you that the patient has not exhibited any discontinuous bubbling noises in his chest?

   _____

4. What was the diagnostic imaging procedure used? _____

5. What term tells you that the patient has a collapsed lung? _____

## DIAGNOSTIC PROCEDURES

The physical examination includes listening to the patient's chest by the process of **auscultation** (os kull TAY shun) (listening) and **percussion** (pur KUH shun) (tapping) (A&P). If the patient's chest is free of fluid or exudates, it is considered *clear to auscultation* (CTA). Further examination of chest sounds may be accomplished through the use of a **stethoscope** (STETH oh scope).

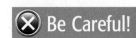

**⊗ Be Careful!**

*A* **stethoscope** *is used to listen, not to look.*

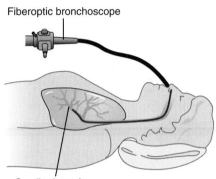

Fig. 11-14 Bronchoscopy.

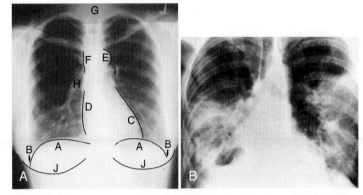

**Fig. 11-15 A,** Normal PA chest x-ray. The backward "L" in the upper right corner is placed on the film to indicate the left side of the patient's chest. *A,* Diaphragm. *B,* Costophrenic angle. *C,* Left ventricle. *D,* Right atrium. *E,* Aortic arch. *F,* Superior vena cava. *G,* Trachea. *H,* Right bronchus. *I,* Left bronchus. *J,* Breast shadows. **B,** X-ray of lung with pneumonia.

## Terms Related to Diagnostic Procedures

| Term | Word Origin | Definition |
|---|---|---|
| arterial blood gases (ABG) | *arteri/o* artery <br> *-al* pertaining to | Blood test that measures the amount of $O_2$ and $CO_2$ in the blood. |
| bronchoscopy <br> brong KOS skuh pee | *bronch/o* bronchus <br> *-scopy* process of viewing | Endoscopic procedure used to examine the bronchial tubes visually (Fig. 11-14). |
| chest x-ray (CXR) | | One of the most common imaging techniques for the respiratory system; used to visualize abnormalities of the respiratory system (Fig. 11-15). X-rays may also include the use of a contrast medium, as in **pulmonary angiography,** which uses a dye injected into the blood vessels of the lung, followed by subsequent x-ray imaging to demonstrate the flow of blood through these vessels. |
| computed tomography (CT) | *tom/o* slice <br> *-graphy* process of recording | Imaging technique that can image the respiratory system and associated structures by creating cross-sections or "slices" of tissue. |
| laryngoscopy <br> lair ing GOS skuh pee | *laryng/o* larynx, voice box <br> *-scopy* process of viewing | Endoscopic procedure used to visualize the interior of the larynx. |
| lung perfusion scan | | Nuclear medicine test that produces an image of blood flow to the lungs; used to detect pulmonary embolism. |

*Continued*

## Terms Related to Diagnostic Procedures—cont'd

| Term | Word Origin | Definition |
|------|-------------|------------|
| lung ventilation scan | | Test using radiopharmaceuticals to produce a picture of how air is distributed in the lungs; measures the ability of the lungs to take in air (Fig. 11-16). |
| magnetic resonance imaging (MRI) | | Computerized imaging that uses radiofrequency pulses to detect lung tumors, embolisms, and chest trauma. |
| Mantoux skin test<br>mon TOO | | Intradermal injection of purified protein derivative (PPD) used to detect the presence of tuberculosis antibodies. |
| mediastinoscopy<br>mee dee ah stih NAH skuh pee | | Endoscopic procedure used for visual examination of the structures contained within the space between the lungs. |
| peak flow meter | | Instrument used in a pulmonary function test (PFT) to measure breathing capacity (Fig. 11-17). |
| pulmonary function tests (PFT) | *pulmon/o* lung<br>*-ary* pertaining to | Procedures for determining the capacity of the lungs to exchange $O_2$ and $CO_2$ efficiently. See the table on the following page for examples of PFTs. |
| pulse oximetry<br>ock SIM uh tree | *ox/i* oxygen<br>*-metry* process of measurement | Noninvasive test to measure oxygen in arterial blood, in which a noninvasive, cliplike device is attached to either the earlobe or the fingertip (Fig. 11-18). |
| quantiferon-TB gold test (QFT) | | Definitive blood test to diagnose tuberculosis. |
| sonography | *son/o* sound<br>*-graphy* process of recording | Use of high-frequency sound waves to image structures within the body. |
| spirometry<br>spy ROM uh tree | *spir/o* breathing<br>*-metry* process of measurement | Test to measure the air capacity of the lungs with a **spirometer**. |
| sputum culture and sensitivity<br>SPYOO tum | | Cultivation of microorganisms from sputum that has been collected from expectoration (spitting). |
| stethoscope<br>STEH tho skohp | *steth/o* chest<br>*-scope* instrument to view | An instrument commonly used to listen to sounds within the body, especially the chest. |
| sweat test | | Method of evaluating sodium and chloride concentration in sweat as a means of diagnosing cystic fibrosis. |
| thoracoscopy<br>thor ah KOSS kuh pee | *thorac/o* chest<br>*-scopy* process of viewing | Visual exam of the chest cavity. |
| throat culture | | Cultivation of microorganisms from a throat swab to determine the type of organism that is causing a disorder. |

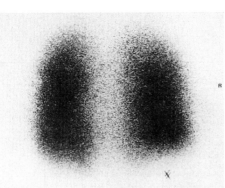

Fig. 11-16 Lung ventilation image of normal lungs.

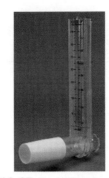

Fig. 11-17 Peak flow meter.

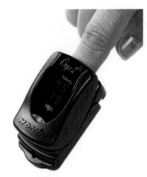

Fig. 11-18 Pulse oximetry.

## Examples of Pulmonary Function Tests

| Function | Abbreviation | Description |
|----------|-------------|-------------|
| Forced expiratory volume | FEV | Amount of air that can be exhaled with force in one breath. |
| Forced residual capacity | FRC | Amount of air remaining after a normal exhalation. |
| Forced vital capacity | FVC | Amount of air that can be exhaled with force after one inhales as deeply as possible. |
| Inspiratory capacity | IC | Amount of air that can be inspired after a normal expiration. |
| Tidal volume | TV | Amount of air normally inspired and expired in one respiration. |
| Total lung capacity | TLC | Amount of air in the lungs after one inhales as deeply as possible. |

## Exercise 7: Diagnostic Procedures

*Fill in the blank.*

1. A test for tuberculosis using purified protein derivation is called _____.

2. A blood test that measures $O_2$ and $CO_2$ is a/an _____.

3. A _____ is used to diagnose cystic fibrosis.

4. A _____ is a test of how air is distributed in the lung.

5. An imaging technique that shows the flow of blood through the vessels of the lungs is called

_____.

*Build the terms.*

6. process of viewing the bronchi _____

7. process of viewing the voice box _____

8. process of measurement of breathing _____

## *Case Study* Ava Derringer

One Saturday afternoon, 3-year-old Ava wakes up feverish and cranky from her nap. She is coughing and has green mucus draining from her nose. Later in the evening, Ava starts to breathe rapidly. Because she had had pneumonia 2 months earlier, her mother decides to take Ava to the ED. The doctor examines Ava and tells her her daughter has an upper respiratory infection with an early lung infection. She is prescribed an antibiotic and ibuprofen.

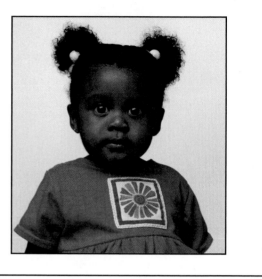

---

DERRINGER, AVA I - 599808 Opened by OBERT, WILLIAM MD

Task   Edit   View   Time Scale   Options   Help

As Of 18:18

**DERRINGER, AVA I**

Age: 3.3 years        Sex: Female        Loc: WHC-SMMC
DOB: 07/03/2008       MRN: 599808        FIN: 3506004

| Reference Text Browser | Form Browser | Medication Profile |
|---|---|---|

Orders | Last 48 Hours | ED | Lab | Radiology | **Assessments** | Surgery | Clinical Notes | Pt. Info | Pt. Schedule | Task List | I & O | MAR

Flowsheet: Assessment   ...   Level: Assessment        ⦿ Table   ◯ Group   ◯ List

**Navigator**

✓ Assessment

This 3-year-old child brought in today by mother with onset of fever and thick greenish drainage from her nose. Also developed a cough again. No history of ear infections and has recently had pneumonia.

T: 101.3      R: 40
P: 89         BP: 110/70

PE:              General appearance of well-developed child in some distress

HEAD:            Flat anterior fontanel

EARS:            Canals small, cleared of cerumen

NECK:            No adenopathy

LUNGS:           Noisy inspiratory respiration for which she had recent bronchoscopy

NOSE:            She does have thick greenish drainage from her nose

ASSESSMENT:      Upper respiratory infection with symptoms of pulmonary infection

PLAN:            Continue with Ibuprofen and decongestants. Placed on Omnicef 250 mg/5 ml.

PROD | MAHAFC | 15 Oct 2011 | 18:18

## Exercise 8: Progress Note

*Using the progress note on p. 428, answer the following questions.*

1. The patient has a history of infection of which organs? _____

2. The term "inspiratory" refers to what? _____

3. What was the recent endoscopic procedure that the patient had? _____

4. Where is the site of the infection? _____

5. What is the abbreviation for the respiratory disorder that this patient is diagnosed with?

_____

## THERAPEUTIC INTERVENTIONS

Therapeutic interventions for the respiratory system involve removal (-ectomy), repair (-plasty), a new opening (-stomy), a surgical puncture to remove fluid (-centesis), or intubation. See examples in the following table.

Patients who need assistance in attaining adequate $O_2$ levels may need a mechanical device called a **ventilator** to provide positive-pressure breathing. The device delivers the $O_2$ in different ways. If a low level of $O_2$ is required, a nasal **cannula** (KAN you lah) (tube) may be adequate. Face masks are another option. The amount of $O_2$ may be monitored more accurately with a **Venturi mask.** If high $O_2$ concentrations are necessary, a nonrebreathing or partial **rebreathing mask** may be used.

**Positive-pressure breathing (PPB)** is a respiratory therapy technique designed to deliver air at greater than atmospheric pressure to the lungs. **Continuous positive airway pressure (CPAP)** may be delivered through a ventilator and endotracheal tube or a nasal cannula, face mask, or hood over the patient's head. See Fig. 11-19 for several examples of oxygenation therapy.

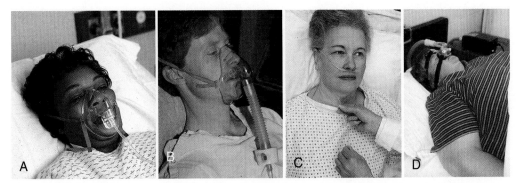

**Fig. 11-19** Routes of oxygen therapy. **A,** Simple face mask. **B,** Venturi mask. **C,** Nasal cannula. **D,** CPAP.

## Terms Related to Therapeutic Interventions

| Term | Word Origin | Definition |
|------|-------------|------------|
| adenoidectomy<br>ad uh noyd ECK tuh mee | *adenoid/o* adenoid<br>*-ectomy* removal, excision | Excision of the pharyngeal tonsils, or adenoids. |
| bronchoplasty<br>BRONG koh plas tee | *bronch/o* bronchus<br>*-plasty* surgical repair | Surgical repair of a bronchial defect. |
| endotracheal intubation<br>en doh TRAY kee ul<br>in too BAY shun | *endo-* within<br>*trache/o* windpipe (trachea)<br>*-al* pertaining to | Passage of a tube through the mouth into the trachea to ensure a patent (open) airway. |
| laryngectomy<br>lair in JECK tuh mee | *laryng/o* voice box (larynx)<br>*-ectomy* removal, excision | Excision of the voice box. |
| pulmonary resection | | Excision of a portion or a lobe of the lung or the entire lung. Called a **lobectomy** when an entire lobe is excised and a **pneumonectomy** when the entire lung is excised (Fig. 11-20). |
| rhinoplasty<br>RYE noh plas tee | *rhin/o* nose<br>*-plasty* surgical repair | Surgical repair of the nose for healthcare or cosmetic reasons. |
| septoplasty<br>SEP toh plas tee | *sept/o* wall, septum<br>*-plasty* surgical repair | Surgical repair of the wall between the nares. |
| sinusotomy<br>sye nuh SOT tuh mee | *sinus/o* sinus<br>*-tomy* incision | Incision of a sinus. |
| thoracocentesis<br>thor ack koh sen TEE sis | *thorac/o* thorax<br>*-centesis* surgical puncture | Aspiration of a fluid from the pleural cavity. Also called **pleurocentesis or thoracentesis**. |
| thoracotomy<br>thor uh KOT uh mee | *thorac/o* chest<br>*-tomy* incision | Incision of the chest as a means of approach for surgery. |
| tonsillectomy<br>ton sih LECK tuh mee | *tonsill/o* tonsil<br>*-ectomy* removal, excision | Excision of the palatine tonsils. |
| tracheostomy<br>tray kee OS tuh mee | *trache/o* trachea (windpipe)<br>*-stomy* new opening | Opening through the neck into the trachea, through which an indwelling tube may be inserted temporarily or permanently (Fig. 11-21). |
| tracheotomy<br>tray kee AH tuh mee | *trache/o* trachea (windpipe)<br>*-tomy* incision | Incision made into the trachea below the larynx to gain access to the airway; usually performed as an emergency procedure. |

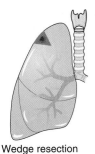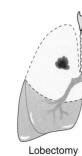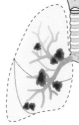

Wedge resection    Lobectomy    Segmental resection    Pneumonectomy

**Fig. 11-20** Pulmonary resections.

┌─┐
└─┘ Portion of tissue surgically removed    ■ Diseased area

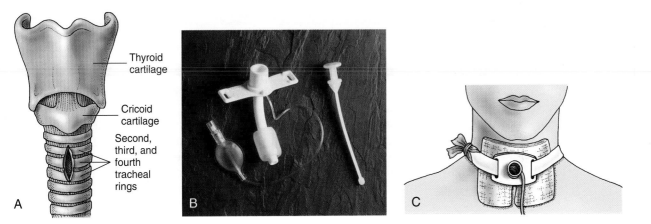

Thyroid cartilage

Cricoid cartilage

Second, third, and fourth tracheal rings

A          B          C

**Fig. 11-21 A,** Vertical tracheal incision for a tracheostomy. **B,** Tracheostomy tube. **C,** Placement of gauze and tie around a tracheostomy tube.

## Exercise 9: Therapeutic Interventions

*Match the terms with their definitions.*

____ 1. excision of the palatine tonsils

____ 2. surgical repair of the wall between the nares

____ 3. incision of a sinus

____ 4. removal of a lobe of the lung

____ 5. removal of the pharyngeal tonsils

____ 6. surgical repair of a bronchus

____ 7. aspiration of fluid from the pleural cavity

____ 8. incision of the windpipe

____ 9. tube within the windpipe

A. thoracocentesis
B. tracheotomy
C. endotracheal intubation
D. bronchoplasty
E. tonsillectomy
F. adenoidectomy
G. lobectomy
H. septoplasty
I. sinusotomy

*Build the terms.*

10. excision of the voice box _____

11. surgical repair of the nose _____

12. new opening in the windpipe _____

> Click on **Hear It, Spell It** to practice spelling the diagnostic and therapeutic terms you have learned in this chapter. To practice pronouncing these terms, click on **Hear It, Say It.**

## PHARMACOLOGY

Routes of administration for respiratory pharmaceuticals include the use of **ventilators,** devices that serve to assist respiration, and intensive positive-pressure breathing. A **hand-held nebulizer (HHN)** is a powered device that converts liquids into a fine spray, such as for inhaled medications. An **inhaler** is a nonmechanical device for administering medications that are inhaled, such as vapors or fine powders. A spacer, a device connected to the inhaler that contains the mist expelled from the inhaler until the user can breathe it, usually is used for children and individuals who have difficulty using the inhaler device alone.

**antihistamines:** block histamine receptors to manage allergies associated with allergic rhinitis or allergy-induced asthma. Examples are clemastine (Tavist), diphenhydramine (Benadryl), loratadine (Claritin), and fexofenadine (Allegra).

**antitussives:** suppress the cough reflex. Examples include dextromethorphan (Delsym), codeine (Robitussin AC), and benzonatate (Tessalon).

**bronchodilators:** relax bronchi to improve ventilation to the lungs. Examples include theophylline (Theo-Dur), ipratropium (Atrovent), and albuterol (Proventil, Ventolin), often administered through inhalers or nebulizers.

**decongestants:** reduce congestion or swelling of mucous membranes. Examples are pseudoephedrine (Sudafed) and phenylephrine (Sudafed PE).

**expectorants:** promote the expulsion of mucus from the respiratory tract. An example is guaifenesin (Mucinex).

**inhaled corticosteroids:** reduce airway inflammation to improve ventilation or reduce nasal congestion. Administered via oral or nasal inhalation accordingly. Examples include fluticasone (Flovent, Flonase), mometasone (Nasonex), and beclomethasone (Qvar).

**mucolytics:** break up thick mucus in respiratory tract. An example is N-acetylcysteine (Mucomyst).

## Exercise 10: Pharmacology

*Matching.*

____ 1. relaxes the bronchi

____ 2. expels mucus

____ 3. reduces congestion

____ 4. blocks histamine receptors to manage allergies

____ 5. suppresses coughs

A. antihistamine
B. antitussive
C. bronchodilator
D. decongestant
E. expectorant

6. What type of mechanical device is used to produce a fine spray for inhaled medications?

_____

7. What type of non-mechanical device is used to administer medications that are inhaled, such as fine

powders or vapors? _____

8. A/An _____ is a device designed to assist in respiration and intensive positive-pressure breathing.

## Abbreviations

| Abbreviation | Definition | Abbreviation | Definition |
|---|---|---|---|
| ABG | arterial blood gases | MDRTB | multidrug-resistant tuberculosis |
| A&P | auscultation and percussion | NSCLC | non–small cell lung cancer |
| AP | anteroposterior | $O_2$ | oxygen |
| ARF | acute respiratory failure | OSA | obstructive sleep apnea |
| CF | cystic fibrosis | PPB | positive-pressure breathing |
| $CO_2$ | carbon dioxide | PPD | purified protein derivative |
| COPD | chronic obstructive pulmonary disease | RAD | reactive airway disease |
| | | RLL | right lower lobe |
| CT | computed tomography | RML | right middle lobe |
| CTA | clear to auscultation | RUL | right upper lobe |
| CWP | coal workers' pneumoconiosis | RSV | respiratory syncytial virus |
| CXR | chest x-ray | SARS | severe acute respiratory syndrome |
| DOE | dyspnea on exertion | | |
| HHN | hand-held nebulizer | SCLC | small cell lung cancer |
| LLL | left lower lobe (of the lung) | SOB | shortness of breath |
| LUL | left upper lobe (of the lung) | TB | tuberculosis |
| MDI | metered dose inhaler | URI | upper respiratory infection |

## Exercise 11: Abbreviations

*Write out the following abbreviations.*

1. A CXR revealed RML pneumonia in the 43-year-old teacher. _____

2. The patient was tested with PPD for suspected TB. _____

3. Solange had rhinorrhea and a productive cough, and she was diagnosed with a URI.

_____

4. The patient with COPD had dyspnea, DOE, and a chronic cough.

_____

5. Years of work in the mines resulted in the patient's diagnosis of CWP. _____

6. The child came to the emergency room and was diagnosed with RSV. _____

# Chapter Review

*Match the word parts to their definitions.*

## WORD PARTS DEFINITIONS

| Prefix/Suffix | Definition |
|---|---|
| a- | 1. _____ healthy, normal |
| dys- | 2. _____ excessive |
| -ectasis | 3. _____ deficient |
| eu- | 4. _____ without |
| hyper- | 5. _____ breathing |
| hypo- | 6. _____ spitting |
| -metry | 7. _____ discharge |
| -pnea | 8. _____ difficult |
| -ptysis | 9. _____ process of measurement |
| -rrhea | 10. _____ dilation |

| Combining Form | Definition |
|---|---|
| capn/o | 11. _____ carbon dioxide |
| cost/o | 12. _____ lung |
| laryng/o | 13. _____ chest |
| muc/o | 14. _____ to breathe |
| nas/o | 15. _____ straight |
| orth/o | 16. _____ pleura |
| ox/i | 17. _____ nose |
| pector/o | 18. _____ septum, wall |
| pharyng/o | 19. _____ chest |
| phren/o | 20. _____ pus |
| pleur/o | 21. _____ throat |
| pneum/o | 22. _____ mucus |
| pulmon/o | 23. _____ oxygen |
| py/o | 24. _____ diaphragm |
| rhin/o | 25. _____ lung |
| salping/o | 26. _____ chest |
| sept/o | 27. _____ rib |
| sin/o | 28. _____ sinus |
| spir/o | 29. _____ tonsil |
| steth/o | 30. _____ eustachian tube |
| thorac/o | 31. _____ voicebox |
| tonsill/o | 32. _____ nose |

# WORDSHOP

| Prefixes | Combining Forms | Suffixes |
|----------|-----------------|----------|
| a- | coni/o | -al |
| brady- | cost/o | -ation |
| dys- | hem/o | -eal |
| endo- | laryng/o | -itis |
| eu- | my/o | -osis |
| ex- | myc/o | -plasty |
| hyper- | pleur/o | -pnea |
| in- | pneum/o | -rrhea |
| inter- | py/o | -scopy |
| para- | rhin/o | -stenosis |
| tachy- | spir/o | -stomy |
| | trache/o | -thorax |
| | thorac/o | -tomy |

Build the following terms by combining the above word parts. Some word parts may be used more than once. Some may not be used at all. The number in parenthesis is the number of word parts needed to build the term.

| Definition | Term |
|------------|------|
| 1. difficult breathing (2) | |
| 2. rapid breathing (2) | |
| 3. abnormal condition of dust in the lungs (3) | |
| 4. discharge from the nose (2) | |
| 5. process of breathing out (3) | |
| 6. pus in the chest (pleural cavity) (2) | |
| 7. inflammation of the pleurae (2) | |
| 8. surgical repair of the nose (2) | |
| 9. blood in the chest (pleural cavity) (2) | |
| 10. abnormal condition of narrowing of the windpipe (2) | |
| 11. incision of the windpipe (2) | |
| 12. pertaining to between the ribs (3) | |
| 13. pertaining to within the windpipe (3) | |
| 14. abnormal condition of fungus in the nose (3) | |
| 15. process of viewing the chest (2) | |

Sort the terms into the correct categories.

## TERM SORTING

| Anatomy and Physiology | Pathology | Diagnostic Procedures | Therapeutic Interventions |
|---|---|---|---|
| | | | |
| | | | |
| | | | |
| | | | |
| | | | |
| | | | |
| | | | |
| | | | |
| | | | |
| | | | |

| | | | |
|---|---|---|---|
| ABG | CXR | mediastinum | SARS |
| alveolus | diaphragm | olfaction | septoplasty |
| aphonia | emphysema | oropharynx | sinusotomy |
| apnea | epiglottis | pleurisy | spirometry |
| bronchiectasis | epistaxis | PFT | thoracocentesis |
| bronchodilator | eustachian tube | pleura | throat culture |
| bronchoplasty | hemoptysis | pulse oximetry | tonsillectomy |
| bronchoscopy | inhalation | QFT | trachea |
| CPAP | laryngectomy | rhinomycosis | tracheostomy |
| CT | mediastinoscopy | rhonchi | tracheotomy |

*Replace the highlighted words with the correct terms.*

## TRANSLATIONS

1. **Difficult and/or painful breathing** and **whistling sound made during breathing** were signs that Sari had asthma.

2. The patient's **difficulty making sounds** and **inflammation of the voice box** were associated with an upper respiratory infection.

3. The baby had **a high-pitched inspiratory sound from the larynx,** which was a sign of **acute viral infection of early childhood marked by stridor caused by spasms of the larynx, trachea, and bronchi.**

4. Dr. Hollander told Ryan's mother that her son's fever and **chest pain** were symptoms of **abnormal accumulation of fluid in the intrapleural space.**

5. The patient underwent a **CXR** to see if she had **an infectious inflammation of the lungs.**

6. After 3 days of **severe inflammation or infection of the pharynx,** Abby had **a cultivation of microorganisms from a throat swab** to determine the pathogen.

7. **A noninvasive test to measure oxygen in arterial blood** and **a test to measure the air capacity of the lungs** were performed on the patient.

8. Marketta's **deflection of the nasal septum** was treated with **a surgical repair of the wall between the nares.**

9. **An aspiration of a fluid from the pleural cavity** was necessary to treat the patient's **blood in the pleural cavity.**

10. The pulmonologist diagnosed Mr. Borasky with **chronic dilation of the bronchi** and **respiratory disorder characterized by a progressive and irreversible diminishment in capacity of the lungs.**

11. After the patient's treatment for **pertaining to the larynx** cancer, she had a temporary **opening through the neck into the trachea.**

12. Monique had **an intradermal injection of PPD,** which revealed that she had **a chronic infectious disorder caused by an acid-fast bacillus.**

13. Mr H. was treated for **abnormal accumulation of coal dust in the lungs,** a type of **loss of lung capacity caused by an accumulation of dust in the lungs** that developed after years of work in a coal mine.

14. The child had a **method of evaluation sodium and chloride concentration in sweat** to see if she had **an inherited disorder of the exocrine glands, resulting in abnormal, thick secretions of mucus.**

# Case Study    Casey Sandoval

Casey Sandoval is a pitcher for her Little League softball team this year, but today on the field, she had so much difficulty catching her breath that now she can barely speak. Her mother has brought her to the emergency department (ED) for help.

Casey has occasionally been short of breath when playing sports before, but not as severely as today. Even in the air-conditioned hospital, she is sweaty, pale, and slightly cyanotic. Her inability to catch her breath is making her panicky.

The ED pediatrician suspects that Casey has exercise-induced asthma. He gives Casey oxygen through a face mask and connects her to a cardiac monitor. He records Casey's heart and respiratory rates and notes the wheezing and bilateral rhonchi.

Casey and her mother are counselled on how to manage Casey's asthma. She is prescribed a bronchodilator to relax the smooth muscle of the airways from the trachea to the bronchioles and inhaled oral steroids to prevent mucus

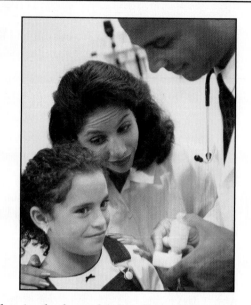

buildup in the bronchioles. She receives instructions on how to use an inhaler with a spacer, a tube that keeps the inhaler mist from scattering in the air. After a couple of tries, Casey is able to manage the inhaler.

## ED Record

*Using the ED Record on p. 439, answer the following questions.*

1. In your own words, explain the meaning of the symptoms "slightly diaphoretic" and "slight nail bed cyanosis." _____

2. How is oxygen measured in pulse oximetry? _____

3. Name and define the two abnormal sounds heard on auscultation in this report.

_____

4. What is the purpose of a peak flow meter? _____

5. What does the abbreviation HHN mean? _____

SANDOVAL, CASEY C - 557248 Opened by HAMILTON, WILLIAM RRT

Task   Edit   View   Time Scale   Options   Help

As Of 17:43

| SANDOVAL, CASEY C | Age: 8 years | Sex: Female | Loc: WHC-SMMC |
| | DOB: 03/31/2004 | MRN: 557248 | FIN: 3506004 |

Reference Text Browser | Form Browser | Medication Profile

Orders | Last 48 Hours | **ED** | Lab | Radiology | Assessments | Surgery | Clinical Notes | Pt. Info | Pt. Schedule | Task List | I & O | MAR

Flowsheet: ED     ...   Level: ED Record     ● Table  ○ Group  ○ List

Navigator

✓   ED Record

Casey Sandoval, an 8-year-old female, came to the ED in moderately severe respiratory distress. She was accompanied by her mother. Pt appeared pale, anxious, and slightly diaphoretic, and had slight nail bed cyanosis. Casey was unable to speak more than two- or three-word phrases between breaths. She was placed on oxygen per face mask and connected to cardiac monitor and pulse oximetry. HR was 125, RR was 33, and labored; oximetry measured 89% on 6 L/min $O_2$. Wheezes were auscultated in all lung fields, with prolonged expiratory phase. Pt has frequent nonproductive cough. Physical exam revealed intercostal retractions and use of accessory muscles on inspiration.

   Pt was given an immediate nebulization treatment via hand-held nebulizer containing 5 mg albuterol and 3 mL NS solution driven by 8 L/min $O_2$. Oximetry increased to 95% by end of nebulization. Peak flows were measured at 100 L/min post-HHN. Respirations had decreased to 25; heart rate was 95. Breath sounds revealed mild, scattered expiratory wheezes and rhonchi bilaterally. Repeat nebulizer treatment was performed 15 minutes later. Peak flow measurements had increased to 175 L/min, and pt was able to wean off supplemental oxygen and maintained oxygen saturation of 94% on room air.

   A third HHN was ordered 30 minutes later, and repeat peak flows measured 210 L/min. Breath sounds were clear, and pt respiratory rate had decreased to 18 breaths/min, heart rate to 87, and saturation was 97% on room air.

   Oral prednisone was prescribed. Pt and parent were instructed on use of metered-dose inhaler with spacer and peak flow meter. MDIs containing albuterol and Flovent 88 mcg b.i.d. were prescribed. Child and parent were instructed to use 4 puffs albuterol every 4 hours, and 2 puffs Flovent b.i.d. Peak flows were to be measured three times daily pre albuterol and post albuterol and graphed on the diary card.

| PROD | MAHAFC | 25 May 2012 | 17:43 |

For more interactive learning, click on:
- **Whack a Word Part** to review respiratory word parts.
- **Wheel of Terminology** and **Word Shop** to practice word building.
- **Tournament of Terminology** to test your knowledge of respiratory terms.
- **Terminology Triage** to practice sorting respiratory terms into categories.

# 12

*Anything's possible if you've got enough nerve.*
**—J. K. Rowling**

## OBJECTIVES

- Recognize and use terms related to the anatomy and physiology of the nervous system.
- Recognize and use terms related to the pathology of the nervous system.
- Recognize and use terms related to the diagnostic procedures for the nervous system.
- Recognize and use terms related to the therapeutic interventions for the nervous system.

# Nervous System

## CHAPTER AT A GLANCE

*Use this list of key word parts and terms to assess your knowledge. Check off the ones you have mastered.*

### ANATOMY AND PHYSIOLOGY

- [ ] autonomic nervous system (ANS)
- [ ] axon
- [ ] brainstem
- [ ] central nervous system (CNS)
- [ ] cerebellum
- [ ] cerebrospinal fluid (CSF)
- [ ] cerebrum
- [ ] cranial nerves
- [ ] meninges
- [ ] myelin sheath
- [ ] nerve root
- [ ] neuron
- [ ] neurotransmitter
- [ ] parasympathetic nervous system
- [ ] peripheral nervous system (PNS)
- [ ] spinal cord
- [ ] spinal nerves
- [ ] sympathetic nervous system
- [ ] synapse

### KEY WORD PARTS

**PREFIX**

- [ ] an-
- [ ] hemi-
- [ ] mono-
- [ ] para-, par-
- [ ] poly-
- [ ] quadri-

**SUFFIX**

- [ ] -al, -ar
- [ ] -ectomy
- [ ] -esthesia
- [ ] -graphy
- [ ] -ia
- [ ] -itis
- [ ] -lepsy
- [ ] -lysis
- [ ] -oma
- [ ] -paresis
- [ ] -plegia
- [ ] -rrhaphy
- [ ] -tomy

**COMBINING FORM**

- [ ] cerebell/o
- [ ] cerebr/o
- [ ] cord/o, chord/o
- [ ] crani/o
- [ ] dur/o
- [ ] electr/o
- [ ] encephal/o
- [ ] esthesi/o
- [ ] hemat/o
- [ ] meningi/o, mening/o
- [ ] myel/o
- [ ] narc/o
- [ ] neur/o
- [ ] osm/o
- [ ] radicul/o
- [ ] rhiz/o
- [ ] somn/o
- [ ] vascul/o

### KEY TERMS

- [ ] anosmia
- [ ] cerebral palsy (CP)
- [ ] cerebrovascular accident (CVA)
- [ ] cordotomy
- [ ] craniotomy
- [ ] electroencephalography
- [ ] encephalitis
- [ ] hemiplegia
- [ ] lumbar puncture (LP)
- [ ] meningitis
- [ ] meningomyelocele
- [ ] multiple sclerosis (MS)
- [ ] myelography
- [ ] narcolepsy
- [ ] neurolysis
- [ ] neurorrhaphy
- [ ] paraparesis
- [ ] paresthesia
- [ ] Parkinson disease (PD)
- [ ] poliomyelitis
- [ ] polysomnography (PSG)
- [ ] quadriplegia
- [ ] rhizotomy
- [ ] transcutaneous electrical nerve stimulation (TENS)
- [ ] transient ischemic attack (TIA)

## FUNCTIONS OF THE NERVOUS SYSTEM

Possibly the most complex and poorly understood system, the nervous system plays a major role in **homeostasis** (hoh mee oh STAY sis), keeping the other body systems coordinated and regulated to achieve optimum performance. It accomplishes this goal by helping the individual respond to his or her internal and external environments.

The nervous and endocrine systems are responsible for communication and control throughout the body. There are three main **neural** functions, which are as follows:

1. Collecting information about the external and internal environment *(sensing)*.
2. Processing this information and making decisions about action *(interpreting)*.
3. Directing the body to put into play the decisions made *(acting)*.

For example, the sensory function begins with a stimulus (e.g., the uncomfortable pinch of tight shoes). That information travels to the brain, where it is interpreted. The return message is sent to react to the stimulus (e.g., remove the shoes).

## SPECIALTIES/SPECIALISTS

Physicians who specialize in the diagnosis, treatment, and prevention of neurologic disorders are called **neurologists.** The specialty is **neurology.**

## ANATOMY AND PHYSIOLOGY

### Organization of the Nervous System

To carry out its functions, the nervous system is divided into two main subsystems. (See Fig. 12-1 for a schematic of the divisions.) The **central nervous system (CNS)** is composed of the brain and the spinal cord. It is the only site of nerve cells called **interneurons** (in tur NOOR ons), which connect sensory and motor neurons. The **peripheral nervous system (PNS)** is composed of the nerves that extend from the brain and spinal cord to the tissues of the body. These are organized into 12 pairs of cranial nerves and 31 pairs of spinal nerves. The PNS is further divided into voluntary and involuntary nerves, which may be **afferent** (or **sensory**), carrying impulses to the brain and spinal cord, or **efferent** (or **motor**), carrying impulses from the brain and spinal cord to either voluntary or involuntary muscles.

PNS nerves are further categorized into two subsystems:

**somatic** (soh MAT ick) **system:** This system is *voluntary* in nature. These nerves collect information from and return instructions to the skin, muscles, and joints.
**autonomic** (ah toh NAH mick) **system:** Mostly *involuntary* functions are controlled by this system as sensory information from the internal environment is sent to the CNS, and, in return, motor impulses from the CNS are sent to involuntary muscles: the heart, glands, and organs.

**homeostasis**
home/o = same
-stasis = stopping, controlling

**nerve** = neur/o

**neurology**
neur/o = nerve
-logy = study of

**body** = somat/o

> ⊗ Be Careful!   *Remember that* **efferent** *means to carry away, while* **afferent** *means to carry toward. In the nervous system, these terms are used to refer to away from and toward the brain.*

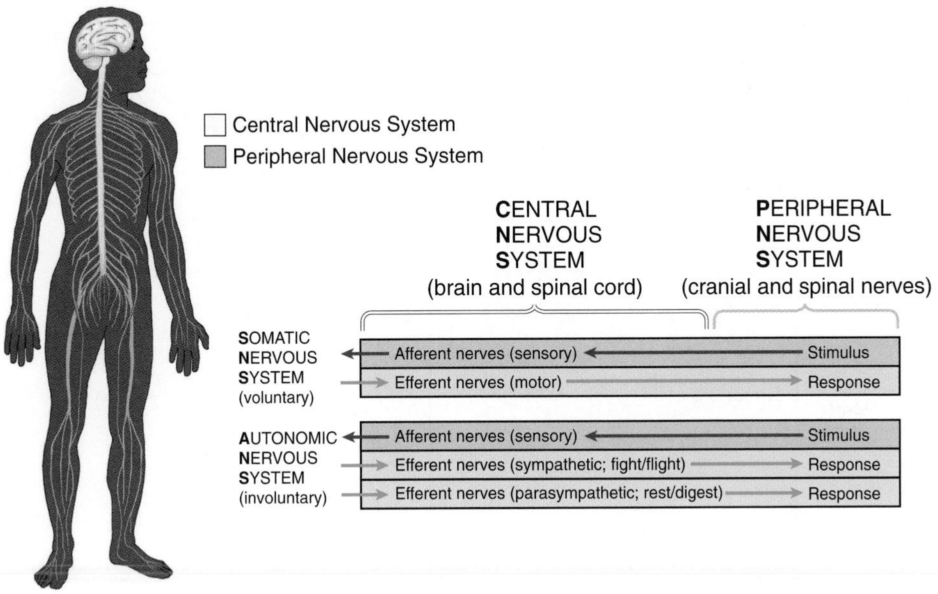

Fig. 12-1 The nervous system. Afferent nerves carry nervous impulses from a stimulus toward the CNS. Efferent nerves carry the impulse away from the CNS to effect a response to the stimulus.

## Exercise 1: Organization of the Nervous System

*Fill in the blanks.*

1. The two main divisions of the nervous system are the _____ and the _____.

*Circle the correct answer.*

2. Sensory neurons *(transmit, receive)* information *(to, from)* the CNS.
3. Motor neurons, also called *(efferent, afferent)* neurons, transmit information *(to, from)* the CNS.
4. The *(somatic, autonomic)* nervous system is voluntary in nature, whereas the *(somatic, autonomic)* nervous system is largely involuntary.

## Cells of the Nervous System

The nervous system is made up of the following two types of cells:

1. Parenchymal cells, or **neurons,** the cells that carry out the work of the system.
2. Stromal cells, or **glia** (GLEE uh), the cells that provide a supportive function.

### Neurons

The basic unit of the nervous system is the nerve cell, or neuron (Fig. 12-2). Not all neurons are the same, but all have the following features in common. **Dendrites** (DEN drytes), projections from the cell body, receive **neural impulses,** also called **action potentials,** from a **stimulus** of some kind. This impulse travels along the dendrite and into the cell body, which is the control center of the cell. This cell body contains the nucleus and surrounding cytoplasm.

From the cell body, the impulse moves out along the **axon** (AX on), a slender, elongated projection that carries the nervous impulse toward the next neuron. The **terminal fibers** result from the final branching of the axon and the site

**neuron**
  neur/o = nerve
  -on = structure

dendrite = dendr/o

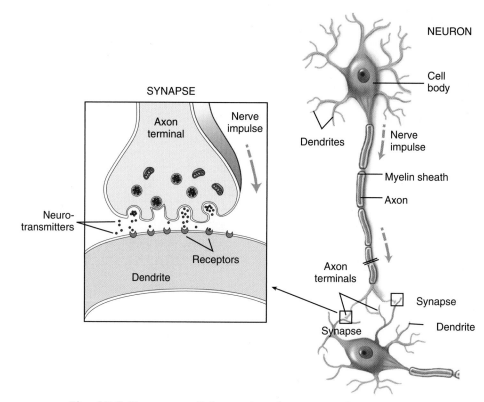

Fig. 12-2 The nerve cell (neuron) with an inset of a synapse.

⊗ Be Careful!

The abbreviation **BBB** can stand for either blood-brain barrier or bundle branch block, a cardiac condition.

**neuroglia**
  **neur/o** = nerve
  **-glia** = glue

**astrocyte**
  **astr/o** = star
  **-cyte** = cell

of the **axon terminals** that store the chemical **neurotransmitters.** In neurons *outside* the CNS, the axon is covered by the **myelin** (MY uh lin) sheath, which is a substance produced by **Schwann** (shvahn) **cells** that coat the axons.

From the axon's terminal fibers, the neurotransmitter is released from the cell to travel across the space between these terminal fibers and the dendrites of the next cell. This space is called the **synapse** (SIN aps) (*see* Fig. 12-2). The impulse continues in this manner until its destination is reached.

### Glia

These supportive, or stromal, cells are also called **neuroglia** (noo RAH glee ah). They accomplish their supportive function by physically holding the neurons together and also protecting them. One type of neuroglia, the **astrocytes** (AS troh sites), connect neurons and blood vessels and form a structure called the **blood-brain barrier (BBB),** which prevents or slows the passage of some drugs and disease-causing organisms to the CNS.

---

⟳ Exercise 2: **Cells of the Nervous System**

1. List words connected by arrows to show the path of the action potential from initial stimulus to

synapse. _____

*Match the terms with their word parts.*

____ 2. star        ____ 5. glue            A. -glia
                                            B. somat/o
____ 3. body        ____ 6. dendrite        C. dendr/o
                                            D. astr/o
____ 4. nerve                               E. neur/o

*Decode the terms.*

7. perineural _____

8. oligodendritic _____

9. microglial _____

## The Central Nervous System

As stated previously, the CNS is composed of the **brain** and the **spinal cord.**

**brain** = encephal/o

### The Brain

The brain is one of the most complex organs of the body. It is divided into four parts: the **cerebrum** (suh REE brum), the **cerebellum** (sair ih BELL um), the **diencephalon** (dye en SEF fuh lon), and the **brainstem** (Fig. 12-3).

**cerebrum** = cerebr/o

**cerebellum** = cerebell/o

### Cerebrum

The largest portion of the brain, the cerebrum, is divided into two halves, or hemispheres (Fig. 12-4). It is responsible for thinking, reasoning, and memory. The surfaces of the hemispheres are covered with **gray matter** and are called the **cerebral cortex.** Arranged into folds, the valleys are referred to as **sulci** (SULL sye) (*sing.* sulcus), and the ridges are **gyri** (JYE rye) (*sing.* gyrus). The cerebrum is further divided into sections called **lobes,** each of which has its own functions:

**cortex** = cortic/o

**lobe** = lob/o

1. The **frontal lobe** contains the functions of speech and the motor area that controls voluntary movement on the contralateral side of the body.
2. The **temporal** (TEM pur rul) **lobe** contains the auditory and olfactory areas.
3. The **parietal** (puh RYE uh tul) **lobe** controls the sensations of touch and taste.
4. The **occipital** (ock SIP ih tul) **lobe** is responsible for vision.

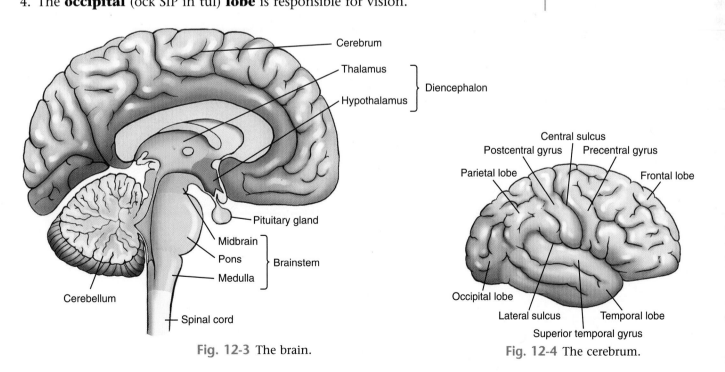

Fig. 12-3 The brain.

Fig. 12-4 The cerebrum.

### Cerebellum

Located inferior to the occipital lobe of the cerebrum, the **cerebellum** coordinates voluntary movement but is involuntary in its function. For example, walking is a voluntary movement. The coordination needed for the muscles and other body parts to walk smoothly is involuntary and is controlled by the cerebellum.

### Diencephalon

The diencephalon is composed of the **thalamus** (THAL uh mus) and the structure inferior to it, the **hypothalamus** (HYE poh thal uh mus). The thalamus is responsible for relaying sensory information (with the exception of smell) and translating it into sensations of pain, temperature, and touch. The hypothalamus activates, integrates, and controls the peripheral autonomic nervous system, along with many functions, such as body temperature, sleep, and appetite.

### Brainstem

The brainstem connects the cerebral hemispheres to the spinal cord. It is composed of three main parts: **midbrain, pons** (ponz), and **medulla oblongata** (muh DOO lah ob lon GAH tah). The midbrain connects the pons and cerebellum with the hemispheres of the cerebrum. It is the site of reflex centers for eye and head movements in response to visual and auditory stimuli. The second part of the brainstem, the pons, serves as a bridge between the medulla oblongata and the cerebrum. Finally, the lowest part of the brainstem, the medulla oblongata, regulates heart rate, blood pressure, and breathing.

### *The Spinal Cord*

The **spinal cord** extends from the medulla oblongata to the first lumbar vertebra (Fig. 12-5). It then extends into a structure called the **cauda equina** (KAH

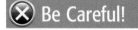

**Be Careful!**

Myel/o *can mean bone marrow or spinal cord; memorization and context will be the student's only methods to determine which meaning applies.*

**spinal cord** = cord/o, chord/o, myel/o

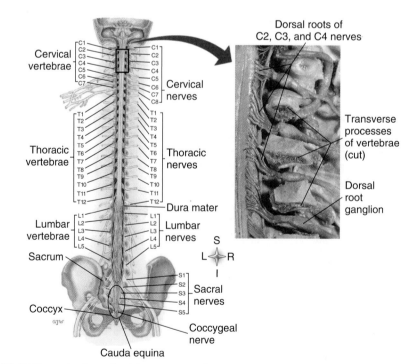

**Fig. 12-5** The spinal cord with an inset of a cervical segment showing emerging cervical nerves.

dah eh KWY nah). The spinal cord is protected by the bony vertebrae surrounding it and the coverings unique to the CNS called **meninges** (meh NIN jeez). The spinal cord is composed of **gray matter,** the cell bodies of motor neurons, and **white matter,** the myelin-covered axons or nerve fibers that extend from the nerve cell bodies. The 31 pairs of spinal nerves emerge from the spinal cord at the **nerve roots.**

### Meninges

Meninges act as protective coverings for the CNS and are composed of three layers separated by spaces (Fig. 12-6). The **dura mater** (DUR ah MAY tur) is the tough, fibrous, outer covering of the meninges; its literal meaning is *hard mother*. The space between the dura mater and arachnoid membrane is called the **subdural space.** Next comes the **arachnoid** (uh RACK noyd) **membrane,** a thin, delicate membrane that takes its name from its spidery appearance. The **subarachnoid space** is the space between the arachnoid membrane and the pia mater, containing **cerebrospinal fluid (CSF).** CSF is also present in cavities in the brain called **ventricles.** Finally, the **pia mater** (PEE uh MAY tur) is the thin, vascular membrane that is the innermost of the three meninges; its literal meaning is *soft mother*.

### The Peripheral Nervous System

The **peripheral nervous system** is divided into 12 pairs of **cranial nerves** that conduct impulses between the brain and the head, neck, thoracic, and abdominal areas, and 31 pairs of **spinal nerves** that closely mimic the organization of the vertebrae and provide innervation to the rest of the body. If the

| | |
|---|---|
| **meninges** = mening/o, meningi/o | |
| **nerve root** = rhiz/o, radicul/o | |
| **dura mater** = dur/o | |
| **ventricle** = ventricul/o | |

Fig. 12-6 The meninges.

nerve fibers from several spinal nerves form a network, it is termed a **plexus** (PLECK sus). Spinal nerves are named by their location (cervical, thoracic, lumbar, sacral, and coccygeal) and by number (Fig. 12-7). Cranial nerves are named by their number and also their function or distribution.

## The Cranial Nerves

| Number | Name | Origin of Sensory Fibers | Effector Innervated by Motor Fibers |
|---|---|---|---|
| I | Olfactory | Olfactory epithelium of nose (smell) | None |
| II | Optic | Retina of eye (vision) | None |
| III | Oculomotor | Proprioceptors* of eyeball muscles | Muscles that move eyeball; muscles that change shape of lens; muscles that constrict pupil |
| IV | Trochlear | Proprioceptors* of eyeball muscles | Muscles that move eyeball |
| V | Trigeminal | Teeth and skin of face | Some muscles used in chewing |
| VI | Abducens | Proprioceptors* of eyeball muscles | Muscles that move eyeball |
| VII | Facial | Taste buds of anterior part of tongue | Muscles used for facial expression; submaxillary and sublingual salivary glands |
| VIII | Vestibulocochlear (Auditory) | | None |
| | Vestibular branch | Semicircular canals of inner ear (senses of movement, balance, and rotation) | |
| | Cochlear branch | Cochlea of inner ear (hearing) | |
| IX | Glossopharyngeal | Taste buds of posterior third of tongue and lining of pharynx | Parotid salivary gland; muscles of pharynx used in swallowing |
| X | Vagus | Nerve endings in many of the internal organs (e.g., lungs, stomach, aorta, larynx) | Parasympathetic fibers to heart, stomach, small intestine, larynx, esophagus, and other organs |
| XI | Spinal accessory | Muscles of shoulder | Muscles of neck and shoulder |
| XII | Hypoglossal | Muscles of tongue | Muscles of tongue |

*Proprioceptors are receptors located in muscles, tendons, or joints that provide information about body position and movement.

**dermatome**
  dermat/o = skin
  -tome = instrument
  used to cut

**Dermatomes** (DUR mah tomes) are skin surface areas supplied by a single afferent spinal nerve. These areas are so specific that it is actually possible to map the body by dermatomes (Fig. 12-8). This specificity can be demonstrated in patients with shingles, who show similar patterns as specific peripheral nerves are affected (*see* Fig. 12-16).

The **autonomic nervous system (ANS)** consists of nerves that regulate involuntary function. Examples include cardiac muscle and smooth muscle. The motor portion of this system is further divided into the sympathetic nervous system and the parasympathetic nervous system, two opposing systems that provide balance in the rest of the body systems:

- The **sympathetic nervous system** is capable of producing a "fight-or-flight" response. This is the one part of the nervous system that helps the individual respond to perceived stress. The heart rate and blood pressure increase, digestive processes slow, and sweat and adrenal glands increase their secretions.

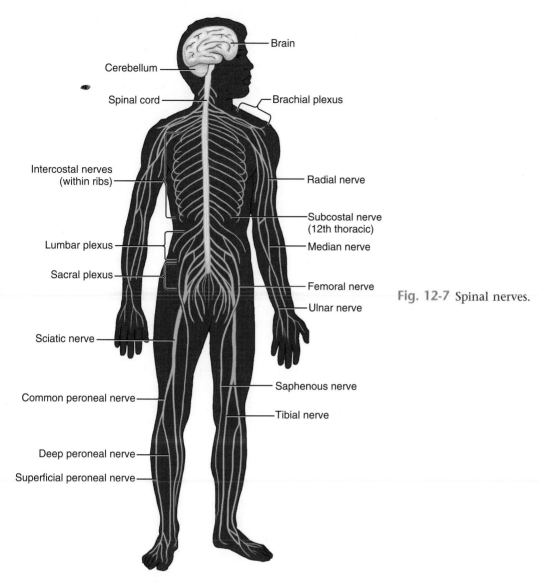

**Fig. 12-7** Spinal nerves.

- The **parasympathetic nervous system** tends to do the opposite of the sympathetic nervous system—slowing the heart rate, lowering blood pressure, increasing digestive functions, and decreasing adrenal and sweat gland activity. This is sometimes called the "rest and digest" system.

Here is an example of a sensory response:

"Eight-year-old Joey is hungry. He decides to sneak some cookies before dinner. Afraid his mother will see him, he surreptitiously takes a handful into the hall closet and shuts the door. As he begins to eat, the closet door flies open. Joey's heart begins to race as he whips the cookies out of sight. When he sees it's only his sister, he relaxes and offers her a cookie as a bribe not to tell on him."

Joey's afferent (sensory) somatic neurons carried the message to his brain that he was hungry. This message was interpreted by his brain as a concern, and the response was to sneak cookies from the jar and hide himself as he ate them. When the closet door flew open, his sensory neurons perceived a danger and triggered a sympathetic "fight-or-flight" response, which raised his heart rate and blood pressure and stimulated his sweat glands. When the intruder was perceived to be harmless, his parasympathetic nervous system took over and reduced his heart rate, bringing it back to normal. The same afferent fibers perceived the intruder in two different ways, with two different sets of autonomic motor responses (sympathetic and parasympathetic).

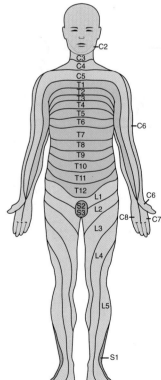

**Fig. 12-8** Dermatomes. Each dermatome is named for the spinal nerve that serves it.

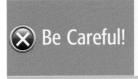

**Be Careful!**

*The term* **dermatome** *can be used to describe an instrument that cuts thin slices of skin for grafting, and the term also signifies a mesodermal layer in early development, which becomes the dermal layers of the skin.*

## Exercise 3: Central and Peripheral Nervous System

*Match the following parts of the brain with their functions.*

____ 1. pons

____ 2. parietal cerebral lobe

____ 3. hypothalamus

____ 4. temporal cerebral lobe

____ 5. midbrain

____ 6. cerebellum

____ 7. occipital cerebral lobe

____ 8. thalamus

____ 9. frontal cerebral lobe

____ 10. medulla oblongata

A. auditory and olfactory activity
B. relays sensory information
C. reflex center for eye and head movements
D. sensation of vision
E. regulates heart rate, blood pressure, and breathing
F. regulates temperature, sleep, and appetite
G. speech and motor activity
H. connects medulla oblongata with cerebrum
I. coordinates voluntary movement
J. sensation of touch and taste

*Match the CNS part with its combining form.*

____ 11. cerebellum

____ 12. spinal cord

____ 13. meninges

____ 14. nerve root

____ 15. dura mater

____ 16. cerebrum

____ 17. brain

____ 18. skin

____ 19. spine

____ 20. ventricle

A. meningi/o, mening/o
B. myel/o, cord/o, chord/o
C. dur/o
D. rhiz/o, radicul/o
E. dermat/o
F. cerebr/o
G. spin/o
H. cerebell/o
I. encephal/o
J. ventricul/o

*Decode the terms.*

21. intraventricular _____

22. epidural _____

23. parasinal _____

24. infracerebellar _____

### Exercise 4: Central and Peripheral Nervous System

*Label the drawings below with the correct anatomic labels.*

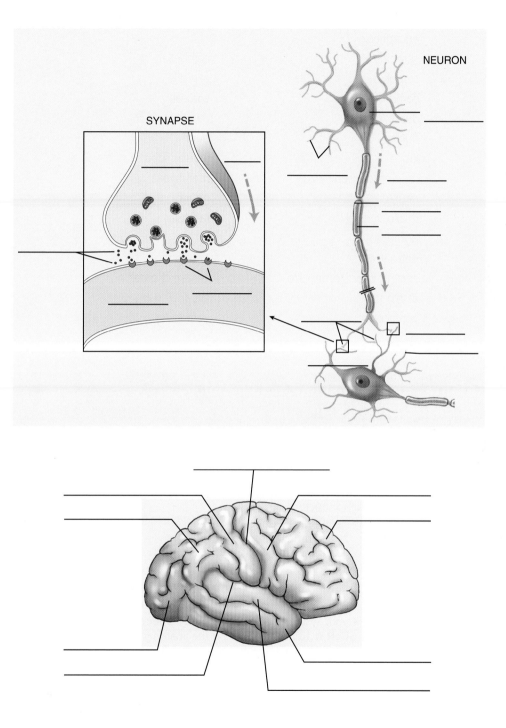

## Combining and Adjective Forms for the Anatomy and Physiology of the Nervous System

| Meaning | Combining Form | Adjective Form |
|---|---|---|
| body | somat/o | somatic |
| brain | encephal/o | |
| cerebellum | cerebell/o | cerebellar |
| cerebrum | cerebr/o | cerebral |
| cortex | cortic/o | cortical |
| dendrite | dendr/o | dendritic |
| dura mater | dur/o | dural |
| lobe | lob/o | lobular, lobar |
| meninges | mening/o, meningi/o | meningeal |
| nerve | neur/o | neural |
| nerve root | rhiz/o, radicul/o | radicular |
| same | home/o | |
| skin | dermat/o | dermatic |
| spinal cord | cord/o, chord/o, myel/o | cordal, chordal |
| star | astr/o | astral |
| ventricle | ventricul/o | ventricular |

## Suffixes for the Anatomy and Physiology of the Nervous System

| Suffix | Meaning |
|---|---|
| -cyte | cell |
| -glia | glue |
| -logy | study of |
| -on | structure |
| -stasis | stopping, controlling |
| -tome | instrument used to cut |

You can review the anatomy of the nervous system by clicking on **Body Spectrum Electronic Anatomy Coloring Book → Nervous.** Choose **Hear It, Spell It** to practice spelling the anatomy and physiology terms, you have learned in this chapter. To practice pronouncing anatomy and physiology terms, choose **Hear it, Say It.**

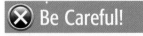

### ⊗ Be Careful!

*Don't confuse* **dysarthria** *(difficulty with speech) and* **dysarthrosis** *(any disorder of a joint).*

## PATHOLOGY

The signs and symptoms for this system encompass many systems because of the nature of the neural function: communicating, or failing to communicate, with other parts of the body.

## Terms Related to Signs and Symptoms

| Term | Word Origin | Definition |
|------|-------------|------------|
| **amnesia**<br>am NEE zsa | | Loss of memory caused by brain damage or severe emotional trauma. |
| **aphasia**<br>ah FAY zsa | *a-* without<br>*phas/o* speech<br>*-ia* condition | Lack or impairment of the ability to form or understand speech. Less severe forms include **dysphasia** (dis FAY zsa) and **dysarthria** (dis AR three ah); dysarthria refers to difficulty in the articulation (pronunciation) of speech. |
| **athetosis**<br>ath uh TOH sis | | Continuous, involuntary, slow, writhing movement of the extremities. |
| **aura**<br>OR uh | | Premonition; sensation of light or warmth that may precede an epileptic seizure or the onset of some types of headache. |
| **dysphagia**<br>dis FAY zsa | *dys-* difficult<br>*phag/o* eat<br>*-ia* condition | Condition of difficulty with swallowing. |
| **dyssomnia**<br>dih SAHM nee ah | *dys-* difficult<br>*somn/o* sleep<br>*-ia* condition | Disorders of the sleep-wake cycles. **Insomnia** is the inability to sleep or stay asleep. **Hypersomnia** is excessive depth or length of sleep, which may be accompanied by daytime sleepiness. |
| **fasciculation**<br>fah sick yoo LAY shun | | Involuntary contraction of small, local muscles. |
| **gait, abnormal** | | Disorder in the manner of walking. An example is **ataxia** (uh TACK see uh), a lack of muscular coordination, as in cerebral palsy. |
| **hypokinesia**<br>hye poh kih NEE sza | *hypo-* deficient<br>*kinesi/o* movement<br>*-ia* condition | Decrease in normal movement; may be due to paralysis. |
| **neuralgia**<br>noor AL jah | *neur/o* nerve<br>*-algia* pain | Nerve pain. If described as a "burning pain," it is called **causalgia.** |
| **paresthesia**<br>pair uhs THEE zsa | *para-* abnormal<br>*esthesi/o* feeling<br>*-ia* condition | Feeling of prickling, burning, or numbness. |
| **seizure**<br>SEE zhur | | Neuromuscular reaction to abnormal electrical activity within the brain (see Fig. 12-21). Causes include fever or epilepsy, a recurring seizure disorder; also called **convulsions.** |
| **spasm**<br>SPAZ um | | Involuntary muscle contraction of sudden onset. Examples are hiccoughs, tics, and stuttering. |
| **syncope**<br>SINK oh pee | | Fainting. A **vasovagal** (VAS soh VAY gul) **attack** is a form of syncope that results from abrupt emotional stress involving the vagus nerve's effect on blood vessels. |
| **tremors**<br>TREH murs | | Rhythmic, quivering, purposeless skeletal muscle movements seen in some elderly individuals and in patients with various neuro-degenerative disorders. |
| **vertigo**<br>VUR tih goh | | Dizziness; abnormal sensation of movement when there is none, either of oneself moving, or of objects moving around oneself. |

## Terms Related to Learning and Perceptual Differences

| Term | Word Origin | Definition |
|---|---|---|
| acalculia<br>ay kal KYOO lee ah | *a-* no, not, without<br>*calcul/o* stone<br>*-ia* condition | Inability to perform mathematical calculations. |
| ageusia<br>ah GOO zsa | *a-* no, not, without<br>*geus/o* taste<br>*-ia* condition | Absence of the ability to taste. **Parageusia** (pair ah GOO zsa) is an abnormal sense of taste or a bad taste in the mouth. |
| agnosia<br>ag NOH zsa | *a-* no, not, without<br>*gnos/o* knowledge<br>*-ia* condition | Inability to recognize objects visually, auditorily, or with other senses. |
| agraphia<br>a GRAFF ee ah | *a-* no, not, without<br>*graph/o* record<br>*-ia* condition | Inability to write. |
| anosmia<br>an NAHS mee ah | *an-* no, not, without<br>*osm/o* sense of smell<br>*-ia* condition | Lack of sense of smell. |
| apraxia<br>ah PRACK see ah | *a-* no, not, without<br>*prax/o* purposeful movement<br>*-ia* condition | Inability to perform purposeful movements or to use objects appropriately. |
| dyslexia<br>dis LECK see ah | *dys-* difficult<br>*lex/o* word<br>*-ia* condition | Inability or difficulty with reading and/or writing. |

### Exercise 5: Neurologic Signs, Symptoms, and Perceptual Differences

*Match the terms with their meanings.*

A. dizziness
B. involuntary contraction of small muscles
C. loss of memory
D. fainting
E. premonition
F. slow, writhing movement of extremities
G. sudden, involuntary muscle contraction
H. decrease in normal movement
I. prickling or burning feeling

____ 1. syncope      ____ 6. aura

____ 2. vertigo      ____ 7. fasciculation

____ 3. amnesia      ____ 8. hypokinesia

____ 4. spasm        ____ 9. paresthesia

____ 5. athetosis

*Build the terms.*

10. Condition of without sense of smell _____

11. Condition of without taste _____

12. Condition of without knowledge _____

13. Condition of difficult sleep _____

14. Condition of difficult eating _____

15. Condition of without speech _____

## Terms Related to Congenital Disorders

| Term | Word Origin | Definition |
|------|-------------|------------|
| **cerebral palsy (CP)**<br>SAIR uh brul<br>PAWL zee | *cerebr/o* cerebrum<br>*-al* pertaining to | Motor function disorder as a result of permanent, nonprogressive brain defect or lesion caused perinatally. Neural deficits may include paralysis, ataxia, athetosis, seizures, and/or impairment of sensory functions. |
| **Huntington chorea**<br>koh REE ah | | Inherited disorder that manifests itself in adulthood as a progressive loss of neural control, uncontrollable jerking movements, and dementia. |
| **hydrocephalus**<br>hye droh SEFF uh lus | *hydr/o* water<br>*-cephalus* head | Condition of abnormal accumulation of fluid in the ventricles of the brain; may or may not result in mental retardation. Although usually diagnosed in babies, may also occur in adults as a result of stroke, trauma, or infection. |
| **spina bifida**<br>SPY nah<br>BIFF uh dah | *spin/o* spine<br>*bi-* two<br>*-fida* split | Condition in which the spinal column has an abnormal opening that allows protrusion of the meninges and/or the spinal cord. This is termed a **meningocele** (meh NIN goh seel) (meninges only) or **meningomyelocele** (meh nin goh MYE eh loh seel) (meninges and spinal cord) (Fig. 12-9). |
| **Tay-Sachs disease**<br>tay sacks | | Inherited disease that occurs mainly in people of Eastern European Jewish origin; caused by an enzyme deficiency that results in CNS deterioration. |

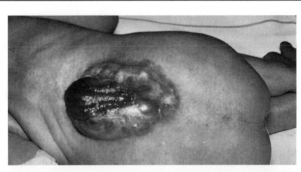

Fig. 12-9 Meningomyelocele.

## Terms Related to Traumatic Conditions

| Term | Word Origin | Definition |
|------|-------------|------------|
| **coma**<br>KOH mah | | Deep, prolonged unconsciousness from which the patient cannot be aroused; usually the result of a head injury, neurologic disease, acute hydrocephalus, intoxication, or metabolic abnormalities. |
| **concussion**<br>kun KUH shun | | Serious head injury characterized by one or more of the following: loss of consciousness, amnesia, seizures, or a change in mental status. |
| **contusion, cerebral**<br>kun TOO zhun | | Head injury of sufficient force to bruise the brain. Bruising of the brain often involves the brain surface and causes extravasation of blood without rupture of the pia-arachnoid; often associated with a concussion. |

*Continued*

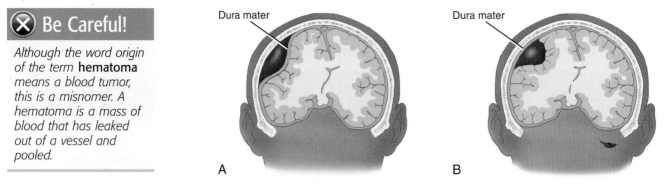

Fig. 12-10 **A,** Epidural hematoma. **B,** Subdural hematoma.

**Be Careful!**

*Although the word origin of the term* **hematoma** *means a blood tumor, this is a misnomer. A hematoma is a mass of blood that has leaked out of a vessel and pooled.*

## Terms Related to Traumatic Conditions—cont'd

| Term | Word Origin | Definition |
|---|---|---|
| hematoma<br>hee muh TOH mah | *hemat/o* blood<br>*-oma* tumor, mass | Localized collection of blood, usually clotted, in an organ, tissue, or space, due to a break in the wall of a blood vessel (Fig. 12-10). |
| herniated intervertebral disk (HIVD) | *inter-* between<br>*vertebr/o* vertebra<br>*-al* pertaining to | A displacement of an intervertebral disk so that it presses on a nerve, causing pain and/or numbness. |

## Exercise 6: Congenital and Traumatic Conditions

*Fill in the blanks with the correct congenital disorder or trauma term listed below.*

**Tay-Sachs, cerebral contusion, cerebral palsy, coma, Huntington chorea, concussion, herniated intervertebral disk**

1. An inherited disorder resulting in dementia and a progressive loss of neural control beginning in

   adulthood. _____

2. An inherited disease of people of Eastern European descent that results in deterioration of the brain

   and spinal cord as a result of an enzyme deficiency. _____

3. Permanent motor function disorder as a result of brain damage during the perinatal period. _____

   _____

4. Prolonged unconsciousness from which the patient cannot be aroused is termed _____.

5. Head injury accompanied by amnesia, loss of consciousness, seizures, and/or change in mental status

   is called a/an _____.

6. Bruising of the brain with hemorrhage and swelling is a/an _____.

7. Displacement of an intervertebral disk is _____.

*Build the terms.*

8. mass of blood _____

9. spine split in two _____

10. water in the head _____

## Terms Related to Degenerative Disorders

| Term | Word Origin | Definition |
|---|---|---|
| **Alzheimer disease (AD)**<br>AHLZ hye mur | | Progressive, neurodegenerative disease in which patients exhibit an impairment of cognitive functioning. The cause of the disease is unknown. Alzheimer is the most common cause of dementia (Fig. 12-11). |
| **amyotrophic lateral sclerosis (ALS)**<br>ay mye oh TROH fick LAT ur ul sklih ROH sis | *a-* no<br>*my/o* muscle<br>*troph/o* development<br>*-ic* pertaining to<br>*later/o* side<br>*-al* pertaining to<br>*sclerosis* condition of hardening | Degenerative, fatal disease of the motor neurons, in which patients exhibit progressive muscle weakness and atrophy; also called **Lou Gehrig disease.** |
| **Guillain-Barré syndrome**<br>GEE on bar AY | | Autoimmune disorder of acute polyneuritis producing profound **myasthenia** (muscle weakness) that may lead to paralysis. |
| **multiple sclerosis (MS)**<br>skleh ROH sis | *sclerosis* condition of hardening | Neurodegenerative disease characterized by destruction of the myelin sheaths on the CNS neurons (demyelination) and their abnormal replacement by the gradual accumulation of hardened plaques. The disease may be progressive or characterized by remissions and relapses. Cause is unknown (Fig. 12-12). |

*Continued*

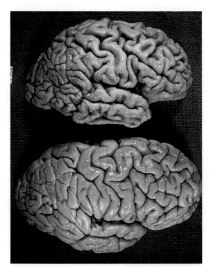

Fig. 12-11 Alzheimer disease. The affected brain *(top)* is smaller and shows narrow gyri and widened sulci compared with the normal, age-matched brain *(bottom)*.

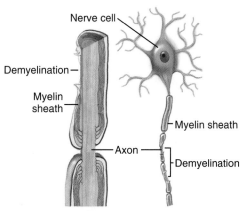

Nerve cell
Demyelination
Myelin sheath
Myelin sheath
Axon
Demyelination

Fig. 12-12 Nerve sheath demyelination seen in multiple sclerosis.

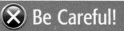

## ⊗ Be Careful!

**MS** *stands for musculoskeletal system, mitral stenosis, and multiple sclerosis.*

## Terms Related to Degenerative Disorders—cont'd

| Term | Word Origin | Definition |
|------|-------------|------------|
| **Parkinson disease (PD)**<br>PAR kin sun | | Progressive neurodegenerative disease characterized by tremors, fasciculations, slow shuffling gait, hypokinesia, dysphasia, and dysphagia. |
| **trigeminal neuralgia**<br>try JEM ih nuhl<br>noo RAL jun | *neur/o* nerve<br>*-algia* pain | Disorder of the 5th cranial nerve (trigemina) characterized by stabbing pain that radiates along the nerve. Also called **tic douloureux** or **prosopalgia** (Fig. 12-13). |

To view an animation of Alzheimer disease, click on **Animations.**

## Terms Related to Nondegenerative Disorders

| Term | Word Origin | Definition |
|------|-------------|------------|
| **Bell palsy**<br>PALL zee | | Paralysis of the facial nerve. Unknown in cause, the condition usually resolves on its own within 6 months (Fig. 12-14). |
| **epilepsy**<br>EP ih lep see | *epi-* above<br>*-lepsy* seizure | Group of disorders characterized by some or all of the following: recurrent seizures, sensory disturbances, abnormal behavior, and/or loss of consciousness. Types of seizures include **tonic clonic (grand mal)**, accompanied by temporary loss of consciousness and severe muscle spasms; **absence seizures (petit mal)**, accompanied by loss of consciousness exhibited by unresponsiveness for short periods without muscle involvement. **Status epilepticus** (STA tis eh pih LEP tih kuss) is a condition of intense, unrelenting, life-threatening seizures. **Pseudoseizures** are false seizures. Causes may be trauma, tumor, intoxication, chemical imbalance, or vascular disturbances. |
| **narcolepsy**<br>NAR koh lep see | *narc/o* sleep<br>*-lepsy* seizure | Disorder characterized by sudden attacks of sleep. |
| **Tourette syndrome**<br>tur ETT | | Abnormal condition characterized by facial grimaces, tics, involuntary arm and shoulder movements, and involuntary vocalizations, including **coprolalia** (kop pro LAYL yah) (the use of vulgar, obscene, or sacrilegious language). |

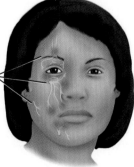

**Fig. 12-13** Trigeminal neuralgia: distribution of trigger zones.

Branches of the trigeminal nerve

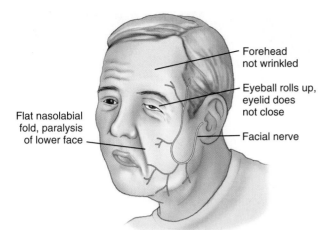

- Forehead not wrinkled
- Eyeball rolls up, eyelid does not close
- Facial nerve
- Flat nasolabial fold, paralysis of lower face

**Fig. 12-14** The facial characteristics of Bell palsy.

## Exercise 7: Degenerative and Nondegenerative Disorders

*Fill in the blank with the correct disorder listed below.*

**Alzheimer disease, Guillain-Barré syndrome, epilepsy, Bell palsy, amyotrophic lateral sclerosis, multiple sclerosis, Parkinson disease, Tourette syndrome, narcolepsy**

1. A paralysis of a facial nerve. _____

2. A disease characterized by tics, facial grimaces, and involuntary vocalizations. _____

3. A progressive disease characterized by a shuffling gait, tremors, and dysphasia. _____

4. A degenerative fatal disorder of motor neurons. _____

5. A progressive, degenerative disorder of impairment of cognitive functioning. _____

6. An autoimmune disorder causing severe muscle weakness, often leading to paralysis.

_____

7. Group of disorders characterized by seizures. _____

8. Neurogenic disease characterized by demyelination. _____

9. Disorder characterized by sudden attacks of sleep. _____

## Terms Related to Infectious Diseases and Inflammations

| Term | Word Origin | Definition |
|------|-------------|------------|
| encephalitis<br>en seff uh LYE tis | *encephal/o* brain<br>*-itis* inflammation | Inflammation of the brain, most frequently caused by a virus transmitted by the bite of an infected mosquito. |
| meningitis<br>men in JYE tis | *mening/o* meninges<br>*-itis* inflammation | Any infection or inflammation of the membranes covering the brain and spinal cord, most commonly due to viral infection, although more severe strains are bacterial or fungal in nature. |
| neuritis<br>noo RYE tis | *neur/o* nerve<br>*-itis* inflammation | Inflammation of the nerves. |

*Continued*

## Terms Related to Infectious Diseases and Inflammations—cont'd

| Term | Word Origin | Definition |
|------|-------------|------------|
| **poliomyelitis**<br>poh lee oh mye uh LYE tiss | *polio-* gray<br>*myel/o* spinal cord<br>*-itis* inflammation | Inflammation of the gray matter of the spinal cord caused by a poliovirus. Severe forms cause paralysis. |
| **polyneuritis**<br>pahl ee noo RYE tis | *poly-* many<br>*neur/o* nerve<br>*-itis* inflammation | Inflammation of several peripheral nerves. |
| **radiculitis**<br>rad ick kyoo LYE tis | *radicul/o* nerve root<br>*-itis* inflammation | Inflammation of the root of a spinal nerve. |
| **sciatica**<br>sye AT ick kah | | Inflammation of the sciatic nerve. Symptoms include pain and tenderness along the path of the nerve through the thigh and leg (Fig. 12-15). |
| **shingles**<br>SHIN guls | | Acute infection caused by the latent varicella zoster virus (chickenpox), characterized by the development of vesicular skin eruption underlying the route of cranial or spinal nerves; also called **herpes zoster** (HER pees ZAH ster) (Fig. 12-16). |

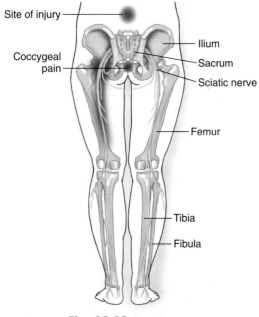

Fig. 12-15 Sciatica.

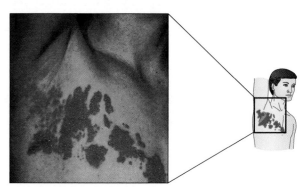

Fig. 12-16 Shingles on dermatome T4.

## Terms Related to Vascular Disorders

| Term | Word Origin | Meaning |
|------|-------------|---------|
| **cerebrovascular accident (CVA)**<br>seh ree broh VAS kyoo lur | *cerebr/o* cerebrum<br>*vascul/o* vessel<br>*-ar* pertaining to | Ischemia of cerebral tissue due to an occlusion (blockage) from a thrombus (*pl.* thrombi) or embolus (*pl.* emboli), or as a result of a cerebral hemorrhage. Results of a stroke depend on the duration and location of the ischemia. These sequelae may include paralysis, weakness, speech defects, sensory changes that last longer than 24 hours, or death. Also called **stroke, brain attack,** and **cerebral infarction** (infarction means tissue death). (Fig. 12-17). |
| **migraine**<br>MYE grain | | Headache of vascular origin. May be classified as *migraine with aura* or *migraine without aura.* |
| **transient ischemic attack (TIA)**<br>TRANS ee ent is KEE mick | *ischem/o* hold back<br>*-ic* condition pertaining to | TIA has the same mechanisms as a CVA, but the sequelae resolve and disappear within 24 hours; also known as a **ministroke.** |

To view an animation of a transient ischemic attack, click on **Animations.**

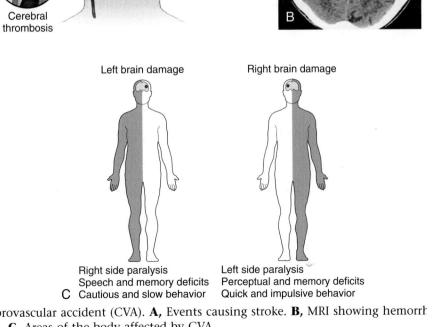

**Fig. 12-17** Cerebrovascular accident (CVA). **A,** Events causing stroke. **B,** MRI showing hemorrhagic stroke in right cerebrum. **C,** Areas of the body affected by CVA.

## Paralysis

**Paralysis** (puh RAL ih sis) is the loss of muscle function, sensation, or both. It may be described according to which side is affected and whether it is the dominant or nondominant side (Fig. 12-18).

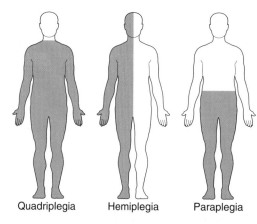

Quadriplegia     Hemiplegia     Paraplegia

**Fig. 12-18** Types of paralysis.

## Terms Related to Paralytic Conditions

| Term | Word Origin | Meaning |
|------|-------------|---------|
| diplegia<br>dye PLEE jee ah | *di-* two<br>*-plegia* paralysis | Paralysis of the same body part on both sides of the body. |
| hemiparesis<br>hem mee pah REE sis | *hemi-* half<br>*-paresis* slight paralysis | Muscular weakness or slight paralysis on the left or right side of the body. |
| hemiplegia<br>hem mee PLEE jee ah | *hemi-* half<br>*-plegia* paralysis | Paralysis on the left or right side of the body (*see* Fig. 12-18). |
| monoparesis<br>mah noh pah REE sis | *mono-* one<br>*-paresis* slight paralysis | Weakness or slight paralysis of one limb on the left or right side of the body. |
| monoplegia<br>mah noh PLEE jee ah | *mono-* one<br>*-plegia* paralysis | Paralysis of one limb on the left or right side of the body. |
| paraparesis<br>pair uh pah REE sis | *para-* abnormal<br>*-paresis* slight paralysis | Slight paralysis of the lower limbs and trunk. |
| paraplegia<br>pair uh PLEE jee ah | *para-* abnormal<br>*-plegia* paralysis | Paralysis of the lower limbs and trunk (*see* Fig. 12-18). |
| quadriparesis<br>kwah drih pah REE sis | *quadri-* four<br>*-paresis* slight paralysis | Weakness or slight paralysis of the arms, legs, and trunk. |
| quadriplegia<br>kwah drih PLEE jee ah | *quadri-* four<br>*-plegia* paralysis | Paralysis of arms, legs, and trunk (*see* Fig. 12-18). |

## Exercise 8: Infectious, Inflammatory, Vascular, and Paralytic Disorders

*Fill in the correct answers.*

1. An acute infection caused by the latent varicella zoster virus is _____ .

2. A headache of vascular origin is a(n) _____ .

3. An inflammation of a nerve in the thigh and leg is called _____.

4. Paralysis on the left or right half of the body is called _____.

5. A ministroke is a _____.

6. A slight paralysis from the waist down is called _____.

7. CVA stands for _____, the medical term for a stroke.

*Match the suffixes and prefixes with their correct meanings.*

____ 8. hemi-      ____ 12. para-

____ 9. -plegia      ____ 13. -paresis

____ 10. mono-      ____ 14. di-

____ 11. quadri-

A. one
B. slight paralysis
C. half
D. abnormal
E. paralysis
F. four
G. two

*Decode the terms.*

15. radiculitis _____

16. encephalitis _____

17. hemiparesis _____

18. quadriplegia _____

*Build the terms.*

19. inflammation of the meninges _____

20. inflammation of a nerve _____

21. inflammation of many nerves _____

## Terms Related to Benign Neoplasms

| Term | Word Origin | Meaning |
| --- | --- | --- |
| **meningioma**<br>meh nin jee OH mah | *meningi/o* meninges<br>*-oma* tumor, mass | Slow growing, usually benign tumor of the meninges. Although benign, may cause problems because of their size and location (Fig. 12-19). |
| **neurofibroma**<br>noor oh fye BROH mah | *neur/o* nerve<br>*fibr/o* fiber<br>*-oma* tumor, mass | Benign fibrous tumors composed of nervous tissue. |
| **neuroma**<br>noor OH mah | *neur/o* nerve<br>*-oma* tumor, mass | Benign tumor of the nerves. |

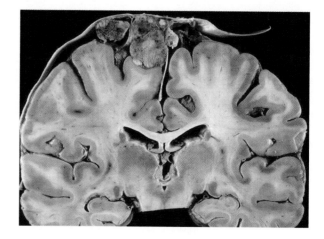

Fig. 12-19 Meningioma.

## Terms Related to Malignant Neoplasms

| Term | Word Origin | Definition |
|------|-------------|------------|
| **astrocytoma**<br>as troh sye TOH mah | *astr/o* star<br>*cyt/o* cell<br>*-oma* tumor, mass | Tumor arising from star-shaped glial cells that is malignant in higher grades. A grade IV astrocytoma is referred to as a **glioblastoma multiforme,** the most common primary brain cancer. |
| **medulloblastoma**<br>med yoo loh blass TOH mah | *medull/o* medulla<br>*blast/o* embryonic<br>*-oma* tumor, mass | Tumor arising from embryonic tissue in the cerebellum. Most commonly seen in children. |
| **neuroblastoma**<br>noor oh blass TOH mah | *neur/o* nerve<br>*blast/o* embryonic<br>*-oma* tumor, mass | Highly malignant tumor arising from either the autonomic nervous system or the adrenal medulla. Usually affects children younger than 10 years of age. |

## Exercise 9: Neoplasms

*Match the neoplasms with their definitions.*

_____ 1. Benign tumor of the meninges

_____ 2. Benign tumor of the nerves

_____ 3. Malignant tumor of star-shaped glial cells

_____ 4. Malignant tumor of embryonic nervous tissue that arises from the autonomic nervous system or the adrenal medulla in children

_____ 5. Benign fibrous tumor composed of nerve tissue

_____ 6. Malignant tumor arising from embryonic cerebellar tissue

A. neurofibroma
B. astrocytoma
C. medulloblastoma
D. neuroma
E. meningioma
F. neuroblastoma

## Case Study   *Celeste Thibeaux*

Celeste is a freshman in college. One evening, her roommate calls 911 because Celeste is acting strangely. Her arms are moving wildly in a jerking motion. She starts and stops this movement four times in the ambulance. The EMTs start IV Valium on Celeste, and she seems to relax. Celeste's mother meets the ambulance at the hospital and asks the ED physician if her daughter is having seizures. She is worried because Celeste is not adjusting well to college and seems depressed. She has been unable to sleep and to concentrate on her studies and has not been eating well. She has been on two different antidepressants in the past 6 months but has recently been taken off them. The physician tells Celeste's mother that he doesn't think Celeste is having seizures.

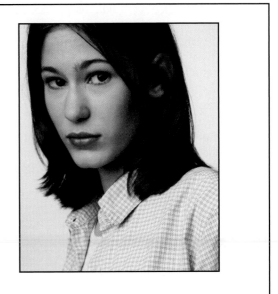

---

THIBEAUX, CELESTE S - 601106 Opened by BIRDSONG, LINDA MD    � ▢ ✕

Task   Edit   View   Time Scale   Options   Help

As Of 10:54

| THIBEAUX, CELESTE S | Age: 19 years | Sex: Female | Loc: WHC-SMMC |
|---|---|---|---|
| | DOB: 02/22/1993 | MRN: 601106 | FIN: 3506004 |

Reference Text Browser    Form Browser    Medication Profile

Orders | Last 48 Hours | **ED** | Lab | Radiology | Assessments | Surgery | Clinical Notes | Pt. Info | Pt. Schedule | Task List | I & O | MAR

Flowsheet: ED    Level: ED Report    ● Table ○ Group ○ List

**Navigator** ✕

✓ ED Report

Physician's Report: 19-year-old female comes in today brought by ambulance with tonic clonic seizure times four. She has been seizing every 1-2 minutes for 30 seconds. Had upper extremity jerking. Gave her some Valium to start an IV and switched to IV Ativan. Seizures do not appear normal. Jerks to the upper extremities in an oddlike fashion with forward flexion and extension of her arms. Talked to her mom out in the hall and questioned whether the seizures were real. Does have some psychological issues. Psych just took her off antidepressants because of drug interactions. Vital signs are stable. Cranial nerves II through XII intact. TMs clear. Pharynx is clear.

IMPRESSION:     Pseudoseizures
Diagnosis:        Pseudoseizures

PROD | MAHAFC | 28 Feb 2012 | 10:54

## ⟳ Exercise 10: Emergency Room Note

*Using the emergency room note on p. 465, fill in the blanks.*

1. This physician is using the term "tonic-clonic seizure." What is another term for that? _____

2. What is a pseudoseizure? _____

3. What action is described by flexion and extension of her arms? _____

4. How do you know that she has no problems with her throat? _____

5. Which cranial nerves are functioning normally? _____

---

## *Age Matters*

### Pediatrics

Most children's neurologic disorders are congenital ones. Cerebral palsy is usually the result of birth trauma, whereas Tay-Sachs is an inherited condition. Hydrocephalus may be detected on an ultrasound before delivery, and intrauterine prenatal procedures can be done to lessen the effects of the disorder. It should be noted that this disorder may, although infrequently, occur in adults after trauma or disease. Spina bifida is yet another congenital disorder that may be detected before birth through prenatal testing. Two pathologic conditions that are not congenital but that are a concern to parents are viral and bacterial meningitis. Although viral meningitis is less severe and usually resolves without treatment, bacterial meningitis can be fatal. The vaccine that is now available and recommended is the Hib, which stands for the bacteria it protects against, *Haemophilus influenzae*, type b.

### Geriatrics

The two major neurologic disorders of concern as we age are cerebrovascular disease and Alzheimer disease. The first disorder manifests itself in two forms: ministrokes (transient ischemic attacks) and strokes (cerebrovascular accidents). The other disorder is Alzheimer disease, a progressive cognitive mental deterioration. It is estimated that by the age of 65, one in 10 individuals will be diagnosed with the disease. By age 85, more than half of the population will carry the diagnosis.

---

⊖ Click on **Hear It, Spell It** to practice spelling the pathology terms you have learned in this chapter. To see how well you pronounce the pathology terms in this chapter, click on **Hear It, Say It.** To review the pathology terms in this chapter, play **Medical Millionaire.**

## DIAGNOSTIC PROCEDURES

### Terms Related to Imaging

| Term | Word Origin | Definition |
|---|---|---|
| brain scan | | Nuclear medicine procedure involving intravenous injection of radioisotopes to localize and identify intracranial masses, lesions, tumors, or infarcts. Photography is done by a scintillator or scanner. |
| cerebral angiography | *cerebr/o* cerebrum <br> *-al* pertaining to <br> *angi/o* vessel <br> *-graphy* process of recording | X-ray of the cerebral arteries, including the internal carotids, taken after the injection of a contrast medium (Fig. 12-20); also called **cerebral arteriography.** |
| computed tomography (CT) scan | *tom/o* slice <br> *-graphy* process of recording | Transverse sections of the CNS are imaged, sometimes after the injection of a contrast medium (unless there is suspected bleeding). Used to diagnose strokes, edema, tumors, and hemorrhage resulting from trauma (Fig. 12-21). |
| echoencephalography <br> eh koh en seh fah LAH gruh fee | *echo-* sound <br> *encephal/o* brain <br> *-graphy* process of recording | Sonography exam of the brain, usually done only on newborns because sound waves do not readily penetrate mature bone. |
| magnetic resonance imaging (MRI) | | Medical imaging that uses radiofrequency pulses in a powerful magnetic field. **Magnetic resonance angiography (MRA)** is imaging of the carotid arteries using injected contrast agents. |
| myelography <br> mye eh LAH gruh fee | *myel/o* spinal cord <br> *-graphy* process of recording | X-ray of the spinal canal after the introduction of a radiopaque substance. |

*Continued*

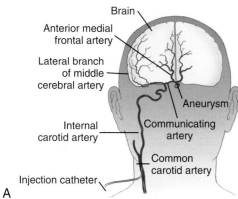

Brain
Anterior medial frontal artery
Lateral branch of middle cerebral artery
Aneurysm
Internal carotid artery
Communicating artery
Common carotid artery
Injection catheter

A

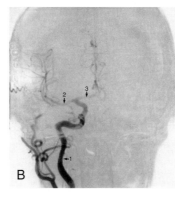

B

Fig. 12-20 Cerebral angiography. **A,** Insertion of dye through a catheter in the common carotid artery outlines the vessels of the brain. **B,** Angiogram showing vessels. *1,* Internal carotid artery; *2,* middle cerebral artery; *3,* middle meningeal artery.

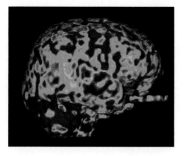

Fig. 12-21 Whole-brain perfusion study using 320 row CT scanner. This 3D scan shows evidence of acute stroke.

## Terms Related to Imaging—cont'd

| Term | Word Origin | Definition |
|------|-------------|------------|
| positron emission tomography (PET) | | Use of radionuclides to visualize brain function. Measurements can be taken of blood flow, volume, and oxygen and glucose uptake, enabling radiologists to determine the functional characteristics of specific parts of the brain (Fig. 12-22). PET scans are used to assist in the diagnosis of Alzheimer disease and stroke. |
| single-photon emission computed tomography (SPECT) | | An injection of a radioactive sugar substance that is metabolized by the brain, which is then scanned for abnormalities. |

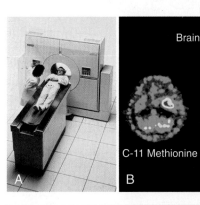
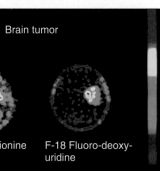

Brain tumor

C-11 Methionine    F-18 Fluoro-deoxy-uridine

A    B

Fig. 12-22 **A,** Clinical setting for PET. **B,** Colorized PET scan showing a brain tumor.

## Terms Related to Electrodiagnostic Procedures

| Term | Word Origin | Definition |
|------|-------------|------------|
| electroencephalography (EEG)<br>ee leck troh en seff fah LAH gruh fee | *electr/o* electricity<br>*encephal/o* brain<br>*-graphy* process of recording | Record of the electrical activity of the brain. May be used in the diagnosis of epilepsy, infection, and coma (Fig. 12-23). |
| evoked potential (EP)<br>ee VOHKT | | Electrical response from the brainstem or cerebral cortex that is produced in response to specific stimuli. This results in a distinctive pattern on an EEG. |
| multiple sleep latency test (MSLT) | | Test that consists of a series of short, daytime naps in the sleep lab to measure daytime sleepiness and how fast the patient falls asleep; used to diagnose or rule out narcolepsy. |
| nerve conduction test | | Test of the functioning of peripheral nerves. Conduction time (impulse travel) through a nerve is measured after a stimulus is applied; used to diagnose polyneuropathies. |
| polysomnography (PSG)<br>pah lee som NAH gruh fee | *poly-* many<br>*somn/o* sleep<br>*-graphy* process of recording | Measurement and record of a number of functions while the patient is asleep (e.g., cardiac, muscular, brain, ocular, and respiratory functions). Most often used to diagnose sleep apnea. |

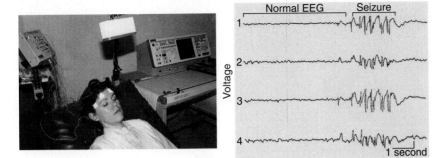

Fig. 12-23 EEG. **A,** Photograph of person with electrodes attached. **B,** EEG tracing showing activity in four different places in the brain. Compare the normal activity with the explosive activity that occurs during a seizure.

## Terms Related to Other Diagnostic Tests

| Term | Word Origin | Definition |
|------|-------------|------------|
| activities of daily living (ADL) | | An ADL assessment may be used to evaluate a patient's ability to live independently after an illness or event (such as a CVA). |
| Babinski reflex <br> bah BIN skee | | In normal conditions, the dorsiflexion of the great toe when the plantar surface of the sole is stimulated. **Babinski sign** is the loss or diminution of the Achilles tendon reflex seen in sciatica. |
| cerebrospinal fluid (CSF) analysis | *cerebr/o* cerebrum <br> *spin/o* spine <br> *-al* pertaining to | Examination of fluid from the CNS to detect pathogens and abnormalities. Useful in diagnosing hemorrhages, tumors, and various diseases. |
| deep tendon reflexes (DTR) | | Assessment of an automatic motor response by striking a tendon. Useful in the diagnosis of stroke. |
| gait assessment rating scale (GARS) | | Inventory of 16 aspects of gait (how one walks) to determine abnormalities. May be used as one method to evaluate cerebellar function. |
| lumbar puncture (LP) | *lumb/o* lower back <br> *-ar* pertaining to | Procedure to aspirate CSF from the lumbar subarachnoid space. A needle is inserted between two lumbar vertebrae to withdraw the fluid for diagnostic purposes. Also called a **spinal tap** (Fig. 12-24). |
| neuroendoscopy <br> noor oh en DOSS kuh pee | *neur/o* nerve <br> *endo-* within <br> *-scopy* process of viewing | Use of a fiberoptic camera to visualize neural structures. Used for placing a shunt in hydrocephalic patients. |

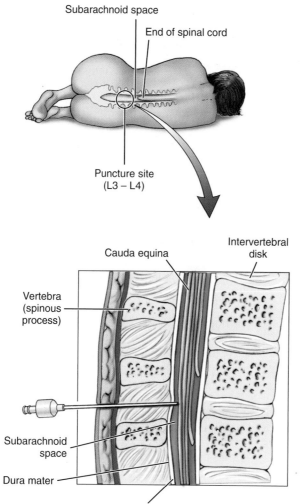

Subarachnoid space

End of spinal cord

Puncture site
(L3 – L4)

**Fig. 12-24** Lumbar puncture.

Cauda equina

Intervertebral
disk

Vertebra
(spinous
process)

Subarachnoid
space

Dura mater

Arachnoid

## Exercise 11: Diagnostic Procedures

*Fill in the blank.*

1. Walking abnormalities are measured by a _____ .

2. Examination of fluid from the CNS is a/an _____ .

3. Aspiration of CSF for diagnostic purposes is a _____ .

4. A finding that indicates loss of Achilles tendon reflex is _____ .

5. _____ is used to diagnose narcolepsy.

6. An x-ray study of cerebral arteries is called _____.

7. _____ is an injection of a radioactive sugar substance to scan for abnormalities.

8. _____ is the use of radionuclides to visualize brain function.

*Decode the terms.*

9. electroencephalography _____

10. echoencephalography _____

11. neuroendoscopy _____

*Build the terms.*

12. process of recording the spinal cord _____

13. process of recording the brain using sound _____

14. process of recording many (functions of) sleep _____

## Case Study   Nellie Shumaker

Nellie is a 72-year-old retired English professor. She volunteers at the local library two mornings a week helping with reading clubs. Two years ago, she had a stroke in that very same library. Her right arm became suddenly weak, and she dropped an armful of books. Her concerned coworkers called for an ambulance, and Nellie was taken to the hospital. After several tests were performed, she was told she had had a stroke. She enrolled in a rehab program and after a month regained most of the strength in the right arm, although some fine movements are still difficult.

Two years go by without additional problems. Nellie makes a lunch date with her daughter and after ordering asks her daughter what she is going to have. She notices her daughter looking at her funny. She tries to ask why but finds that she can't say what she wants to. Frustrated and

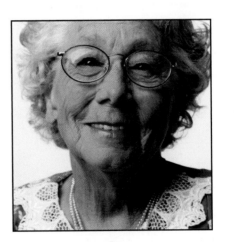

angry, she keeps trying, but no words come out. Her daughter becomes alarmed and takes her straight to the hospital for evaluation. They find that Nellie has had another stroke.

# Case Study   Nellie Shumaker

SHUMAKER, ELEANOR R - 673016 Opened by RAIS, ROBERT MD

Task   Edit   View   Time Scale   Options   Help

As Of 12:58

| SHUMAKER, ELEANOR R | Age: 72 years<br>DOB: 08/29/1940 | Sex: Female<br>MRN: 673016 | Loc: WHC-SMMC<br>FIN: 3506004 |

Reference Text Browser | Form Browser | Medication Profile

Orders | Last 48 Hours | **ED** | Lab | Radiology | Assessments | Surgery | Clinical Notes | Pt. Info | Pt. Schedule | Task List | I & O | MAR

Flowsheet: ED          Level: ED Record          ● Table  ○ Group  ○ List

**Navigator**

✓ ED Record

**REASON FOR VISIT:**  Difficulty with speech

This 72-year-old female with past history of CVA comes in for symptoms that started on Friday. Apparently, she had an episode, which lasted approximately 15 minutes, of not being able to express her words. She says her thoughts were clear, but she was unable to say the words she wanted to say. In conjunction with that, she had some pain along the left temporal and parietal region. No visual symptoms. No obvious facial drooping according to witnesses. No weakness or paresthesias in her arms or legs. Since then has felt excessively tired and has a very mild dull headache across the frontal area.

**CURRENT MEDS:**  Coumadin 4.5 mg po every day

**PAST MEDICAL HISTORY:**  Significant for CVA involving her right hand. She was involved in PT for approximately 1 month. Back to about 90% to 95% function. Work-up at that time included an echocardiogram and carotid Dopplers, which she says are normal. No symptoms since that time.

**REVIEW OF SYSTEMS:**  Otherwise unremarkable. No upper respiratory problems. Did have an eye infection and was treated with antibiotics a couple of weeks ago. No chest pain, palpitations, shortness of breath. No abdominal complaints. No dysuria or joint pain.

**PHYSICAL EXAM:**  On exam, patient is alert and oriented. Memory is intact to conversation. HEENT exam reveals pupils equal, round, and reactive to light. Extraocular eye movements are intact. No obvious facial asymmetry is noted. Oropharynx is pink and moist. Uvula and tongue midline. Neck supple, no carotid bruits appreciated. Carotid upstrokes are of good quality and equal bilaterally. Lungs are clear to auscultation bilaterally. Heart sounds are regular, no murmurs, rubs, or gallops.

Neurologic exam: cranial nerves II through XII grossly intact. Motor exam reveals good strength in both upper and lower extremities. No gross sensory deficits. Deep tendon reflexes are of good quality and equal bilaterally. Patient able to do tandem finger to nose and to move her heel up and down without difficulty. Rapid alternating movements were not tested. Able to ambulate without difficulty. No ataxia or limp.

**ASSESSMENT:**  Expressive aphasia most likely caused by transient ischemic attack or small stroke. Symptoms have resolved at this time. Remains fatigued but no neurologic symptoms.

**PLAN:**  She does have a residual headache; however, if neurologic symptoms reemerge or worsen, she should have a CT scan done emergently.

Continue Coumadin 4.5 mg po every day.

PROD | MAHAFC | 27 Dec 2012 | 12:58

# Exercise 12: Emergency Room Record

*Using the emergency room record on previous page, answer the following questions.*

1. This patient has a history of what disorder? _____

2. What term tells you that she has had no prickling, burning, or numbness in her legs? _____

3. In the Review of Systems, what term tells you that she had no lack of muscular coordination?

_____

4. How did her aphasia manifest itself? _____

5. Why would a CT be done emergently if her neurologic symptoms worsen or reemerge?

_____

## THERAPEUTIC INTERVENTIONS

### Terms Related to Brain and Skull Interventions

| Term | Word Origin | Definitions |
|------|-------------|-------------|
| craniectomy<br>kray nee ECK tuh mee | *crani/o* skull, cranium<br>*-ectomy* removal | Removal of part of the skull. |
| craniotomy<br>kray nee AH tuh mee | *crani/o* skull, cranium<br>*-tomy* incision | Incision into the skull as a surgical approach or to relieve intracranial pressure; also called **trephination** (treff fin NAY shun). |
| stereotaxic radiosurgery<br>stair ee oh TACK sick | *stere/o* 3-D<br>*tax/o* order, arrangement<br>*-ic* pertaining to | Surgery using radiowaves to localize structures within 3-D space. |
| ventriculoperitoneal shunt<br>ven trick yoo loh pair ih tuh nee uhl | *ventricul/o* ventricle<br>*peritone/o* peritoneum<br>*-al* pertaining to | A tube used to drain fluid from brain ventricles into the abdominal cavity (Fig. 12-25). |
| ventriculostomy, endoscopic<br>ven trick yoo LAH stuh mee | *endo-* within<br>*-scopic* pertaining to viewing<br>*ventricul/o* ventricle<br>*-stomy* new opening | A new opening between the third ventricle and the subarachnoid space used to relieve pressure and to treat one type of hydrocephalus. |

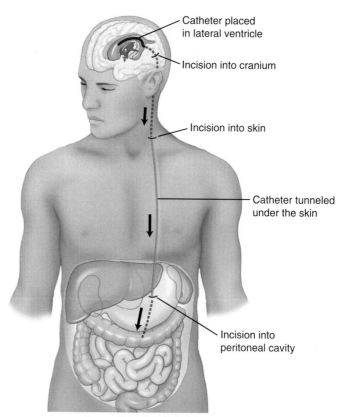

**Fig. 12-25** Ventriculoperitoneal shunt.

## Terms Related to Peripheral Nervous System Interventions

| Term | Word Origin | Definition |
|------|-------------|------------|
| **vagotomy**<br>vay GAH tuh mee | *vag/o* vagus nerve<br>*-tomy* incision | Cutting of a branch of the vagus nerve to reduce the secretion of gastric acid. |

## Terms Related to General Interventions

| Term | Word Origin | Definition |
|------|-------------|------------|
| **microsurgery** | *micro-* small, tiny | Surgery in which magnification is used to repair delicate tissues. |
| **nerve block** | | Use of anesthesia to prevent sensory nerve impulses from reaching the CNS. |
| **neurectomy**<br>noo RECK tuh mee | *neur/o* nerve<br>*-ectomy* removal | Excision of part or all of a nerve. |
| **neurolysis**<br>noo RAH lih sis | *neur/o* nerve<br>*-lysis* destruction | Destruction of a nerve. |
| **neuroplasty**<br>NOO roh plas tee | *neur/o* nerve<br>*-plasty* surgical repair | Surgical repair of a nerve. |
| **neurorrhaphy**<br>noo ROAR ah fee | *neur/o* nerve<br>*-rrhaphy* suture | Suture of a severed nerve. |
| **neurotomy**<br>noo RAH tuh mee | *neur/o* nerve<br>*-tomy* incision | Incision of a nerve. |

## Terms Related to Pain Management

| Term | Word Origin | Definition |
|------|-------------|------------|
| cordotomy<br>kore DAH tuh mee | *cord/o* spinal cord<br>*-tomy* incision | Incision of the spinal cord to relieve pain. Also spelled **chordotomy.** |
| rhizotomy<br>rye ZAH tuh mee | *rhiz/o* spinal nerve root<br>*-tomy* incision | Resection of the dorsal root of a spinal nerve to relieve pain. |
| sympathectomy<br>sim puh THECK tuh mee | *sympath/o* to feel with<br>*-ectomy* removal | Surgical interruption of part of the sympathetic pathways for the relief of chronic pain or to promote vasodilation. |
| transcutaneous electrical nerve stimulation (TENS) | *trans-* through<br>*cutane/o* skin<br>*-ous* pertaining to | Method of pain control effected by the application of electrical impulses to the skin (Fig. 12-26). |

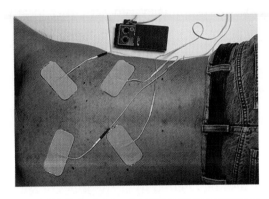

Fig. 12-26 TENS treatment.

## Exercise 13: Therapeutic Interventions

*Match the terms with their meanings.*

____ 1. neuroplasty

____ 2. TENS

____ 3. sympathectomy

____ 4. rhizotomy

____ 5. neurotomy

____ 6. microsurgery

____ 7. nerve block

____ 8. endoscopic ventriculostomy

____ 9. stereotaxic radiosurgery

____ 10. craniotomy

____ 11. neurectomy

A. surgical repair of a nerve
B. pain control using electronic impulses
C. incision of a nerve
D. incision of the skull
E. excision of a dorsal nerve root
F. anesthesia to prevent sensory impulses from reaching the CNS
G. new opening in brain to relieve the pressure of CSF fluid in hydrocephalus
H. surgery using radiowaves within 3-D space
I. excision of a sympathetic pathway
J. surgery in which magnification is used to repair delicate tissues
K. removal of a nerve

*Decode the terms.*

12. cordotomy _____

13. neurolysis _____

14. ventriculoperitoneal shunt _____

*Build the terms.*

15. suture of a severed nerve _____

16. incision of the vagus nerve _____

17. removal of part or all of the skull _____

## PHARMACOLOGY

**analgesics:** reduce pain. Narcotic analgesics have a CNS effect. NSAIDs (non-steroidal antiinflammatory drugs), opioids, or COX-2 inhibitors. Examples include morphine (MS Contin), hydrocodone (Vicodin or Lortab, in combination with acetaminophen), sumatriptan (Imitrex), acetaminophen (Tylenol), and naproxen (Anaprox).

**anesthetics:** cause a loss of feeling or sensation. They can act either locally (local anesthetic) or systemically (general anesthetic), and a general anesthetic can induce unconsciousness. Examples include propofol (Diprivan) and lidocaine (Xylocaine, Lidoderm).

**anticonvulsants:** reduce the frequency and severity of epileptic or other convulsive seizures. Examples include clonazepam (Klonopin), carbamazepine (Tegretol), and phenytoin (Dilantin).

**antiparkinsonian drugs:** effective against Parkinson disease. Examples include levodopa and carbidopa (Sinemet) and tolcapone (Tasmar).

**antipyretics:** reduce fever. Examples include aspirin (Bayer), acetaminophen (Tylenol), and ibuprofen (Advil, Motrin).

**hypnotics:** promote sleep. They may also be referred to as soporifics or somnifacients. Many hypnotics have a sedative effect also. Examples include temazepam (Restoril), zolpidem (Ambien), and flurazepam (Dalmane).

**neuromuscular blockers:** drugs that block the action of acetylcholine at the motor nerve end plate to cause paralysis. May be used in surgery to minimize patient movement. Examples include pancuronium (Pavulon), vecuronium (Norcuron), and succinylcholine (Anectine).

**sedatives:** inhibit neuronal activity to calm and relax. Many sedatives also have hypnotic effects. Examples include alprazolam (Xanax), lorazepam (Ativan), and phenylbarbitol (Luminal).

**stimulants:** increase synaptic activity of targeted neurons in the CNS to treat narcolepsy, attention-deficit disorder with hyperactivity, and fatigue, and to suppress the appetite. Examples include dextroamphetamine (Dexedrine), methylphenidate (Ritalin), caffeine, and phentermine (Adipex-P).

## Exercise 14: Pharmacology

*Match the drug type with its effect.*

____ 1. treats PD

____ 2. relieves pain

____ 3. calms and relaxes

____ 4. induces sleep

____ 5. reduces fever

____ 6. reduces severity of seizures

____ 7. causes paralysis

____ 8. causes loss of sensation

A. anesthetic
B. antipyretic
C. soporific
D. anticonvulsant
E. sedative
F. neuromuscular blocker
G. analgesic
H. antiparkinsonian drug

Click on **Hear It, Spell It** to practice spelling the diagnostic and therapeutic terms you have learned in this chapter. To practice pronouncing these terms, click on **Hear It, Say it.**

## Abbreviations

| Abbreviation | Definition | Abbreviation | Definition |
|---|---|---|---|
| AD | Alzheimer disease | LP | lumbar puncture |
| ADL | activities of daily living | MRI | magnetic resonance imaging |
| ALS | amyotrophic lateral sclerosis | MS | multiple sclerosis |
| ANS | autonomic nervous system | MSLT | multiple sleep latency test |
| BBB | blood-brain barrier | PD | Parkinson disease |
| C1-C8 | cervical nerves | PET scan | positron emission tomography scan |
| CNS | central nervous system | PNS | peripheral nervous system |
| CP | cerebral palsy | PSG | polysomnography |
| CSF | cerebrospinal fluid | S1-S5 | sacral nerves |
| CT scan | computerized tomography scan | SNS | somatic nervous system |
| CVA | cerebrovascular accident | SPECT | single-photon emission computed tomography |
| DTR | deep tendon reflex | | |
| EEG | electroencephalogram | T1-T12 | thoracic nerves |
| EP | evoked potential | TENS | transcutaneous electrical nerve stimulation |
| GARS | gait assessment rating scale | | |
| HIVD | herniated intervertebral disk | TIA | transient ischemia |
| L1-L5 | lumbar nerves | | |

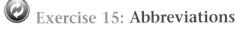

## Exercise 15: Abbreviations

*Spell out the following abbreviations.*

1. Barry had an LP to analyze his CSF for meningitis.

_____

2. Maria became a quadriplegic when she sustained a C2 fracture while diving into the shallow end of a swimming pool.

_____

3. Ms. Damjanov had an MRI to aid in the diagnosis of her MS.

_____

4. The patient underwent PSG to detect abnormalities related to hypersomnia.

_____

5. Walter needed help with his ADL after a CVA that left him with right hemiparesis.

_____

# Chapter Review

Match the word parts to their definitions.

## WORD PARTS DEFINITIONS

| Prefix/Suffix | Definition |
|---|---|
| -esthesia | 1. _____ four |
| hemi- | 2. _____ slight paralysis |
| -lepsy | 3. _____ half |
| mono- | 4. _____ many |
| -oma | 5. _____ one |
| para- | 6. _____ seizure |
| -paresis | 7. _____ tumor, mass |
| -plegia | 8. _____ abnormal |
| poly- | 9. _____ feeling |
| quadri- | 10. _____ paralysis |

| Combining Form | Definition |
|---|---|
| blast/o | 11. _____ cortex |
| cerebell/o | 12. _____ eat |
| cerebr/o | 13. _____ taste |
| cord/o | 14. _____ nerve root |
| cortic/o | 15. _____ cerebellum |
| dendr/o | 16. _____ feeling |
| dur/o | 17. _____ embryonic |
| encephal/o | 18. _____ spinal cord |
| esthesi/o | 19. _____ dura mater |
| geus/o | 20. _____ speech |
| gnos/o | 21. _____ ventricle |
| mening/o | 22. _____ brain |
| myel/o | 23. _____ spinal cord |
| narc/o | 24. _____ dendrite |
| neur/o | 25. _____ sleep |
| osm/o | 26. _____ nerve |
| phag/o | 27. _____ cerebrum |
| phas/o | 28. _____ knowledge |
| radicul/o | 29. _____ nerve root |
| rhiz/o | 30. _____ sleep |
| somn/o | 31. _____ sense of smell |
| ventricul/o | 32. _____ meninges |

# WORDSHOP

| Prefixes | Combining Forms | Suffixes |
|---|---|---|
| a- | ambul/o | -algia |
| an- | encephal/o | -graphy |
| di- | esthesi/o | -ia |
| dys- | geus/o | -ism |
| echo- | gnos/o | -itis |
| hemi- | mening/o | -lysis |
| hyper- | myel/o | -paresis |
| in- | neur/o | -plegia |
| mono- | osm/o | -somnia |
| par- | radicul/o | -stomy |
| para- | rhiz/o | -tomy |
| poly- | somn/o | |
| quadri- | vag/o | |
| | ventricul/o | |

Build the following terms by combining the above word parts. Some word parts may used more than once. Some may not be used at all. The number in parentheses is the number of word parts needed to build the terms.

| Definition | Term |
|---|---|
| 1. inflammation of many nerves (3) | _____ |
| 2. inflammation of the brain (2) | _____ |
| 3. paralysis of four (limbs) (2) | _____ |
| 4. process of recording the brain using sound (3) | _____ |
| 5. incision of a nerve (2) | _____ |
| 6. condition of no recognition (3) | _____ |
| 7. condition of without sense of smell (3) | _____ |
| 8. nerve pain (2) | _____ |
| 9. condition of abnormal sensation (3) | _____ |
| 10. process of (many) sleep recording (3) | _____ |
| 11. resection of the dorsal root of a spinal nerve (2) | _____ |
| 12. destruction of a nerve to relieve pain (2) | _____ |
| 13. condition of no ability to taste (3) | _____ |
| 14. condition of difficult sleep (3) | _____ |
| 15. slight paralysis of four (limbs) (2) | _____ |

*Sort the terms into the correct categories.*

## TERM SORTING

| Anatomy and Physiology | Pathology | Diagnostic Procedures | Therapeutic Interventions |
|---|---|---|---|
| | | | |
| | | | |
| | | | |
| | | | |
| | | | |
| | | | |
| | | | |
| | | | |
| | | | |
| | | | |

| | | | |
|---|---|---|---|
| ADL | craniectomy | meninges | rhizotomy |
| agraphia | CSF | MRI | sciatica |
| ALS | echoencephalography | nerve block | SPECT |
| amnesia | evoked potential | neuroendoscopy | spina bifida |
| axon | fasciculation | neurolysis | synapse |
| Babinski reflex | GARS | neuron | syncope |
| cauda equina | HIVD | neuroplasty | TENS |
| cerebellum | hydrocephalus | neurorrhaphy | TIA |
| CNS | hypnotic | neurotransmitter | vagotomy |
| cordotomy | LP | polysomnography | ventricle |

*Replace the highlighted words with the correct terms.*

## TRANSLATIONS

1. Mr. Sharif had a right-sided **ischemia of cerebral tissue due to an occlusion or a cerebral hemorrhage** that affected the **pertaining to the opposite side.**

2. After Roberto's CVA, he suffered **slight paralysis on the left or right side of the body** and **condition of lack of the ability to form or understand speech.**

3. As a result of a blow to the head, the patient sustained an epidural **localized collection of blood** and **resultant loss of memory caused by brain damage.**

4. Ms. C reported **dizziness** and **fainting** before her arrival at the emergency department.

5. The baby's **condition in which there is an abnormal opening in the spinal column** resulted in a **saclike protrusion of the meninges.**

6. The neonate's **condition of abnormal accumulation of fluid in the ventricles of the brain** was treated with a **tube used to drain fluid from brain ventricles into the abdominal cavity.**

7. Mrs. Aubrum was experiencing **rhythmic, quivering, purposeless skeletal muscle movements** and **decrease in normal movement** and was ultimately diagnosed with Parkinson disease.

8. The physician suspected that the patient had **a disorder characterized by sudden attacks of sleep** and ordered a **test that measures daytime sleepiness and how fast the patient falls asleep.**

9. A **procedure to aspirate CSF from the lumbar subarachnoid space** was done to rule out **an infection or inflammation of the membranes covering the brain and spinal cord.**

10. Helen O'Neal underwent **measurement and record of a number of functions while patient is asleep** to determine why she was experiencing **excessive depth or length of sleep.**

11. Alice underwent a **resection of the dorsal root of a spinal nerve to relieve pain** to stop the pain resulting from **a disorder of the 5th cranial nerve.**

12. Hector told his doctor that his **headache of vascular origin** was preceded by a/an **sensation of light.**

13. The neurologist asked Bella if she was experiencing **nerve pain** or **a feeling or prickling, burning, or numbness.**

14. Mike's doctor told him that his **inflammation of the sciatic nerve** was caused by **a displacement of an intervertebral disk so that it presses on a nerve.**

## *Case Study*  Max Janovski

While visiting his son's family 65-year-old Max Janovski became dizzy and fainted. He quickly regained consciousness, only to find that he had difficulty using the right side of his body, and his speech was slurred. The symptoms were of brief duration, and Max insisted that he was fine. However, his son insisted he go to the emergency department (ED). Max was admitted to the hospital and subsequently suffered a stroke while there.

It is likely that one of the arteries in Max's brain was initially temporarily deprived of its blood flow, and hence, its oxygen. This is termed a transient ischemic attack (TIA). The first blood clot either dislodged or disintegrated, only to be replaced by another while Max was in the hospital. This blood clot did not dissolve and subsequently caused his stroke, or cerebrovascular accident (CVA). Depending on the area affected, a neural deficit will develop when a clot lodges in the brain area. In Max's case, the clot on the left side of his brain caused weakness on his right side and slurred speech.

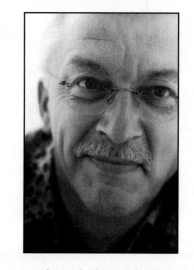

Intravenous thrombolytic (clot buster) therapy was begun soon after Max's stroke to prevent more serious damage. Max is referred for physical and occupational therapy to help improve his motor skills, strength, and coordination on the right side of his body.

*Using the report on p. 483, answer the following questions.*

### Discharge Summary

1. Patient was admitted for vertigo and syncope. Define each.

   _____

2. What is an MRA? _____

3. On what part of the head were the MRAs performed? _____

4. Ataxia refers to _____ .

JANOVSKI, MAXWELL W - 693269 Opened by SMYTHE JM, MD          [_] [⊟] [X]

Task   Edit   View   Time Scale   Options   Help

[toolbar icons]   As Of 21:01

| JANOVSKI, MAXWELL W | Age: 65 years | Sex: Male | Loc: WHC-SMMC |
| | DOB: 01/12/1947 | MRN: 693269 | FIN: 3506004 |

Reference Text Browser | Form Browser | Medication Profile

Orders | Last 48 Hours | ED | Lab | Radiology | Assessments | Surgery | **Clinical Notes** | Pt. Info | Pt. Schedule | Task List | I & O | MAR

Flowsheet: Clinical Notes [▼] [...]   Level: Discharge Summary [▼]      ⦿ Table  ○ Group  ○ List

[◄][►]                                                                      [◄][►]

Navigator                    [X]

✓   Discharge Summary

Admission Diagnosis: Rule out cerebrovascular accident
Discharge Diagnoses: (1) Cerebrovascular accident; (2) emphysema; (3) CAD.

**History**
This patient is a 65-year-old white male with a history of emphysema, coronary artery disease, and benign prostatic hyperplasia. His BPH was treated with a TURP in 2005. He had a triple CABG in 2007. Patient reports smoking two packs per day until 2 years ago. Denies any recent tobacco or alcohol use. He has benefited from oxygen therapy for the past 2 months.

He was admitted for an episode of vertigo and several episodes of syncope that occurred as he was visiting his son's family over the fourth of July holiday. His son brought him to the ED when he reported a loss of feeling on his right side, and his speech became slurred. These symptoms resolved before he arrived at the hospital. He has no history of headaches, but has admitted to continued dizziness. Patient was admitted and experienced a right-sided CVA the following morning. Intravenous thrombolytic therapy was administered immediately, but patient remains with a right hemiparesis.

**Physical Examination on Admission**
Physical examination was largely negative. The patient is quiet, mildly anxious yet cooperative. Pupils are equal and reactive. Neck is negative. There is a normal sinus rhythm with no significant murmurs. Abdomen is negative. There is no peripheral edema. Patient exhibits a minimal amount of ataxia on walking, but there are no other neurologic findings.

The neurologist ordered and reviewed CT scans of head, MRIs, intracranial and extracranial MRAs, and Holter monitor readings. Cerebral hemorrhage was ruled out.
Laboratory findings included mild hypercholesterolemia and a hemoglobin of 12.1. Chest x-ray demonstrated hyperinflation, with vascular markings diminished at the apices. EEG was normal.
Patient appears to be stable at the present time and is discharged to his son's home while continuing his physical and occupational therapy. He has demonstrated a good understanding of his condition and of the need for full cooperation with his therapists to work toward regaining his independence.
An appointment has been scheduled for followup in 2 weeks.

| PROD | MAHAFC | 04 July 2012 | 21:01 |

---

ℯ   For more interactive learning, click on:
- **Whack a Word Part** to review nervous system word parts.
- **Wheel of Terminology** and **Word Shop** to practice word building.
- **Tournament of Terminology** to test your knowledge of nervous system terms.
- **Terminology Triage** to practice sorting nervous system terms into categories.

# 13

*Health … is not a static condition, but rather is manifested in dynamic responses to the stresses and challenges of life. The more complete the human freedom, the greater the likelihood that new stresses will appear— organic and psychic—because man himself continuously changes his environment through technology, and because endlessly he moves into new conditions during his restless search for adventure.*
**—René Jules Dubos**

## CHAPTER OUTLINE

## OBJECTIVES

- Understand the role of DSM-IV TR and definitions of mental and behavioral health.
- Recognize and use terms related to the pathology of mental and behavioral health.
- Recognize and use terms related to the diagnostic procedures for mental and behavioral health.
- Recognize and use terms related to the therapeutic interventions for mental and behavioral health.

# Mental and Behavioral Health

## CHAPTER AT A GLANCE

*Use the list of word parts and key terms to assess your knowledge. Check off the ones you have mastered.*

### KEY WORD PARTS

**PREFIXES**
- [ ] acro-
- [ ] agora-
- [ ] an-
- [ ] bi-
- [ ] dys-
- [ ] para-

**SUFFIXES**
- [ ] -ia
- [ ] -mania
- [ ] -phobia
- [ ] -thymia

**COMBINING FORMS**
- [ ] anthrop/o
- [ ] claustr/o
- [ ] cycl/o
- [ ] hedon/o
- [ ] iatr/o
- [ ] klept/o
- [ ] nymph/o
- [ ] orex/o
- [ ] ped/o
- [ ] phil/o
- [ ] phor/o
- [ ] pol/o
- [ ] psych/o
- [ ] pyr/o
- [ ] somat/o
- [ ] somn/o

### KEY TERMS

- [ ] acrophobia
- [ ] amnesia
- [ ] anhedonia
- [ ] anorexia nervosa
- [ ] attention-deficit/hyperactivity disorder (ADHD)
- [ ] autism
- [ ] bipolar disorder (BP)
- [ ] borderline personality disorder
- [ ] bulimia nervosa
- [ ] claustrophobia

- [ ] cyclothymia
- [ ] dementia
- [ ] depressive disorder
- [ ] dysphoria
- [ ] generalized anxiety disorder (GAD)
- [ ] kleptomania
- [ ] nymphomania
- [ ] obsessive-compulsive disorder (OCD)
- [ ] panic disorder (PD)

- [ ] paraphilia
- [ ] parasomnia
- [ ] posttraumatic stress disorder (PTSD)
- [ ] psychotic disorders
- [ ] pyromania
- [ ] schizophrenic disorders
- [ ] somatoform disorder

## INTRODUCTION TO MENTAL AND BEHAVIORAL HEALTH

Recent national statistics reveal the following:

- One out of every four American adults and children has a mental disorder.
- More than 25% of the 100 top-selling medications are for psychiatric disorders.
- The fourth most common diagnostic category for inpatient admissions is substance-related mental disorders.
- Approximately 40 million Americans are diagnosed with anxiety.
- The number of discharges for patients with substance-related mental health disorders has more than doubled in the past 10 years.
- Approximately 7.5 million Americans are classified as mentally retarded.*

Given these statistics, behavioral health is a content area that cannot be ignored.

The term *behavioral health* reflects an integration of the outdated concept of the separate nature of the body (physical health/illness) and the mind (mental health/illness). Advances in research continually acknowledge the roles of culture, environment, and spirituality in influencing physical and behavioral health. The use of the term *behavior* refers to observable, measurable activities that may be used to evaluate the progress of treatment.

Similar to previous chapters, this chapter examines disorders that result when an individual has a maladaptive response to his or her environment (internal or external). (See Chapter 12 for an explanation of the anatomy and physiology of the brain and nervous system.) However, even though some mental illnesses have organic causes in which neurotransmitters and other known brain functions play a role, there is no mental "anatomy" per se. Instead, behavioral health is a complex interaction among an individual's emotional, physical, mental, and behavioral processes in an environment that includes cultural and spiritual influences.

*Mental health* may be defined as a relative state of mind in which a person who is healthy is able to cope with and adjust to the recurrent stresses of everyday living in a culturally acceptable way. Thus mental illness may be generally defined as a functional impairment that substantially interferes with or limits one or more major life activities for a significant duration.

The American Psychiatric Association (APA) publishes the official listing of diagnosable mental disorders: the *Diagnostic and Statistical Manual of Mental Disorders* (DSM). The codes that are used within the DSM are coordinated with the International Classification of Diseases (ICD), which provides acceptable billing codes in the United States. Major revisions to the DSM occur at approximately 10-year intervals, with minor updates about every 5 years. The current edition as this book goes to press is DSM IV-TR (text revision), published in the year 2000. DSM-V is scheduled for release in 2013.

## SPECIALTIES/SPECIALISTS

**Psychologists** work with the diagnosis and treatment of mental health disorders. Most psychologists will have a doctoral degree (PhD or PsyD). Their specialty is psychology. **Psychiatrists** are medical doctors who specialize in the treatment of mental health disorders. Their discipline is **psychiatry.**

---

*It should be noted that mental retardation is not an illness; it is a condition characterized by developmental delays and difficulty with learning and social situations.

---

**mind** = psych/o, thym/o, phren/o

**treatment** = iatr/o

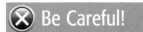 **Be Careful!**

*Don't confuse* **psychiatry,** *the treatment of mental disorders, with* **physiatry,** *the treatment of physical disorders.*

**psychologist**
  psych/o = mind
  -logist = one who specializes in the study of

**psychiatrist**
  psych/o = mind
  -iatrist = one who specializes in treatment

## Combining and Adjective Forms for Mental Health

| Meaning | Combining Form | Adjective Form |
|---------|----------------|----------------|
| attraction | phil/o | |
| mind | psych/o, thym/o, phren/o | psychic, thymic |
| treatment | iatr/o | |

## Suffixes for Mental Health

| Suffix | Meaning |
|--------|---------|
| -ia, -ism | condition |
| -iatrist | one who specializes in treatment |
| -mania | condition of madness |
| -phobia | condition of fear |

## PATHOLOGY

### Terms Related to General Symptoms

| Term | Word Origin | Definition |
|------|-------------|------------|
| **akathisia**<br>ack uh THEE zsa | *a-* lack of<br>*kathis/o* sitting<br>*-ia* condition | Inability to remain calm, still, and free of anxiety. |
| **amnesia**<br>am NEE zsa | | Inability to remember either isolated parts of the past or one's entire past; may be caused by brain damage or severe emotional trauma. |
| **anhedonia**<br>an hee DOH nee ah | *an-* without<br>*hedon/o* pleasure<br>*-ia* condition | Absence of the ability to experience either pleasure or joy, even in the face of causative events. |
| **catatonia**<br>kat tah TOH nee ah | *cata-* down<br>*ton/o* tension<br>*-ia* condition | Paralysis or immobility from psychological or emotional rather than physical causes. |
| **confabulation**<br>kon fab byoo LAY shun | | Effort to conceal a gap in memory by fabricating detailed, often believable stories. Associated with alcohol abuse. |
| **defense mechanism** | | Unconscious mechanism for psychological coping, adjustment, or self-preservation in the face of stress or a threat. Examples include **denial** of an unpleasant situation or condition and **projection** of intolerable aspects onto another individual. |

*Continued*

## Terms Related to General Symptoms—cont'd

| Term | Word Origin | Definition |
|------|-------------|------------|
| delirium<br>dih LEER ree um | | Condition of confused, unfocused, irrational agitation. In mental disorders, agitation and confusion may also be accompanied by a more intense disorientation, incoherence, or fear, and illusions, hallucinations, and delusions. |
| delusion<br>dih LOO zhun | | Persistent belief in a demonstrable untruth or a provable inaccurate perception despite clear evidence to the contrary. |
| dementia<br>dih MEN shah | | Mental disorder in which the individual experiences a progressive loss of memory, personality alterations, confusion, loss of touch with reality, and **stupor** (seeming unawareness of, and disconnection with, one's surroundings). |
| echolalia<br>eh koh LAYL yuh | *echo-* reverberation<br>*-lalia* condition of babbling | Repetition of words or phrases spoken by others. |
| hallucination<br>hah loo sih NAY shun | | Any unreal sensory perception that occurs with no external cause. |
| illusion<br>ill LOO zhun | | Inaccurate sensory perception based on a real stimulus; examples include mirages and interpreting music or wind as voices. |
| libido<br>lih BEE doh | | Normal psychological impulse drive associated with sensuality, expressions of desire, or creativity. Abnormality occurs only when such drives are excessively heightened or depressed. |
| psychosis<br>sye KOH sis | *psych/o* mind<br>*-osis* abnormal condition | Disassociation with or impaired perception of reality; may be accompanied by hallucinations, delusions, incoherence, akathisia, and/or disorganized behavior. |
| somnambulism<br>som NAM byoo liz um | *somn/o* sleep<br>*ambul/o* walking<br>*-ism* condition | Sleepwalking. |

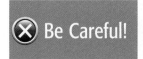 **Be Careful!** *Don't confuse **delusion**, a persistent belief in an untruth, with **illusion**, an inaccurate sensory perception based on a real stimulus.*

### Affects

Affects are observable demonstrations of emotion that can be described in terms of quality, range, and appropriateness. The following list defines the most significant affects encountered in behavioral health:

**blunted:** moderately reduced range of affect.
**flat:** the diminishment or loss of emotional expression sometimes observed in schizophrenia, mental retardation, and some depressive disorders.
**labile:** multiple, abrupt changes in affect seen in certain types of schizophrenia and bipolar disorder.
**full/wide range of affect:** generally appropriate emotional response.

## Terms Related to Moods

| Term | Word Origin | Definition |
|------|-------------|------------|
| anxiety | | Anticipation of impending danger and dread accompanied by restlessness, tension, tachycardia, and breathing difficulty not associated with an apparent stimulus. |
| dysphoria<br>dis FOR ree ah | *dys-* abnormal<br>*phor/o* to carry, to bear<br>*-ia* condition | Generalized negative mood characterized by depression. |
| euphoria<br>yoo FOR ree ah | *eu-* good, well<br>*phor/o* to carry, to bear<br>*-ia* condition | Exaggerated sense of physical and emotional well-being not based on reality, disproportionate to the cause, or inappropriate to the situation. |
| euthymia<br>yoo THIGH mee ah | *eu-* good, well<br>*-thymia* condition of the mind | Normal range of moods and emotions. |

**⊗ Be Careful!**   *The suffix -thymia means a condition of the mind, but thym/o refers to the thymus gland or to the mind.*

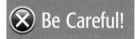 **Exercise 1: Symptoms, Affects, and Moods of Mental Illness**

*Matching.*

| | | |
|---|---|---|
| _____ 1. delusion | _____ 7. confabulation | A. paralysis from psychological causes |
| | | B. lack of memory |
| _____ 2. hallucination | _____ 8. delirium | C. restlessness, inability to sit still |
| | | D. normal drive of sensuality, creativity, desire |
| _____ 3. dementia | _____ 9. catatonia | E. mental condition characterized by confusion and agitation |
| _____ 4. dysphoria | _____ 10. illusion | F. inaccurate sensory perception based on a real stimulus |
| _____ 5. amnesia | _____ 11. libido | G. belief in a falsehood |
| | | H. negative mood characterized by depression |
| _____ 6. akathisia | | I. making up stories to conceal lack of memory |
| | | J. unreal sensory perception |
| | | K. condition characterized by loss of memory, personality changes, confusion, and loss of touch with reality |

*Circle the correct answer.*

12. Anger, anxiety, and dysphoria are examples of a patient's *(affect, mood)*.

13. Individuals whose emotions change rapidly are said to have a *(labile, blunted)* affect.

14. Patients who subconsciously blame another person for their own problems are using a defense mechanism called *(denial, projection)*.

*Build the term.*

15. abnormal condition of the mind  _____

16. condition of sleep walking  _____

17. condition of well mind  _____

18. condition of no pleasure  _____

## Terms Related to Disorders Usually First Diagnosed in Childhood

| Term | Word Origin | Definition |
|---|---|---|
| **attention-deficit/hyperactivity disorder (ADHD)** | | Series of syndromes that includes impulsiveness, inability to concentrate, and short attention span. |
| **conduct disorder** | | Any of a number of disorders characterized by patterns of persistent aggressive and defiant behaviors. **Oppositional defiant disorder (ODD),** an example of a conduct disorder, is characterized by hostile, disobedient behavior. |
| **mental retardation (MR)** | | Condition of subaverage intellectual ability, with impairments in social and educational functioning. The "intelligence quotient" (IQ) is a measure of an individual's intellectual functioning compared with the general population. **Mild mental retardation:** IQ range of 50-69; learning difficulties result. **Moderate mental retardation:** IQ range of 35-49; support needed to function in society. **Severe mental retardation**: IQ of 20-34; continuous need for support to live in society. **Profound mental retardation:** IQ <20; severe self-care limitations. |
| **pervasive developmental disorder (PDD)** <br> pur VAY siv | | A group of developmental delay disorders characterized by impairment of communication skills and social interactions. Also called **autistic spectrum disorder**. |
| **autistic disorder** <br> ah TISS tick | *auto-* self <br> *-istic* pertaining to | Condition of abnormal development of social interaction, impaired communication (including delayed language acquisition), and repetitive behaviors. |
| **Asperger disorder** <br> AS pur gur | | Disorder characterized by impairment of social interaction and repetitive patterns of inappropriate behavior without the delays of language acquisition and cognitive functions of autistic disorder. |

| Term | Word Origin | Definition |
|------|-------------|------------|
| **Rett disorder**<br>reht | | Condition usually diagnosed in female children only. It is characterized by initial normal functioning followed by loss of social and intellectual functioning, ataxia, and seizures. |
| **Tourette syndrome**<br>too RETT | | Group of involuntary behaviors that includes the vocalization of words or sounds (sometimes obscene) and repetitive movements; vocal and multiple tic disorder. |

**Terms Related to Disorders Usually First Diagnosed in Childhood—cont'd**

## Exercise 2: Disorders Usually First Diagnosed In Childhood

*Choose the correct answer from the following list.*

**attention-deficit/hyperactivity disorder, mild mental retardation, severe mental retardation, autistic disorder, Rett disorder, Asperger disorder, conduct disorder, oppositional defiant disorder, moderate mental retardation, Tourette syndrome**

1. Type of mental retardation in which the IQ range is 20 to 34. _____

2. Disorder characterized by impairment of social interaction caused by repetitive patterns of inappropriate behavior without language delay. _____

3. Group of involuntary behaviors that include tics, vocalizations, and repetitive movements.

   _____

4. Group of disorders characterized by persistent aggressive and defiant behaviors. _____

5. IQ range of 50 to 69. Most prevalent form of mental retardation, which manifests itself in learning difficulties. _____

6. IQ range of 35 to 49. Adults will need support to live in society. _____

7. A series of syndromes that include impulsiveness, inability to concentrate, and a short attention span. _____

8. Condition of pathologic social withdrawal, impairment of communication, and repetitive behaviors, along with language delay. _____

9. Persistent negative behavior characterized by hostile, disobedient behavior. _____

10. Condition characterized by initial normal functioning followed by loss of social and intellectual functioning in female children. _____

## Substance-Related Disorders

The most rapidly increasing group of disorders are substance-related disorders. These include abuse of a number of substances, including alcohol, opioids, cannabinoids, sedatives or hypnotics, cocaine, stimulants (including caffeine), hallucinogens, tobacco, and volatile solvents (inhalants). Classifications for substance abuse include psychotic, amnesiac, and late-onset disorders. It is important to be aware that addiction is not a character flaw. Rather, addiction has a neurologic basis; the effects of specific drugs are localized to equally specific areas of the brain.

An individual is considered an "abuser" if he or she uses substances in ways that threaten health or impair social or economic functioning. Levels of abuse vary.

### Terms Related to Substance Abuse

| Term | Word Origin | Definition |
|---|---|---|
| acute intoxication | *in-* in<br>*toxic/o* poison<br>*-ation* process of | Episode of behavioral disturbance following ingestion of alcohol or psychotropic drugs. |
| delirium tremens (DTs)<br>deh LEER ee um TREM uns | | Acute and sometimes fatal delirium induced by the cessation of ingesting excessive amounts of alcohol over a long period of time. |
| dependence syndrome | | Difficulty in controlling use of a drug. |
| harmful use | | Pattern of drug use that causes damage to health. |
| tolerance | | State in which the body becomes accustomed to the substances ingested; hence the user requires greater amounts to create the desired effect. |
| withdrawal state | | Group of symptoms that occur during cessation of the use of a regularly taken drug. |

## Schizophrenic, Schizotypal, and Delusional Disorders

These disorders are not always easy to classify but carry with them some common characteristics. Roughly, these disorders can be grouped as follows:

**acute and transient psychotic disorders:** heterogeneous group of disorders characterized by the acute onset of psychotic symptoms, such as delusions, hallucinations, and perceptual disturbances, and by the severe disruption of ordinary behavior. *Acute onset* is defined as a crescendo from a normal perceptual state to a clearly abnormal clinical picture in about 2 weeks or less. For these disorders, there is no evidence of organic causation. Perplexity and puzzlement are often present, but disorientation to time, place, and person is not persistent or severe enough to justify a diagnosis of organically caused delirium. The disorder may or may not be associated with acute stress (usually defined as stressful events preceding onset by 1 or 2 weeks).

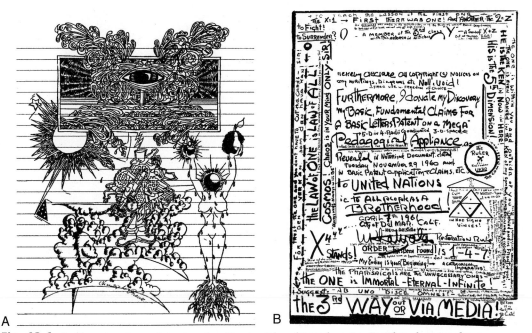

Fig. 13-1 **A,** Drawing by a delusional patient with schizophrenia. **B,** This drawing by a patient with schizophrenia demonstrates thought disorder.

**persistent delusional disorders:** variety of disorders in which long-standing delusions constitute the only, or the most conspicuous, clinical characteristic and cannot be classified as organic, schizophrenic, or affective.

**schizophrenia:** disorders characterized by fundamental distortions of thinking and perception, coupled with affects that are inappropriate or blunted. The patient exhibits characteristic inability to recognize an appropriate perception of reality (Fig. 13-1). The patient's intellectual capacity is usually intact. Symptoms may include hallucinations, delusions, and thought disorder.

- **catatonic schizophrenia** (kat tah TAH nick skit zoh FREH nee uh) is dominated by prominent psychomotor disturbances that may alternate between extremes, such as hyperkinesis and stupor, and may be accompanied by a dreamlike (oneiric) state and hallucinations.
- **disorganized schizophrenia** is characterized by prominent affective changes, fleeting and fragmentary delusions and hallucinations, and irresponsible and unpredictable behavior. Shallow, inappropriate mood, flighty thoughts, social isolation, and incoherent speech are also present.
- **paranoid schizophrenia** is dominated by relatively stable, persistent delusions, usually accompanied by auditory hallucinations and perceptual disturbances in affect, volition (will), and speech.
- **schizotypal** (skiz zoh TIE pull) **disorder,** although sometimes described as borderline schizophrenia, has none of the characteristic schizophrenic anomalies. Patients may exhibit anhedonia, eccentric behavior, cold affect, and social isolation.

**schizophrenia**
schiz/o = split
phren/o = mind
-ia = condition, state of

⊗ Be Careful!

*The combining form*
**phren/o** *can mean*
*mind or diaphragm.*

## Exercise 3: Substance Abuse and Schizophrenic Disorders

*Fill in the blanks with the following terms.*

**schizophrenia, hallucinations, persistent delusional, disorganized, delusions, alcohol, inhalants, dream, controlling substance use**

1. A patient with the DTs is showing withdrawal symptoms from _____.

2. Volatile solvents are included under the category of _____.

3. Dependence syndrome is a condition in which the patient has difficulty _____.

4. Auditory hallucinations, delusions, and thought disturbances are characteristic of _____.

5. A patient with oneiric symptoms acts as if he or she is in a _____ like state.

6. The difference between schizophrenic and schizotypal disorders is that the schizotypal patient does

   not have sustained _____ or _____.

7. The only, or most conspicuous, clinical characteristic of patients with _____
   disorders is the presence of long-standing aberrant beliefs or perceptions.

8. Shallow, inappropriate mood, flighty thought, social isolation, and incoherent speech are all

   symptoms of which type of schizophrenia? _____

## Mood Disorders

Patients with mood disorders, also called *affective disorders*, show a disturbance of affect ranging from depression (with or without associated anxiety) to elation. The mood change is usually accompanied by a change in the overall level of activity; most of the other symptoms are either secondary to, or easily understood in the context of, the change in mood and activity. Most of these disorders tend to be recurrent, and the onset of individual episodes can often be related to stressful events or situations.

### Terms Related to Mood Disorders

| Term | Word Origin | Definition |
|------|-------------|------------|
| **bipolar disorder (BP)**<br>bye POH lur | *bi-* two<br>*pol/o* pole<br>*-ar* pertaining to | Disorder characterized by swings between an elevation of mood, increased energy and activity (hypomania and mania), and a lowering of mood and decreased energy and activity (depression). |
| **cyclothymia**<br>sye kloh THIGH mee ah | *cycl/o* recurring<br>*-thymia* condition of the mind | Disorder characterized by recurring episodes of mild elation and depression that are not severe enough to warrant a diagnosis of bipolar disorder. |

## Terms Related to Mood Disorders—cont'd

| Term | Word Origin | Definition |
|---|---|---|
| depressive disorder | | Depression typically characterized by its degree (minimal, moderate, severe) or number of occurrences (single or recurrent, persistent). Patient exhibits dysphoria, reduction of energy, and decrease in activity. Symptoms include anhedonia, lack of ability to concentrate, and fatigue. Patient may experience **parasomnias** (abnormal sleep patterns), diminished appetite, and loss of self-esteem. |
| dysthymia<br>dis THIGH mee ah | *dys-* difficult<br>*-thymia* condition of the mind | Mild, chronic depression of mood that lasts for years but is not severe enough to justify a diagnosis of depression. |
| hypomania<br>hye poh MAY nee ah | *hypo-* decreased<br>*-mania* condition of madness | Disorder characterized by an inappropriate elevation of mood that may include positive and negative aspects. Patient may report increased feelings of well-being, energy, and activity, but may also report irritability and conceit. |
| persistent mood disorders | | Group of long-term, cyclic mood disorders in which the majority of the individual episodes are not sufficiently severe to warrant being described as hypomanic or mild depressive episodes. |
| seasonal affective disorder (SAD) | | Weather-induced depression resulting from decreased exposure to sunlight in autumn and winter. |

## Terms Related to Anxiety Disorders

| Term | Word Origin | Definition |
|---|---|---|
| acrophobia<br>ack roh FOH bee ah | *acro-* heights, extremes<br>*-phobia* condition of fear | Fear of heights. |
| agoraphobia<br>ah gore uh FOH bee ah | *agora-* marketplace<br>*-phobia* condition of fear | Fear of leaving home and entering crowded places. |
| anthropophobia<br>an throh poh FOH bee ah | *anthrop/o* man<br>*-phobia* condition of fear | Fear of scrutiny by other people; also called **social phobia.** |
| claustrophobia<br>klos troh FOH bee ah | *claustr/o* a closing<br>*-phobia* condition of fear | Fear of enclosed spaces. |
| generalized anxiety disorder (GAD) | | One of the most common diagnoses assigned, but not specific to any particular situation or circumstance. Symptoms may include persistent nervousness, trembling, muscular tensions, sweating, lightheadedness, palpitations, dizziness, and epigastric discomfort. |
| obsessive-compulsive disorder (OCD) | | Characterized by recurrent, distressing, and unavoidable preoccupations or irresistible drives to perform specific rituals (e.g., constantly checking locks, excessive hand washing) that the patient feels will prevent some harmful event. |

*Continued*

## Terms Related to Anxiety Disorders—cont'd

| Term | Word Origin | Definition |
|------|-------------|------------|
| panic disorder (PD) | | Recurrent, unpredictable attacks of severe anxiety (panic) that are not restricted to any particular situation. Symptoms may include vertigo, chest pain, and heart palpitations. |
| posttraumatic stress disorder (PTSD) | | Extended emotional response to a traumatic event. Symptoms may include flashbacks, recurring nightmares, anhedonia, insomnia, hypervigilance, anxiety, depression, suicidal thoughts, and emotional blunting. |

## Terms Related to Adjustment Disorder, Dissociative Identity Disorder, and Somatoform Disorder

| Term | Word Origin | Definition |
|------|-------------|------------|
| adjustment disorder | | Disorder that tends to manifest during periods of stressful life changes (e.g., divorce, death, relocation, job loss). Symptoms include anxiety, impaired coping mechanisms, social dysfunction, and a reduced ability to perform normal daily activities. |
| dissociative identity disorder | | Maladaptive coping with severe stress by developing one or more separate personalities. A less severe form, **dissociative disorder** or **dissociative reaction,** results in identity confusion accompanied by amnesia, a dreamlike state, and somnambulism. |
| somatoform disorder<br>soh MAT toh form | *somat/o* body | Any disorder that has unfounded physical complaints by the patient, despite medical assurance that no physiologic problem exists. One type of somatoform disorder is **hypochondriacal disorder,** which is the preoccupation with the possibility of having one or more serious and progressive physical disorders. |

## Terms Related to Eating Disorders

| Term | Word Origin | Definition |
|------|-------------|------------|
| anorexia nervosa<br>an oh RECKS see ah<br>nur VOH sah | *an-* without<br>*orex/o* appetite<br>*-ia* condition | Prolonged refusal to eat adequate amounts of food and an altered perception of what constitutes a normal minimum body weight caused by an intense fear of becoming obese. Primarily affects adolescent females; emaciation and amenorrhea result (Fig. 13-2). |
| bulimia nervosa<br>boo LIM ee ah<br>nur VOH sah | | Eating disorder in which the individual eats large quantities of food and then purges the body through self-induced vomiting or inappropriate use of laxatives. |

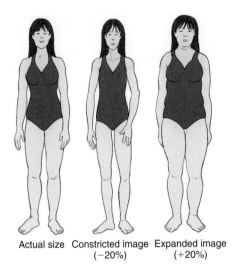

Actual size    Constricted image    Expanded image
(−20%)      (+20%)

**Fig. 13-2** The perception of body shape and size can be evaluated with the use of special computer drawing programs that allow a subject to distort (increase or decrease) the width of an actual picture of a person's body by as much as 20%. Subjects with anorexia consistently adjusted their own body picture to a size 20% larger than its true form, which suggests that they have a major problem with the perception of self-image.

## Terms Related to Sleep Disorders

| Term | Word Origin | Definition |
|---|---|---|
| **parasomnia** <br> pair ah SAHM nee ah | **para-** abnormal <br> **somn/o** sleep <br> **-ia** condition | Abnormal activation of physiologic functions during the sleep cycle. Examples include **sleep terrors,** in which repeated episodes of sudden awakening are accompanied by intense anxiety, agitation, amnesia, and somnambulism. |

## Terms Related to Sexual Dysfunction

| Term | Word Origin | Definition |
|---|---|---|
| **hypoactive sexual disorder** | | Indifference or unresponsiveness to sexual stimuli; inability to achieve orgasm during intercourse. Formerly called **frigidity.** |
| **nymphomania** <br> nim foh MAY nee ah | **nymph/o** woman <br> **-mania** condition of madness | Relentless drive to achieve sexual orgasm in the female. In the male, the condition is called **satyriasis** (sat tih RYE ah sis). |
| **premature ejaculation** | | Involuntary, anxiety-induced ejaculation of semen during sexual activity. |
| **sexual anhedonia** <br> an hee DOH nee ah | **an-** without <br> **hedon/o** pleasure <br> **-ia** condition | Inability to enjoy sexual pleasure. |

## Personality Disorders

Personality disorders have several common characteristics, including longstanding, inflexible, dysfunctional behavior patterns and personality traits that result in an inability to function successfully in society. These characteristics are not caused by stress, and affected patients have very little to no insight into their disorder.

## Terms Related to Personality Disorders

| Term | Word Origin | Definition |
| --- | --- | --- |
| borderline personality disorder | | Disorder characterized by impulsive, unpredictable mood and self-image, resulting in unstable interpersonal relationships and a tendency to see and respond to others as unwaveringly good or evil. |
| dissocial personality disorder | | Disorder in which the patient shows a complete lack of interest in social obligations, to the extreme of showing antipathy for other individuals. Patients frustrate easily, are quick to display aggression, show a tendency to blame others, and do not change their behavior even after punishment. Also called **dyssocial personality disorder.** |
| paranoid personality disorder | | State in which the individual exhibits inappropriately suspicious thinking, self-importance, a lack of ability to forgive perceived insults, and an extreme sense of personal rights. |
| schizoid personality disorder | | Condition in which the patient withdraws into a fantasy world, with little need for social interaction. Most patients have a limited capacity to experience pleasure or to express their feelings. |

## Terms Related to Habit and Impulse Disorders

| Term | Word Origin | Definition |
| --- | --- | --- |
| kleptomania<br>klep toh MAY nee ah | *klept/o* steal<br>*-mania* condition of madness | Uncontrollable impulse to steal. |
| pyromania<br>pye roh MAY nee ah | *pyr/o* fire<br>*-mania* condition of madness | Uncontrollable impulse to set fires. |
| trichotillomania<br>trick oh till oh MAY nee ah | *trich/o* hair<br>*till/o* pulling<br>*-mania* condition of madness | Uncontrollable impulse to pull one's hair out by the roots. |

## Terms Related to Paraphilias (Sexual Perversion) or Disorders of Sexual Preference

| Term | Word Origin | Definition |
| --- | --- | --- |
| exhibitionism<br>eck sih BISH uh niz um | | Condition in which the patient derives sexual arousal from the exposure of his or her genitals to strangers. |
| fetishism<br>FET ish iz um | | Reliance on an object as a stimulus for sexual arousal and pleasure. |
| pedophilia<br>ped oh FILL ee ah | *ped/o* child<br>*phil/o* attraction<br>*-ia* condition | Sexual preference, either in fantasy or actuality, for children as a means of achieving sexual excitement and gratification. |
| sadomasochism<br>say doh MASS oh kiz um | | Preference for sexual activity that involves inflicting or receiving pain and/or humiliation. |
| voyeurism<br>VOY yur iz um | | Condition in which an individual derives sexual pleasure and gratification from surreptitiously looking at individuals engaged in intimate behavior. |

## Exercise 4: Miscellaneous Behavioral Disorders

*Fill in the blanks with the following terms.*

**acrophobia, posttraumatic stress disorder, anorexia nervosa, hypomania, satyriasis, somnambulism, sadomasochism, dysthymia, bipolar disorder, obsessive-compulsive disorder, social phobia, cyclothymia, panic disorder, paranoid personality disorder, premature ejaculation, pyromania, depressive disorder, hypochondriacal disorder, dissociative identity disorder, generalized anxiety disorder, claustrophobia**

1. An alternative name for anthropophobia is _____.

2. Fear of enclosed spaces is called _____.

3. Patients who experience symptoms of persistent nervousness, trembling, muscular tension, sweating, lightheadedness, palpitations, dizziness, and epigastric discomfort may be given the diagnosis of

   _____.

4. Patients who are compelled to have repetitive thoughts or to repeat specific rituals may have a

   diagnosis of _____.

5. Extreme trauma that may result in flashbacks, nightmares, hypervigilance, or reliving the trauma is

   called _____.

6. Patients who develop separate personalities as a result of a severely stressful situation are given the

   diagnosis of what disorder? _____

7. Patients who continually express physical complaints that have no real basis have a type of

   _____.

8. Episodes of mood change from depression to mania are called _____.

9. Patients who have a loss of energy, of pleasure, and of interest in life may be experiencing

   _____.

10. An inappropriate, persistent elevation of mood that may include irritability is called

    _____.

11. Recurring episodes of mild elation and depression not severe enough to warrant diagnosis of bipolar

    disorder is called _____.

12. A chronic depression that lasts for years but does not warrant a diagnosis of depression may be

    termed _____.

13. What is the healthcare term for walking in one's sleep? _____

14. What is the term for an insatiable sexual desire in men? _____

15. Male patients who experience uncontrollable ejaculation caused by anxiety may be given the diagnosis of _____.

16. What are recurrent unpredictable attacks of severe anxiety? _____

17. What is the disorder in which patients refuse to maintain a body weight that is a minimum weight for height? _____

18. What is the healthcare term for the pathologic impulse to set fires? _____

19. What is the healthcare term for a severe, enduring personality disorder with paranoid tendencies?

_____

20. A preference for sexual activity that involves pain and humiliation is called _____.

21. Fear of heights is called _____.

*Decode the term.*

22. pedophilia _____

23. parasomnia _____

24. kleptomania _____

25. agoraphobia _____

26. trichotillomania _____

---

Click on **Hear It, Spell It** to practice spelling the pathology terms you have learned in this chapter. To see how well you pronounce the pathology terms in this chapter, click on **Hear It, Say It.** To review the pathology terms in this chapter, play **Medical Millionaire.**

## Age Matters

### Pediatrics

Aside from the disorders first diagnosed in childhood—Asperger, ADHD, autism, conduct disorders, mental retardation, and Rett disorder—children are being diagnosed in increasing numbers for depressive disorders, substance abuse, and eating disorders.

### Geriatrics

Seniors are seen with disorders associated with depression and anxiety, along with those caused by dementia.

## DIAGNOSTIC PROCEDURES

Behavioral diagnoses must take into account underlying healthcare abnormalities that may cause or influence a patient's mental health. Some of the common laboratory and imaging procedures are mentioned here, along with procedures that are traditionally considered to be psychological.

### Diagnostic Criteria

**DSM-IV-TR multiaxial assessment diagnosis:** diagnostic tool measuring mental health of the individual across five axes. The first three (if present) are stated as diagnostic codes, whereas Axis IV is a statement of factors influencing the patient's mental health (e.g., lack of social supports, unemployment), and Axis V is a numerical score that summarizes a patient's overall functioning.
  1. Axis I: Clinical Disorders
  2. Axis II: Personality Disorders and/or Mental Retardation
  3. Axis III: General Medical Conditions
  4. Axis IV: Psychosocial and Environmental Problems
  5. Axis V: Global Assessment of Functioning Scale (GAF)
**Mental status examination:** a diagnostic procedure to determine a patient's current mental state. It includes assessment of the patient's appearance, affect, thought processes, cognitive function, insight, and judgment.

### Laboratory Tests

Patients may have blood counts (complete blood cell count [CBC] with differential), blood chemistry, thyroid function panels, screening tests for syphilis (rapid plasma reagin [RPR] or microhemagglutination assay-*Treponema pallidum* [MHA-TP]), urinalyses with drug screen, urine pregnancy checks for females with childbearing potential, blood alcohol levels, serum levels of medications, and human immunodeficiency virus (HIV) tests in high-risk patients.

### Imaging

Imaging is most helpful in ruling out neurologic disorders and in research; it is less helpful in diagnosing or treating psychiatric problems. Computed tomography (CT) scans and magnetic resonance imaging (MRI) can be used to screen for brain lesions. Positron emission tomography (PET) scans can be used to examine and map the metabolic activity of the brain (Figure 13-3).

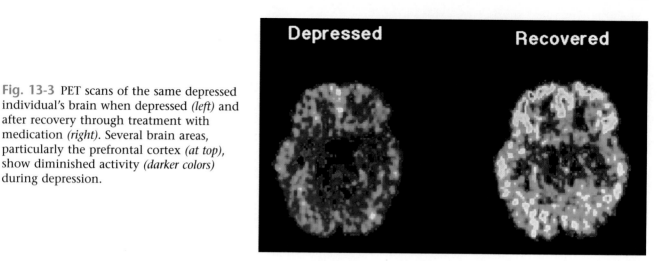

Fig. 13-3 PET scans of the same depressed individual's brain when depressed *(left)* and after recovery through treatment with medication *(right)*. Several brain areas, particularly the prefrontal cortex *(at top)*, show diminished activity *(darker colors)* during depression.

## Psychological Testing

**Bender Gestalt Test:** a test of visuomotor and spatial abilities; useful for children and adults.

**Draw-a-Person (DAP) Test:** analysis of patient's drawings of male and female individuals. Used to assess personality.

**Minnesota Multiphasic Personality Inventory (MMPI):** assessment of personality characteristics through a battery of forced-choice questions.

**Rorschach:** a projective test using inkblots to determine the patient's ability to integrate intellectual and emotional factors into his or her perception of the environment.

**Thematic Apperception Test (TAT):** test in which patients are asked to make up stories about the pictures they are shown. This test may provide information about a patient's interpersonal relationships, fantasies, needs, conflicts, and defenses.

**Wechsler Adult Intelligence Scale (WAIS):** measure of verbal IQ, performance IQ, and full-scale IQ.

 Exercise 5: Diagnostic Procedures

*Match the diagnostic procedures with their definitions.*

_____ 1. WAIS         _____ 5. Rorschach

_____ 2. TAT          _____ 6. GAF

_____ 3. PET scan     _____ 7. Bender Gestalt

_____ 4. MMPI

A. numerical measure of overall mental health
B. provides information about needs, fantasies, and interpersonal relationships
C. measures personality characteristics
D. IQ test
E. test of visuomotor and spatial skills
F. imaging of metabolic activity (in brain)
G. examines integration of emotional and intellectual factors

# *Case Study*   *Leah Wellor*

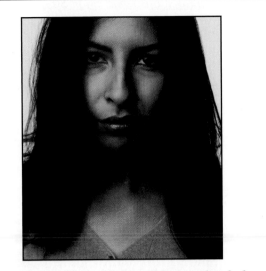

Leah Wellor is a 26-year-old female who presented at the Women's Shelter last year seeking help. She tells a counselor that her husband has been repeatedly beating her over the past 6 months. At first, he only slapped her and shouted abuse. But the slapping had changed to punching, and after a particularly brutal assault, she left him and moved in with her friend. She breaks down while talking to the counselor, telling her that she has been having nightmares and has started viewing all men as physical threats. The counselor refers her to a psychiatrist who, after several sessions, helps calm her anxiety. She knows that she still is unable to trust a man enough to have a romantic relationship, but she is now able to work and interact with men without fear.

Her last appointment with her psychiatrist involves a kind of test where she is asked what she feels are odd questions—things like counting backward by sevens and repeating rhymes and talking local politics. She is told that this helps her psychiatrist evaluate how well she has progressed. She will not have to return to see her again for 6 months unless she starts to have new nightmares or her anxiety becomes worse.

---

WELLOR, LEAH H - 818077  Opened by JEZIK, LATISHA    _ ⊡ ☒

Task   Edit   View   Time Scale   Options   Help

| WELLOR, LEAH H | Age: 26 years<br>DOB: 12/18/1985 | Sex: Female<br>MRN: 818077 | Loc: WHC-SMMC<br>FIN: 3506004 |
| --- | --- | --- | --- |

Reference Text Browser | Form Browser | Medication Profile

Orders | Last 48 Hours | ED | Lab | Radiology | **Assessments** | Surgery | Clinical Notes | Pt. Info | Pt. Schedule | Task List | I & O | MAR

Flowsheet: Assessment ▼ ...   Level: Mental Health Exam ▼    ⦿ Table ○ Group ○ List

◀ ▶      ◀ ▶

Navigator ☒
✓   Mental Health Exam

Patient was a pleasant, alert, well-groomed woman who showed no evidence of distractibility. Orientation was intact for person, time, and place. Eye contact was appropriate. There were no abnormalities of gait, posture, or demeanor. Vocabulary and grammar skills were suggestive of intellectual functioning within the high average range.

The patient's attitude was warm, open, and cooperative. Her mood was euthymic. Affect was appropriate to verbal content and showed broad range. Memory functions were grossly intact with respect to immediate and remote recall of events and factual information. Her thought processes were intact, goal oriented, and well organized. Thought content revealed no evidence of delusions, paranoia, or suicidal/homicidal ideation. There was no evidence of perceptual disorder. Her level of personal insight appeared to be very good, as evidenced by her ability to state her current diagnosis of PTSD and to identify events that contributed to its exacerbations. Social judgment appeared good, as evidenced by appropriate interactions with other patients in the waiting room.

PROD | MAHAFC | 03 Nov 2012 | 14:41

## Exercise 6: Mental Status Report

*Using the mental status report on p. 503, answer the following questions.*

1. What term indicates that the patient exhibited a normal range of emotions?

   _____

2. What term indicates that the patient exhibited a variety of moods that were appropriate to the conversation? _____

3. How do you know that the patient did not exhibit any persistent beliefs in things that are untrue?

   _____

4. What is her current diagnosis? _____

## THERAPEUTIC INTERVENTIONS

### Terms Related to Psychotherapy

| Term | Word Origin | Definition |
|------|-------------|------------|
| behavioral therapy | | Therapeutic attempt to alter an undesired behavior by substituting a new response or set of responses to a given stimulus. |
| cognitive therapy | | Wide variety of treatment techniques that attempt to help the individual alter inaccurate or unhealthy perceptions and patterns of thinking. |
| psychoanalysis<br>sye koh uh NAL ih sis | *psych/o* mind<br>*ana-* up, apart<br>*-lysis* breakdown | Behavioral treatment developed initially by Sigmund Freud to analyze and treat any dysfunctional effects of unconscious factors on a patient's mental state. This therapy uses techniques that include analysis of defense mechanisms and dream interpretation. |

### Terms Related to Other Therapeutic Methods

| Term | Word Origin | Definition |
|------|-------------|------------|
| detoxification<br>dee tock sih fih KAY shun | *de-* lack of, removal<br>*toxic/o* poison<br>*-ation* process of | Removal of a chemical substance (drug or alcohol) as an initial step in treatment of a chemically dependent individual. |
| electroconvulsive therapy (ECT)<br>ee leck troh kun VUHL siv | | Method of inducing convulsions to treat affective disorders in patients who have been resistant or unresponsive to drug therapy. |
| hypnosis<br>hip NOH sis | *hypn/o* sleep<br>*-sis* state | The induction of an altered state of consciousness to change an unwanted behavior or emotional response. |
| light therapy | | Exposure of the body to light waves to treat patients with depression due to seasonal fluctuations (Fig. 13-4). |
| narcosynthesis<br>nar koh SIN thih sis | *narc/o* sleep, stupor<br>*-synthesis* bring together | The use of intravenous barbiturates to elicit repressed memories or thoughts. |
| pharmacotherapy<br>far mah koh THAIR uh pee | *pharmac/o* drugs<br>*-therapy* treatment | The use of medication to affect behavior and/or emotions. |

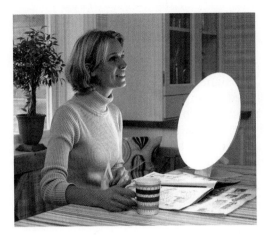

**Fig. 13-4** Broad-spectrum, fluorescent lamps, such as this one, are used in daily therapy sessions from autumn into spring for individuals with SAD. Patients report that they feel less depressed within 3 to 7 days. (Courtesy Apollo Light Systems.)

## Exercise 7: Therapeutic Interventions

*Fill in the blanks with the following terms.*

**hypnosis, cognitive therapy, ECT, behavioral, pharmacotherapy, light therapy, psychoanalysis, narcosynthesis**

1. Patients are treated with _____ therapy when an attempt is made to replace maladjusted patterns with a new response to a given stimulus.

2. What type of therapy uses exposure of the body to light waves to treat patients with depression caused by seasonal fluctuations?

   _____

3. What is a method of inducing convulsions to treat affective disorders in patients who have been resistant or unresponsive to drug therapy?

   _____

4. What therapy is used to analyze and treat any dysfunctional effects of unconscious factors or a patient's mental state?

   _____

5. What are any of the various methods of treating mental and emotional disorders that help a person change attitudes, perceptions, and patterns of thinking?

   _____

6. What therapy induces an altered state of unconsciousness to change an unwanted behavior or

   emotional response? _____

7. The use of intravenous barbiturates to elicit repressed memories or thoughts.

   _____

8. The use of medication to affect behavior and/or emotions. _____

## PHARMACOLOGY

A major part of treatment for behavioral disorders is the use of drug therapy. Various neurotransmitters may be out of balance in the brain, causing mental disorders. Many drugs have been developed to improve this balance and minimize symptoms of these disorders. The psychiatric medications described appear in the top 100 prescribed medications in the United States. Medications are continually being developed and reevaluated and are closely regulated by the Food and Drug Administration. Examples include the following:

**antialcoholics:** discourage use of alcohol. Naltrexone (ReVia) can be used for alcohol and narcotic withdrawal. Disulfiram (Antabuse) is used to deter alcohol consumption.

**antidepressants:** relieve symptoms of depressed mood. Many drug classes are available, including SSRIs, tricyclic antidepressants (TCAs), monoamine oxidase inhibitors (MAOIs), and some newer unclassified agents. Examples include fluoxetine (Prozac), sertraline (Zoloft), mirtazapine (Remeron), bupropion (Wellbutrin), and venlafaxine (Effexor).

**antipsychotics or neuroleptics:** control psychotic symptoms such as hallucinations and delusions. Haloperidol (Haldol) and chlorpromazine (Thorazine) are examples of typical antipsychotics; olanzapine (Zyprexa) and risperidone (Risperdal) are examples of the newer atypical antipsychotics.

**anxiolytics:** relieve symptoms of anxiety. These drugs are often used as sedatives or sedative-hypnotics as well. Examples are lorazepam (Ativan), buspirone (BuSpar), and alprazolam (Xanax).

**cholinesterase inhibitors:** combat the cognitive deterioration seen in disorders characterized by dementia, such as Alzheimer disease. Also known as acetylcholinesterase inhibitors (AChEIs). Examples are donepezil (Aricept) and galantamine (Reminyl, Razadyne).

**hypnotics:** promote sleep. Hypnotics, sedatives, sedative–hypnotics, and anxiolytics are often similar in effect and may be used interchangeably. Zolpidem (Ambien), zaleplon (Sonata), and flurazepam (Dalmane) are examples of hypnotics.

**mood stabilizers:** balance neurotransmitters in the brain to reduce or prevent acute mood swings (mania or depression). Lithium (Lithobid) is the most well-known mood stabilizer. Some anticonvulsants such as valproic acid (Depakote) and lamotrigine (Lamictal) are also considered mood stabilizers.

**NMDA receptor antagonists:** preserve cognitive function in patients suffering from progressive memory loss. Memantine (Namenda) is the first available drug of this new class.

**sedatives and sedative-hypnotics:** exert a calming effect with or without inducing sleep. The most commonly used agents are benzodiazepines and barbiturates.

**stimulants:** generally increase synaptic activity of targeted neurons to increase alertness. Examples include methylphenidate (Ritalin) and caffeine.

## Exercise 8: Pharmacology

*Match the drug class with the drug action.*

_____ 1. mood stabilizer        _____ 5. anxiolytic

_____ 2. antidepressant         _____ 6. stimulant

_____ 3. cholinesterase         _____ 7. antialcoholic
        inhibitor
                                _____ 8. hypnotic

_____ 4. sedative

A. discourages use of alchol
B. increases CNS synaptic activity
C. relieves symptoms of depression
D. reduces anxiety
E. improves cognition from effects of dementia
F. promotes sleep
G. prevents acute mood swings
H. calms and relaxes

## *Case Study*    Sherry Prichet

Sherry Prichet is a 54-year-old businesswoman who visits her physician with complaints of insomnia. She states that she has racing thoughts that keep her awake, and that if she does fall asleep, she wakes up with nightmares. She has a history of being sexually abused as a child by a close family member. She is having trouble now at work because she is overly tired, and she feels overwhelmed by her responsibilities. Her 17-year-old son has been skipping school, and she found marijuana in his room over the weekend. To make things worse, their house has been broken into twice in the past 2 months. She has lost weight and is not eating well. She asks her physician for something to make her sleep.

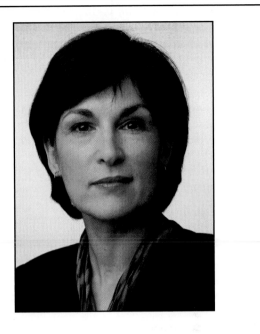

---

PRICHET, SHERILYN B - 620018 Opened by REXFORD, CHRISTIANA MD

Task   Edit   View   Time Scale   Options   Help

As Of 11:52

| **PRICHET, SHERILYN B** | Age: 54 years | Sex: Female | Loc: WHC-SMMC |
| | DOB: 05/07/1958 | MRN: 620018 | FIN: 3506004 |

Reference Text Browser | Form Browser | Medication Profile

Orders | Last 48 Hours | ED | Lab | Radiology | Assessments | Surgery | **Clinical Notes** | Pt. Info | Pt. Schedule | Task List | I & O | MAR

Flowsheet: Clinical Notes       Level: Progress Note          ⦿ Table   ○ Group   ○ List

Navigator
✓ Progress Note

54-year-old female has stress, says she just can't handle any more.

Issues circle around behavior of son age 17 and excessive workload at her job. Past history includes molestation and house robberies. Last several nights has been waking up with sleep terrors. Is having nightmares of being robbed. She just can't take it anymore and would like a sleeping pill.

IMPRESSION:    Insomnia associated with nightmares/anxiety disorder

PLAN:          Issued trazodone 25 mg to take 1-2 hours before bed for the next several nights. She is to schedule visit with a psychologist to begin to resolve these issues on a more prolonged basis.

PROD | MAHAFC | 08 May 2012 | 11:52

## Exercise 9: Progress Note

*Using the progress note on p. 503, answer the following questions.*

1. The impression notes that the patient has "insomnia." What is the meaning of the term?

   _____

2. What healthcare professional is she scheduled to visit? _____

3. What class of drug do you expect trazodone to be in? _____

4. She is diagnosed with a disorder in which the mood may be described as an "anticipation of impending danger and dread accompanied by restlessness, tension, tachycardia, and breathing difficulty not associated with the general stimulus." What is it? _____

---

Click on **Hear It, Spell It** to practice spelling the diagnostic and therapeutic terms you have learned in this chapter. To practice pronouncing these terms, click on **Hear It, Say It.**

---

## Abbreviations

| Abbreviation | Definition | Abbreviation | Definition |
|---|---|---|---|
| ADHD | attention-deficit/hyperactivity disorder | MMPI | Minnesota Multiphasic Personality Inventory |
| APA | American Psychiatric Association | MR | mental retardation |
| BP | bipolar disorder | OCD | obsessive-compulsive disorder |
| DAP | Draw-a-Person test | ODD | oppositional defiant disorder |
| DSM | Diagnostic and Statistical Manual of Mental Disorders | PD | panic disorder |
|  |  | PDD | pervasive developmental disorder |
| DTs | delirium tremens | PTSD | posttraumatic stress disorder |
| ECT | electroconvulsive therapy | SAD | seasonal affective disorder |
| GAD | generalized anxiety disorder | SSRI | selective serotonin reuptake inhibitor |
| GAF | Global Assessment of Functioning |  |  |
| ICD | International Classification of Diseases | TAT | Thematic Apperception Test |
|  |  | WAIS | Wechsler Adult Intelligence Scale |
| IQ | intelligence quotient |  |  |

---

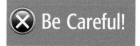 **Be Careful!**    *The abbreviation **BP** can stand for both bipolar disorder and blood pressure.*

## Exercise 10: Abbreviations

*Write out the abbreviations in the following sentences.*

1. Michele was being treated with light therapy for her SAD. _____

2. John was diagnosed with GAD after exhibiting symptoms of difficulty concentrating, excessive worry, and disturbed sleep over the last year. _____

3. The patient had a diagnosis of mild MR, with an IQ of 55, as determined by the WAIS.

   _____

4. Roger was referred to the school psychologist by his teacher to be evaluated for the possibility of an ADHD diagnosis after many behavioral problems at school and at home.

   _____

5. The patient was diagnosed with PTSD after she was assaulted. _____

Match the word parts to their definitions.

## WORD PART DEFINITIONS

| Prefix/Suffix | Definition |
| --- | --- |
| acro- | 1. _____ babbling |
| agora- | 2. _____ condition of madness |
| an- | 3. _____ without |
| bi- | 4. _____ condition of fear |
| dys- | 5. _____ condition of mind |
| eu- | 6. _____ marketplace |
| -ia | 7. _____ good, well |
| -iatrist | 8. _____ one who specializes in the study of |
| -lalia | 9. _____ two |
| -logist | 10. _____ condition |
| -mania | 11. _____ heights |
| -phobia | 12. _____ one who specializes in treatment |
| -thymia | 13. _____ difficult |

| Combining Form | Definition |
| --- | --- |
| anthrop/o | 14. _____ pleasure |
| claustr/o | 15. _____ recurring |
| cycl/o | 16. _____ appetite |
| hedon/o | 17. _____ mind |
| iatr/o | 18. _____ body |
| kathis/o | 19. _____ man |
| klept/o | 20. _____ woman |
| nymph/o | 21. _____ sitting |
| orex/o | 22. _____ pole |
| ped/o | 23. _____ mind |
| phil/o | 24. _____ steal |
| phor/o | 25. _____ child |
| phren/o | 26. _____ treatment |
| pol/o | 27. _____ sleep |
| psych/o | 28. _____ mind |
| pyr/o | 29. _____ attraction |
| somat/o | 30. _____ fire |
| somn/o | 31. _____ a closing |
| thym/o | 32. _____ to carry, bear |

# WORDSHOP

| Prefixes | Combining Forms | Suffixes |
|----------|-----------------|----------|
| a- | ambul/o | -ia |
| acro- | anthrop/o | -ism |
| agora- | claustr/o | -lalia |
| an- | cycl/o | -logy |
| dys- | hedon/o | -mania |
| echo- | klept/o | -osis |
| eu- | orex/o | -phobia |
| para- | phren/o | -thymia |
|  | psych/o |  |
|  | pyr/o |  |
|  | schiz/o |  |
|  | somn/o |  |
|  | till/o |  |
|  | trich/o |  |

Build the following terms by combining the above word parts. Some word parts may be used more than once. Some may not be used at all. The number in parentheses is the number of word parts needed to build the terms.

| Definition | Term |
|------------|------|
| 1. condition of no pleasure (3) | |
| 2. study of the mind (2) | |
| 3. fear of men (people) (2) | |
| 4. abnormal condition of the mind (2) | |
| 5. condition of compulsion (to set) fires (2) | |
| 6. fear of closed spaces (2) | |
| 7. condition of a healthy state of mind (2) | |
| 8. fear of heights (2) | |
| 9. condition of split mind (3) | |
| 10. condition of sleep walking (3) | |
| 11. condition of compulsion to pull (one's own) hair (3) | |
| 12. condition of abnormal sleep (3) | |
| 13. fear of the marketplace (2) | |
| 14. condition of babbling repetition of words spoken by others (2) | |
| 15. condition of no appetite (3) | |

*Sort the terms into the correct categories.*

## TERM SORTING

| Pathology | Pathology | Diagnostic Procedures | Therapeutic Interventions |
|---|---|---|---|
| | | | |
| | | | |
| | | | |
| | | | |
| | | | |
| | | | |
| | | | |
| | | | |
| | | | |
| | | | |

| | | | |
|---|---|---|---|
| acrophobia | confabulation | GAF | PTSD |
| ADHD | cyclothymia | hallucination | pyromania |
| akathisia | DAP | hypomania | Rorschach |
| anhedonia | delusion | hyponosis | schizophrenia |
| antidepressants | detoxification | MMPI | sedative |
| anxiety | DSM-IV-TR | OCD | somnambulism |
| anxiolytics | DTs | PD | stimulants |
| Bender Gestalt | ECT | psychoanalysis | TAT |
| catatonia | GAD | psychosis | WAIS |

*Replace the highlighted words with the correct terms.*

## TRANSLATIONS

1. The patient had a **moderately reduced range of affect** and **mild, chronic depression of mood.**

2. Amy was admitted with a diagnosis of **prolonged refusal to eat adequate amounts of food** and **fear of leaving home and entering crowded places.**

3. The patient was referred to a sleep therapist for **abnormal activation of physiologic functions during the sleep cycle** and **sleepwalking.**

4. Marielle was diagnosed with **a weather-induced depression** after telling her doctor that she had a loss of **normal psychological impulse drive associated with sensuality or creativity** and **absence of the ability to experience pleasure or joy.**

5. Because Mr. Ballestero was experiencing **generalized negative mood characterized by depression** and **an exaggerated sense of well-being not based on reality**, he was diagnosed with **a disorder characterized by elevation and lowering of mood.**

6. After Andrew McKlin returned home from Iraq, he suffered from **anticipation of impending danger and dread** and **extended emotional response to a traumatic event.**

7. Cho Ling told her **one who specializes in the study of the mind** that she thought she had **fear of heights** and **fear of enclosed spaces.**

8. Adam was washing his hands 40 times a day and his **one who specializes in treatment of the mind** diagnosed **recurrent, distressing, and unavoidable preoccupation to perform specific rituals.**

9. The patient's **impaired perception of reality** was accompanied by **unreal sensory perceptions that occur with no external cause.**

10. Tiffany showed signs of **a syndrome that includes impulsiveness, inability to concentrate and short attention span.**

11. Sixteen-year-old Ray Huggins was diagnosed with **a conduct disorder characterized by hostile, disobedient behavior** and **an uncontrollable impulse to set fires.**

12. By the time Brooke was 20 years old, she had no eyelashes because she had suffered from **an uncontrollable impulse to pull one's hair out by the roots** since she was 8 years old.

13. Dr. Linder used **the use of medication to affect behavior and/or emotions** to treat Sylvia's depression.

## Case Study   Walter Hu

Walter Hu's wife of 46 years died last spring after a long stay in a nursing home. Walter has been unable to adjust to life without her. According to his daughter, Walter is no longer interested in his friends, family or hobbies. He hasn't been sleeping well and eats very little. Today he is meeting with a psychotherapist, Andrew Lachlan, to whom he was referred to by his family physician. Andrew has read Walter Hu's chart, which contains a SOAP note from Dr. McGuire. Dr. McGuire notes that Mr Hu's generally flattened affect has been punctuated by bouts of tearfulness and anxiety. He recognizes that Mr. Hu has been exhibiting classic signs of depression: fatigue, anhedonia, insomnia, and the inability to concentrate.

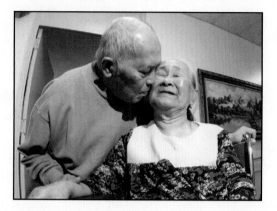

During the session Andrew gently question Mr. Hu about how his life is different now, after his wife's death. In a voice barely above a whisper and devoid of emotion, he states that his is unable to be happy anymore. "We weren't together for the last three years because Zhang was in the nursing home, but I visted her every day and we talked about the kids and the grandkids. Up until the end, she thought she would get to come home, but I knew was too ill."

Andrew empathizes with him about how hard it is to accept the death of a loved one, especially a life partner. "I want you to know that your symptoms are not unusual or untreatable. I think I can help you get back on track and enjoy life again. Talking about your loss is the first step."

At the end of the session, Andrew suggests that along with weekly counseling sessions, Mr Hu participate in a bereavement group for me who have lost their partner. "I think you'll find it useful to hear how other people are coping with their grief."

After a moment Mr Hu nods sadly. "I need to learn to live without Zhang."

---

The problem-oriented medical record (POMR) was proposed by Lawrence Weed, MD in the New England Journal of Medicine in the late 1960s. The record is composed of a problem list of health concerns organized by SOAP notes:

**S**  subjective (the patient's complaints)
**O**  objective (the physician's findings)
**A**  assessment (interpretation by the physician)
**P**  plan (action plan for what can be done for that particular problem)

This method is still being used, and applications have been extended to all disciplines, including veterinary medicine.

**Castlewood Clinic**
14037 Marion St.

Reno, NV 89512
Patient: Walter Hu
DOB: 3/24/46
MR#: 234569
Date: 8/12/12

**S:** This 76-year-old Asian male was brought here today by his daughter. He has a history of hypertension, GERD, and constipation. His daughter states, "Dad has been eating very poorly and seems uninterested in life since my mom's death." The patient says that he has come only because his daughter insisted and admits that he has not been eating or sleeping well. He has been using Correctol for his constipation, but says that it causes runny stools.

**O:** General: The patient is an older Asian male who appears to be fatigued and somewhat sad and tearful. HEENT: Tympanic membranes were clear bilaterally. Nose had some pale mucosa, otherwise clear. Throat was clear. Neck was supple. Lungs: Clear to auscultation. Cardiovascular: Regular rate and rhythm without murmur. Abdomen: Soft and diffusely tender to a mild degree. Bowel sounds were active.

**A:** (1) Depression. (2) Hypertension. (3) GERD. (4) Constipation.

**P:** (1) He will be referred to a psychotherapist for cognitive therapy. If he does not seem improved within the month, a prescription for Zoloft or Prozac will be considered. (2) His hypertension has been controlled through diet and is within normal limits today. (3) His GERD is being treated with Tagamet. (4) For his constipation, I recommended Citrucel or some similar type of fiber, increasing his fluid intake, and closely monitoring his diet for additional roughage.

*Patrick McGuire, MD*

**SOAP Note**

1. If the multiaxial format had been used, which diagnosis would have been included in Axis I?

   _____

2. Would the patient have had a diagnosis appropriate for Axis II (with the information you have been given)? _____

3. What is the meaning of GERD? _____

4. Zoloft and Prozac are what types of medications? _____

5. What type of therapy has been suggested for Mr. Hu? _____

For more interactive learning, click on:
- **Whack a Word Part** to review mental and behavioral health word parts.
- **Wheel of Terminology** and **Word Shop** to practice word building.
- **Tournament of Terminology** to test your knowledge of mental and behavioral health terms.
- **Terminology Triage** to practice sorting mental and behavioral health terms into categories.

# 14

*A beautiful eye makes silence eloquent, a kind eye makes contradiction an assent, an enraged eye makes beauty deformed. This little member gives life to every part about us.*
**—Joseph Addison**

## OBJECTIVES

- Recognize and use terms related to the anatomy and physiology of the eyes and ears.
- Recognize and use terms related to the pathology of the eyes and ears.
- Recognize and use terms related to the diagnostic procedures for the eyes and ears.
- Recognize and use terms related to the therapeutic interventions for the eyes and ears.

# Special Senses: Eye and Ear

## CHAPTER AT A GLANCE

Use the list of word parts and key terms to assess your knowledge. Check off the ones you have mastered.

### ANATOMY AND PHYSIOLOGY: THE EYE

- ☐ accommodation
- ☐ aqueous humor
- ☐ cones
- ☐ conjunctiva
- ☐ cornea
- ☐ extraocular muscle
- ☐ fovea
- ☐ iris
- ☐ lacrimal gland
- ☐ lacrimation
- ☐ lens
- ☐ macula lutea
- ☐ meibomian gland
- ☐ optic disk
- ☐ orbit
- ☐ palpebral fissure
- ☐ pupil
- ☐ refraction
- ☐ retina
- ☐ rods
- ☐ sclera
- ☐ uvea
- ☐ vitreous humor

### KEY WORD PARTS

#### PREFIX
- ☐ a, an-
- ☐ bi-, bin-
- ☐ ex-, exo-
- ☐ extra-
- ☐ hemi-
- ☐ presby-

#### SUFFIX
- ☐ -ar
- ☐ -edema
- ☐ -ia
- ☐ -itis
- ☐ -metry
- ☐ -opia
- ☐ -opsia
- ☐ -pathy
- ☐ -plasty
- ☐ -ptosis
- ☐ -scopy

#### COMBINING FORM
- ☐ ambly/o
- ☐ blephar/o
- ☐ choroid/o
- ☐ chromat/o
- ☐ conjunctiv/o
- ☐ cor/o, core/o
- ☐ corne/o
- ☐ cycl/o
- ☐ dacry/o
- ☐ dipl/o
- ☐ goni/o
- ☐ ir/o, irid/o
- ☐ kerat/o
- ☐ lacrim/o
- ☐ macul/o
- ☐ ocul/o
- ☐ ophthalm/o
- ☐ opt/o, optic/o
- ☐ palpebr/o
- ☐ papill/o
- ☐ phac/o, phak/o
- ☐ pupill/o
- ☐ retin/o
- ☐ scler/o
- ☐ ton/o
- ☐ trop/o
- ☐ uve/o
- ☐ vitre/o
- ☐ xer/o

### KEY TERMS

- ☐ achromatopsia
- ☐ age-related macular degeneration (ARMD)
- ☐ amblyopia
- ☐ aphakia
- ☐ blepharedema
- ☐ blepharoptosis
- ☐ cataract
- ☐ conjunctivitis
- ☐ coreoplasty
- ☐ dacryoadenitis
- ☐ diabetic retinopathy
- ☐ diplopia
- ☐ exophthalmia
- ☐ exotropia
- ☐ extraocular
- ☐ goniotomy
- ☐ hemianopsia
- ☐ keratitis
- ☐ keratoplasty
- ☐ ophthalmoscopy
- ☐ presbyopia
- ☐ strabismus
- ☐ tonometry
- ☐ vitrectomy
- ☐ xerophthalmia

# CHAPTER AT A GLANCE—cont'd

## ANATOMY AND PHYSIOLOGY: THE EAR

- ☐ auricle
- ☐ cerumen
- ☐ cochlea
- ☐ crista ampullaris
- ☐ eustachian tube
- ☐ external auditory canal
- ☐ external auditory meatus
- ☐ incus
- ☐ labyrinth
- ☐ macula
- ☐ malleus
- ☐ organ of Corti
- ☐ ossicular chain
- ☐ oval window
- ☐ pinna
- ☐ saccule
- ☐ stapes
- ☐ tympanic membrane
- ☐ utricle
- ☐ vestibule

## KEY WORD PARTS

**PREFIX**
- ☐ an-
- ☐ macro-
- ☐ micro-
- ☐ para-
- ☐ presby-

**SUFFIX**
- ☐ -acusis
- ☐ -algia
- ☐ -ectomy
- ☐ -ia
- ☐ -itis
- ☐ -metry
- ☐ -oma
- ☐ -plasty
- ☐ -scopy
- ☐ -stomy

**COMBINING FORM**
- ☐ acous/o
- ☐ audi/o
- ☐ aur/o, auricul/o
- ☐ cerumin/o
- ☐ cochle/o
- ☐ labyrinth/o
- ☐ myring/o
- ☐ ossicul/o
- ☐ ot/o
- ☐ salping/o
- ☐ staped/o
- ☐ tympan/o

## KEY TERMS

- ☐ anacusis
- ☐ audiometry
- ☐ ceruminoma
- ☐ infectious myringitis
- ☐ mastoiditis
- ☐ microtia
- ☐ myringostomy
- ☐ otalgia
- ☐ otitis media (OM)
- ☐ otoplasty
- ☐ otosclerosis
- ☐ otoscopy
- ☐ paracusis
- ☐ presbycusis
- ☐ stapedectomy
- ☐ tinnitus
- ☐ tympanometry
- ☐ tympanoplasty
- ☐ vertigo

## FUNCTIONS OF THE SPECIAL SENSES

When we want to relate our understanding of how someone is feeling, we say, "I hear you" or even "I see what you're saying!" Our experience in the world is filtered through our senses and our interpretations of them.

The senses include vision, hearing, taste, smell, and touch. They allow us to experience our environment through specific nervous tissue that transmits, processes, and then acts on our perceptions. This chapter covers the eyes and ears. Disorders of taste and touch are covered in Chapter 12, and olfaction (smell) is discussed in Chapter 11.

## SPECIALTIES/SPECIALISTS

**Ophthalmology** (Ophth) is the diagnosis and treatment of disorders and diseases of the eye. The specialist is an **ophthalmologist.** An **optometrist** is a healthcare professional who measures vision and prescribes corrective solutions as needed. Although glasses and contact lenses used to be the only options to correct vision, corrective surgery is now accepted practice.

**Audiology** is the diagnosis, treatment, and prevention of hearing disorders. An **audiologist** is the healthcare specialist in this field.

**Otorhinolaryngology** is the diagnosis and treatment of disorders of the ears, nose, and throat (ENT). The specialist is an **otorhinolaryngologist.**

## THE EYE

## ANATOMY AND PHYSIOLOGY

The **eye** can be divided into the ocular adnexa—the structures that surround and support the function of the eyeball—and the structures of the globe of the eye itself.

### Ocular Adnexa

Each of our paired eyes is encased in a protective, bony socket called the **orbit.** Our **binocular** vision sends two slightly different images to the brain that produce depth of vision. The right eye is called the *oculus dextra,* the left eye is called the *oculus sinistra,* and the term for "each eye" is *oculus uterque.* Within the orbit, the eyeball is protected by a cushion of fatty tissue. The **eyebrows** mark the supraorbital area and provide a modest amount of protection from perspiration and sun glare. Further protection is provided by the upper and lower eyelids and the eyelashes that line their edges (Fig. 14-1).

The corners of the eyes are referred to as the **canthi** (KAN thy) (*sing.* canthus); the inner canthus is termed *medial* (toward the middle of the body), and the outer canthus is *lateral.* The area where the upper and lower eyelids meet is referred to as the **palpebral fissure** (PAL puh brul FISH ur). This term comes from the function of blinking, called **palpebration** (pal puh BRAY shun). The eyelids are lined with a protective, thin mucous membrane called the **conjunctiva** (kun jungk TYE vuh) (*pl.* conjunctivae) that spreads to coat the anterior surface of the eyeball as well.

Also surrounding the eye are two types of glands. Sebaceous glands in the eyelid secrete oil to lubricate the eyelashes, and lacrimal glands above the eyes produce **tears.** The sebaceous glands for the eyelashes are called **meibomian** (mye BOH mee un) **glands.** These glands can be a source of complaint when they become blocked or infected. The other type of gland, the **lacrimal** (LACK

### Be Careful!

*The Joint Commission has designated the former abbreviations for right eye (OD), left eye (OS), and each eye (OU) as "dangerous" abbreviations. The recommendation is to write out the full term, e.g., "right eye."*

**vision** = opt/o, optic/o

**hearing** = audi/o, acous/o

**otorhinolaryngology**
  ot/o = ear
  rhin/o = nose
  laryng/o = throat
  -logy = study of

**eye** = ocul/o, ophthalm/o

**orbit** = orbit/o

**binocular**
  bin- = two
  ocul/o = eye
  -ar = pertaining to

**supraorbital**
  supra- = above
  orbit/o = orbit
  -al = pertaining to

**eyelid** = blephar/o, palpebr/o

**canthus** = canth/o

**conjunctiva** = conjunctiv/o

**tears** = lacrim/o, dacry/o

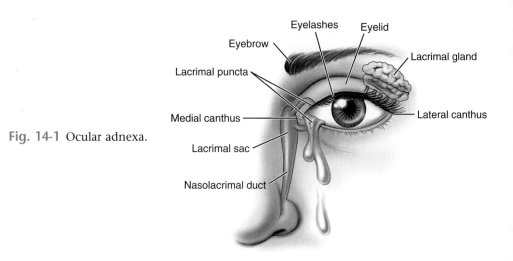

**Fig. 14-1** Ocular adnexa.

 **Be Careful!**

*The term* **palpebrate** *means to blink or wink. Do not confuse this with the terms* **palpate** *or* **palpitate***.*

---

**lacrimal gland** =
dacryoaden/o

**lacrimal sac** =
dacryocyst/o

**nasolacrimal**
  nas/o = nose
  lacrim/o = tear
  -al = pertaining to

**extraocular**
  extra- = outside
  ocul/o = eye
  -ar = pertaining to

---

rih mul) **gland,** or tear gland, provides a constant source of cleansing and lubrication for the eye. The process of producing tears is termed **lacrimation** (lack rih MAY shun). The lacrimal glands are located in the upper outer corners of the orbit. The constant blinking of the eyelids spreads the tears across the eyeball. They then drain into two small holes (the lacrimal puncta) in the medial canthus, into the **lacrimal sacs,** and then into the **nasolacrimal ducts,** which carry the tears to the nasal cavity.

The **extraocular** (eck strah OCK yoo lur) **muscles** attach the eyeball to the orbit and, on impulse from the cranial nerves, move the eyes. These six voluntary (skeletal) muscles are made up of four rectus (straight) and two oblique (diagonal) muscles.

## Exercise 1: Accessory Eye Structures

*Match the term with its correct combining form or prefix. More than one answer may be correct.*

_____ 1. membrane that lines eyelids and covers the surface of the eyes

_____ 2. eyelid

_____ 3. tear

_____ 4. vision

_____ 5. two

_____ 6. eye

_____ 7. outside

_____ 8. above

A. lacrim/o
B. conjunctiv/o
C. optic/o, opt/o
D. ophthalm/o
E. palpebr/o
F. ocul/o

G. blephar/o
H. bin-
I. dacry/o
J. supra-
K. extra-

*Build the terms.*

9. pertaining to two eyes _____

10. pertaining to above the orbit _____

11. pertaining to outside the eye _____

## Exercise 2: Accessory Eye Structures

*Label the drawing below with the correct anatomic terms and combining forms where appropriate.*

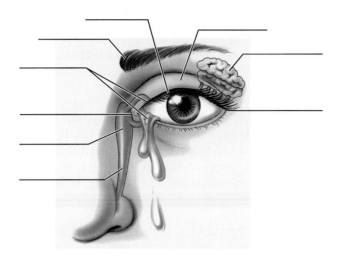

## The Eyeball

The anatomy of the eyeball itself is traditionally described as being three layers, or **tunics** (TOO nicks) (Fig. 14-2). The outer layer, or **fibrous tunic,** consists of the **sclera** (SKLAIR uh) and **cornea** (KOR nee uh). The middle layer, or **vascular tunic,** consists of the **uvea** (YOO vee uh), which is made up of the **choroid** (KOR oyd), **ciliary** (SILL ih air ee) **body,** and **iris** (EYE ris). The inner layer, or **nervous tunic,** consists of the **retina** (RET in uh). These three layers are essential to the process of seeing. All parts work together with impressive

**sclera** = scler/o

**cornea** = corne/o, kerat/o

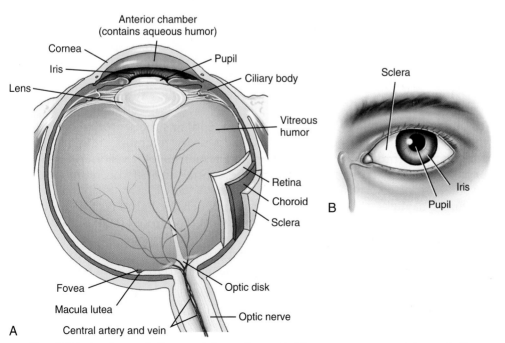

Fig. 14-2 **A,** The eyeball viewed from above. **B,** The anterior view of the eyeball.

harmony. The eye muscles coordinate their movements with one another; the cornea and pupil control the amount of light that enters the eye; the lens focuses the image on the retina; and the optic nerve transmits the image to the brain.

Two important mechanisms also contribute to the ability to see. As light hits the eye, it passes first through the cornea, which bends the rays of light **(refraction)** so that they are projected properly onto receptor cells in the eye. Then, muscles in the ciliary body adjust the shape of the lens to aid in this refraction. The lens flattens to adjust to something seen at a distance, or thickens for close vision—a process called **accommodation.** Errors of refraction are the most common reason for lens prescriptions.

### The Sclera

The outermost lateral and posterior portion of the eye, the white of the eye, is called the **sclera,** which means *hard*. The portion of the sclera that covers the anterior section of the eye is transparent and is called the **cornea.** The border of the cornea, between it and the sclera, is called the **limbus** (LIM bus). The cornea is where refraction (the bending of light) begins.

### The Uvea

The **uvea** is the middle, highly vascular layer of the eye. It includes the **iris,** the **ciliary body,** and the **choroid.** The iris (*pl.* irides), pupil, lens (*pl.* lenses), and ciliary body are located directly behind the cornea. The iris is a smooth muscle that contracts and relaxes to moderate the amount of light that enters the eye. In most individuals, this is the colored part of the eye (brown, gray, hazel, blue) because of its pigmentation. Individuals with albinism, however, have reddish-pink irides (*sing.* iris) because a lack of pigment makes visible the blood cells traveling through the vessels supplying the iris.

The **pupil** is the dark area in the center of the iris where the light continues its progress through to the lens. The **lens** is an avascular structure made of protein and covered by an elastic capsule. It is held in place by the thin strands of muscle that make up the ciliary body. The fluid produced by the capillaries of the ciliary body is called the **aqueous** (AY kwee us) **humor.** It nourishes the cornea, gives shape to the anterior eye, and maintains an optimum intraocular pressure. It normally drains through tiny veins called the canals of Schlemm. The aqueous humor circulates in both the anterior chamber, between the cornea and the iris, and the posterior chamber, behind the iris and in front of the lens. Between the lens and the retina is a jellylike substance, the **vitreous** (VIT ree us) **humor** (also called the **vitreous body),** which holds the choroid membrane against the retina to ensure an adequate blood supply. The choroid is the vascular membrane between the sclera and the retina.

### The Retina

The inner layer of the eye, called the **retina,** contains the sensory receptors for the images carried by the light rays. These sensory receptors are either **rods,** which appear throughout the retina and are responsible for vision in dim light, or **cones,** which are concentrated in the central area of the retina and are responsible for color vision.

During daylight, the area of the retina on which the light rays focus is called the **macula lutea** (MACK yoo lah LOO tee uh). The **fovea** (FOH vee uh) **centralis** is an area within the macula that contains only cones and provides the sharpest image. The area that allows a natural blind spot in our vision is the **optic disk,** where the optic nerve leaves the retina to travel to the brain. There are no light receptors there.

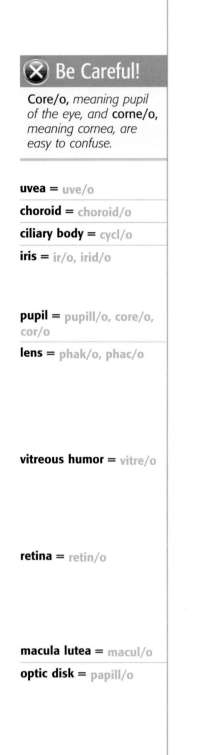

**⊗ Be Careful!**

Core/o, *meaning pupil of the eye, and* **corne/o,** *meaning cornea, are easy to confuse.*

**uvea =** uve/o

**choroid =** choroid/o

**ciliary body =** cycl/o

**iris =** ir/o, irid/o

**pupil =** pupill/o, core/o, cor/o

**lens =** phak/o, phac/o

**vitreous humor =** vitre/o

**retina =** retin/o

**macula lutea =** macul/o

**optic disk =** papill/o

## Exercise 3: The Eyeballs

*Match the parts of the eye with the correct combining forms. More than one answer may be correct.*

_____ 1. ir/o, irid/o          _____ 8. choroid/o

_____ 2. papill/o             _____ 9. cycl/o

_____ 3. retin/o              _____10. uve/o

_____ 4. cor/o, core/o        _____11. kerat/o

_____ 5. pupill/o             _____12. scler/o

_____ 6. macul/o              _____13. vitre/o

_____ 7. phac/o, phak/o

A. hard, outer covering of the eye
B. dark center of iris
C. substance between retina and lens
D. middle, highly vascular layer of the eye
E. choroid
F. ciliary body
G. transparent, anterior portion of sclera
H. lens
I. made up of rods and cones
J. pigmented muscle that allows light in eye
K. light focuses on this retinal structure
L. optic disk
M. inner layer of eye

*Decode the adjective forms.*

14. extraocular _____

15. preretinal _____

16. intrascleral _____

## Exercise 4: The Eyeballs

*Label the drawings below with correct anatomic terms and combining forms where appropriate.*

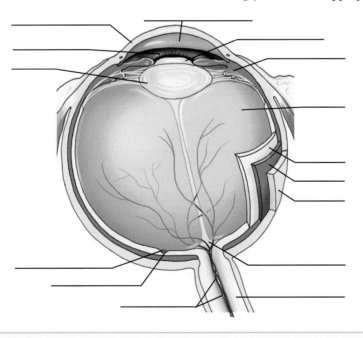

You can review the anatomy of the eye by going to Evolve at http://evolve.elsevier.com/Shiland and clicking on **Body Spectrum Electronic Anatomy Coloring Book** → **Senses** → **Eye**. Choose **Hear It, Spell It** to practice spelling the anatomy and physiology terms for the eye. To practice pronouncing these terms, click on **Hear It, Say it.**

## Combining and Adjective Forms for the Anatomy and Physiology of the Eye

| Meaning | Combining Form | Adjective Form |
|---|---|---|
| canthus | canth/o | canthal |
| choroid | choroid/o | choroidal |
| ciliary body | cycl/o | cyclic |
| conjunctiva | conjunctiv/o | conjunctival |
| cornea | corne/o, kerat/o | corneal, keratic |
| eye | ocul/o, ophthalm/o | ocular, ophthalmic |
| eyelid | blephar/o, palpebr/o | palpebral |
| iris | ir/o, irid/o | iridic |
| lacrimal gland | dacryoaden/o | dacryoadenal |
| lacrimal sac | dacryocyst/o | dacryocystic |
| lens | phak/o, phac/o | |
| macula lutea | macul/o | macular |
| optic disk | papill/o | papillary |
| orbit | orbit/o | orbital |
| pupil | pupill/o, core/o, cor/o | pupillary |
| retina | retin/o | retinal |
| sclera | scler/o | scleral |
| tears | lacrim/o, dacry/o | lacrimal |
| uvea | uve/o | uveal |
| vision | opt/o, optic/o | optic, optical |
| vitreous humor | vitre/o, vitr/o | vitreous |

## Prefixes for Anatomy of the Eye

| Prefix | Meaning |
|---|---|
| bin- | two |
| extra- | outside |
| supra- | above |

## PATHOLOGY

### Terms Related to Eyelid Disorders

| Term | Word Origin | Definition |
|---|---|---|
| **blepharedema**<br>bleff ah ruh DEE mah | *blephar/o* eyelid<br>*-edema* swelling | Swelling of the eyelid. |
| **blepharitis**<br>bleff ah RYE tis | *blephar/o* eyelid<br>*-itis* inflammation | Inflammation of the eyelid. |

## Terms Related to Eyelid Disorders—cont'd

| Term | Word Origin | Definition |
|------|-------------|------------|
| blepharochalasis<br>bleff ah roh KAL luh sis | *blephar/o* eyelid<br>*-chalasis* relaxation, slackening | Hypertrophy of the skin of the eyelid. |
| blepharoptosis<br>bleff ah rop TOH sis | *blephar/o* eyelid<br>*-ptosis* drooping | Drooping of the upper eyelid. |
| ectropion<br>eck TROH pee on | *ec-* out<br>*trop/o* turning<br>*-ion* process of | Turning outward (eversion) of the eyelid, exposing the conjunctiva (Fig. 14-3). |
| entropion<br>en TROH pee on | *en-* in<br>*trop/o* turning<br>*-ion* process of | Turning inward of the eyelid toward the eye (Fig. 14-4). |

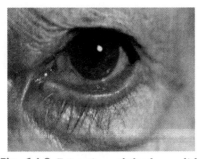

Fig. 14-3 Ectropion of the lower lid.

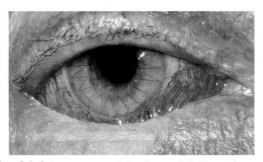

Fig. 14-4 Entropion of the lower lid. Note that this patient has undergone corneal transplantation.

## Terms Related to Eyelash Disorders

| Term | Word Origin | Definition |
|------|-------------|------------|
| chalazion<br>kuh LAY zee on | | Hardened swelling of a meibomian gland resulting from a blockage. Also called **meibomian cyst** (Fig. 14-5). |
| hordeolum<br>hor DEE uh lum | | Stye; infection of one of the sebaceous glands of an eyelash (Fig. 14-6). |

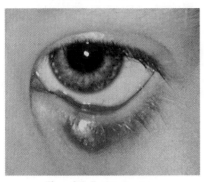

Fig. 14-5 Chalazion.

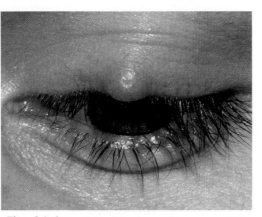

Fig. 14-6 Acute hordeolum of upper eyelid.

## Terms Related to Tear Gland Disorders

| Term | Word Origin | Definition |
|------|-------------|------------|
| dacryoadenitis<br>dack ree oh add eh NYE tis | *dacryoaden/o* lacrimal gland<br>*-itis* inflammation | Inflammation of a lacrimal gland. |
| dacryocystitis<br>dack ree oh sis TYE tis | *dacryocyst/o* lacrimal sac<br>*-itis* inflammation | Inflammation of a lacrimal sac. |
| epiphora<br>eh PIFF or ah | | Overflow of tears; excessive lacrimation. |
| xerophthalmia<br>zeer off THAL mee ah | *xer/o* dry<br>*ophthalm/o* eye<br>*-ia* condition | Dry eye; lack of adequate tear production to lubricate the eye. Usually the result of vitamin A deficiency. |

## Terms Related to Conjunctiva Disorders

| Term | Word Origin | Definition |
|------|-------------|------------|
| conjunctivitis<br>kun junk tih VYE tis | *conjunctiv/o* conjunctiva<br>*-itis* inflammation | Inflammation of the conjunctiva, commonly known as **pinkeye,** a highly contagious disorder (Fig. 14-7). |
| ophthalmia neonatorum<br>off THAL mee uh<br>nee oh nay TORE um | *ophthalm/o* eye<br>*-ia* condition<br>*neo-* new<br>*nat/o* born<br>*-um* structure | Severe, purulent conjunctivitis in the newborn, usually due to gonorrheal or chlamydial infection. Routine introduction of an antibiotic ophthalmic ointment (erythromycin) prevents most cases. |

❌ **Be Careful!**

*Do not confuse these similar terms:* **esotropia, exotropia, entropion,** *and* **ectropion**.

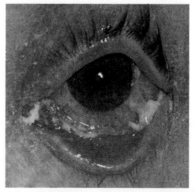

Fig. 14-7 Acute purulent conjunctivitis.

## Terms Related to Eye Muscle and Orbital Disorders

| Term | Word Origin | Definition |
|------|-------------|------------|
| amblyopia<br>am blee OH pee ah | *ambly/o* dull, dim<br>*-opia* vision condition | Dull or dim vision due to disuse. |
| diplopia<br>dih PLOH pee ah | *dipl/o* double<br>*-opia* vision condition | Double vision. **Emmetropia** (EM, Em) means normal vision. |

## Terms Related to Eye Muscle and Orbital Disorders—cont'd

| Term | Word Origin | Definition |
|------|-------------|------------|
| esotropia<br>eh soh TROH pee ah | *eso-* inward<br>*trop/o* turning<br>*-ia* condition | Turning inward of one or both eyes. |
| exophthalmia<br>eck soff THAL mee ah | *ex-* out<br>*ophthalm/o* eye<br>*-ia* condition | Protrusion of the eyeball from its orbit; may be congenital or the result of an endocrine disorder (Fig. 14-8). |
| exotropia<br>eck so TROH pee ah | *exo-* outward<br>*trop/o* turning<br>*-ia* condition | Turning outward of one or both eyes. |
| photophobia<br>foh toh FOH bee ah | *phot/o* light<br>*-phobia* condition of fear | Extreme sensitivity to light. The suffix -phobia here means "aversion," not fear. |
| strabismus<br>strah BISS mus | | General term for a lack of coordination between the eyes, usually due to a muscle weakness or paralysis. Sometimes called a "squint," which refers to the patient's effort to correct the disorder. |

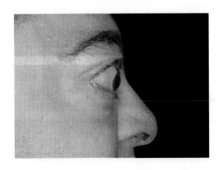

**Fig. 14-8** Exophthalmia.

## Exercise 5: Disorders of the Ocular Adnexa

*Match the disorders with their definitions.*

____ 1. epiphora      ____ 7. chalazion

____ 2. strabismus      ____ 8. exotropia

____ 3. hordeolum      ____ 9. conjunctivitis

____ 4. ectropion      ____ 10. exophthalmia

____ 5. diplopia      ____ 11. blepharedema

____ 6. amblyopia      ____ 12. ophthalmia neonatorum

A. severe conjunctivitis in the newborn
B. eversion of the eyelid
C. swelling of the eyelid
D. excessive lacrimation
E. dull or dim vision
F. stye
G. meibomian cyst
H. outward protrusion of the eyeball
I. squint
J. outward turning of the eye
K. pinkeye
L. double vision

*Decode the terms.*

13. xerophthalmia _____

14. esotropia _____

15. blepharochalasis _____

16. dacryocystitis _____

*Build the terms.*

17. inflammation of the eyelids _____

18. inflammation of a tear gland _____

19. drooping of an eyelid _____

20. process of inward turning (of the eyelid) _____

## Terms Related to Refraction and Accommodation Disorders

| Term | Word Origin | Definition |
|---|---|---|
| **astigmatism (Astig, As, Ast)**<br>ah STIG mah tiz um | | Malcurvature of the cornea leading to blurred vision. If uncorrected, asthenopia (a condition in which the eyes tire easily) may result (Fig. 14-9, *A*). |
| **hyperopia**<br>hye pur OH pee ah | *hyper-* excessive<br>*-opia* vision condition | Farsightedness; refractive error that does not allow the eye to focus on nearby objects (Fig. 14-9, *B*). |
| **myopia (MY)**<br>mye OH pee ah | *my/o* to shut<br>*-opia* vision condition | Nearsightedness; refractive error that does not allow the eye to focus on distant objects (Fig. 14-9, *C*). |
| **presbyopia**<br>press bee OH pee ah | *presby-* old age<br>*-opia* vision condition | Progressive loss of elasticity of the lens (usually accompanies aging), resulting in hyperopia. |

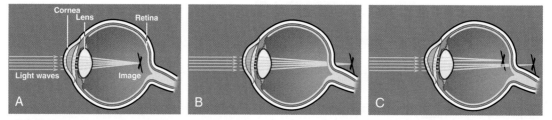

Fig. 14-9 Refraction errors. **A,** Myopia (nearsightedness). **B,** Hyperopia (farsightedness). **C,** Astigmatism.

## Terms Related to Sclera Disorders

| Term | Word Origin | Definition |
|---|---|---|
| **corneal ulcer**<br>KORE nee uhl<br>UHL sur | *corne/o* cornea<br>*-al* pertaining to | Trauma to the outer covering of the eye, resulting in an abrasion. |
| **keratitis**<br>kair uh TYE tis | *kerat/o* cornea<br>*-itis* inflammation | Inflammation of the cornea. |

## Terms Related to Uvea Disorders

| Term | Word Origin | Definition |
|------|-------------|------------|
| **anisocoria**<br>an nye soh KORE ee ah | *an-* no, not, without<br>*is/o* equal<br>*cor/o* pupil<br>*-ia* condition | Condition of unequally sized pupils, sometimes due to pressure on the optic nerve as a result of trauma or lesion (Fig. 14-10). |
| **hyphema**<br>hye FEE mah | *hypo-* under<br>*hem/o* blood<br>*-a* noun ending | Blood in the anterior chamber of the eye as a result of hemorrhage due to trauma. |
| **uveitis**<br>yoo vee EYE tis | *uve/o* uvea<br>*-itis* inflammation | Inflammation of the uvea (iris, ciliary body, and choroids). |

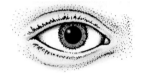
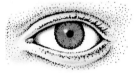

Fig. 14-10 Anisocoria.

## Terms Related to Lens Disorders

| Term | Word Origin | Definition |
|------|-------------|------------|
| **aphakia**<br>ah FAY kee ah | *a-* no, not, without<br>*phak/o* lens<br>*-ia* condition | Condition of no lens, either congenital or acquired. |
| **cataract**<br>KAT ur ackt | | Progressive loss of transparency of the lens of the eye (Fig. 14-11). |
| **glaucoma**<br>glah KOH mah | *glauc/o* gray, bluish green<br>*-oma* mass | Group of disorders characterized by abnormal intraocular pressure due to obstruction of the outflow of the aqueous humor. **Chronic** or **primary open-angle glaucoma** (Fig. 14-12) is characterized by an open anterior chamber angle. **Angle-closure** or **narrow-angle glaucoma** is characterized by an abnormally narrowed anterior chamber angle. |

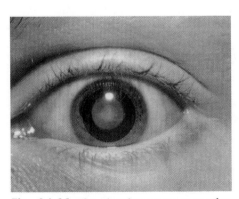

Fig. 14-11 The cloudy appearance of a lens affected by a cataract.

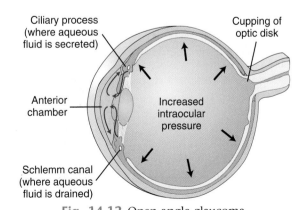

Ciliary process (where aqueous fluid is secreted)

Cupping of optic disk

Anterior chamber

Increased intraocular pressure

Schlemm canal (where aqueous fluid is drained)

Fig. 14-12 Open-angle glaucoma.

## Terms Related to Retina Disorders

| Term | Word Origin | Definition |
|------|-------------|------------|
| achromatopsia<br>ah kroh mah TOP see ah | *a-* no, not, without<br>*chromat/o* color<br>*-opsia* vision condition | Impairment of color vision. Inability to distinguish between certain colors because of abnormalities of the photopigments produced in the retina. Also called **color blindness**. |
| age-related macular degeneration (ARMD or AMD)<br>MACK kyoo luhr dee jen ur RAY shun | | Progressive destruction of the macula, resulting in a loss of central vision. This is the most common visual disorder after the age of 75 (Fig. 14-13). |
| diabetic retinopathy<br>dye ah BET ick ret in OP ah thee | *retin/o* retina<br>*-pathy* disease | Damage of the retina due to diabetes; the leading cause of blindness (Fig. 14-14). Classified according to stages from mild, nonproliferative diabetic retinopathy (NPDR) to proliferative diabetic retinopathy (PDR). |
| hemianopsia<br>hem ee an NOP see ah | *hemi-* half<br>*an-* no, not, without<br>*-opsia* vision condition | Loss of half the visual field, often as the result of a cerebrovascular accident. |
| nyctalopia<br>nick tuh LOH pee ah | *nyctal/o* night<br>*-opia* vision condition | Inability to see well in dim light. May be due to a vitamin A deficiency, retinitis pigmentosa, or choroidoretinitis. |
| retinal tear, retinal detachment | | Separation of the retina from the choroid layer. May be due to trauma, inflammation of the interior of the eye, or aging. A hole in the retina allows fluid from the vitreous humor to leak between the two layers. |
| retinitis pigmentosa<br>ret in EYE tis pig men TOH sah | *retin/o* retina<br>*-itis* inflammation | Hereditary, degenerative disease marked by nyctalopia and a progressive loss of the visual field. |
| scotoma<br>skoh TOH mah | *scot/o* darkness<br>*-oma* mass, tumor | Area of decreased vision in the visual field. Commonly called a **blind spot**. |

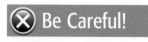 To view a video of a retinal detachment, click on **Animations**.

## ⊗ Be Careful!

*Nyctalopia* means night blindness, not night vision.

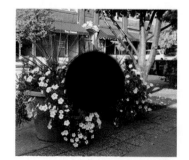

Fig. 14-13 Macular degeneration.

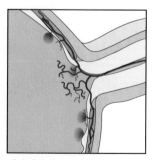

Fig. 14-14 Diabetic retinopathy.

## Terms Related to Optic Nerve Disorders

| Term | Word Origin | Definition |
|---|---|---|
| **nystagmus**<br>nye STAG mus | | Involuntary, back-and-forth eye movements due to a disorder of the labyrinth of the ear and/or parts of the nervous system associated with rhythmic eye movements. |
| **optic neuritis**<br>OP tick<br>nyoo RYE tis | *opt/o* vision<br>*-ic* pertaining to<br>*neur/o* nerve<br>*-itis* inflammation | Inflammation of the optic nerve resulting in blindness; often mentioned as a predecessor to the development of multiple sclerosis. |

## Exercise 6: Disorders of the Eyeball

*Match the terms with their definitions.*

____ 1. cataract

____ 2. ARMD

____ 3. glaucoma

____ 4. anisocoria

____ 5. aphakia

____ 6. myopia

____ 7. hyperopia

____ 8. corneal ulcer

____ 9. astigmatism

____ 10. hyphema

____ 11. scotoma

____ 12. nystagmus

____ 13. retinal detachment

A. abrasion of the outer eye
B. nearsightedness
C. involuntary back-and-forth movements of the eye
D. hemorrhage within the eye
E. malcurvature of the cornea
F. increased intraocular pressure
G. unequally sized pupils
H. blind spot
I. loss of central vision
J. loss of transparency of the lens
K. lack of a lens
L. farsightedness
M. separation of retina from choroid layer

*Decode the terms.*

14. nyctalopia _____

15. achromatopsia _____

16. aphakia _____

17. hemianopsia _____

18. optic neuritis _____

*Build the terms.*

19. inflammation of the cornea _____

20. (lack of) vision due to old age _____

21. inflammation of the uvea _____

22. disease of the retina _____

## Terms Related to Benign Neoplasms

| Term | Word Origin | Definition |
|---|---|---|
| **choroidal hemangioma**<br>koh ROY dul<br>hee man jee OH mah | *choroid/o* choroid<br>*-al* pertaining to<br>*hemangi/o* blood vessel<br>*-oma* tumor, mass | Tumor of the blood vessel layer under the retina (the choroid layer). May cause visual loss or retinal detachment. |

## Terms Related to Malignant Neoplasms

| Term | Word Origin | Definition |
|---|---|---|
| **intraocular melanoma**<br>in trah AHK yoo lur<br>mell uh NOH mah | *intra-* within<br>*ocul/o* eye<br>*-ar* pertaining to<br>*melan/o* dark, black<br>*-oma* tumor, mass | Malignant tumor of the choroid, ciliary body, or iris that usually occurs in individuals in their 50s or 60s. |
| **retinoblastoma**<br>reh tih noh blas TOH mah | *retin/o* retina<br>*blast/o* embryonic, immature<br>*-oma* tumor, mass | An inherited condition present at birth that arises from embryonic retinal cells (Fig. 14-15). |

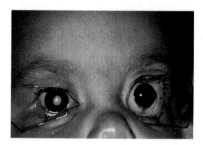

Fig. 14-15 Retinoblastoma. White pupil is a classic sign.

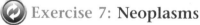

## Exercise 7: Neoplasms

*Fill in the blank.*

1. What is an inherited malignant condition of the eye? _____

2. What is a malignant tumor of the choroids, iris, or ciliary body? _____

3. What is a benign tumor of the vascular layer of the eye? _____

# Age Matters

### Pediatrics

The most prevalent disorder of the eyes is conjunctivitis, which accounts for a large number of pediatric visits. Because it is highly contagious, entire classrooms may be infected as a result of one student's infection. Routine introduction of erythromycin has severely limited the number of cases of ophthalmia neonatorum, conjunctivitis of the newborn that is usually due to gonorrhea or chlamydial infection.

### Geriatrics

Age-related macular degeneration and cataracts are the most common causes of blindness in the elderly, although there are several successful procedures to treat cataracts. Currently there are no treatments to cure ARMD. Diabetic retinopathy is the most common cause of blindness, but it may also occur much earlier in life. Presbyopia is a visual disorder that usually accompanies aging, resulting in farsightedness.

## DIAGNOSTIC PROCEDURES

### Terms Related to Diagnostic Procedures

| Term | Word Origin | Definition |
|---|---|---|
| **Amsler grid**<br>AMZ lur | | Test to assess central vision and to assist in the diagnosis of age-related macular degeneration. |
| **diopters**<br>DYE op turs | | Level of measurement that quantifies **refraction errors,** including the amount of nearsightedness (negative numbers), farsightedness (positive numbers), and astigmatism. |
| **fluorescein angiography**<br>FLOO reh seen<br>an jee AH gruh fee | *angi/o* vessel<br>*-graphy* process of recording | Procedure to confirm suspected retinal disease by injection of a fluorescein dye into the eye and use of a camera to record the vessels of the retina. |
| **fluorescein staining**<br>FLOO reh seen | | Use of a dye dropped into the eyes that allows differential staining of abnormalities of the cornea. |
| **gonioscopy**<br>goh nee AH skuh pee | *goni/o* angle<br>*-scopy* process of viewing | Visualization of the angle of the anterior chamber of the eye; used to diagnose glaucoma and to inspect ocular movement. |
| **ophthalmic sonography**<br>off THALL mick | *ophthalm/o* eye<br>*-ic* pertaining to<br>*son/o* sound<br>*-graphy* process of recording | Use of high-frequency sound waves to image the interior of the eye when opacities prevent other imaging techniques. May be used for diagnosing retinal detachments, inflammatory conditions, vascular malformations, and suspicious masses. |
| **ophthalmoscopy**<br>off thal MAH skuh pee | *ophthalm/o* eye<br>*-scopy* process of viewing | Any visual examination of the interior of the eye with an ophthalmoscope. |
| **Schirmer tear test**<br>SHURR mur | | Test to determine the amount of tear production; useful in diagnosing dry eye (xerophthalmia). |

*Continued*

## Terms Related to Diagnostic Procedures—cont'd

| Term | Word Origin | Definition |
|------|-------------|------------|
| slit lamp examination | | Part of a routine eye examination; used to examine the various layers of the eye. Medications may be used to dilate the pupils (mydriatics), numb the eye (anesthetics), or dye the eye (fluorescein staining). |
| tonometry<br>toh NAH meh tree | *ton/o* tone, tension<br>*-metry* process of measurement | Measurement of intraocular pressure (IOP); used in the diagnosis of glaucoma. In **Goldmann applanation tonometry,** the eye is numbed and measurements are taken directly on the eye. In **air-puff tonometry,** a puff of air is blown onto the cornea. |
| visual acuity (VA)<br>    assessment<br>ah KYOO ih tee | | Test of the clearness or sharpness of vision; also called the **Snellen test.** Normal vision is described as being 20/20. The top figure is the number of feet the examinee is standing from the Snellen chart (Fig. 14-16); the bottom figure is the number of feet a normal person would be from the chart and still be able to read the smallest letters. Thus if the result is 20/40, the highest line that the individual can read is what a person with normal vision can read at 40 feet. |
| visual field (VF) test | | Test to determine the area of physical space visible to an individual. A normal visual field is 65 degrees upward, 75 degrees downward, 60 degrees inward, and 90 degrees outward (Fig. 14-17). |

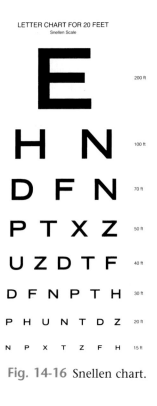

Fig. 14-16 Snellen chart.

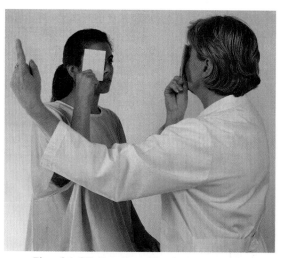

Fig. 14-17 Assessment of visual fields.

## ⟳ Exercise 8: Diagnostic Procedures

*Matching.*

____ 1. measure of the area of physical space visible to an individual

____ 2. exam of intraocular pressure

____ 3. visual exam of interior of eye

____ 4. test of sharpness of vision

____ 5. visualization of angle of anterior chamber

____ 6. test to measure central vision

____ 7. test to determine amount of tear production

____ 8. exam of abnormalities of cornea

____ 9. part of routine eye exam of layers of the eye

____ 10. use of injected dye to record suspected retinal disease

____ 11. measurement units used to determine refraction errors

A. slit lamp exam
B. VA test
C. Schirmer test
D. fluorescein staining
E. VF test
F. ophthalmoscopy
G. Amsler grid
H. tonometry
I. gonioscopy
J. fluorescein angiography
K. diopters

## THERAPEUTIC INTERVENTIONS

### Terms Related to Interventions of the Eyeball and Adnexa

| Term | Word Origin | Definition |
|---|---|---|
| blepharoplasty<br>BLEFF or uh plas tee | *blephar/o* eyelid<br>*-plasty* surgical repair | Surgical repair of the eyelids. May be done to correct blepharoptosis or blepharochalasis (Fig. 14-18). |
| blepharorrhaphy<br>BLEFF ar oh rah fee | *blephar/o* eyelid<br>*-rrhaphy* suture | Suture of the eyelids. |
| dacryocystorhinostomy<br>dak ree oh sis toh rye NOSS tuh mee | *dacryocyst/o* lacrimal sac<br>*rhin/o* nose<br>*-stomy* new opening | Creation of an opening between the tear sac and the nose. |
| enucleation of the eye<br>eh noo klee AY shun | *e-* out<br>*nucle/o* nucleus<br>*-ation* process of | Removal of the entire eyeball. |
| evisceration of the eye<br>eh vis uh RAY shun | *e-* out<br>*viscer/o* organ<br>*-ation* process of | Removal of the contents of the eyeball, leaving the outer coat (the sclera) intact. |
| exenteration of the eye<br>eck sen tur RAY shun | | Removal of the entire contents of the orbit. |

## Terms Related to Scleral and Corneal Procedures

| Term | Word Origin | Definition |
|------|-------------|------------|
| anterior ciliary sclerotomy (ACS)<br>sklair AH tuh mee | *scler/o* sclera<br>*-tomy* incision | Incision in the sclera to treat presbyopia. |
| corneal incision procedure | | Any keratotomy procedure in which the cornea is cut to change shape, thereby correcting a refractive error. |
| astigmatic keratotomy (AK)<br>as tig MAT ick<br>kair uh TAH tuh mee | *kerat/o* cornea<br>*-tomy* incision | Corneal incision process that treats astigmatism by effecting a more rounded cornea. |
| photorefractive keratectomy (PRK)<br>foh toh ree FRACK tiv<br>kair uh TECK tuh mee | *kerat/o* cornea<br>*-ectomy* removal | Treatment for astigmatism, hyperopia, and myopia that uses an excimer laser to reshape the cornea. |
| corneal transplant | | Transplantation of corneal tissue from a donor or the patient's own (autograft) cornea. May be either full- or partial-thickness grafts; also called **keratoplasty** (KAIR uh toh plas tee). |
| flap procedure | | Any procedure in which a segment of the cornea is cut as a means of access to the structures below (LASIK). |
| laser-assisted in-situ keratomileusis (LASIK)<br>kair uh toh mih LOO sis | *kerat/o* cornea | Flap procedure in which an excimer laser is used to remove material under the corneal flap. Corrects astigmatism, myopia, and hyperopia (Fig. 14-19). |

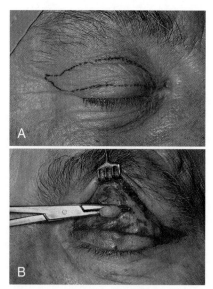

Fig. 14-18 Upper-lid blepharoplasty. **A,** Incision marked where skin will be removed. **B,** Prolapsed fat is snipped.

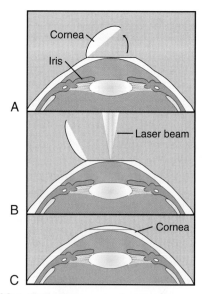

Fig. 14-19 LASIK surgery. **A,** A microkeratome is used to create a hinged cap of tissue, which is lifted off the cornea. **B,** Anexcimer laser is used to vaporize and reshape underlying tissue. **C,** Tissue cap is replaced.

## Terms Related to Lens Interventions

| Term | Word Origin | Definition |
|------|-------------|------------|
| cataract extraction | *ex-* out<br>*tract/o* pull<br>*-ion* process of | Removal of the lens to treat cataracts. May be **intracapsular** (ICCE), in which the entire lens and capsule are removed, or **extracapsular** (ECCE), in which the lens capsule is left in place (Fig. 14-20). |
| intraocular lenses (IOLs) | *intra-* within<br>*ocul/o* eye<br>*-ar* pertaining to | Use of an artificial lens implanted behind the iris and in front of the natural abnormal lens to treat myopia and hyperopia. Also called **implantable contact lenses (ICLs)**. |
| phacoemulsification and<br>  aspiration of cataract<br>fay koh ee mull sih fih KAY shun | *phac/o* lens | Vision correction accomplished through the destruction and removal of the contents of the capsule by breaking it into small pieces and removing them by suction. |

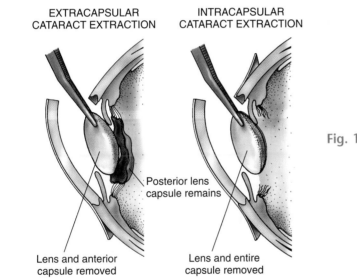

EXTRACAPSULAR
CATARACT EXTRACTION

INTRACAPSULAR
CATARACT EXTRACTION

Posterior lens
capsule remains

Lens and anterior
capsule removed

Lens and entire
capsule removed

Fig. 14-20 Lens removal.

## Terms Related to Iris Interventions

| Term | Word Origin | Definition |
|------|-------------|------------|
| coreoplasty<br>KORE ee oh plas tee | *core/o* pupil<br>*-plasty* surgical repair | Surgical repair to form an artificial pupil. |
| goniotomy<br>goh nee AH tuh mee | *goni/o* angle<br>*-tomy* incision | Incision of the Schlemm canal to correct glaucoma by providing an exit for the aqueous humor. |
| trabeculotomy<br>truh beck kyoo LAH tuh mee | *trabecul/o* little beam<br>*-tomy* incision | Incision of the orbital network of the eye to promote intraocular circulation and decrease intraocular pressure (IOP). |

## Terms Related to Retina Interventions

| Term | Word Origin | Definition |
|------|-------------|------------|
| **retinal photocoagulation**<br>RET in ul<br>foh toh koh agg yoo LAY shun | *retin/o* retina<br>*-al* pertaining to<br>*phot/o* light<br>*-coagulation* to clot | Destruction of retinal lesions using light rays to solidify tissue. |
| **scleral buckling**<br>SKLAIR ul<br>BUCK ling | *scler/o* sclera<br>*-al* pertaining to | Reattachment of the retina with a cryoprobe and the use of a silicone sponge to push the sclera in toward the retinal scar; includes the removal of fluid from the subretinal space (Fig. 14-21). |
| **vitrectomy**<br>vih TRECK tuh mee | *vitr/o* vitreous humor, glassy<br>*-ectomy* removal | Removal of part or all of the vitreous humor. |

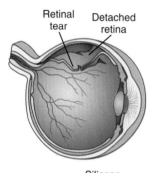

Retinal tear    Detached retina

Silicone sponge

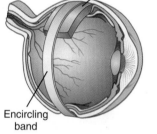

Encircling band

**Fig. 14-21** Scleral buckling procedure.

 ## Exercise 9: Therapeutic Interventions

*Match the interventions with their definitions.*

____ 1. suture of the eyelids

____ 2. removal of vitreous humor

____ 3. surgical repair of a pupil defect

____ 4. destruction of retinal lesions with light

____ 5. incision of the Schlemm canal to correct glaucoma

____ 6. removal of contents of eyeball, except for outer coat

____ 7. any keratotomy procedure to correct a refractive error

____ 8. procedure to cut cornea to access deeper structures

____ 9. implantable contact lenses

____ 10. corneal transplant

____ 11. removal of entire orbital contents

____ 12. reattachment of retina

____ 13. removal of entire eyeball

A. retinal photocoagulation
B. scleral buckling
C. enucleation of eye
D. intraocular lenses
E. exenteration of the eye
F. flap procedure
G. vitrectomy
H. blepharorrhaphy
I. corneal incision procedure
J. goniotomy
K. evisceration of eye
L. coreoplasty
M. keratoplasty

*Decode the terms.*

14. trabeculotomy _____

15. dacryocystorhinostomy _____

16. vitrectomy _____

## PHARMACOLOGY

**antibiotics:** medications used to treat bacterial infections. Examples include gentamicin (Garamycin) and ciprofloxacin (Ciloxan).

**antiglaucoma drugs:** decrease the intraocular pressure by decreasing the amount of fluid in the eye or increasing the drainage. Examples include carbonic anhydrase (dorzolamide), cholinergics (pilocarpine), prostaglandin agonists (latanoprost), beta blockers (levobunolol) and alpha-2 agonists (brimonidine).

**antihistamines:** drugs used to treat allergic conditions such as itchy or watery eyes. Diphenhydramine (Benadryl) is a common oral OTC product used to treat allergies. Ketotifen (Zaditor) is an example of OTC eyedrops.

**cycloplegics:** induce paralysis of the ciliary body to allow examination of the eye. One example is atopical atropine eye drops.

**lubricants:** keep the eyes moist, mimicking natural tears.

**miotics:** cause the pupils to constrict; often used to treat glaucoma.

**mydriatics:** cause the pupils to dilate; used in diagnostic and refractive examination of the eye.

**ophthalmics:** drugs applied directly to the eye. These may be in the form of solutions or ointments.

**topical anesthetics:** temporarily anesthetize the eye for the purpose of examination.

## Exercise 10: Pharmacology

*Matching.*

____ 1. used to treat allergic conditions

____ 2. used to constrict pupils

____ 3. used to allow examination of eye by paralyzing ciliary body

____ 4. used to dilate pupils

____ 5. used to keep eyes moist

A. mydriatics
B. cycloplegics
C. antihistamines
D. lubricants
E. miotics

# Case Study  *Alfred Olson*

Alfred Olson is a 75-year-old retired postman who has been enjoying his retirement. He has stayed active both physically and mentally. Lately, however, he has noticed that his vision has been getting worse. Things look blurry in the day, and at night, when the street lights come on, they seem to have rings around them. Even car lights hurt his eyes. His physician refers him to an ophthalmologist, who tells Alfred that he has a cataract on his right eye and one starting to develop on his left eye. He is scheduled for surgery to remove the cataract on the right eye.

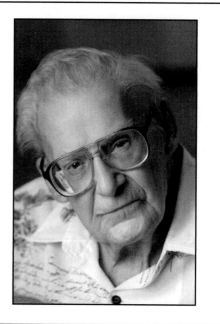

---

OLSON, ALFRED U - 600048 Opened by WESTGATE, ADAM MD     _ ⬜ ✕

Task    Edit    View    Time Scale    Options    Help

As Of 09:22

**OLSON, ALFRED U**

| | | | |
|---|---|---|---|
| | Age: 75 years | Sex: Male | Loc: WHC-SMMC |
| | DOB: 11/11/1936 | MRN: 600048 | FIN: 3506004 |

Reference Text Browser | Form Browser | Medication Profile

Orders | Last 48 Hours | ED | Lab | Radiology | Assessments | **Surgery** | Clinical Notes | Pt. Info | Pt. Schedule | Task List | I & O | MAR

Flowsheet: Surgery ▾ ...    Level: Operative Report ▾    ◉ Table ◯ Group ◯ List

◀▶                                                                                                    ◀▶

| Navigator ✕ |
|---|
| ✓  Operative Report |

Patient is a 75-year-old gentleman with a visually significant cataract of the right eye. He was seen preoperatively by his family physician and cleared for local anesthetic. Patient was brought into the outpatient surgical suite and underwent uncomplicated phacoemulsification and posterior lens implant of the right eye under local standby using topical anesthetic.

He was taken to the recovery room in good condition.

PROD | MAHAFC | 25 April 2011 | 09:22

## Exercise 11: Operative Report

*Using the operative report on p. 540, answer the following questions.*

1. What is the condition that the procedure is intended to correct? _____

2. When was he seen by his family physician? _____

3. Phacoemulsification means that the lens was _____ .

4. How do you know that he received a new lens? _____

5. What type of anesthetic was used during the surgery? _____

## Abbreviations

| Abbreviation | Meaning | Abbreviation | Meaning |
|---|---|---|---|
| Acc | accommodation | IOL | intraocular lens |
| ACS | anterior ciliary sclerotomy | IOP | intraocular pressure |
| AK | astigmatic keratotomy | LASIK | laser-assisted in-situ keratomileusis |
| ARMD, AMD | age-related macular degeneration | MY | myopia |
| Astigm, As, Ast | astigmatism | NPDR | nonproliferative diabetic retinopathy |
| ECCE | extracapsular cataract extraction | Ophth | ophthalmology |
| EM, Em | emmetropia | PDR | proliferative diabetic retinopathy |
| EOM | extraocular movements | PRK | photorefractive keratectomy |
| ICCE | intracapsular cataract extraction | VA | visual acuity |
| ICL | implantable contact lens | VF | visual field |

## Exercise 12: Abbreviations

*Write out the following abbreviations.*

1. Jonathan Sobel was diagnosed with MY in his left eye. _____

2. Marlena decided to consider the merits of LASIK and PRK before she had her prescription filled.

_____

3. Katsuko's vision was described as 20/300 on his VA test. _____

4. The patient had ARMD. _____

5. Arielle was referred to Ophth. _____

6. The patient's IOP is described as being within normal limits. _____

7. An Amsler grid is used to test the patient's VF. _____

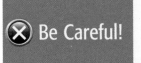 **Be Careful!**    *The abbreviations for left eye (OS), right eye (OD), and each eye (OU) have been declared "dangerous" by the Joint Commission. Write out the full term instead of using an abbreviation.*

# THE EAR

## ANATOMY AND PHYSIOLOGY

**ear** = ot/o, aur/o, auricul/o

The ear is regionally divided into the outer, middle, and inner **ear** (Fig. 14-22). Sound is conducted through air, bone, and fluid through these divisions. The majority of the ear is contained within the **petrous** (PEH trus) portion of the temporal bone. Petrous refers to the hard (petr/o = stone) nature of the temporal bone that protects the ear. The **mastoid process** is a hard, small projection of the temporal bone that is behind the opening of the auditory canal.

**mastoid process** = mastoid/o

### Outer (External) Ear

Sound waves are initially gathered by the flesh-covered cartilage of the outer ear called the **pinna** (PIN nuh), or **auricle** (ORE ick kul). The gathered sound is then funneled into the **external auditory canal**. Earwax, or **cerumen** (sih ROO mun), is secreted by modified sweat glands within the external auditory canal and protects the ear with its antiseptic property and its stickiness, trapping foreign debris and moving it out of the ear. The opening of the outer ear is the **external auditory meatus** (AH dih tor ee mee AY tus). The **tympanic** (tim PAN ick) **membrane** (TM), or **eardrum**, marks the end of the external ear and the beginning of the middle ear.

**cerumen, earwax** = cerumin/o

**meatus** = meat/o

**eardrum** = tympan/o, myring/o

### Middle Ear

The eardrum conducts sound to three tiny bones in the middle ear called the **ossicles** (AH sick kuls), or the **ossicular chain.** These ossicles are named for their shapes: the **malleus** (MAL ee us), or hammer; the **incus** (ING kus), or anvil; and the **stapes** (STAY peez) (*pl.* stapedes), or stirrup. The ossicles transmit the sound to the **oval window** through the stapes. Within the middle ear is the opening for the **eustachian** (yoo STAY shun) **tube,** also called the auditory tube, a mucous membrane–lined connection between the ears and the throat that equalizes pressure within the middle ear.

**ossicle** = ossicul/o

**stapes** = staped/o

**eustachian tube** = salping/o

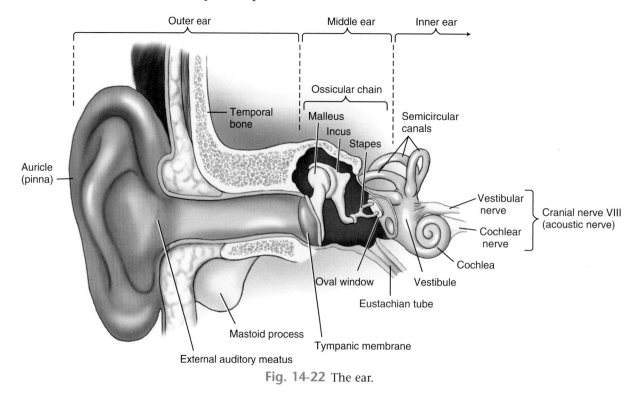

**Fig. 14-22** The ear.

**⊗ Be Careful!**   *The combining form* **salping/o** *means both fallopian tube and eustachian tube.*

**⊗ Be Careful!**   **Malleus** *means one of the ossicles in the ear.* **Malleolus** *means one of the processes on the distal tibia and fibula.*

## Inner Ear

Once sound is conducted to the oval window, it is transmitted to a structure called the **labyrinth** (LAB uh rinth), or the **inner ear.** The labyrinth is the organ of receptors for hearing and balance. A membranous labyrinth is enclosed within a bony labyrinth. Between the two, and surrounding the inner labyrinth, is a fluid called **perilymph** (PAIR ee limf). Within the membranous labyrinth is a fluid called **endolymph** (EN doh limf). Hair cells within the inner ear fluids act as nerve endings that function as sensory receptors for hearing and equilibrium. The outer, bony labyrinth is composed of three parts: the vestibule, the semicircular canals, and the cochlea. The **vestibule** (VES tih byool) and **semicircular canals** function to provide information about the body's sense of equilibrium, whereas the **cochlea** (KAH klee ah) is an organ of hearing.

Within the vestibule, two saclike structures called the **utricle** (YOO trick ul) and the **saccule** (SACK yool) function to determine the body's static equilibrium. A specialized patch of epithelium called the **macula** (MACK yoo lah), found in both the utricle and the saccule, provides information about the position of the head and a sense of acceleration and deceleration. The semicircular canals detect dynamic equilibrium, or a sense of sudden rotation, through the function of a structure called the **crista ampullaris** (KRIS tah am pyoo LAIR is).

The cochlea receives the vibrations from the perilymph and transmits them to the cochlear duct, which is filled with endolymph. The transmission of sound continues through the endolymph to the **organ of Corti,** where the hearing receptor cells (hairs) stimulate a branch of the eighth cranial nerve, the vestibulocochlear nerve, to transmit the information to the temporal lobe of the brain.

**labyrinth, inner ear =** labyrinth/o

**perilymph**
   peri- = surrounding
   lymph/o = lymph

**endolymph**
   endo- = within
   lymph/o = lymph

**vestibule =** vestibul/o

**cochlea =** cochle/o

**macula =** macul/o

**hearing =** audi/o, acous/o

**⊗ Be Careful!**

*Do not confuse* **oral,** *meaning pertaining to the mouth, with* **aural,** *meaning pertaining to the ear.*

---

⊖ To view an animation of the pathway of sound waves, click on **Animations.**

---

⟳ Exercise 13: **Anatomy of the Ear**

*Match the combining forms with the correct parts of the ear. More than one answer may be correct.*

____ 1. eardrum        ____ 5. hearing            A. labyrinth/o
                                                   B. ossicul/o
____ 2. bones of the ear   ____ 6. eustachian tube   C. cerumin/o
                                                   D. staped/o
____ 3. earwax         ____ 7. ear               E. myring/o
                                                   F. salping/o
____ 4. inner ear      ____ 8. stirrup-shaped ear bone   G. ot/o
                                                   H. audi/o
                                                   I. tympan/o
                                                   J. aur/o

*Decode the terms.*

9. preauricular _____

10. supratympanic _____

11. circumaural _____

## Exercise 14: Anatomy of the Ear

*Label the drawing below with the correct anatomic labels and combining forms where appropriate.*

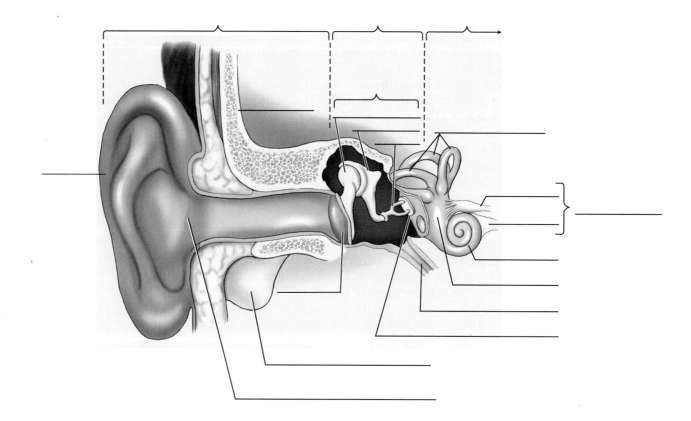

You can review the anatomy of the ear by clicking on **Body Spectrum Electronic Anatomy Coloring Book →
Senses → Ear.** Choose **Hear It, Spell It** to practice spelling the anatomy and physiology terms for the ear. Practice
pronouncing anatomy and physiology terms by Clicking on **Hear It, Say It.**

## Combining and Adjective Forms for the Anatomy and Physiology of the Ear

| Meaning | Combining Form | Adjective Form |
|---|---|---|
| cerumen, earwax | cerumin/o | ceruminous |
| cochlea | cochle/o | cochlear |
| ear | ot/o, aur/o, auricul/o | otic, aural, auricular |
| eardrum | tympan/o, myring/o | tympanic |
| eustachian tube | salping/o | salpingeal |
| hearing | audi/o, acous/o | acoustic |
| labyrinth, inner ear | labyrinth/o | labyrinthine |
| lymph | lymph/o, lymphat/o | lymphatic |
| macula | macul/o | macular |
| mastoid process | mastoid/o | mastoidal |
| meatus | meat/o | meatal |
| ossicle | ossicul/o | ossicular |
| stapes | staped/o | stapedial |
| vestibule | vestibul/o | vestibular |

## Prefixes for Anatomy of the Ear

| Prefix | Meaning |
|---|---|
| endo- | within |
| peri- | surrounding |

## PATHOLOGY

### Terms Related to Symptomatic Disorders

| Term | Word Origin | Definition |
|---|---|---|
| otalgia<br>oh TAL juh | *ot/o* ear<br>*-algia* pain | Earache, pain in the ear; also called **otodynia** (oh toh DIN nee ah). |
| otorrhea<br>oh tuh REE ah | *ot/o* ear<br>*-rrhea* discharge | Discharge from the auditory canal; may be serous, bloody, or purulent. |
| tinnitus<br>tin EYE tis | | Abnormal sound heard in one or both ears caused by trauma or disease; may be a ringing, buzzing, or jingling. |
| vertigo<br>VUR tih goh | | Dizziness; abnormal sensation of movement when there is none, either of one's self moving, or of objects moving around oneself. May be caused by middle ear infections or the toxic effects of alcohol, sunstroke, and certain medications. |

## Terms Related to Outer Ear Disorders

| Term | Word Origin | Definition |
|------|-------------|------------|
| **impacted cerumen**<br>sur ROO mun | | Blockage of the external auditory canal with cerumen. |
| **macrotia**<br>mah KROH sha | *macro-* large<br>*ot/o* ear<br>*-ia* condition | Condition of abnormally large auricles. |
| **microtia**<br>mye KROH sha | *micro-* small<br>*ot/o* ear<br>*-ia* condition | Condition of abnormally small auricles. |
| **otitis externa**<br>oh TYE tis<br>eck STER nah | *ot/o* ear<br>*-itis* inflammation<br>*externa* outer | Inflammation of the outer ear and ear canal. Also called **swimmer's ear**. |

## Terms Related to Middle Ear Disorders

| Term | Word Origin | Definition |
|------|-------------|------------|
| **cholesteatoma**<br>koh less tee ah TOH mah | *chol/e* bile<br>*steat/o* fat<br>*-oma* tumor | Cystic mass composed of epithelial cells and cholesterol. Mass may occlude middle ear and destroy adjacent bones. |
| **infectious myringitis**<br>meer in JYE tis | *myring/o* eardrum<br>*-itis* inflammation | Inflammation of the eardrum due to a bacterial or viral infection. |
| **mastoiditis**<br>mass toy DYE tis | *mastoid/o* mastoid process<br>*-itis* inflammation | Inflammation of the mastoid process of the temporal bone (Fig. 14-23). |
| **otitis media (OM)**<br>oh TYE tis<br>MEE dee ah | *ot/o* ear<br>*-itis* inflammation<br>*media* middle | Inflammation of the middle ear. **Suppurative OM** is characterized by a pus-filled fluid. **Secretory OM** is characterized by clear fluid discharge (Fig. 14-24). |
| **otosclerosis**<br>oh toh sklair ROH sis | *ot/o* ear<br>*-sclerosis* condition of hardening | Development of bone around the oval window with resulting ankylosis of the stapes to the oval window; usually results in progressive deafness. |

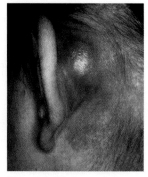

Fig. 14-23 Mastoiditis.

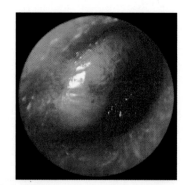

Fig. 14-24 Otitis media. Tympanic membrane is erythematous, opaque, and bulging.

## Terms Related to Inner Ear Disorders

| Term | Word Origin | Definition |
|------|-------------|------------|
| labyrinthitis<br>lab uh rinth EYE tis | *labyrinth/o* labyrinth<br>*-itis* inflammation | Inflammation of the inner ear that may be due to infection or trauma; symptoms may include vertigo, nausea, and nystagmus. |
| Meniere disease<br>may nee UR | | Chronic condition of the inner ear characterized by vertigo, hearing loss, and tinnitus. The cause is unknown. |
| ruptured tympanic membrane | | Tear (perforation) of the eardrum due to trauma or disease process (Fig. 14-25). |

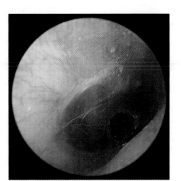

Fig. 14-25 Tympanic membrane perforation.

## Terms Related to Hearing Loss Disorders

| Term | Word Origin | Definition |
|------|-------------|------------|
| anacusis<br>an uh KYOO sis | *an-* no, not, without<br>*-acusis* hearing | General term for hearing loss or deafness. |
| conductive hearing loss | | Hearing loss resulting from damage to or malformation of the middle or outer ear. |
| paracusis<br>pair uh KYOO sis | *para-* abnormal<br>*-cusis* hearing | Abnormality of hearing. |
| presbycusis<br>prez bee KYOO sis | *presby-* old age<br>*-cusis* hearing | Loss of hearing common in old age. |
| sensorineural hearing loss<br>sen suh ree NOOR uhl | | Hearing loss resulting from damage to the inner ear (cochlea) or the auditory nerve. |

## Exercise 15: Disorders of the Ear

*Matching.*

____ 1. cholesteatoma      ____ 7. tinnitus

____ 2. vertigo            ____ 8. presbycusis

____ 3. otorrhea           ____ 9. Meniere disease

____ 4. macrotia           ____ 10. anacusis

____ 5. labyrinthitis      ____ 11. otitis externa

____ 6. otitis media       ____ 12. paracusis

A. cystic mass in the middle ear composed of cholesterol
B. ringing in the ears
C. inner ear condition characterized by vertigo, hearing loss, and tinnitus
D. loss of hearing typical of aging
E. hearing loss
F. inflammation of inner ear
G. abnormally large auricles
H. abnormal sense of movement
I. middle ear infection
J. inflammation of outer ear
K. discharge from the ear
L. abnormality of hearing

*Build the terms.*

13. ear pain _____

14. condition of small ears _____

15. condition of hardening of the ear _____

| Terms Related to Benign Neoplasms | | |
|---|---|---|
| Term | Word Origin | Definition |
| **acoustic neuroma**<br>ah KOO stik<br>noo ROH mah | *acous/o* hearing<br>*-tic* pertaining to<br>*neur/o* nerve<br>*-oma* tumor, mass | A benign tumor of the eighth cranial nerve (vestibulocochlear) that causes tinnitus, vertigo, and hearing loss. Also called **vestibular schwannoma**. |
| **ceruminoma**<br>seh roo min NOH mah | *cerumin/o* cerumen, ear wax<br>*-oma* tumor, mass | A benign adenoma of the glands that produce earwax. |

## Exercise 16: Neoplasms

*Fill in the blank.*

1. What is a benign tumor of the eighth cranial nerve? _____

2. What is a benign adenoma of the glands that produce earwax? _____

Click on **Hear It, Spell It** to practice spelling the pathology terms you have learned in this chapter. To see how well you pronounce the pathology terms in this chapter, click on **Hear It, Say It.** To review the pathology terms in this chapter, play **Medical Millionaire.**

# *Case Study* *Luis Pujols*

Two-year-old Luis has had quite a few ear infections in his short life, and today his mother brings him to the PA because she is sure he has another one. He has been running a slight fever for the past 2 days and has not been eating or drinking much. Last night he didn't sleep well, and today he woke up complaining that his right ear hurts.

The PA notes that his right ear is inflamed and that he has copious amounts of yellow nasal drainage. As Luis' mother suspected, her son has another ear infection. The PA writes a prescription for an oral antibiotic and tells his mother to place anesthetic drops in his ear as needed for pain.

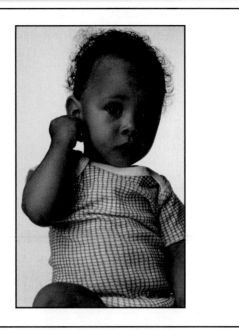

---

PUJOLS, LUIS A - 645233 Opened by WASHINGTON, FELIX MD     ▬ ⬜ ✕

Task   Edit   View   Time Scale   Options   Help

As Of 15:20

| PUJOLS, LUIS A | Age: 2 years | Sex: Male | Loc: WHC-SMMC |
|---|---|---|---|
| | DOB: 05/24/2010 | MRN: 645233 | FIN: 3506004 |

| Reference Text Browser | Form Browser | Medication Profile |
|---|---|---|

Orders | Last 48 Hours | ED | Lab | Radiology | Assessments | Surgery | **Clinical Notes** | Pt. Info | Pt. Schedule | Task List | I & O | MAR

Flowsheet: Clinical Notes ▼ ... Level: Progress Note ▼    ⦿ Table ⃝ Group ⃝ List

Navigator ✕

✓ Progress Note

This 2-year-old male comes in with a temperature of 101.1 F. In some pain, and mother has noted him to be lethargic. Patient has had frequent ear infections in the past. He also has history of strep throat.

PHYSICAL EXAM:   Alert male, lethargic, but responsive
Not in acute respiratory distress

Temperature:   101.1, Pulse 120, BP 120/80

Neck:   No lymphadenopathy or stiffness. Full ROM

Lungs:   Clear with upper respiratory sounds, but no wheezing

Cardiac:   Regular rate and rhythm

HEENT:   Reveals dull red right TM. Oropharyngeal exam normal.

ASSESSMENT:   Right otitis media
Treat with Zithromax 200 per 5/mL. Given Auralgan suspension, 3 drops to right ear.

PROD | MAHAFC | 05 Jun 2012 | 15:20

## Exercise 17: Progress Note

*Using the progress note on p. 549, answer the following questions.*

1. How do you know that the patient had no disease of his lymph glands? _____

2. What term tells you that the patient did not exhibit a whistling sound made during breathing?

   _____

3. The patient's right eardrum is examined and is found to be dull and red. What do you think TM

   stands for? _____

4. What area of the throat appears normal on exam? _____

5. The diagnosis is an inflammation of the middle ear. What is the term? _____

## *Age Matters*

### Pediatrics

Although very few babies are born with a hearing loss, the Universal Newborn Hearing Screening test is a means to detect deafness in infancy. Once given the diagnosis, the parents can begin to plan for how to best handle the condition.

Otitis media is the most frequently diagnosed childhood ear disease.

### Geriatrics

Hearing loss that may accompany the aging process is termed presbycusis.

## DIAGNOSTIC PROCEDURES

### Terms Related to Hearing Tests

| Term | Word Origin | Definition |
|---|---|---|
| **audiometric testing**<br>ah dee oh MEH trick | *audi/o* hearing<br>*-metric* pertaining to measurement | Measurement of hearing, usually with an instrument called an **audiometer** (ah dee AH met tur). The graphic representation of the results is called an **audiogram** (Fig. 14-26). |
| **otoscopy**<br>oh TAH skuh pee | *ot/o* ear<br>*-scopy* process of viewing | Visual examination of the external auditory canal and the tympanic membrane using an **otoscope.** |
| **pure tone audiometry**<br>ah dee AH meh tree | *audi/o* hearing<br>*-metry* process of measuring | Measurement of perception of pure tones with extraneous sound screened out. |
| **Rinne tuning fork test**<br>RIH nuh | | Method of distinguishing conductive from sensorineural hearing loss. |

## Terms Related to Hearing Tests—cont'd

| Term | Word Origin | Definition |
|------|-------------|------------|
| speech audiometry | *audi/o* hearing<br>*-metry* process of measuring | Measurement of ability to hear and understand speech. |
| tympanometry<br>tim pan NAH muh tree | *tympan/o* eardrum<br>*-metry* process of measuring | Measurement of the condition and mobility function of the eardrum. The resultant graph is called a **tympanogram.** |
| Universal Newborn Hearing Screening (UNHS) test | | Test that uses **otoacoustic emissions (OAEs)** measured by the insertion of a probe into the baby's ear canal, and **auditory brainstem response (ABR)**, which involves the placement of four electrodes on the baby's head to measure the change in electrical activity of the brain in response to sound while the baby is sleeping. |
| Weber tuning fork test<br>WEB ur | | Method of testing auditory acuity. |

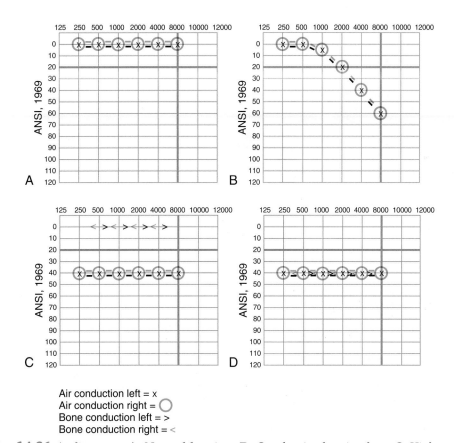

Air conduction left = x
Air conduction right = ◯
Bone conduction left = >
Bone conduction right = <

**Fig. 14-26** Audiograms. **A,** Normal hearing. **B,** Conductive hearing loss. **C,** High-frequency hearing loss. **D,** Sensorineural hearing loss.

## Exercise 18: Diagnostic Procedures

*Matching.*

____ 1. instrument to measure hearing

____ 2. test of auditory acuity

____ 3. record of function of eardrum

____ 4. instrument to visually examine the ears

____ 5. test to distinguish between conductive and sensorineural hearing loss

____ 6. measurement of ability to hear and understand speech

A. otoscope
B. Rinne tuning fork test
C. speech audiometry
D. Weber tuning fork test
E. audiometer
F. tympanogram

*Decode the terms.*

7. otoscopy _____

8. tympanometry _____

9. audiometric _____

## THERAPEUTIC INTERVENTIONS

### Terms Related to Therapeutic Interventions

| Term | Word Origin | Definition |
|------|-------------|------------|
| **cochlear implant** KAH klee ur | *cochle/o* cochlea -*ar* pertaining to | Implanted device that assists those with hearing loss by electrically stimulating the cochlea (Fig. 14-27). |
| **hearing aid** | | Electronic device that amplifies sound. |
| **mastoidectomy** mass toyd ECK tuh mee | *mastoid/o* mastoid process -*ectomy* removal | Removal of the mastoid process, usually to treat intractable mastoiditis. |
| **otoplasty** OH toh plas tee | *ot/o* ear -*plasty* surgical repair | Surgical or plastic repair and/or reconstruction of the external ear. |
| **stapedectomy** stay puh DECK tuh mee | *staped/o* stapes -*ectomy* removal | Removal of the third ossicle, the stapes, from the middle ear. |
| **tympanoplasty** TIM pan oh plas tee | *tympan/o* eardrum -*plasty* surgical repair | Surgical repair of the eardrum, with or without ossicular chain reconstruction. Some patients may require a prosthesis (an artificial replacement) for one or more of the ossicles. |
| **tympanostomy** tim pan AH stuh mee | *tympan/o* eardrum -*stomy* new opening | Surgical creation of an opening through the eardrum to promote drainage and/or allow the introduction of artificial tubes to maintain the opening (Fig. 14-28); also called a **myringostomy** (mir ring AH stuh mee). |
| **tympanotomy** tim pan AH tuh mee | *tympan/o* eardrum -*tomy* incision | Incision of an eardrum; also called a **myringotomy** (mir ring AH toh mee). |

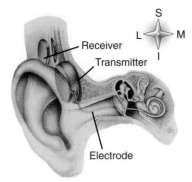

Fig. 14-27 Cochlear implant.

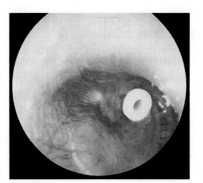

Fig. 14-28 Tympanostomy tube in place.

## Exercise 19: Therapeutic Interventions

*Match the interventions with their definitions.*

____ 1. incision of eardrum

____ 2. surgical reconstruction of the external ear

____ 3. surgical creation of a new opening through the eardrum

____ 4. device implanted in inner ear to stimulate hearing

____ 5. excision of ossicle that strikes the oval window

A. cochlear implant
B. otoplasty
C. tympanostomy
D. stapedectomy
E. myringotomy

Click on **Hear It, Spell It** to practice spelling the diagnostic and therapeutic terms you have learned in this chapter. To practice pronouncing these terms, click on **Hear it, Say It.**

## PHARMACOLOGY

**antibiotics:** treat bacterial infections. A commonly used oral agent to treat ear infections is amoxicillin (Amoxil). A topical example is ciprofloxacin with hydrocortisone (Cipro HC Otic).

**ceruminolytics:** soften and break down earwax. An example is carbamide peroxide (Debrox).

**decongestants:** relieve congestion associated with a cold, allergy, or sinus pressure. These drugs may be available as a nasal spray or an oral product. Examples include pseudoephedrine (Sudafed) and oxymetazoline (Afrin, Visine LR).

**otics:** drugs applied directly to the external ear canal. These may be administered in the form of solutions, suspensions, or ointments.

## Exercise 20: Pharmacology

*Matching.*

_____ 1. otics

_____ 2. ceruminolytics

_____ 3. antibiotics

_____ 4. decongestants

A. drugs used to treat infection
B. drugs used to relieve congestion
C. drugs applied to the external ear canal
D. medications to soften and break down earwax

## Abbreviations

| Abbreviation | Meaning | Abbreviation | Meaning |
|---|---|---|---|
| ABR | auditory brain response | OM | otitis media |
| ASL | American sign language | oto | otology |
| ENT | ear, nose, throat | TM | tympanic membrane |
| OAE | otoacoustic emission | UNHS | Universal Newborn Hearing Screening test |

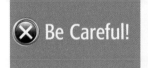 Exercise 21: **Abbreviations**

*Matching.*

| | | | |
|---|---|---|---|
| ____ 1. OM | ____ 4. ENT | A. | tympanic membrane |
| | | B. | otoacoustic emission |
| ____ 2. ASL | ____ 5. OAE | C. | American sign language |
| | | D. | ear, nose, throat |
| ____ 3. TM | | E. | otitis media |

**⊗ Be Careful!** *The abbreviations for left ear (AS), right ear (AD), and each ear (AU) have been declared "dangerous" by the Joint Commission. Write out the full term instead of using an abbreviation.*

# Chapter Review

Match the word parts to their definitions.

## WORD PART DEFINITIONS

| Prefix/Suffix | Definition |
|---|---|
| an- | 1. _____ surgical repair |
| -cusis | 2. _____ outside |
| exo- | 3. _____ inflammation |
| extra- | 4. _____ outward |
| -itis | 5. _____ hearing |
| macro- | 6. _____ not |
| micro- | 7. _____ old age |
| -opsia | 8. _____ vision condition |
| -plasty | 9. _____ large |
| presby- | 10. _____ small |

| Combining Form | Definition |
|---|---|
| acous/o | 11. _____ tears |
| audi/o | 12. _____ cornea |
| auricul/o | 13. _____ earwax |
| blephar/o | 14. _____ eardrum |
| cerumin/o | 15. _____ lacrimal sac |
| core/o | 16. _____ ear |
| dacryoaden/o | 17. _____ vision |
| dacryocyst/o | 18. _____ hearing |
| irid/o | 19. _____ eyelid |
| kerat/o | 20. _____ inner ear |
| labyrinth/o | 21. _____ eardrum |
| lacrim/o | 22. _____ eye |
| myring/o | 23. _____ pupil |
| ocul/o | 24. _____ eye |
| ophthalm/o | 25. _____ hearing |
| opt/o | 26. _____ optic disk |
| ot/o | 27. _____ eyelid |
| palpebr/o | 28. _____ iris |
| papill/o | 29. _____ ear |
| phac/o | 30. _____ lens |
| salping/o | 31. _____ eustachian tube |
| tympan/o | 32. _____ lacrimal gland |

## WORDSHOP

| Prefixes | Combining Forms | Suffixes |
|---|---|---|
| a- | blephar/o | -opia |
| an- | phak/o | -ia |
| par- | chromat/o | -opsia |
| para- | dacryoaden/o | -rrhea |
| presby- | dacryocyst/o | -ptosis |
| micro- | nas/o | -ectomy |
| | rhin/o | -cusis |
| | lacrim/o | -tomy |
| | phot/o | -sclerosis |
| | ton/o | -itis |
| | labyrinth/o | -metry |
| | ot/o | -stomy |
| | audi/o | -al |
| | tympan/o | -phobia |

Build the following terms by combining the above word parts. Some word parts may be used more than once. Some may not be used at all The number in parentheses is the number of word parts needed to build the terms.

| Definition | Term |
|---|---|
| 1. condition of small ear (3) | |
| 2. condition of no lens (3) | |
| 3. discharge from the ear (2) | |
| 4. (loss of) hearing due to old age (2) | |
| 5. incision of the eardrum (2) | |
| 6. abnormal hearing (2) | |
| 7. abnormal condition of hardening of the ear (2) | |
| 8. inflammation of the inner ear (2) | |
| 9. condition of no color vision (3) | |
| 10. process of measurement of hearing (2) | |
| 11. inflammation of the tear glands (2) | |
| 12. drooping of the eyelids (2) | |
| 13. pertaining to the nose and tears (3) | |
| 14. condition of aversion to light (2) | |
| 15. process of measurement of pressure (of the eye) (2) | |

*Sort the terms into the correct categories.*

## TERM SORTING

| Anatomy and Physiology | Pathology | Diagnostic Procedures | Therapeutic Interventions |
|---|---|---|---|
|  |  |  |  |
|  |  |  |  |
|  |  |  |  |
|  |  |  |  |
|  |  |  |  |
|  |  |  |  |
|  |  |  |  |
|  |  |  |  |
|  |  |  |  |
|  |  |  |  |

| | | | |
|---|---|---|---|
| accommodation | fovea | otoplasty | slit lamp |
| Amsler grid | gonioscopy | otorrhea | stapedectomy |
| anacusis | IOLs | otosclerosis | stapes |
| audiometer | iridotomy | otoscopy | strabismus |
| cerumen | labyrinth | phacoemulsification | tinnitus |
| chalazion | lacrimation | pinna | tonometry |
| cochlea | miotics | refraction | tympanometry |
| coreoplasty | nyctalopia | sclera | tympanostomy |
| diopters | ophthalmoscopy | scleral buckling | tympanotomy |
| exophthalmia | otalgia | scotoma | VA |

*Replace the highlighted words with the correct terms.*

## TRANSLATIONS

1. Maria was complaining of **extreme sensitivity to light** and **excessive lacrimation**.

2. The pediatrician used an **instrument to view the ear** to diagnose baby Grace's **inflammation of the middle ear**.

3. The auto accident victim came to the ED with **a condition of unequally sized pupils** and **blood in the anterior chamber of the eye**.

4. During Michael's eye examination, it was discovered that he had red/green **impairment of color vision** and slight **nearsightedness**.

5. The 80-year-old patient was evaluated by **one who specializes in the study of hearing** and was found to have **loss of hearing common in old age**.

6. Rose's **disorder characterized by abnormal intraocular pressure** was tested with **measurement of intraocular pressure**.

7. Terrance had **a surgical repair of the eyelids** to correct his **drooping of the upper eyelid**.

8. The patient had **reattachment of the retina with a cryoprobe** to correct a **separation of the retina from the choroid layer**.

9. Mrs. M came to the ED complaining of **an abnormal sound heard in the ear** and **dizziness**.

10. The patient had **a creation of an opening between the tear sac and the nose** to correct a blockage in her **pertaining to tears** sac.

11. A **test to determine the amount of tear production** was used to determine the degree of the patient's **dry eye**.

12. Mary Kate's **inability to see well in dim light** was a result of **a hereditary degenerative disease marked by nyctalopia and a progressive loss of visual field**.

13. A bilateral **surgical repair of the external ear** was performed to correct the patient's **condition of abnormally large auricles**.

14. Carl's **hearing loss** was caused by a **development of bone around the oval window**.

## *Case Study*  Mary Ellen Wright

Mary Ellen Wright has had moderate vision problems for much of her life. She has worn glasses since she was 10 years old. She tried contacts a couple of times, but could not get used to them. Today she is visiting her optometrist, Dr. Roland O'Connor, for her annual checkup. She is planning to ask him if he thinks she is a candidate for LASIK surgery.

Mary Ellen has astigmatism. Because it has always been diligently treated with eyeglasses, she has no muscle weakening, but her blurred vision is beginning to get worse. Dr. O'Connor performs routine ophthalmoscopy and slit lamp exam on Mary Ellen. Then the doctor uses fluorescein staining to visualize the abnormalities on Mary Ellen's cornea.

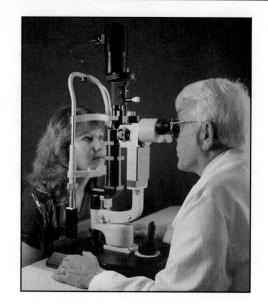

After a thorough examination, Dr. O'Connor talks to Mary Ellen about LASIK. He thinks she is an excellent candidate for such a procedure. He gives her a list of recommended doctors that perform LASIK and other procedures. Mary Ellen has the procedure done and very soon is seeing 20/20 again. She gratefully donates her glasses to charity.

### ⟳ Medical Letter

*Using the medical letter on p. 561, answer the following questions.*

1. Mary Ellen denies diplopia and cephalgia. Explain these terms.

   _____

   _____

2. Mary Ellen has been diagnosed with myopic astigmatism. In your own words, explain this visual disorder.

   _____

3. What is the name of the test for glaucoma? _____

4. Explain the term paralimbal. _____

---

For more interactive learning, click on:
- **Whack-a-Word**-Part to review eye and ear word parts.
- **Wheel of Terminology** and **Word Shop** to practice word building.
- **Tournament of Terminology** to test your knowledge of eye and ear terms.
- **Terminology Triage** to practice sorting eye and ear terms into categories.

**O'Connor Eye Associates**
456 Humphrey St.
Philadelphia, PA 19117

Morgan Ophthalmology Associates
789 Henry Ave.
Philadelphia, PA 19118

August 12, 2012

Re: Mary Ellen Wright, DOB: 4/1/1974

Dear Dr. Morgan:

I have had the pleasure of treating Mary Ellen Wright for the past 11 years. She has asked me to summarize her treatment for you.

Ms. Wright had received comprehensive optometric care from her previous optometrist from 1995 to 2001. Her previous records reflected good binocular oculomotor function and good ocular health, including the absence of posterior vitreous detachment, retinal breaks, or peripheral retinal degeneration in either eye. She specifically denies any incidence of trauma, diplopia, or cephalgia. She also denies any personal or family history of glaucoma, strabismus, retinal disease, diabetes, hypertension, heart disease, or breathing problems. She is on no medications. Entrance tests, such as EOMs, pupils, color vision, confrontation fields, and cover test, appeared unchanged from previously reported exams. Refractive correction for compound myopic astigmatism contained the following parameters:

Spectacle Correction: Right eye −7.50−1.00 × 165 20/20
                                    Left eye −7.50−1.00 × 180 20/20

Contact Lenses: Right eye 20/15; Left eye 20/15

The contact lens fit showed a stable paralimbal soft lens fit with good centration, 360 degree corneal coverage, and 0.50 mm movement in each eye. Each lens surface contained a trace amount of scattered protein deposits.

She came for her last comprehensive examination without any visual or ocular complaints. She desired a new supply of disposable contact lenses. She reported clear and comfortable vision at distance, intermediate, and near with both her glasses and contact lenses.

Eye Health Assessment: Slit lamp examination revealed clean lids with good tonicity and apposition to the globe. The lashes and lid margins were clear of debris. There was no discharge either eye. The corneas were clear with no fluorescein staining either eye. Pupils were equal, round, and reactive to light and accommodation without afferent defect. Intraocular pressures measured 10 mm Hg right eye, left eye at 1:30 pm with Goldmann applanation tonometry.

If any further information is needed, please feel free to contact me regarding this patient.

Sincerely,

*Roland O'Connor, OD*

# 15

*If I'd known I was gonna live this long, I'd have taken better care of myself.*
**—Eubie Blake at age 100**

## OBJECTIVES

- Recognize and use terms related to the anatomy and physiology of the endocrine system.
- Recognize and use terms related to the pathology of the endocrine system.
- Recognize and use terms related to the diagnostic procedures for the endocrine system.
- Recognize and use terms related to the therapeutic interventions for the endocrine system.

# Endocrine System

## CHAPTER AT A GLANCE

*Use this list of word parts and key terms to assess your knowledge. Check off the ones you have mastered.*

### ANATOMY AND PHYSIOLOGY

- [ ] adenohypophysis
- [ ] adrenal cortex
- [ ] adrenal medulla
- [ ] endocrine gland
- [ ] hormones
- [ ] insulin
- [ ] islets of Langerhans
- [ ] neurohypophysis
- [ ] oxytocin
- [ ] pancreas
- [ ] parathyroid gland
- [ ] parathyroid hormone
- [ ] pituitary gland
- [ ] thymus gland
- [ ] thyroid gland
- [ ] vasopressin

### KEY WORD PARTS

#### PREFIXES
- [ ] an-
- [ ] endo-
- [ ] exo-, ex-
- [ ] hypo-
- [ ] poly-

#### SUFFIXES
- [ ] -crine
- [ ] -ia
- [ ] -oma

#### COMBINING FORMS
- [ ] aden/o
- [ ] adren/o
- [ ] calc/o
- [ ] crin/o
- [ ] gluc/o, glyc/o
- [ ] gonad/o
- [ ] hypophys/o
- [ ] kal/i
- [ ] lob/o
- [ ] natr/o
- [ ] ophthalm/o
- [ ] orex/o
- [ ] pancreat/o
- [ ] thalam/o
- [ ] thym/o
- [ ] thyr/o, thyroid/o
- [ ] trop/o

### KEY TERMS

- [ ] A1c
- [ ] acromegaly
- [ ] anorexia
- [ ] Cushing disease
- [ ] diabetes insipidus (DI)
- [ ] diabetes mellitus (DM)
- [ ] exophthalmia
- [ ] fasting plasma glucose (FPG)
- [ ] glucometer
- [ ] glucosuria
- [ ] growth hormone deficiency (GHD)
- [ ] hypercalcemia
- [ ] hyperthyroidism
- [ ] hypoglycemia
- [ ] hypokalemia
- [ ] hyponatremia
- [ ] hypothyroidism
- [ ] ketonuria
- [ ] pancreatectomy
- [ ] paresthesia
- [ ] polydipsia
- [ ] polyphagia
- [ ] polyuria
- [ ] thymoma
- [ ] thyroid function tests (TFTs)
- [ ] thyroidectomy
- [ ] type 1 diabetes
- [ ] type 2 diabetes

**endocrine**
    **endo-** = within
    **-crine** = to secrete

**endocrinology**
    **endo-** = within
    **crin/o** = to secrete
    **-logy** = study of

⊗ Be Careful!

*Do not confuse **aden/o**, which means gland, with **adren/o**, which means the adrenal gland.*

**pituitary gland** =
hypophys/o, pituitar/o

**gland** = aden/o

## FUNCTIONS OF THE ENDOCRINE SYSTEM

The **endocrine** (EN doh krin) system assists in the function of achieving the delicate physiologic balance necessary for survival. The endocrine system uses the circulatory system and chemical messengers called **hormones** to regulate a number of body functions, including metabolism, growth, reproduction, and water and electrolyte balances.

## SPECIALISTS/SPECIALTIES

**Endocrinology** is the study of the glands that secrete hormones within the body. An **endocrinologist** is a medical doctor who diagnoses and treats diseases and disorders of the endocrine system.

## ANATOMY AND PHYSIOLOGY

The endocrine system is composed of several single and paired ductless glands that secrete hormones into the bloodstream. The hormones regulate specific body functions by acting on target cells with receptor sites for those particular hormones only. See Fig. 15-1 for an illustration of the body with the locations of the endocrine glands.

### Pituitary Gland

The **pituitary** (pih TOO ih tare ree) **gland**, also known as the **hypophysis** (hye POFF ih sis), is a tiny gland located behind the optic nerve in the cranial cavity. Sometimes called the *master gland* because of its role in controlling the

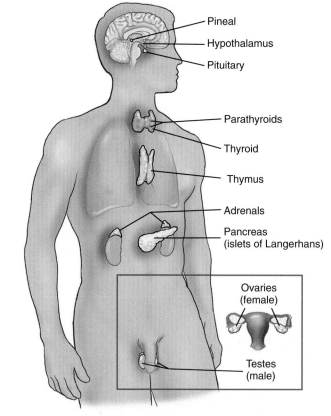

**Fig. 15-1** Locations of the endocrine glands.

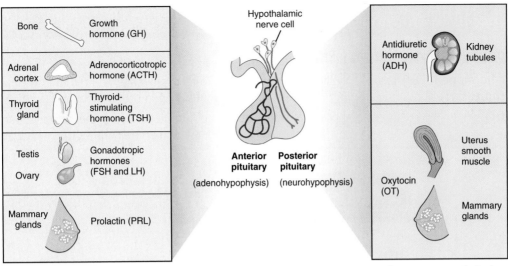

**Fig. 15-2** Pituitary hormones. Principal anterior and posterior pituitary hormones and their target organs.

## Adenohypophysis Hormones and Their Effects

| Adenohypophysis Hormone | Effect |
|---|---|
| **Adrenocorticotropic hormone (ACTH)** | Stimulates the adrenal cortex to release steroids. |
| **Gonadotropic hormones** (include **follicle-stimulating hormone [FSH]**, **luteinizing hormone [LH]**, and **interstitial cell-stimulating hormone [ICSH]**) | FSH stimulates the development of gametes in the respective sexes. LH stimulates ovulation in the female and the secretion of sex hormones in both the male and the female. ICSH stimulates production of reproductive cells in the male. |
| **Growth hormone (GH)** (also called **human growth hormone [hGH]** or **somatotropin hormone [STH]**) | Stimulates growth of long bones and skeletal muscle; converts proteins to glucose. |
| **Prolactin (PRL)** (also called **lactogenic hormone**) | Stimulates milk production in the breast. |
| **Thyrotropin** (also called **thyroid-stimulating hormone [TSH]**) | Stimulates thyroid to release two other thyroid hormones. |

**⊗ Be Careful!**    *The combining form* **trop/o** *means turning, whereas* **troph/o** *means development or nourishment.*

functions of other endocrine glands, it is composed of anterior and posterior lobes, each with its own functions.

The **anterior lobe**, or **adenohypophysis** (add uh noh hye POFF ih sis), is composed of glandular tissue and secretes myriad hormones in response to stimulation by the hypothalamus. The **hypothalamus** sends hormones through blood vessels, which cause the adenohypophysis either to release or to inhibit the release of specific hormones. The adenohypophysis has a wide range of effects on the body, as Fig. 15-2 and the table above illustrate.

The **posterior lobe (neurohypophysis)** of the pituitary gland is composed of nervous tissue. The hormones that it secretes are produced in the hypothalamus, transported to the neurohypophysis directly through the tissue connecting the organs, and released from storage in the posterior lobe by neural stimulation from the hypothalamus. The two hormones released by this lobe are **antidiuretic hormone (ADH)** and **oxytocin (OT).** See the following table and Fig. 15-2 for the hormones secreted by the neurohypophysis and their effects.

**turning** = trop/o

**lobe** = lob/o

**hypothalamus**
  hypo- = under
  thalam/o = thalamus
  -us = structure

## Neurohypophysis Hormones and Their Effects

| Neurohypophysis Hormone | Effect |
|---|---|
| Antidiuretic hormone (ADH) (also called **vasopressin**) | Stimulates the kidneys to reabsorb water and return it to circulation; is also a vasoconstrictor, resulting in higher blood pressure. |
| Oxytocin (OT) | Stimulates the muscles of the uterus during the delivery of an infant and the muscles surrounding the mammary ducts to contract, releasing milk. |

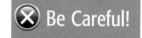 **Be Careful!**  *Oxytocin* should not be confused with **oxytocia**, which means a rapid delivery.

### Thyroid Gland

**thyroid gland** = thyr/o, thyroid/o

**calcium** = calc/o

The **thyroid gland** is a single organ located in the anterior part of the neck. It regulates the metabolism of the body and normal growth and development, and controls the amount of calcium (Ca) deposited into bone. The following table describes the hormones secreted by the thyroid and their effects.

## Thyroid Gland Hormones and Their Effects

| Thyroid Gland Hormone | Effect |
|---|---|
| Calcitonin | Regulates the amount of calcium in the bloodstream. |
| Tetraiodothyronine (also called **thyroxine [T4]**) | Increases cell metabolism. |
| Triiodothyronine (T3) | Increases cell metabolism. |

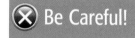 **Be Careful!**  *Don't confuse* **calc/o**, *meaning calcium, with* **calic/o**, *meaning calyx, and* **kal/i**, *meaning potassium.*

### Parathyroid Glands

**parathyroid gland** = parathyroid/o

The **parathyroids** (pair uh THIGH royds) are four small glands located on the posterior surface of the thyroid gland in the neck. They secrete **parathyroid hormone (PTH)** in response to a low level of calcium in the blood. When low calcium is detected, the PTH increases calcium by causing it to be released from the bone, which results in calcium reabsorption by the kidneys and the digestive system. PTH is inhibited by high levels of calcium.

### Adrenal Glands (Suprarenals)

**adrenal gland** = adren/o

**suprarenal**
  supra- = above
  ren/o = kidney
  -al = pertaining to

**cortex** = cortic/o

**medulla** = medull/o

The **adrenal** (uh DREE nul) **glands,** also called the **suprarenals,** are paired, one on top of each kidney. Different hormones are secreted by the two different parts of these glands: the external portion called the **adrenal cortex** (uh DREE nul KORE tecks) and an internal portion called the **adrenal medulla** (uh DREE nul muh DOO lah).

The adrenal cortex secretes three hormones that are called steroids.

The adrenal medulla is the inner portion of the adrenal gland. It produces sympathomimetic hormones that stimulate the fight-or-flight response to stress, similar to the action of the sympathetic nervous system.

To view an animation of adrenal gland functions, click on **Animations.**

## Adrenal Cortex Hormones and Their Effects

| Adrenal Cortex Hormones | Effect |
|---|---|
| Glucocorticoids (e.g., cortisol [hydrocortisone]) | Respond to stress; have antiinflammatory properties. |
| Mineralocorticoids (e.g., aldosterone) | Regulate blood volume, blood pressure, and electrolytes. |
| Sex hormones (e.g., estrogen, androgen) | Responsible for secondary sex characteristics. |

## Adrenal Medulla Hormones and Their Effects

| Adrenal Medulla Hormones (Catecholamines) | Effect |
|---|---|
| Dopamine | Dilates arteries and increases production of urine, blood pressure, and cardiac rate. Acts as a neurotransmitter in the nervous system. |
| Epinephrine (also called **adrenaline**) | Dilates bronchi, increases heart rate, raises blood pressure, dilates pupils, and elevates blood sugar levels. |
| Norepinephrine (also called **noradrenaline**) | Increases heart rate and blood pressure and elevates blood sugar levels for energy use. |

## Pancreas

The pancreas, located inferior and posterior to the stomach, is a gland with both exocrine and endocrine functions. The **exocrine function** is to release digestive enzymes through a duct into the small intestines. The **endocrine function,** accomplished through a variety of types of cells called **islets of Langerhans** (EYE lets of LANG gur hahnz), is to regulate the level of glucose in the blood by stimulating the liver. The two main types of islets of Langerhans cells are alpha and beta cells. Alpha cells produce the hormone glucagon that increases the level of glucose in the blood when levels are low. Beta cells secrete **insulin** (IN suh lin) that decreases the level of glucose in the blood when levels are high. Insulin is needed to transport glucose out of the bloodstream and into the cells. In the absence of glucose in the cells, proteins and fats are broken down, causing excessive fatty acids and **ketones** in the blood. Normally, these hormones regulate glucose levels through the metabolism of fats, carbohydrates, and proteins.

**pancreas** = pancreat/o

**exocrine**
    exo- = outward
    -crine = to secrete

**glucose, sugar** = gluc/o, glyc/o

## Thymus Gland

The **thymus** (THIGH mus) gland is located in the mediastinum above the heart. It releases a hormone called **thymosin** that is responsible for stimulating key cells in the immune response. For more detail, see Chapter 9 on the blood, lymphatic, and immune systems.

**thymus gland** = thym/o

**ketone** = ket/o, keton/o

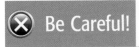 Be Careful!   *Do not confuse **thyr/o**, which means thyroid, and **thym/o,** which means thymus.*

**gonads** = gonad/o

### Ovaries and Testes

The **ovaries** and **testes,** the female and male **gonads,** also act as endocrine glands, which influence reproductive functions.

### Pineal Gland

The **pineal** (PIH nee ul) gland is located in the center of the brain, functioning to secrete the hormone **melatonin,** thought to be responsible for inducing sleep.

## Exercise 1: Endocrine Anatomy and Physiology

*Fill in the blanks.*

1. The pituitary gland, or the _____, is called the master gland because of its control over other endocrine glands.

2. The pituitary gland is controlled by the _____.

3. The anterior lobe of the pituitary gland is also known as the _____.

4. The thyroid gland is responsible for regulation of the body's _____ and

   controls the amount of _____ deposited into bone.

5. Adrenal glands are named for their location above the _____.

6. The inner part of the adrenal gland is the adrenal _____, whereas the

   outer part of the adrenal gland is the adrenal _____.

7. The endocrine function of the pancreas is to regulate glucose in the blood through its hormones

   _____ and _____.

8. Fatty acids and _____ are produced if glucose cannot pass out of the

   bloodstream and into the cells to be metabolized.

9. The thymus gland is located in the _____ above the heart and is

   responsible for stimulating key cells in the _____ response.

10. The _____ gland is located in the center of the brain, functioning to

   secrete the hormone _____, thought to be responsible for inducing _____.

*Match the endocrine word parts with their definitions.*

____ 11. -al

____ 12. aden/o

____ 13. hypophys/o

____ 14. lob/o

____ 15. thalam/o

____ 16. thyr/o

____ 17. calc/o

____ 18. parathyroid/o

____ 19. adren/o

____ 20. ren/o

____ 21. cortic/o

____ 22. medull/o

____ 23. pancreat/o

____ 24. gluc/o

____ 25. thym/o

____ 26. ket/o

____ 27. gonad/o

____ 28. trop/o

____ 29. endo-

____ 30. supra-

____ 31. exo-

____ 32. hypo-

____ 33. -crine

____ 34. -logy

____ 35. -us

A. kidney
B. above
C. to secrete
D. calcium
E. outside
F. turning
G. sugar
H. structure
I. gland with exocrine and endocrine functions
J. reproductive organ
K. gland
L. the study of
M. medulla
N. within
O. ketone
P. gland in mediastinum
Q. pertaining to
R. master gland
S. under
T. suprarenal gland
U. cortex
V. gland regulating metabolism
W. glands regulating calcium in the blood
X. lobe
Y. thalamus

*Decode the terms.*

36. perithyroidal _____

37. hypoglycemic _____

38. retropancreatic _____

39. interlobar _____

Choose **Hear It, Spell It** to practice spelling the anatomy and physiology terms you have learned in this chapter. To practice pronouncing anatomy and physiology terms choose **Hear It, Say It.**

## Exercise 2: Endocrine Glands

*Label the drawing below with the correct anatomic terms and accompanying combining forms where appropriate.*

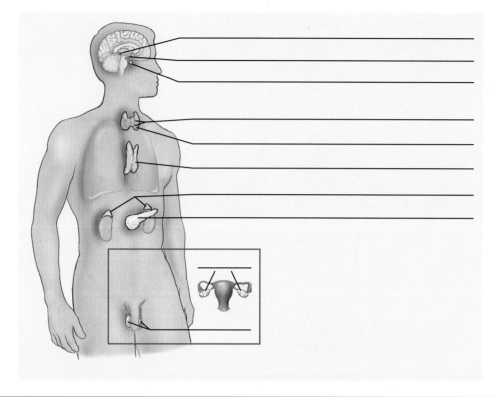

## Combining and Adjective Forms for the Anatomy and Physiology of the Endocrine System

| Meaning | Combining Form | Adjective Form |
|---|---|---|
| adrenal gland | adren/o, adrenal/o | adrenal |
| calcium | calc/o | |
| cortex | cortic/o | cortical |
| gland | aden/o | |
| glucose, sugar | gluc/o, glyc/o, glucos/o | |
| gonads | gonad/o | gonadal |
| ketone | ket/o, keton/o | |
| kidney | ren/o, nephr/o | renal |
| lobe | lob/o | lobar |
| medulla | medull/o | medullary |
| pancreas | pancreat/o | pancreatic |
| parathyroid gland | parathyroid/o | parathyroidal |
| pituitary gland | hypophys/o, pituitar/o | hypophyseal |
| thalamus | thalam/o | thalamic |
| thymus gland | thym/o | thymic |
| thyroid gland | thyr/o, thyroid/o | thyroidal |
| to secrete | crin/o | |
| turning | trop/o | tropic |

## Prefixes for the Anatomy of the Endocrine System

| Prefix | Meaning |
|--------|---------|
| endo- | within |
| exo- | outward |
| hypo- | under |
| supra- | above |

## Suffixes for the Anatomy of the Endocrine System

| Suffix | Meaning |
|--------|---------|
| -al | pertaining to |
| -crine | to secrete |
| -logy | study of |
| -us, -is | structure |

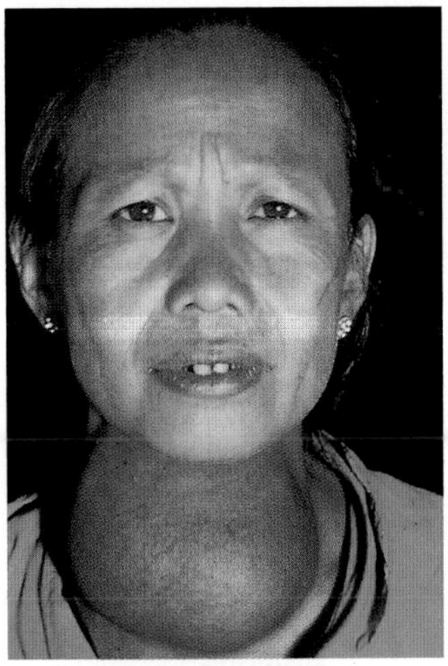

Fig. 15-3 Goiter.

## PATHOLOGY

Most of the pathology of the endocrine system is the result of either *hyper-* (too much) or *hypo-* (too little) hormonal secretion. Developmental issues also play a role in determining when the malfunction occurs and what the results will be.

## Terms Related to Signs and Symptoms of Endocrine Disorders

| Term | Word Origin | Definition |
|------|-------------|------------|
| **anorexia**<br>an oh RECK see ah | *an-* without<br>*orex/o* appetite<br>*-ia* condition | Lack of **appetite**. Anorexia nervosa is an eating disorder. |
| **exophthalmia**<br>eck soff THAL mee ah | *ex-* out<br>*ophthalm/o* eye<br>*-ia* condition | Protrusion of eyeballs from their orbits (see Fig. 14-8). |
| **glucosuria**<br>gloo koh SOOR ee ah | *glucos/o* sugar, glucose<br>*-uria* urinary condition | Presence of glucose in the urine. May indicate diabetes mellitus. Also called **glycosuria**. |
| **goiter**<br>GOY tur | | Enlargement of the thyroid gland, not due to a tumor (Fig. 15-3). |

*Continued*

## Terms Related to Signs and Symptoms of Endocrine Disorders—cont'd

| Term | Word Origin | Definition |
|------|-------------|------------|
| **hirsutism**<br>HUR soo tiz um | | Abnormal hairiness, especially in women (Fig. 15-4). Also called **hypertrichosis**. |
| **hypocalcemia**<br>hye poh kal SEE mee ah | *hypo-* deficient<br>*calc/o* calcium<br>*-emia* blood condition | Condition of deficient calcium (Ca) in the blood. The opposite would be **hypercalcemia**—excessive calcium in the blood. |
| **hypoglycemia**<br>hye poh gly SEE mee ah | *hypo-* deficient<br>*glyc/o* sugar, glucose<br>*-emia* blood condition | Condition of deficient sugar in the blood. The opposite would be **hyperglycemia**—excessive sugar in the blood. |
| **hypokalemia**<br>hye poh kuh LEE mee ah | *hypo-* deficient<br>*kal/i* potassium<br>*-emia* blood condition | Condition of deficient potassium (K) in the blood. The opposite would be **hyperkalemia**—excessive potassium in the blood. |
| **hyponatremia**<br>hye poh nuh TREE mee ah | *hypo-* deficient<br>*natr/o* sodium<br>*-emia* blood condition | Condition of deficient sodium (Na) in the blood. The opposite would be **hypernatremia**—excessive sodium in the blood. |
| **ketoacidosis**<br>kee toh ass ih DOH sis | *ket/o* ketone<br>*acid/o* acid<br>*-osis* abnormal condition | Excessive number of ketone acids in the bloodstream. |
| **ketonuria**<br>kee toh NOOR ee ah | *keton/o* ketone<br>*-uria* urinary condition | Presence of ketones in urine. |
| **paresthesia**<br>pair uh STHEE zsa | *par-* abnormal<br>*esthesi/o* feeling<br>*-ia* condition | Abnormal sensation, such as prickling. |
| **polydipsia**<br>pah lee DIP see ah | *poly-* excessive<br>*-dipsia* condition of thirst | Condition of excessive thirst. |
| **polyphagia**<br>pah lee FAY jee ah | *poly-* excessive<br>*phag/o* to eat, swallow<br>*-ia* condition | Condition of excessive appetite. |
| **polyuria**<br>pah lee YOO ree ah | *poly-* excessive<br>*ur/o* urine<br>*-ia* condition | Condition of excessive urination. |
| **tetany**<br>TET uh nee | | Continuous muscle spasms. |

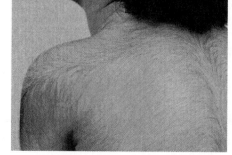

**Fig. 15-4** Hirsutism.

## Exercise 3: Signs and Symptoms

___ 1. goiter     ___ 6. anorexia

___ 2. hirsutism     ___ 7. polyphagia

___ 3. tetany     ___ 8. polyuria

___ 4. polydipsia     ___ 9. ketonuria

___ 5. exophthalmia     ___ 10. ketoacidosis

A. condition of excessive appetite
B. presence of ketones in urine
C. condition of excessive urination
D. enlargement of thyroid gland
E. abnormal hairiness
F. condition of excessive thirst
G. lack of appetite
H. protrusion of eyeballs from orbits
I. excessive quantity of ketone acids in blood
J. continuous muscle spasms

*Decode the terms.*

11. hypoglycemia _____

12. paresthesia _____

13. hypercalcemia _____

*Build the terms.*

14. condition of deficient sodium in the blood _____

15. condition of excessive potassium in the blood _____

16. condition of glucose in the urine _____

## Terms Related to Pituitary Gland Disorders

| Term | Word Origin | Definition |
|---|---|---|
| **acromegaly**<br>ack roh MEG uh lee | *acro-* extremities<br>*-megaly* enlargement | Hypersecretion of somatotropin from the adenohypophysis during adulthood; leads to an enlargement of the extremities (hands and feet), jaw, nose, and forehead (Fig. 15-5). Usually caused by an adenoma of the pituitary gland. |
| **diabetes insipidus (DI)**<br>dye ah BEE teez in SIP ih dus | | Deficiency of antidiuretic hormone (ADH), which causes the patient to excrete large quantities of urine **(polyuria)** and exhibit excessive thirst **(polydipsia)**. |

*Continued*

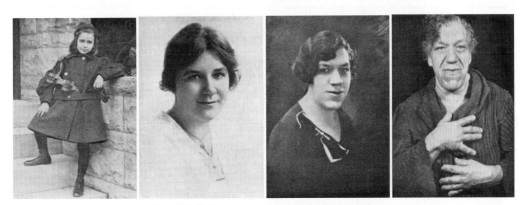

**Fig. 15-5** The progression of acromegaly.

## Terms Related to Pituitary Gland Disorders—cont'd

| Term | Word Origin | Definition |
|---|---|---|
| **gigantism**<br>jye GAN tiz um | | Hypersecretion of somatotropin from adenohypophysis during childhood, leading to excessive growth. |
| **growth hormone deficiency (GHD)** | | Somatotropin deficiency due to dysfunction of adeno-hypophysis during childhood results in dwarfism (Fig. 15-6). If during adulthood, patients may develop obesity and may experience weakness and cardiac difficulties. |
| **panhypopituitarism**<br>pan hye poh pih TOO ih tur iz um | *pan-* all<br>*hypo-* deficient<br>*pituitar/o* pituitary<br>*-ism* condition | Deficiency or lack of all pituitary hormones causing hypotension, weight loss, weakness, and loss of libido; also called **Simmonds disease**. |
| **syndrome of inappropriate antidiuretic hormone (SIADH)** | | Oversecretion of ADH from the neurohypophysis leading to severe hyponatremia and the inability to excrete diluted urine. |

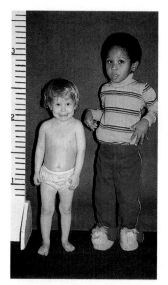

**Fig. 15-6** The normal 3½-year-old boy is in the 50th percentile for height. The short, 3-year-old girl exhibits the characteristic "kewpie doll" appearance, suggesting a diagnosis of growth hormone (GH) deficiency.

## Terms Related to Thyroid Disorders

| Term | Word Origin | Definition |
|------|-------------|------------|
| **hyperthyroidism** <br> hye pur THIGH roy diz um | *hyper-* excessive <br> *thyroid/o* thyroid gland <br> *-ism* condition | Excessive thyroid hormone production; also called **thyrotoxicosis**, the most common form of which is **Graves disease**, which may be accompanied by exophthalmia. Ketonuria is a diagnostic sign. |
| **hypothyroidism** <br> hye poh THIGH roy diz um | *hypo-* deficient <br> *thyroid/o* thyroid gland <br> *-ism* condition | Deficient thyroid hormone production. If it occurs during childhood, it causes a condition called **cretinism**, which results in stunted mental and physical growth. The extreme adult form is called **myxedema** (mick suh DEE mah), which is characterized by facial and orbital edema. |

## Terms Related to Parathyroid Disorders

| Term | Word Origin | Definition |
|------|-------------|------------|
| **hyperparathyroidism** <br> hye pur pair uh THIGH roy diz um | *hyper-* excessive <br> *parathyroid/o* parathyroid gland <br> *-ism* condition | Overproduction of parathyroid hormone; symptoms include polyuria, hypercalcemia, hypertension, and kidney stones. |
| **hypoparathyroidism** <br> hye poh pair uh THIGH roy diz um | *hypo-* deficient <br> *parathyroid/o* parathyroid gland <br> *-ism* condition | Deficient parathyroid hormone production results in tetany, hypocalcemia, irritability, and muscle cramps. |

## Terms Related to Adrenal Gland Disorders

| Term | Word Origin | Definition |
|------|-------------|------------|
| **Addison disease** <br> ADD ih sun | | Insufficient secretion of adrenal cortisol from the adrenal cortex is manifested by gastric complaints, hypotension, fatigue, and hyperpigmentation of skin and mucous membranes (Fig. 15-7). |
| **Cushing disease** <br> CUSH ing | | Excessive secretion of cortisol by the adrenal cortex causes symptoms of obesity, leukocytosis, hirsutism, hypokalemia, hyperglycemia, and muscle wasting (Fig. 15-8). |

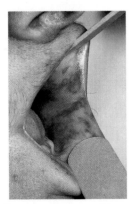

Fig. 15-7 Pigmentation of buccal membranes caused by Addison disease.

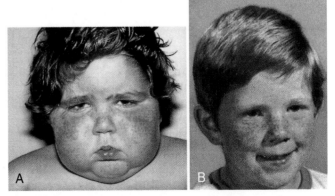

Fig. 15-8 Cushing disease. **A,** First diagnosed with Cushing disease. **B,** Four months later after treatment.

## Terms Related to Pancreas (Islets of Langerhans) Disorders

| Term | Word Origin | Definition |
| --- | --- | --- |
| diabetes mellitus (DM) | | Diabetes mellitus is a group of metabolic disorders characterized by high glucose levels that result from inadequate amounts of insulin, resistance to insulin, or a combination of both. |
| gestational diabetes | | Insulin resistance acquired during pregnancy. Usually resolves after birth, although some women develop type 2 diabetes later in life. |
| hyperinsulinism<br>hye pur IN suh lin iz um | *hyper-* excessive<br>*insulin/o* insulin<br>*-ism* condition | Oversecretion of insulin; seen in some newborns of diabetic mothers. Causes severe hypoglycemia. |
| prediabetes | | A condition in which an individual's blood glucose level is higher than normal, but not high enough for a diagnosis of type 2 diabetes. |
| type 1 diabetes | | Total lack of insulin production resulting in glycosuria, polydipsia, polyphagia, polyuria, blurred vision, fatigue, and frequent infections. Thought to be an autoimmune disorder. Previously called **insulin-dependent diabetes mellitus (IDDM)**. |
| type 2 diabetes | | Deficient insulin production, with symptoms similar to type 1 diabetes. Cause unknown but associated with obesity and family history; previously called **non–insulin-dependent diabetes mellitus (NIDDM)**. |

## Nutritional Recommendations for Persons With Diabetes

| Recommendation | Description |
| --- | --- |
| Calories | Sufficient to achieve and maintain reasonable weight. |
| Carbohydrates | May be up to 45%-55% of total calories. Emphasis is on unrefined carbohydrates with fiber; modest amounts of sucrose and other refined sugars may be acceptable contingent on diabetes control and body weight. |
| Protein | Usual intake is double the amount needed; exact ideal percentage of total calories is unknown; usually, intake is 10%-20%. |
| Fat | Ideally, less than 30% of total calories; must be individualized because 30% may be too low for some individuals.<br>• Polyunsaturated fats: 6%-8%<br>• Saturated fats: <10%<br>• Monounsaturated fats: remaining percentage |
| Fiber | Up to 40 g/day; 25 g/1000 cal for low-calorie diet. |
| Alternative sweeteners | Use of various nutritive and nonnutritive sweeteners is acceptable. |
| Sodium | 1000 mg/1000 cal, not to exceed 3000 mg/day; modified for those with special medical conditions. |
| Vitamins/minerals | No evidence that diabetes influences vitamin/mineral needs. |

## Exercise 4: Diseases and Disorders of the Endocrine System

*Fill in the blanks with the following choices.*

**type 2 diabetes, pituitary, cortex, SIADH, hypoparathyroidism, thyroid, hormones, cretinism, myxedema, type 1 diabetes**

1. Most endocrine disorders are the result of an abnormal secretion of _____.

2. Graves disease is a disorder of the _____ gland.

3. Addison and Cushing diseases are endocrine disorders of the adrenal _____.

4. Diabetes insipidus is a disorder of the _____.

5. _____ is characterized by tetany.

6. Hypothyroidism in childhood results in _____ and _____ in adults.

7. _____ is the result of oversecretion of ADH.

8. Lack of insulin leads to _____. Deficient insulin production leads to _____.

*Decode the terms.*

9. hyperinsulinism _____

10. hypothyroidism _____

11. acromegaly _____

## Terms Related to Benign Neoplasms

| Term | Word Origin | Definition |
|---|---|---|
| **pheochromocytoma** <br> fee oh kroh mah sye TOH mah | *phe/o* dark <br> *chrom/o* color <br> *cyt/o* cell <br> *-oma* tumor, mass | Usually benign tumor of the adrenal medulla. |
| **prolactinoma** <br> pro lack tih NOH mah | *prolactin/o* prolactin <br> *-oma* tumor, mass | Most common type of pituitary tumor (Fig. 15-9). Causes the pituitary to oversecrete prolactin. |
| **thymoma** <br> thigh MOH mah | *thym/o* thymus <br> *-oma* tumor, mass | Noncancerous tumor of epithelial origin that is often associated with myasthenia gravis. |

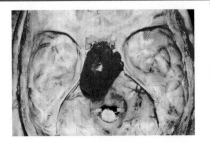

Fig. 15-9 Pituitary tumor.

## Terms Related to Malignant Neoplasms

| Term | Word Origin | Definition |
|------|-------------|------------|
| **islet cell carcinoma**<br>EYE let | *carcin/o* epithelial cancer<br>*-oma* tumor, mass | Pancreatic cancer; fourth leading cause of cancer death in the United States. Treated with a Whipple procedure (pancreatoduodenectomy). |
| **malignant thymoma**<br>thigh MOH mah | *thym/o* thymus gland<br>*-oma* tumor, mass | Rare cancer of the thymus gland. |
| **thyroid carcinoma**<br>kar sih NOH mah | *carcin/o* epithelial cancer<br>*-oma* tumor, mass | The most common types of thyroid carcinoma are follicular and papillary. Both have high 5-year survival rates. |

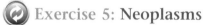

## Exercise 5: Neoplasms

*Match the neoplasms with their definitions.*

____ 1. malignant thymoma

____ 2. islet cell carcinoma

____ 3. pheochromocytoma

____ 4. thyroid carcinoma

____ 5. thymoma

____ 6. prolactinoma

A. most common type of pituitary tumor
B. rare cancer of the thymus gland
C. most common thyroid cancer
D. benign tumor of adrenal medulla
E. benign thymus tumor
F. pancreatic cancer

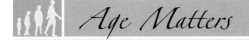

## Age Matters

### Pediatrics

On the whole, children do not suffer from many endocrine disorders. Congenitally, growth hormone deficiency and gigantism cause extremes in height, and some children are born with type 1 diabetes.

### Geriatrics

The major impact of the endocrine system on the elderly is seen in the consequences of the complications of diabetes. Uncontrolled diabetes can lead to amputations and blindness, which severely limit a senior's mobility.

## Case Study    Omanike Mwangi

Omanike Mwangi is a 54-year-old newspaper editor who is 5'6' and weighs 186 lbs. She has been type 2 diabetic for 15 years and recently has had to begin taking insulin to try to keep her glucose level under control. Because she has had difficulty in the past controlling her blood sugars, and because she smokes, she has begun to have problems with her vision and has suffered from periodic foot ulcers. In the past, she has not been compliant with her medications or diet, but the loss of vision has spurred her to try to keep her blood sugars under control and to exercise more, although she is finding it hard to stop smoking.

Omanike calls her doctor one day and tells him that the ulcerous sore on her left foot refuses to heal, even with the antibiotic therapy he had prescribed, and that the foot is now red and swollen. He tells her that she needs to be admitted to the hospital to have the ulcer treated.

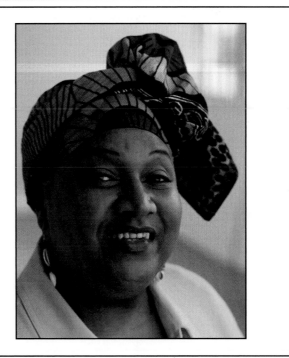

## Case Study    Omanike Mwangi

MWANGI, OMANIKE - 640597 Opened by SUSINO, MARIA MD    ☐ ☐ ☒

Task   Edit   View   Time Scale   Options   Help

[toolbar icons]    As Of 13:11

**MWANGI, OMANIKE**          Age: 54 years      Sex: Female      Loc: WHC-SMMC
                             DOB: 07/18/1958    MRN: 640597      FIN: 3506004

| Reference Text Browser | Form Browser | Medication Profile |

| Orders | Last 48 Hours | ED | Lab | Radiology | **Assessments** | Surgery | Clinical Notes | Pt. Info | Pt. Schedule | Task List | I & O | MAR |

Flowsheet:  Assessments  ▼  ...   Level:  History and Physical  ▼        ⦿ Table   ○ Group   ○ List

◀ ▶                                                                                                    ◀ ▶

| Navigator                    ✕ |
| ✓    History and Physical      |

**HISTORY OF PRESENT ILLNESS:** Patient has chief complaint of pain and redness in the left foot with underlying history of peripheral vascular disease, insulin-dependent diabetes.

**SUMMARY:** Patient with complex history of slow healing ulcers and pain between the left fourth and fifth toes has been followed with débridement and antibiotic coverage. She has been treated with oral antibiotics without success. Cultures that were drawn have now reported *Pseudomonas*, and she was advised to come in for admission and treatment of her foot ulcer.

**PAST MEDICAL HISTORY:** Significant for insulin-dependent diabetes with subsequent diabetic retinopathy. Patient has also had venous thrombosis in the past.

**HABITS:** Patient has continued to smoke, having quit once in 1995.

**CURRENT MEDICATIONS:** Percocet for pain, Silvadene, Norvasc 5 mg b.i.d. Catapres TTS 2 patch, prednisone 5 mg, Zocor 20 mg day, calcium carbonate, and Keflex 500.

**PHYSICAL EXAM:** She is afebrile with pulse of 110, respirations 20, BP 190/88. HEENT, respirations, cardiac, abdomen all appear normal. Extremities remarkable for erythema on the left foot up to the ankle. Has purulent discharge and open sore between fourth and fifth digits on left foot. Skin otherwise intact on left foot.

**LAB:** Glucose 263, creatinine 0.9, potassium 4.3. Patient's wound culture grew numerous *Pseudomonas*.

**ASSESSMENT:** Patient with vascular disease and now deep nonhealing ulcer of the left foot. Initiate broad-spectrum antibiotic IV therapy while watching her diabetes status cautiously during treatment.

| PROD | MAHAFC | 02 March 2011 | 13:11 |

Click on **Hear It, Spell It** to practice spelling the pathology terms you have learned in this chapter. To see how well you pronounce the pathology terms in this chapter, click on **Hear It, Say It**. To review the pathology terms in this chapter, play **Medical Millionaire**.

## Exercise 6: Admission History & Physical

*Using the form on p. 580, answer the following questions.*

1. Which type (number) of diabetes does this patient have? _____

2. What is the term for the eye disease that the patient has in her past history? _____

3. What particular complication of diabetes mellitus is this patient being seen for? _____

4. What does the term *afebrile* tell you about the patient's temperature? _____

## DIAGNOSTIC PROCEDURES

### Terms Related to Laboratory Tests

| Term | Word Origin | Definition |
|------|-------------|------------|
| A1c | | Measure of average blood glucose during a 3-month time span. Used to monitor response to diabetes treatment. Also called **glycosylated hemoglobin** or **HbA1c**. |
| fasting plasma glucose (FPG) | | After a period of fasting, blood is drawn. The amount of glucose present is used to measure the body's ability to break down and use glucose. 100–125 mg/dL = prediabetes; >126 = diabetes. Previously called **fasting blood sugar (FBS)**. |
| glucometer<br>gloo KAH muh tur | *gluc/o* sugar, glucose<br>*-meter* instrument to measure | An instrument for measurement of blood sugar. |
| hormone tests | | Measure the amount of antidiuretic hormone (ADH), cortisol, growth hormone, or parathyroid hormone in the blood. |
| oral glucose tolerance test (OGTT) | | Blood test to measure the body's response to a concentrated glucose solution. May be used to diagnose diabetes mellitus or gestational diabetes. |
| radioimmunoassay studies (RIA)<br>ray dee oh ih myoo noh ASS say | | Nuclear medicine tests used to tag and detect hormones in the blood through the use of radionuclides. |
| thyroid function tests (TFTs) | | Blood tests done to assess $T_3$, $T_4$, and calcitonin. May be used to evaluate abnormalities of thyroid function. |
| total calcium | | Measures the amount of calcium in the blood. Results may be used to assess parathyroid function, calcium metabolism, or cancerous conditions. |
| urinalysis (UA)<br>yoor in AL ih sis | *urin/o* urine<br>*-lysis* breaking down | Physical, chemical, and microscopic examination of urine. |

*Continued*

## Terms Related to Laboratory Tests—cont'd

| Term | Word Origin | Definition |
| --- | --- | --- |
| urine glucose | | Used as a screen for or to monitor diabetes mellitus; a urine specimen is tested for the presence of glucose. |
| urine ketones<br>KEE tones | | Test to detect presence of ketones in a urine specimen; may indicate diabetes mellitus or hyperthyroidism. |

## Terms Related to Imaging

| Term | Word Origin | Definition |
| --- | --- | --- |
| computed tomography (CT) scan | *tom/o* slice<br>*-graphy* process of recording | May be used to test for bone density in hypoparathyroidism and the size of the adrenal glands in Addison disease. |
| magnetic resonance imaging (MRI) | | May be used to examine changes in the size of soft tissues, for example, the pituitary, pancreas, or hypothalamus. |
| radioactive iodine uptake (RAIU) scan | | May be used to test thyroid function by measuring the gland's ability to concentrate and retain iodine. Useful to test for hyperthyroidism (Fig. 15-10). |
| radiography | *radi/o* ray<br>*-graphy* process of recording | X-rays are done to examine suspected endocrine changes that affect the density or thickness of bone; also may reveal underlying causes of an endocrine disorder. |
| sonography | *son/o* sound<br>*-graphy* process of recording | Aside from visualizing the pancreas (Fig. 15-11), sonography may be used to guide biopsies of the thyroid gland to discern the differences between solid and fluid-filled cysts. |

## Exercise 7: Diagnostic Procedures

*Fill in the blank.*

1. High-frequency sound waves may be used to image the pancreas, adrenals, or thyroid in a procedure called a/an _____.

2. Detailed images of soft tissues, such as the pituitary, pancreas, or hypothalamus, may be acquired through a technique called _____.

3. A test used to monitor a patient's response to diabetes treatment is _____.

4. Parathyroid dysfunction may be detected through a blood test for parathyroid hormone or a test for _____.

5. Which type of test can be used to screen for diabetes mellitus? _____

6. Blood sugar can be measured using a _____.

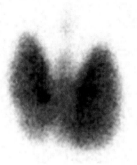

**Fig. 15-10** RAIU demonstrating hyperthyroidism. The thyroid gland absorbed 65% of the iodine.

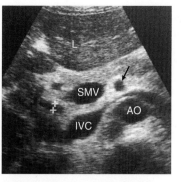

**Fig. 15-11** Transverse scan over the epigastric region of the abdomen, demonstrating a normal pancreas *(cross marks)*. *L*, left lobe of the liver; *AO*, aorta; *IVC*, inferior vena cava; *SMV*, superior mesenteric vein; *arrow*, superior mesenteric artery.

## THERAPEUTIC INTERVENTIONS

Most of the therapeutic interventions for endocrine system disorders are excisions. Unlike the case with other body systems, incisions, repairs, or new openings are not as helpful as the removal of part, or all, of the malfunctioning gland.

### Terms Related to Excisions

| Term | Word Origin | Definition |
|------|-------------|------------|
| **adrenalectomy** uh dree nuh LECK tuh mee | *adrenal/o* adrenal gland *-ectomy* excision | Bilateral removal of the adrenal glands to reduce excess hormone secretion. |
| **hypophysectomy** hye poff uh SECK tuh mee | *hypophys/o* pituitary gland *-ectomy* excision | Excision of the pituitary gland; usually done to remove a pituitary tumor (Fig. 15-12). |
| **pancreatectomy** pan kree uh TECK tuh mee | *pancreat/o* pancreas *-ectomy* excision | Excision of all or part of the pancreas to remove a tumor or to treat an intractable inflammation of the pancreas. |
| **pancreatoduodenectomy** pan kree ah toh doo ah den ECK tuh mee | *pancreat/o* pancreas *duoden/o* duodenum *-ectomy* excision | Excision of the head of the pancreas together with the duodenum; used to treat pancreatic cancer. Also called **Whipple procedure**. |
| **parathyroidectomy** pair uh thigh roy DECK tuh mee | *parathyroid/o* parathyroid gland *-ectomy* excision | Removal of the parathyroid gland, usually to treat hyperparathyroidism. |
| **thyroidectomy** thigh roy DECK tuh mee | *thyroid/o* thyroid gland *-ectomy* excision | Removal of part or all of the thyroid gland to treat goiter, tumors, or hyperthyroidism that does not respond to medication. Removal of most, but not all, of this gland will result in a regrowth of the gland with normal function. If cancer is detected, a total thyroidectomy is performed. |

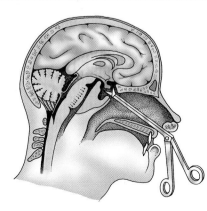

**Fig. 15-12** Hypophysectomy.

## ⊘ Exercise 8: Therapeutic Interventions

*Build the terms.*

1. excision of the pancreas _____

2. excision of the adrenal gland _____

3. excision of the pituitary gland _____

4. excision of the parathyroid gland _____

5. excision of the thyroid gland _____

## PHARMACOLOGY

Most of the pharmacologic interventions for endocrine disorders are provided to correct imbalances, either inhibiting or replacing abnormal hormone levels.

**antidiabetics:** manage glucose levels in the body when the pancreas or insulin receptors are no longer functioning properly. These drugs are also known as hypoglycemic agents and encompass various oral agents and replacement insulin. Type 1 diabetes mellitus typically requires insulin therapy, and management of type 2 diabetes mellitus begins with oral antidiabetics such as metformin (Glucophage), glipizide (Glucotrol), or pioglitazone (Actos); insulin is used as a last resort. See Figs. 15-13 and 15-14 for sites of insulin injection and an insulin pump.

**antithyroid agents:** treat hyperthyroidism. Examples include methimazole (Tapazole) and propylthiouracil (PTU).

**corticosteroids:** mimic or replace the body's steroids normally produced by the adrenal glands. Underfunctioning adrenal cortices (Addison disease) may be treated with prednisone (Deltasone). Corticosteroids are classified as glucosteroids and mineralocorticoids, depending on structure and function.

**growth hormones:** treat various disease-causing growth inhibitions. Examples include somatropin (Genotropin, Nutropin) and somatrem (Protropin).

**posterior pituitary hormones:** vasopressin and desmopressin acetate are used to treat diabetes insipidus.

**thyroid hormones:** treat hypothyroidism. Examples include natural thyroid hormones (Armour Thyroid) and levothyroxine (Levoxyl, Synthroid).

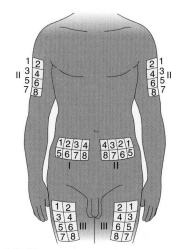

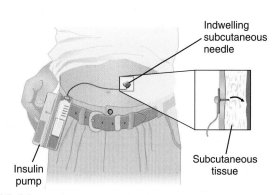

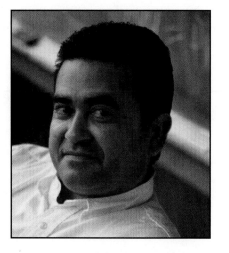

Fig. 15-13 Sites for insulin injection.

Fig. 15-14 Insulin pump. The device is worn externally and is connected to an indwelling subcutaneous needle, usually inserted into the abdomen.

Labels in Fig. 15-14: Indwelling subcutaneous needle; Insulin pump; Subcutaneous tissue.

 Exercise 9: **Pharmacology**

*Match the pharmacologic agent with the correct disease or disorder.*

____ 1. insulin

____ 2. prednisone

____ 3. vasopressin

____ 4. Synthroid

A. Addison disease
B. hypothyroidism
C. diabetes mellitus
D. diabetes insipidus

## *Case Study* *Hector Ramirez*

Hector Ramirez is a 59-year-old business owner who was diagnosed 2 weeks ago with type 2 diabetes. He was prescribed Glucophage and was instructed to work with a dietitian on improving his diet. He has been taking his medication faithfully 4 times a day and has been trying to eat better, although he dislikes counting carbs and misses his pasta and breads.

Last night, he woke up feeling nauseated and vomited twice. He was thirsty but was unable to drink anything because of the nausea. The next morning, he checked his blood sugar and was astounded to see that it was over 600. His wife immediately took him to the ED, where he was diagnosed with uncontrolled type 2 diabetes and was admitted to the hospital so he could be rehydrated and his blood sugars could be brought under control.

## *Case Study*   Hector Ramirez

RAMIREZ, HECTOR J - 500109 Opened by FORESTER, HALLE MD      _ ☐ ✕

Task   Edit   View   Time Scale   Options   Help

As Of 00:12

| **RAMIREZ, HECTOR J** | Age: 59 years | Sex: Male | Loc: WHC-SMMC |
|---|---|---|---|
| | DOB: 02/13/1952 | MRN: 500109 | FIN: 3506004 |

Reference Text Browser  |  Form Browser  |  Medication Profile

Orders | Last 48 Hours | ED | Lab | Radiology | **Assessments** | Surgery | Clinical Notes | Pt. Info | Pt. Schedule | Task List | I & O | MAR

Flowsheet: Assessments    ...    Level: History and Physical     ⦿ Table   ○ Group   ○ List

Navigator      ✕

✓   Assessments

| | |
|---|---|
| **CHIEF COMPLAINT:** | 59-year-old with dehydration and uncontrolled type 2 diabetes. |
| **HISTORY OF PRESENT ILLNESS:** | This 59-year-old male was seen on an outpatient basis approximately 2 weeks ago and was diagnosed with type 2 diabetes. He was started on Glucophage, and he was to see a dietitian. Last night, he reported nausea and emesis × 2. He continues to be quite thirsty and has had polyuria and dry mouth. He started checking his blood sugar with the presentation of these symptoms, and he reports his monitor showed a blood glucose greater than 600 this morning. |
| **PAST MEDICAL HISTORY:** | Hypertension. |
| **CURRENT MEDS:** | Glucophage 500 mg p.o. b.i.d<br>Zestoretic: bid, 20 mg AM/25 mg PM. |
| **FAMILY HISTORY:** | Patient's mother died of congestive heart failure as did his father. Two brothers have died of coronary artery disease. One surviving brother is in good health. |
| **SOCIAL HISTORY:** | Patient owns a business in the area. He was a smoker until approximately 6 weeks ago, at which time he reports he stopped. No alcohol intake. |
| **REVIEW OF SYSTEMS:** | No fever or chills. HEENT, dry mouth. Cardiac: no complaints. Respiratory: no complaints. No other complaints other than those listed in chief complaint. |
| **PHYSICAL EXAMINATION:** | Pleasant man in no acute distress. Vital signs as noted. HEENT, PERRLA, TMs clear bilaterally. Neck supple without lymphadenopathy. Lungs clear to auscultation bilaterally. Abdomen, soft nontender. No clubbing, cyanosis, or edema. Normal reflexes. |
| **ASSESSMENT AND PLAN:** | 1. Dehydration—will rehydrate with IV fluids.<br>2. Uncontrolled type 2 diabetes. This is probably causing his dehydration. Will put on sliding insulin scale to bring his blood sugar under control. |

PROD | MAHAFC | 01 June 2011 | 00:12

Click on **Hear It, Spell It** to practice spelling the diagnostic and therapeutic terms you have learned in this chapter. To practice pronouncing these terms, click on **Hear It, Say It.**

# Exercise 10: Admission History & Physical

*Using the form on p. 586, answer the following questions.*

1. What type of diabetes does this patient have? _____

2. What is the complication that he has? _____

3. What medication is he taking for his diabetes? _____

4. What treatment is being performed for his complication? _____

## Abbreviations

| Abbreviation | Meaning | Abbreviation | Meaning |
|---|---|---|---|
| A1c | average glucose level | OGTT | oral glucose tolerance test |
| ACTH | adrenocorticotropic hormone | OT | oxytocin |
| ADH | antidiuretic hormone | PGH | pituitary growth hormone |
| Ca | calcium | PRL | prolactin |
| DI | diabetes insipidus | PTH | parathyroid hormone |
| FBS | fasting blood sugar | RAIU | radioactive iodine uptake scan |
| FPG | fasting plasma glucose | RIA | radioimmunoassay |
| FSH | follicle-stimulating hormone | SIADH | syndrome of inappropriate anti-diuretic hormone |
| GH | growth hormone | | |
| GHD | growth hormone deficiency | STH | somatotropic hormone |
| hGH | human growth hormone | T₃ | triiodothyronine |
| ICSH | interstitial cell-stimulating hormone | T₄ | thyroxine |
| IDDM | insulin-dependent diabetes mellitus | TFT | thyroid function test |
| K | potassium | TSH | thyroid-stimulating hormone |
| LH | luteinizing hormone | UA | urinalysis |
| Na | sodium | | |
| NIDDM | non–insulin-dependent diabetes mellitus | | |

# Exercise 11: Abbreviations

*Match the abbreviations with their definitions.*

_____ 1. Ca     _____ 5. DI

_____ 2. K     _____ 6. OGTT

_____ 3. Na     _____ 7. ADH

_____ 4. OT

A. diabetes insipidus
B. oxytocin
C. potassium
D. oral glucose tolerance test
E. calcium
F. sodium
G. antidiuretic hormone

# Chapter Review

Match the word parts to their definitions.

## WORD PART DEFINITIONS

| Prefix/Suffix | Definition |
|---|---|
| *acro-* | 1. _____ process of recording |
| *-crine* | 2. _____ all |
| *-ectomy* | 3. _____ within |
| *-emia* | 4. _____ excessive |
| *endo-* | 5. _____ above |
| *exo-* | 6. _____ deficient |
| *-graphy* | 7. _____ blood condition |
| *hyper-* | 8. _____ outward |
| *hypo-* | 9. _____ to secrete |
| *pan-* | 10. _____ extremities |
| *poly-* | 11. _____ excessive |
| *supra-* | 12. _____ excision |

| Combining Form | Definition |
|---|---|
| *aden/o* | 13. _____ potassium |
| *adren/o* | 14. _____ pituitary gland |
| *calc/o* | 15. _____ color |
| *crin/o* | 16. _____ sodium |
| *chrom/o* | 17. _____ glucose, sugar |
| *cyt/o* | 18. _____ gonads |
| *gluc/o* | 19. _____ parathyroid gland |
| *glyc/o* | 20. _____ turning |
| *gonad/o* | 21. _____ gland |
| *hypophys/o* | 22. _____ thymus gland |
| *kal/i* | 23. _____ sugar, glucose |
| *natr/o* | 24. _____ dark |
| *pancreat/o* | 25. _____ to secrete |
| *parathyroid/o* | 26. _____ thyroid gland |
| *phe/o* | 27. _____ thalamus |
| *pituitar/o* | 28. _____ adrenal gland |
| *thalam/o* | 29. _____ calcium |
| *thym/o* | 30. _____ pancreas |
| *thyr/o* | 31. _____ cell |
| *trop/o* | 32. _____ pituitary gland |

# WORDSHOP

| Prefixes | Combining Forms | Suffixes |
|---|---|---|
| acro- | acid/o | -dipsia |
| an- | crin/o | -ectomy |
| endo- | esthesi/o | -emia |
| ex- | gluc/o | -ia |
| hyper- | glucos/o | -logy |
| hypo- | glyc/o | -megaly |
| par- | kal/i | -meter |
| para- | ket/o | -osis |
| poly- | keton/o | -tomy |
|  | natr/o | -uria |
|  | ophthalm/o |  |
|  | parathyroid/o |  |
|  | phag/o |  |

*Build the following terms by combining the above word parts. Some word parts may be used more than once. Some may not be used at all. The number in parentheses is the number of word parts needed to build the terms.*

| Definition | Term |
|---|---|
| 1. condition of excessive sodium in the blood (3) | |
| 2. enlargement of the extremities (2) | |
| 3. condition of sugar in the urine (2) | |
| 4. condition of an eye (that protrudes) outward (3) | |
| 5. instrument to measure (blood) sugar (2) | |
| 6. condition of excessive urination (2) | |
| 7. condition of ketones in the urine (2) | |
| 8. abnormal condition of acidity due to ketones (3) | |
| 9. condition of excessive eating (3) | |
| 10. condition of abnormal sensation (2) | |
| 11. removal of the parathyroid gland (2) | |
| 12. condition of excessive thirst (2) | |
| 13. study of the glands that secrete within (3) | |
| 14. condition of excessive blood sugar (3) | |
| 15. condition of deficient potassium in the blood (3) | |

*Sort the terms into the correct categories.*

## TERM SORTING

| Anatomy and Physiology | Pathology | Diagnostic Procedures | Therapeutic Interventions |
|---|---|---|---|
|  |  |  |  |
|  |  |  |  |
|  |  |  |  |
|  |  |  |  |
|  |  |  |  |
|  |  |  |  |
|  |  |  |  |
|  |  |  |  |
|  |  |  |  |
|  |  |  |  |

| | | | |
|---|---|---|---|
| A1c | GHD | OGTT | RIA |
| ACTH | gigantism | orchiectomy | SIADH |
| adrenalectomy | glucagon | oxytocin | sonography |
| anorexia | glucometer | pancreas | TFT |
| antidiabetics | goiter | pancreatectomy | thymectomy |
| cortex | hirsutism | pancreatoduodenectomy | thymoma |
| diabetes insipidus | hyperinsulinism | parathyroidectomy | thyroidectomy |
| endocrineepinephrine | hypophysectomy | polydipsia | urinalysis |
| FPG | hypophysis | prednisone | vasopressin |
| GH | MRI | RAIU | |

*Replace the highlighted words with the correct terms.*

## TRANSLATIONS

1. After experiencing **condition of excessive thirst** and **condition of excessive urination**, Tilda was diagnosed with diabetes insipidus.

2. Victor's **protrusion of eyeballs from their orbits** was caused by **condition of excessive thyroid production**.

3. Moira went to the endocrinologist with symptoms of **condition of deficient calcium production** and **continuous muscle spasms**. She was diagnosed with **condition of deficient parathyroid hormone production**.

4. The child suffered from **deficient thyroid hormone production that occurs in childhood**. Her aunt suffered from the **extreme adult form of deficient hormone production**.

5. Soo Lin had **abnormal hairiness**, easy bruising, **condition of excessive sugar in the blood** and **condition of deficient potassium in the blood**, which led to a diagnosis of Cushing disease.

6. The patient's **condition of oversecretion of insulin** caused a **severe condition of deficient sugar in the blood**.

7. Franco had **a pancreatic cancer**, which was treated with an **excision of the head of the pancreas and the duodenum**.

8. The patient with **total lack of insulin production** was instructed to purchase **an instrument for measurement of blood sugar**.

9. A **partial removal of the thyroid gland** was performed to treat the patient's **enlargement of the thyroid gland not due to a tumor**.

10. Severe **condition of deficient sodium in the blood** and the inability to excrete diluted urine were two symptoms of **oversecretion of ADH from the neurohypophysis**.

11. Kyonia's **insulin resistance acquired during pregnancy** developed into **deficient insulin production** when she was in her forties.

12. After undergoing **a blood test done after fasting**, Mrs. Brown was diagnosed with a **condition in which an individual's blood glucose level is higher than normal, but not high enough for type 2 diabetes**.

13. When she was an adult, Martha developed **enlargement of the extremities** due to hypersecretion of somatotropin from the **anterior part of her pituitary gland**.

14. Maria suffered from **lack of appetite** and **abnormal sensation of prickling**.

# Case Study     Darren Williams

Darren Williams has just been diagnosed with type 2 diabetes mellitus. Besides prescribing oral medication, his physician has referred Darren to a dietician to discuss necessary diet and lifestyle changes.

The dietician explains the nutritional recommendations for persons with diabetes as she talks to Darren about his new diet. She tells him that his new diet will take some time to get used to, but that his health will depend on adhering as closely as possible to it. She tells him that if he follows the diet, it is possible that he will lose enough weight that he will no longer need medication.

Darren releases his pent-up breath, "That's enough for me," he says. "I'll do it."

---

**WILLIAMS, DARREN D - 492891 Opened by BURNS, CHRISTOPHER MD**     _  🗗  X

Task    Edit    View    Time Scale    Options    Help

As Of 10:23

**WILLIAMS, DARREN D**

| | | | |
|---|---|---|---|
| | Age: 57 years | Sex: Male | Loc: WHC-SMMC |
| | DOB: 08/13/1953 | MRN: 492891 | FIN: 3506004 |

Reference Text Browser | Form Browser | Medication Profile

Orders | Last 48 Hours | ED | Lab | Radiology | Assessments | Surgery | **Clinical Notes** | Pt. Info | Pt. Schedule | Task List | I & O | MAR

Flowsheet: Clinical Notes ▼ ...    Level: Office Visit ▼        ⦿ Table  ○ Group  ○ List

| Navigator | X |
|---|---|
| ✓ | Office Visit |

Mr. Williams returned today to review results of a previous visit. At that time, he had complaints of polyuria over the last few months, a significant increase in thirst, and unusual fatigue. He has a family history of diabetes mellitus (father and paternal grandmother). Weight at that time was 198 lb, an increase of 12 lb over last office visit on 1/20/11. Patient admitted to increased appetite and an "abandonment" of his exercise program because of the addition of a second job.

Patient underwent FPG, OGTT, and UA and was diagnosed with type 2 diabetes mellitus. Glucophage was prescribed. Patient was referred to our dietitian, who will help him develop a management plan. Patient has been advised to call if difficulties develop or symptoms do not lessen.

PROD | MAHAFC | 05 Feb 2011 | 10:23

**Office Visit Summary**

*Using the office visit summary on p. 592, answer the following questions.*

1. Mr. Williams initially complained of a symptom called polyuria. What is that? _____

2. What is the healthcare term for his other symptom of "increased thirst"? _____

3. Explain the abbreviations used for testing in this note: _____

   A. FPG _____

   B. OGTT _____

   C. UA _____

4. Glucophage is being prescribed to replace which missing (or ineffective) hormone? _____

---

For more interactive learning, click on:
- **Whack a Word Part** to review endocrine word parts.
- **Wheel of Terminology** and **Word Shop** to practice word building.
- **Tournament of Terminology** to test your knowledge of endocrine terms.
- **Terminology Triage** to practice sorting endocrine terms into categories.

# 16

*While there are several chronic diseases more destructive to life than cancer, none is more feared.*
**—Charles Horace Mayo**

## OBJECTIVES

- Recognize and use terms related to the physiology of neoplasms.
- Recognize and use terms related to neoplasm pathology.
- Recognize and use terms related to the diagnostic procedures for detecting neoplasms.
- Recognize and use terms related to the therapeutic interventions for treating neoplasms.

# Oncology

## CHAPTER AT A GLANCE

*Use this list of word parts and key terms to assess your knowledge. Check off the ones you have mastered.*

### KEY WORD PARTS

#### PREFIX
- [ ] ana-
- [ ] apo-
- [ ] brachy-
- [ ] dys-
- [ ] ecto-
- [ ] endo-
- [ ] hyper-
- [ ] meta-
- [ ] neo-

#### SUFFIX
- [ ] -genesis
- [ ] -oma
- [ ] -plasia
- [ ] -plasm
- [ ] -ptosis
- [ ] -sarcoma
- [ ] -stasis
- [ ] -therapy

#### COMBINING FORMS
- [ ] carcin/o
- [ ] mut/a
- [ ] nod/o
- [ ] onc/o
- [ ] sarc/o

### KEY TERMS

- [ ] anaplasia
- [ ] apoptosis
- [ ] benign
- [ ] biopsy
- [ ] bone marrow transplant (BMT)
- [ ] brachytherapy
- [ ] carcinogenesis
- [ ] carcinoma
- [ ] carcinoma in situ (CIS)
- [ ] chemotherapy

- [ ] dedifferentiation
- [ ] grading
- [ ] immunotherapy
- [ ] leukemia
- [ ] lymphoma
- [ ] malignant
- [ ] mammogram
- [ ] metastasis
- [ ] mixed tumor
- [ ] mutation

- [ ] myeloma
- [ ] neoplasm
- [ ] oncology
- [ ] osteosarcoma
- [ ] radiotherapy
- [ ] sarcoma
- [ ] sentinel node
- [ ] staging
- [ ] tumor marker

**cancer** = carcin/o

Where there is life, there is cancer. Although the types of cancer and their incidence (the number of new types diagnosed each year) may vary by geography, sex, race, age, and ethnicity, cancer exists in every population and has since ancient times. Archeologists have found evidence of cancer in dinosaur bones and human mummies. Written descriptions of cancer treatment have been discovered dating back to 1600 BC. The name itself comes from the Greek word for crab, used by Hippocrates to describe the appearance of the most common type of cancer, carcinoma.

## SPECIALTIES/SPECIALISTS

**oncologist**
   onc/o = tumor
   -logist = one who studies

**Oncology** is the study of tumors, both benign (noncancerous) and malignant (cancerous). An **oncologist** is a specialist in the diagnosis, treatment, and prevention of tumors.

   **Cancer registrars** (also called **tumor registrars**) are specialists in cancer data management. Their primary responsibility is to report and track patients with cancer who are diagnosed and/or treated at the registrar's healthcare facility.

## CARCINOGENESIS

Cancer is not *one* disease but a group of hundreds of diseases with similar characteristics. The shared characteristics are uncontrolled cell growth and a spread of altered cells. Different types of cancers have different occurrence rates and different causes.

   Current research suggests that there is no single cause of cancer. Radiation, bacteria, viruses, genetics, diet, smoking (or exposure to tobacco smoke), alcohol, and other factors all contribute to the development of cancer termed **carcinogenesis.** Each of these factors is instrumental in disrupting the normal balance of cell growth and destruction within the body by causing a mutation in the DNA of cells (Fig. 16-1). Once this **mutation** takes place, a process of uncontrolled cell growth may begin. It is important to note that the cancer cells that replace normal cells no longer function to keep the body working. The only mission of cancer cells is to reproduce. Fig. 16-2 illustrates the process of **apoptosis** (a pop TOH sis), the body's normal restraining function to keep cell growth in check. Fig. 16-3 shows the progression from normally functioning skin tissue to **hyperplasia,** to **dysplasia,** and finally to carcinoma in situ (CIS). Cancer

**carcinogenesis**
   carcin/o = cancer
   -genesis = production, origin

**mutation**
   mut/a = change
   -tion = process of

**apoptosis**
   apo- = away from
   -ptosis = falling

**hyperplasia**
   hyper- = excessive
   -plasia = condition of formation

**dysplasia**
   dys- = abnormal
   -plasia = condition of formation

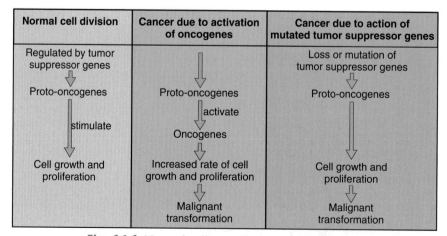

Fig. 16-1 Normal cell growth vs. oncogenesis.

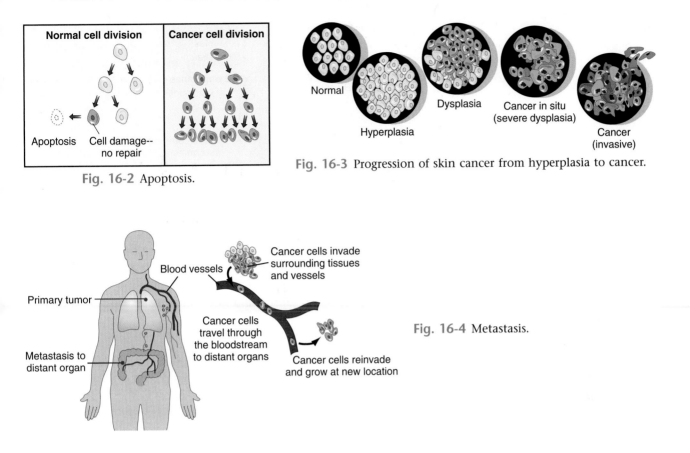

Fig. 16-2 Apoptosis.

Fig. 16-3 Progression of skin cancer from hyperplasia to cancer.

Fig. 16-4 Metastasis.

is a continuum—from tissue made up of normally functioning cells fulfilling their role to keep the body healthy, to tissue replaced by cancerous cells that no longer perform the work of the tissue and now perform only the function of reproducing themselves. Cancers are capable of destroying not only the tissue in which they originate (the primary site), but also other tissues, through the process of **metastasis,** the spread of cancer. Metastasis can occur by direct extension to contiguous organs and tissues or to distant sites through blood (Fig. 16-4) or lymphatic involvement.

## NAMING MALIGNANT TUMORS

All cancers are **neoplasms** (new growths), but not all neoplasms are cancerous. Cancerous **tumors** are termed *malignant,* whereas noncancerous tumors are termed *benign.*

Although the hundreds of known types of malignant tumors commonly share the characteristics listed previously, the names that they are given reflect their differences. All tissues (and hence organs) are derived from the progression of three embryonic germ layers that differentiate into specific tissues and organs. Tumors are generally divided into two broad categories and a varying number of other categories, based on their **embryonic** origin. Fig. 16-5 illustrates the different types of cancers and where they occur.

- **Carcinomas:** Approximately 80% to 90% of malignant tumors are derived from the outer **(ectodermal)** and inner **(endodermal)** layers of the embryo that develop into epithelial tissue that either covers or lines the surfaces of the body. This category of cancer is divided into two main types. If derived from an organ or gland, it is an adenocarcinoma; if derived from squamous

**metastasis**
    meta- = beyond, change
    -stasis = controlling, stopping

**tumor** = onc/o, -oma

**neoplasm**
    neo- = new
    -plasm = formation

**embryonic** = blast/o, -blast

**ectodermal**
    ecto- = outer
    derm/o = skin
    -al = pertaining to

**endodermal**
    endo- = within
    derm/o = skin
    -al = pertaining to

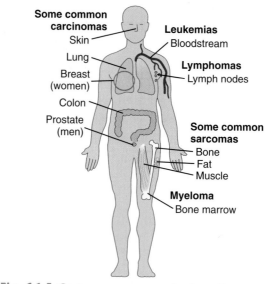

Fig. 16-5 Common cancers and where they occur.

epithelium, it is a squamous cell carcinoma. Examples include gastric adenocarcinoma and squamous cell carcinoma of the lung.

- **Sarcomas** are derived from the middle **(mesodermal)** layer, which becomes connective tissue (bones, muscle, cartilage, blood vessels, and fat). Most end in the suffix **-sarcoma.** Examples include osteosarcoma, chondrosarcoma, hemangiosarcoma, mesothelioma, and glioma.
- **Lymphomas** develop in lymphatic tissue (vessels, nodes, and organs, including the spleen, tonsils, and thymus gland). Lymphomas are solid cancers and may also appear outside of the sites of lymphatic organs in the stomach, breast, or brain; these are called **extranodal lymphomas.** All lymphomas may be divided into two categories: Hodgkin lymphoma and non-Hodgkin lymphoma.
- **Leukemia** is cancer of the bone marrow. An example is acute myelocytic leukemia.
- **Myelomas** arise from the plasma cells in the bone marrow. An example is multiple myeloma.
- **Mixed tumors** are a combination of cells from within one category or between two cancer categories. Examples are **teratocarcinoma** and **carcinosarcoma.**

## STAGING AND GRADING

To treat cancer, the treating physician must determine the severity of the cancer, the grade, and its stage, or size and spread. Cancers at different grades and stages react differently to various treatments.

**Grading** is the first means of affixing a value to a clinical opinion of the degree of **dedifferentiation (anaplasia)** of cancer cells, or how much the cells appear different from their original form. Healthy cells are well differentiated; cancer cells are poorly differentiated. The pathologist determines this difference and assigns a grade ranging from I to IV. The higher the grade, the more cancerous, or dedifferentiated, is the tissue sample. Grading is a measure of the cancer's *severity.*

The other means of determining the *size and spread* of the cancer from its original site, which is called **staging.** A number of systems are used to describe staging. Some are specific to the type of cancer; others are general systems. If staging is determined by various diagnostic techniques, it is referred to as **clinical staging.** If it is determined by the pathologist's report, it is called

---

**mesodermal**
    meso- = middle
    derm/o = skin
    -al = pertaining to

**connective tissue cancer**
    = sarc/o, -sarcoma

**extranodal**
    extra- = outside
    nod/o = node
    -al = pertaining to

**myeloma**
    myel/o = bone marrow, spinal cord
    -oma = tumor, mass

**teratocarcinoma**
    terat/o = deformity
    -carcinoma = cancer of epithelial origin

**carcinosarcoma**
    carcin/o = cancer
    -sarcoma = connective tissue cancer

**anaplasia**
    ana- = up, apart
    -plasia = condition of formation

**pathologic**
    path/o = disease
    -logic = pertaining to studying

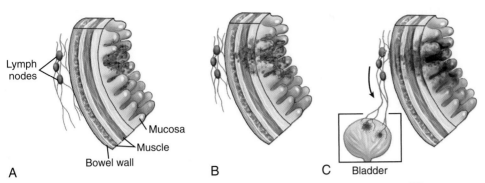

Fig. 16-6 Staging of colon cancer. **A,** Stage I; **B,** stage II; **C,** stage III.

**pathologic staging.** An example is TNM staging. In this system, **T** stands for the size of the **tumor, N** stands for the number of lymph **nodes** positive for cancer, and **M** stands for the presence of distant **metastasis** (meh TAS tuh sis). Summary staging puts together the TNM to give one number as a stage. Again, this helps the clinician to determine the type of treatment that is most effective. Fig. 16-6 illustrates a staging system. If the cancer cells appear only at the original site and have not invaded the organ of origin, it is called **carcinoma in situ (CIS).**

Cancer that begins in an organ is referred to as a primary tumor. When a cancer spreads to another site in the body from that primary tumor, the new tumor is referred to as secondary, or **metastatic.** The cells in the metastatic tumor are composed of the same tissue as the cancer at the original site. For example, a patient can have a primary liver cancer that begins in the liver, or a metastatic brain tumor that is composed of cells from a primary liver cancer that has spread.

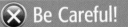 **Be Careful!**

*Don't confuse **sarc/o,** meaning flesh, and **sacr/o,** meaning sacrum.*

## Exercise 1: **General Oncology Terms**

*Match the word part with its correct meaning.*

| | | |
|---|---|---|
| ____ 1. -stasis | ____ 6. -carcinoma | A. up, apart |
| | | B. abnormal |
| ____ 2. -oma | ____ 7. ana- | C. connective tissue tumor |
| | | D. new |
| ____ 3. -plasia | ____ 8. hyper- | E. cancer of epithelial tissue origin |
| | | F. stopping, controlling |
| ____ 4. meta- | ____ 9. neo- | G. beyond, change |
| | | H. tumor |
| ____ 5. dys- | ____ 10. sarcoma | I. excessive |
| | | J. formation |

*Underline the correct answer.*

11. Tumors that are cancerous are considered to be *(benign, malignant).*

12. The most common type of malignant cancer is *(carcinoma, sarcoma, leukemia, lymphoma, myeloma, mixed cell cancer).*

13. Cancer composed of connective tissue is classified as *(carcinoma, sarcoma, leukemia, lymphoma, myeloma, mixed cell cancer).*

14. Cancer cells that derive from plasma cells in the bone marrow are classified as *(carcinoma, sarcoma, leukemia, lymphoma, myeloma, mixed cell cancer).*

15. Healthy cells are *(well, poorly)* differentiated.

16. A determination of the degree of dedifferentiation of cancer cells is called *(grading, staging)*.

17. A system of determining how far a cancer has spread from its original site is called *(grading, staging)*.

18. The site where the cancer originates is referred to as the *(primary, metastatic site)*.

---

Choose **Hear It, Spell It** to practice spelling the staging and grading terms you have learned in this chapter. To practice pronouncing staging and grading terms, choose **Hear It, Say It**.

---

## Combining and Adjective Forms for Oncology

| Meaning | Combining Form | Adjective Form |
|---------|----------------|----------------|
| change | mut/a | |
| disease | path/o | embryonic |
| embryo | blast/o | |
| node | nod/o | nodal |
| tumor | onc/o | |

## Prefixes for Oncology

| Prefix | Meaning |
|--------|---------|
| ana- | up, apart |
| apo- | away from |
| dys- | abnormal |
| ecto- | outer |
| endo- | within |
| extra- | outside |
| hyper- | excessive |
| meso- | middle |
| meta- | beyond, change |
| neo- | new |

## Suffixes for Oncology

| Suffix | Meaning |
|--------|---------|
| -carcinoma | cancer of epithelial origin |
| -genesis | production, origin |
| -oma | tumor, mass |
| -plasia | condition of formation |
| -plasm | formation |
| -ptosis | falling |
| -sarcoma | connective tissue cancer |
| -stasis | controlling, stopping |

## PATHOLOGY

### Signs and Symptoms

The signs and symptoms of cancer are manifestations of how cancer cells replace the functions of healthy tissue. Some examples include anorexia (lack of appetite), bruising, leukocytosis (slight increase of white blood cells), fatigue, cachexia (wasting), and thrombocytopenia (deficiency of clotting cells).

### Neoplasia by Body System

The following tables summarize characteristics of benign and malignant tumors by body system. Note that a particular system does not always have all one type of cancer because organs are composed of a variety of tissues with different embryonic origins. The integumentary system has both carcinomas and sarcomas.

## Comparison of Benign and Malignant Neoplasms

| Characteristics | Benign | Malignant |
|---|---|---|
| Mode of growth | Relatively slow growth by expansion; encapsulated; cells adhere to each other | Rapid growth; invades surrounding tissue by infiltration |
| Cells under microscopic examination | Resemble tissue of origin; well differentiated; appear normal | Do not resemble tissue of origin; vary in size and shape; abnormal appearance and function |
| Spread | Remains isolated | Metastasis; cancer cells carried by blood and lymphatics to one or more other locations; secondary tumors occur |
| Other properties | No tissue destruction; not prone to hemorrhage; may be smooth and freely movable | Ulceration and/or necrosis; prone to hemorrhage; irregular and less movable |
| Recurrence | Rare after excision | A common characteristic |
| Pathogenesis | Symptoms related to location with obstruction and/or compression of surrounding tissue or organs; usually not life threatening unless inaccessible | Cachexia; pain; fatal if not controlled |

From Frazier MS, Drzymkowski JW: Essentials of human diseases and conditions, ed 4, Philadelphia, 2008, Saunders.

## Examples of Neoplasms by Body System*

| Body System | Organ | Benign Neoplasms | Malignant Neoplasms |
|---|---|---|---|
| Musculoskeletal | bone<br>cartilage<br>muscle | osteoma<br>chondroma<br>rhabdomyoma, leiomyoma | Ewing sarcoma, osteosarcoma<br>chondrosarcoma<br>rhabdomyosarcoma, leiomyosarcoma |
| Integumentary | skin | dermatofibroma | basal cell carcinoma, squamous cell carcinoma, malignant melanoma, Kaposi sarcoma |

Continued

## Examples of Neoplasms by Body System—cont'd

| Body System | Organ | Benign Neoplasms | Malignant Neoplasms |
|---|---|---|---|
| Gastrointestinal | esophagus | leiomyoma | adenocarcinoma of the esophagus, stomach, pancreas, colon, and/or rectum |
| | stomach<br>pancreas<br>colon/rectum | polyp<br>gastric adenoma | |
| Urinary | kidney | nephroma | hypernephroma/renal cell carcinoma, Wilms tumor/nephroblastoma |
| | bladder | | transitional cell carcinoma (bladder cancer) |
| Male reproductive | testis<br>prostate | benign prostatic hyperplasia | seminoma, teratoma<br>adenocarcinoma of the prostate |
| Female reproductive | breast | fibrocystic changes in the breast | infiltrating ductal adenocarcinoma of the breast |
| | uterus<br>ovaries<br>cervix | fibroids<br>ovarian cyst<br>cervical dysplasia | stromal endometrial carcinoma<br>epithelial ovarian carcinoma<br>squamous cell carcinoma of the cervix |
| Blood/ lymphatic/ immune | blood<br>lymph vessels | | leukemia<br>non-Hodgkin lymphoma, Hodgkin lymphoma |
| | thymus gland | thymoma | malignant thymoma |
| Cardiovascular | blood vessels<br>heart | hemangioma<br>myxoma | hemangiosarcoma<br>myxosarcoma |
| Respiratory | epithelial tissue of respiratory tract, lung, bronchus | papilloma of lung | adenocarcinoma of the lung, small cell carcinoma, mesothelioma, bronchogenic carcinoma |
| Nervous | CNS (brain, spinal cord, meninges)<br>PNS | neuroma, neurofibroma, meningioma | glioblastoma multiforme |
| Endocrine | pituitary<br>thyroid<br>adrenal medulla | benign pituitary tumor<br><br>pheochromocytoma | thyroid carcinoma |
| Eyes and ears | retina<br>choroid<br>acoustic nerve | choroidal hemangioma<br>acoustic neuroma | retinoblastoma |

*See also neoplasm tables in Chapters 3-15.

---

Click on **Hear It, Spell It** to practice spelling the pathology terms you have learned in this chapter. To hear well you pronounce the pathology terms in this chapter, click on **Hear It, Say It.** To review the pathology terms in this chapter, play **Medical Millionaire.**

## Age Matters

### Pediatrics

Childhood cancer is such a rarity that incidence rates are routinely expressed as the number of cases per million, instead of per 100,000 as with adult cancers. Still, certain cancers have a childhood form. Wilms tumor (children's kidney cancer), acute lymphocytic leukemia, retinoblastoma, and Ewing sarcoma are examples of cancers that seldom occur outside of childhood.

### Geriatrics

The cumulative exposure to a lifetime of carcinogens reveals itself in cancer statistics that show cancer rates to increase as age increases. Lung, prostate, breast, colon, and skin cancers are common in elderly patients. Researchers estimate that 97% of men who have the prostate cancer gene will develop prostate cancer by the time they are 85.

## DIAGNOSTIC PROCEDURES

### Patient History

Along with the various clinical techniques described, the patient's history is especially important, including information regarding family history (for genetic information) and social history, such as tobacco and alcohol use, diet, and sexual history. A patient's smoking history is described in terms of "pack years." Pack years equals the average number of packs smoked per day multiplied by the number of years of smoking. For example: 1 pack/day × 25 years of smoking represents 25 pack years. A patient's current or former occupation may also shed light on the type of cancer. For example, exposure to asbestos, through an occupation of ship building or working with brake repair, may lead to a rare type of lung cancer, mesothelioma.

### Tumor Markers

Tumor marker tests measure the levels of a variety of biochemical substances detected in the blood, urine, or body tissues that often appear in higher than normal amounts in individuals with certain neoplasms. Because other factors may influence the amount of the tumor marker present, they are not intended to be used as a sole means of diagnosis. Examples include the following:

**AFP:** increased levels may indicate liver or testicular cancer.
**B2M (beta-2 microglobulin):** levels are elevated in multiple myeloma and chronic lymphocytic leukemia.
**BTA (bladder tumor antigen):** present in the urine of patients with bladder cancer.
**CA125:** used for ovarian cancer detection and management.
**CA15-3:** levels are measured to determine the stage of breast cancer.
**CA19-9:** levels are elevated in stomach, colorectal, and pancreatic cancers.
**CA27-29:** used to monitor breast cancer; especially useful in testing for recurrences.
**CEA:** monitors colorectal cancer when the disease has spread or after treatment to measure the patient's response.
**hCG:** used as a screen for choriocarcinoma and testicular and ovarian cancers.
**NSE:** used to measure the stage and/or patient's response to treatment of small cell cancer and neuroblastoma.
**PSA:** increased levels may be due to BPH or prostate cancer.
**TA-90:** used to detect the spread of malignant melanoma.

### Biopsy (bx)

See Chapter 4 for additional information on types of biopsies.

### Imaging

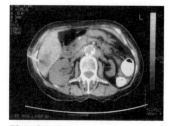

**Fig. 16-7** Computed tomography (CT) scan of needle biopsy of the liver clearly shows the needle in the liver on the left. (Courtesy Riverside Methodist Hospitals, Columbus, Ohio.)

**computed tomography (CT) scans:** CT scans provide information about a tumor's shape, size, and location, along with the source of its blood supply. They are useful in detecting, evaluating, and monitoring cancer, especially liver, pancreatic, bone, lung, and adrenal gland cancers. CT scans are also useful in staging cancer and guiding needles for aspiration biopsy (Fig. 16-7).

**magnetic resonance imaging (MRI):** areas of the body that are often difficult to image are possible to see with MRI because of its three-dimensional capabilities. MRI is useful in detecting cancer in the central nervous system (CNS) and the musculoskeletal (MS) system. It is also used to stage breast and endometrial cancer before surgery and to detect metastatic spread of cancer to the liver.

**nuclear scans:** nuclear scans are useful in locating and staging cancer of the thyroid and the bone. A **positron emission tomography (PET) scan** provides information about the metabolism of an internal structure, along with its size and shape. It is primarily used for images of the brain, neck, colon, rectum, ovary, and lung. It may also help to identify more aggressive tumors (Fig. 16-8). **Single-photon emission computed tomography (SPECT)** uses a rotating camera to create three-dimensional images with the use of radioactive substances. It is useful in identifying metastases to the bone. *Monoclonal antibodies* are used to evaluate cancer of the prostate, colon, breast, and ovaries, and melanoma.

**radiography:** because tumors are usually more dense than the tissue surrounding them, they may appear as a lighter shade of gray (blocking more radiation). Abdominal x-rays may reveal tumors of the stomach, liver, kidneys, and so on, whereas chest x-rays are useful in detecting lung cancer. If a contrast medium is used, as in an upper or lower gastrointestinal (GI) series or intravenous urogram (IVU), tumors of the esophagus, rectum, colon, or kidneys may be detected. Another special type of x-ray is a **mammogram,** which is useful in the early detection of breast cancer. **Stereotactic (3-D) mammography** may be used for an image-guided biopsy.

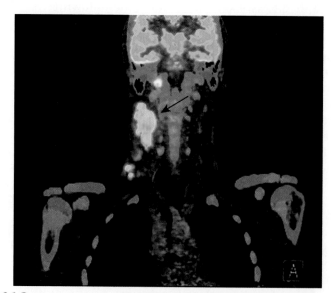

**Fig. 16-8** High resolution PET scan showing neck cancer *(arrow)*.

## Self-Detection

Self-detection remains the most important method of discovering cancer. The American Cancer Society (ACS) has developed a series of reminders and rules to help individuals become aware of cancer signs and symptoms. For general detection of cancer, they have developed the following CAUTION criteria:

### CAUTION Criteria

**C**hange in bowel or bladder habits
**A** sore that does not heal
**U**nusual bleeding or discharge
**T**hickening or lump in the breast, testicles, or elsewhere
**I**ndigestion or difficulty swallowing
**O**bvious change in the size, shape, color, or thickness of a wart, mole, or mouth sore
**N**agging cough or hoarseness

For discovering skin cancer, the ACS has come up with the following ABCDE rule:

### ABCDE Rule

**A** for **asymmetry:** a mole that, when divided in half, does not look the same on both sides.
**B** for **border:** a mole with edges that are blurry or jagged.
**C** for **color:** changes in the color of a mole, including darkening, spread of color, loss of color, or the appearance of multiple colors, such as blue, red, white, pink, purple, or gray.
**D** for **diameter:** a mole larger than $\frac{1}{4}$ inch in diameter.
**E** for **elevation:** a mole that is raised above the skin and has an uneven surface.

The ACS also has criteria for breast self-examination (BSE) and testicular self-examination (TSE).

## Exercise 2: Diagnostic Procedures

*Fill in the blank.*

1. A patient's history of smoking may be described as pack years, which is the number of

   _____ smoked per day × the number of years of smoking.

2. Information regarding previous diet, alcohol use, and family members with cancer may be found in

   the _____ section of a patient's medical record.

3. Levels of biochemical substances present in the blood that may indicate neoplastic activity are referred

   to as _____.

4. Removal of a sample of tissue to be examined for signs of cancer is a _____.

5. Mammography may be done to test for cancer of the _____.

*Case Study* Terrence McAffee

Terrence McAffee is a 68-year-old real estate broker who has a wonderful marriage, two successful daughters, and a new grandson. He enjoys his job and his hobbies and is looking forward to his and his wife's retirement to their home in Florida in a couple of years. Four years ago, a routine colonoscopy revealed polyps in his colon, some of which turned out to be cancerous. He had successful surgery for the cancer and has had normal colonoscopies for the past 3 years. He is back today for his 3-year follow-up and colonoscopy, which unfortunately reveals more polyps, some of which are inflamed. The surgeon removes them and sends samples to pathology for cancer analysis.

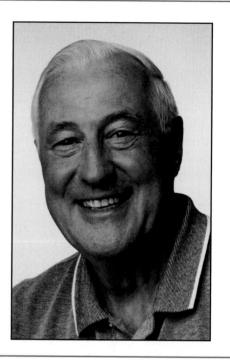

McAFFEE, TERRENCE C - 599999 Opened by CLINTON, ANNALIESE MD

Task   Edit   View   Time Scale   Options   Help

As Of 08:27

**McAFFEE, TERRENCE C**

| Age: 68 years | Sex: Male | Loc: WHC-SMMC |
| DOB: 01/27/1943 | MRN: 599999 | FIN: 3506004 |

Reference Text Browser   Form Browser   Medication Profile

Orders | Last 48 Hours | ED | Lab | Radiology | Assessments | **Surgery** | Clinical Notes | Pt. Info | Pt. Schedule | Task List | I & O | MAR

Flowsheet: Surgery      Level: Operative Report      ⦿ Table  ○ Group  ○ List

Navigator

✓ Operative Report

| Preoperative diagnosis: | History of colon cancer, multiple colon polyps |
| Postoperative diagnosis: | History of colon cancer, multiple colon polyps |
| Surgery: | Colonoscopy with polypectomy ×5 |

This 68-year-old male has colon polyps and a previous history of colon carcinoma. Patient was taken to the endoscopy suite and in the left lateral position, the long colonoscope was inserted without difficulty. The perirectal area was normal. Rectal ampulla was normal. The left colon showed a few diverticula. The right colon had multiple polyps, five of which were removed with hot forceps. The patient tolerated the procedure well and went to the recovery room in stable condition.

PROD | MAHAFC | 26 April 2011 | 08:27

## Exercise 3: Operative Report

*Using the operative report on p. 606, fill in the blanks.*

1. What are "polyps" and why do you think they were removed? _____

2. What is the medical term for "colon cancer"? _____

3. Give example of procedures done in an endoscopy suite. _____

4. What is a colonoscope? _____

5. Explain the meaning of the procedure "colonoscopy with polypectomy ×5."

_____

## THERAPEUTIC INTERVENTIONS

### Surgery

The primary treatment for cancer has always been and remains removal of the tumor. When the tumor is relatively small and is present only in the organ that is removed, surgery is most effective.

The amount of tissue removed varies with the stage and grade of the cancer. In breast cancer surgery, for example, the types of surgery are as follows:

**en bloc resection:** removal of the cancerous tumor and the lymph nodes.
**lumpectomy:** removal of the tumor only.
**lymph node dissection:** the removal of clinically involved lymph nodes. **Lymph node mapping** determines a pattern of spread from the primary tumor site through the lymph nodes. The **sentinel node** is the first node in which lymphatic drainage occurs in a particular area. If this node is negative for cancer upon dissection, then the lymph system is free of cancer, and no other nodes need to be excised.
**radical mastectomy:** removal of the breast containing the cancer, along with the lymph nodes and the muscle under the breast. When the surgical report discusses **margins,** it refers to the borders of normal tissue surrounding the cancer. A **wide margin resection** means that the cancer is removed with a significant amount of tissue around the tumor to ensure that all cancer cells are removed. If the margins are reported as negative, no cancer cells are seen. If positive, cancer cells have been detected by the pathologist.
**simple mastectomy:** removal of the breast containing the cancer.

To view an animation of radiation therapy, click on **Animations.**

### Radiotherapy

Approximately half of all cancer patients receive radiation. The goal of radiation therapy is to destroy the nucleus of the cancer cells, thereby destroying their ability to reproduce and spread.

Although radiation is usually started after removal of the tumor, sometimes it is done before removal to shrink the tumor. Some cancers may be treated solely with radiation.

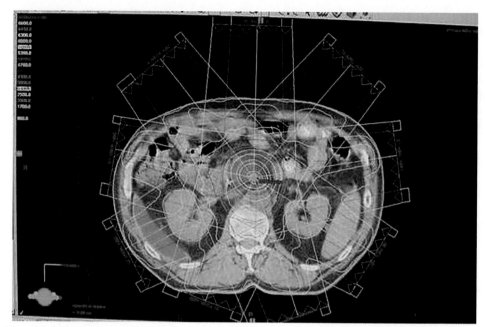

**Fig. 16-9** Dosimetry plan showing nine different radiation fields used to treat a pancreatic tumor.

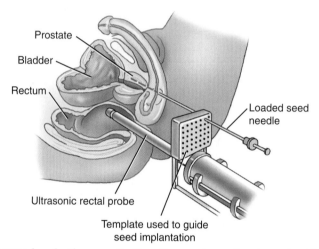

Prostate

Bladder

Rectum

Loaded seed needle

Ultrasonic rectal probe

Template used to guide seed implantation

**Fig. 16-10** Prostate brachytherapy. Radioactive seeds are implanted with a needle guided by sonography and a template grid.

**brachytherapy**

brachy- = short
-therapy = treatment

**3-dimensional conformal radiation therapy (3DCRT):** targeted radiation therapy that uses digital diagnostic imaging and specialized software to treat tumors without damaging surrounding tissue (Fig. 16-9).

**brachytherapy** (brah kee THAYR uh pee): the use of radiation placed directly on or within the cancer through the use of needles or beads containing radioactive gold, cobalt, or radium (Fig. 16-10).

**gamma knife surgery:** a noninvasive type of surgery that uses gamma radiation to destroy a brain tumor.

**intensity-modulated radiation therapy (IMRT):** high-dosage radiation delivered via a beam that changes its dosage and shape.

## Systemic Therapy

**bone marrow transplant (BMT):** patients who are incapable of producing healthy blood cells are given bone marrow from a matching donor to stimulate normal blood cell growth. Patients with specific types of leukemia may receive bone marrow transplants after chemotherapy has effectively destroyed the functioning of their own bone marrow.

**chemotherapy:** chemotherapy is the circulation of cancer-destroying medicine throughout the body. Chemotherapy may also be used as an adjuvant (aid) to other forms of treatment to relieve symptoms or slow down the spread of cancer. Combination chemotherapy is the use of two or more anticancer drugs at one time. See the Pharmacology section for more details on chemotherapy drugs.

**chemotherapy**
chem/o = drug, chemical
-therapy = treatment

**complementary and alternative medicine (CAM) techniques:** prayer, massage, diet, exercise, and mind-body techniques constitute the majority of CAM methods used in cancer treatment. The U.S. government has established the National Center for Complementary and Alternative Medicine, which reports on results of research studies on the use of CAM techniques for various disorders (http://www.nccam.nih.gov).

**immunotherapy:** immunotherapy is the use of the body's own defense system to attack cancer cells. See the description of interleukins in the Pharmacology section.

## Preventive Measures

**vaccines:** Two vaccines are currently in use to prevent specific cancers. The hepatitis B vaccine prevents hepatitis B with its sequelae of liver cancer and cirrhosis. The cervical cancer vaccine protects a woman against strains 16 and 18 of the human papilloma virus (HPV).

## Exercise 4: Therapeutic Interventions

*Fill in the blank.*

1. Treatment with radioactive beads near or inside the cancer is called _____.

2. A determination of the spread of the primary tumor through the lymph nodes is referred to as lymph

   node _____.

3. The first node in which lymphatic drainage occurs is the _____ node.

4. Removal of the tumor and lymph nodes is called_____.

5. The borders of normal tissue surrounding the cancer are called _____.

6. Use of the body's own defense system to attack cancer cells is called _____.

7. Prayer, massage, exercise, and mind-body techniques are examples of _____.

8. Three-dimensional targeted radiation treatment to treat tumors without damaging surrounding tissue

   is _____.

## PHARMACOLOGY

**Chemotherapy** works by disrupting the cycle of cell replication. All cells go through a cycle of reproducing themselves, but, unlike cancer cells, they have a built-in mechanism that limits their growth. The side effects of cancer therapy, such as hair loss or nausea, are due to the inability of chemotherapeutic agents to differentiate between normal and cancerous cells. Thus cells that reproduce rapidly, such as hair cells or those that line the stomach, are also affected. It should also be noted that two or more chemotherapeutic agents usually are used together to effectively attack the cancer at various stages. This is referred to as a drug *protocol* or plan.

Most of the pharmaceuticals prescribed to treat cancer are referred to as *antineoplastic agents*. They accomplish the goal of slowing or stopping the progression of cancer in different ways:

**alkylating agents:** interfere with DNA replication to lead to cancer cell death or dysfunction. Examples include cisplatin (Platinol AQ), nitrosoureas like carmustine (Gliadel), and nitrogen mustards like cyclophosphamide (Cytoxan).
**antimetabolites:** replace compounds that cancer cells need to grow and/or replicate. Examples are methotrexate and fluorouracil (5-FU).
**antineoplastic antibiotics:** prevent or delay cell replication. Examples include doxorubicin (Rubex, Adriamycin) and dactinomycin (Cosmegen).
**antineoplastic hormones:** interfere with receptors for growth-stimulating proteins. Examples include flutamide (Eulexin) and tamoxifen (Nolvadex).
**interleukins:** stimulate cells of the immune system to boost attacks on cancer cells. An example is aldesleukin (Proleukin).
**mitotic inhibitors:** prevent cell division. An example is paclitaxel (Taxol).
**vinca alkaloids:** prevent formation of chromosome spindles necessary for cell duplication. Examples include vincristine (Oncovin) and vinblastine.

## Exercise 5: Pharmacology

*Underline the correct answer.*

1. Patients who are prescribed chemotherapy receive a drug *(protocol, adjuvent)*.

2. Side effects of chemotherapy frequently occur because the drugs used to kill cancer cells often *(stimulate, kill)* normal cells.

3. Most chemotherapeutic agents work by disrupting a phase of the cell *(cycle, movement)*.

4. Drugs that interfere with receptors for growth-stimulating proteins are *(antineoplatic hormones, antimetabolites)*.

5. Drugs that interfere with DNA replication are called *(antineoplastic, antibiotics, alklating agents)*.

6. Drugs that replace compounds that cancer cells need to grow or replicate are *(interleukins, antimetabolites)*.

7. Cell division is prevented by *(vinca alkaloids, miotic inhibitors)*.

Click on **Hear It, Spell It** to practice spelling the diagnostic and therapeutic terms you have learned in this chapter. To practice pronouncing these terms, click on **Hear It, Say It.**

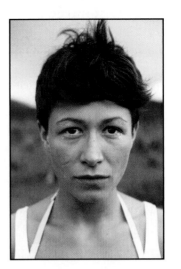

Stella is a 40-year-old nurse who had been in excellent health until a year ago, when a routine mammogram revealed a cancerous mass in her upper left breast. She underwent a lumpectomy and chemotherapy, and her 6-month mammogram was normal. However, her 1-year follow-up exam revealed metastases in her neck and liver. Her original cancer had spread in spite of her surgery and treatments. The oncologist tells Stella that surgery and chemotherapy will not cure her but will only deter the advance of the cancer. She tries chemo again, but it makes her so ill that she decides to stop. She continues to feel ill and is unable to eat or drink, so she is admitted to the hospital for tests and treatment for dehydration and a possible infection.

---

YATES, STELLA M - 618022 Opened by SINGH, SHEPHALI    _ 🗗 ✕

Task   Edit   View   Time Scale   Options   Help

🗎🏛◆➔🔥🖐📉📉🔄🗘■🗝🖵💾📑🔗🖨⁉️🗒✒️    As Of 20:25    📊🔍📑

| **YATES, STELLA M** | **Age: 40 years** | **Sex: Female** | **Loc: WHC-SMMC** |
|---|---|---|---|
| | **DOB: 03/02/1972** | **MRN: 618022** | **FIN: 3506004** |

Reference Text Browser | Form Browser | **Medication Profile**

Orders | Last 48 Hours | ED | Lab | Radiology | Assessments | Surgery | **Clinical Notes** | Pt. Info | Pt. Schedule | Task List | I & O | MAR

Flowsheet: Clinical Notes ▾ …   Level: Discharge Summary ▾    ⦿ Table ○ Group ○ List

◄►

Navigator ✕

✓ Discharge Summary

Final Diagnosis: 1. Metastatic breast cancer

2. Dehydration with confusion

SUMMARY:   This is a 40-year-old woman who developed breast cancer approximately 1 year ago. She had surgery and chemotherapy, seemed to be doing well, but this fall developed recurrence. This was present in the neck and liver. She underwent cycles of chemotherapy. Although the nodes in her neck subsided, she has had advancing cancer in the liver and does not seem to be responding to chemotherapy, and in fact, the chemotherapy is making her quite ill. This has been discussed with her family, and because this therapy is not going to cure her and is making her ill, she has decided to forego any more chemotherapy at this time, which seems appropriate.

She has had some right flank pain, I presume from the liver metastases. She has had a very poor appetite and poor oral intake, and has become quite dehydrated and confused. She came to the hospital in an extremely weak and confused condition. She was noted to have hyponatremia with sodium down to 125, extremely dry mucous membranes. White count was elevated to 16.5. Hemoglobin has been right around 10. Initial labs also suggested a urinary tract infection, although the culture did not grow anything.

She was admitted and treated with IV fluids and nausea medication, and started on Cipro for presumed UTI. Her condition improved so that she became mentally clear. She continues to have poor oral intake and needs a lot of encouragement, but is discharged home to be followed by hospice. Her long-term prognosis is poor, probably in the range of months.

Discharge medications include Cipro 500 mg for an additional 7 days. Compazine 10 mg po every 6 hr for nausea, Ultram 1 to 2 tablets t.i.d. for pain, and Senokot 1 to 2 tablets p.r.n. for constipation. Plan of care was discussed with her and her family, and hospice will be following her.

| PROD | MAHAFC | 04/07/2012 | 20:25 |

# Exercise 6: Discharge Summary

*Using the discharge summary on p. 611, fill in the blanks.*

1. This patient has "metastatic breast cancer." What does this mean? _____

2. Where has the cancer spread to? _____

3. What type of treatment has she received? _____

4. The patient is dehydrated and hyponatremia is noted. What is hyponatremia? _____

5. Explain what "her long-term prognosis is poor, probably in the range of months" means.

_____

## Abbreviations

| Abbreviations | Meaning | Abbreviations | Meaning |
| --- | --- | --- | --- |
| 3DCRT | 3-dimensional conformal radiotherapy | CT | computed tomography |
| ACS | American Cancer Society | CTR | certified tumor registrar |
| AFP | alpha-fetoprotein test | FOBT | fecal occult blood test |
| B2M | beta-2 microglobulin | G | grade |
| BMT | bone marrow transplant | GI | gastrointestinal |
| BSE | breast self-examination | hCG | human chorionic gonadotropin |
| BTA | bladder tumor antigen | IMRT | intensity-modulated radiation therapy |
| bx | biopsy | IVU | intravenous urogram |
| CA | cancer | mets | metastases |
| CA125 | tumor marker primarily for ovarian cancer | MS | musculoskeletal |
| CA15-3 | tumor marker to monitor breast cancer | NSE | neuron-specific enolase (used to detect neuroblastoma, small cell cancer) |
| CA19-9 | tumor marker for pancreatic, stomach, and bile duct cancer | Pap | Papanicolaou test for cervical/vaginal cancer |
| CA27-29 | tumor marker to check for recurrence of breast cancer | PET | positron emission tomography |
| CAM | complementary and alternative medicine | PSA | prostate-specific antigen |
| | | SPECT | single-photon emission computed tomography |
| CEA | carcinoembryonic antigen (used to monitor colorectal cancer) | TA-90 | tumor marker for spread of malignant melanoma |
| CIS | carcinoma in situ | TNM | tumor-nodes-metastases |
| CNS | central nervous system | TSE | testicular self-examination |

## Exercise 7: Abbreviations

*Write the meaning of the following abbreviations.*

1. The patient appeared for a bx of a suspicious mole.

   _____

2. The prognosis was poor for the lung cancer patient with a G IV finding on his pathology report.

   _____

3. The 50-year-old woman made an appointment for a colonoscopy to check for CA after she had a positive finding on a home FOBT.

   _____

4. The CTR at Montgomery Memorial recorded the TNM stage for the patient's abstract.

   _____

5. SPECT was used to detect bone mets in the patient with advanced breast cancer.

   _____

For more interactive learning, go to Evolve and click on:
- **Whack a Word Part** to review oncology word parts.
- **Wheel of Terminology** and **Word Shop** to practice word building.
- **Tournament of Terminology** to test your knowledge of oncology terms.
- **Terminology Triage** to practice sorting oncology terms into categories.

# Chapter Review

*Match the word parts to their definitions.*

## WORD PART DEFINITIONS

| Prefix/Suffix | | Definition |
|---|---|---|
| ana- | 1. _____ | new |
| apo- | 2. _____ | condition of formation |
| -blast | 3. _____ | tumor |
| -carcinoma | 4. _____ | away from |
| dys- | 5. _____ | abnormal |
| ecto- | 6. _____ | production, origin |
| -genesis | 7. _____ | up, apart |
| hyper- | 8. _____ | embryonic |
| meta- | 9. _____ | cancer of epithelial origin |
| neo- | 10. _____ | outer |
| -oma | 11. _____ | controlling, stopping |
| -plasia | 12. _____ | connective tissue cancer |
| -plasm | 13. _____ | beyond, change |
| -ptosis | 14. _____ | formation |
| -sarcoma | 15. _____ | excessive |
| -stasis | 16. _____ | falling |

| Combining Form | | Definition |
|---|---|---|
| blast/o | 17. _____ | change |
| carcin/o | 18. _____ | embryonic |
| derm/o | 19. _____ | connective tissue cancer |
| mut/a | 20. _____ | tumor |
| nod/o | 21. _____ | disease |
| onc/o | 22. _____ | node |
| path/o | 23. _____ | skin |
| sarc/o | 24. _____ | cancer |

## WORDSHOP

| Prefixes | Combining Forms | Suffixes |
|---|---|---|
| ana- | aden/o | -oma |
| apo- | astr/o | -plasia |
| brachy- | blast/o | -ptosis |
|  | chrom/o | -sarcoma |
|  | cyt/o | -therapy |
|  | hemangi/o | -tion |
|  | meningi/o |  |
|  | mut/a |  |
|  | nephr/o |  |
|  | neur/o |  |
|  | oste/o |  |
|  | phe/o |  |
|  | retin/o |  |

Build the following terms by combining the above word parts. Some word parts will be used more than once. Some may not be used at all. The number in parentheses indicates the number of word parts needed to build the terms.

| Definition | Term |
|---|---|
| 1. tumor of a nerve (2) |  |
| 2. tumor of a blood vessel (2) |  |
| 3. malignant tumor of bone (2) |  |
| 4. tumor of a gland (2) |  |
| 5. tumor of embryonic retinal (cells) (3) |  |
| 6. treatment using short distance (radiation) (2) |  |
| 7. condition of formation apart (dedifferentiation) (2) |  |
| 8. falling away (cell suicide) (2) |  |
| 9. process of change (2) |  |
| 10. tumor of the meninges (2) |  |
| 11. star cell tumor (3) |  |
| 12. kidney tumor (2) |  |
| 13. dark color cell tumor (4) |  |

*Sort the terms into the correct categories.*

## TERM SORTING

| Benign Neoplasms | Malignant Neoplasms | Diagnostic Procedures | Therapeutic Interventions |
|---|---|---|---|
| | | | |
| | | | |
| | | | |
| | | | |
| | | | |
| | | | |
| | | | |
| | | | |
| | | | |
| | | | |

| | | | |
|---|---|---|---|
| 3DCRT | chemotherapy | IMRT | osteoma |
| acoustic neuroma | CT scan | Kaposi sarcoma | PET |
| adenocarcinoma | dermatofibroma | leiomyoma | pheochromocytoma |
| AFP | Ewing sarcoma | leukemia | PSA |
| biopsy | fibroids | lumpectomy | radiotherapy |
| BMT | gamma knife | mammogram | retinoblastoma |
| BPH | hcG | mastectomy | seminoma |
| brachytherapy | hemangiosarcoma | meningioma | SPECT |
| BTA | hypernephroma | myxosarcoma | thymoma |
| CA125 | immunotherapy | neuroma | Wilms tumor |

*Replace the highlighted words with the correct terms.*

## TRANSLATIONS

1. The cancer registry student had four cases to abstract: one **testicular cancer,** one **cancer of the bone marrow,** and **two glandular cancers of the lung.**

2. The pathologist described the cancer as **appearing to have cells that retain most of their intended function.**

3. The patient was diagnosed with **spreading beyond control** of breast cancer.

4. The **test for vaginal and cervical cancer** revealed severe **abnormal condition of formation** of the cervical cells.

5. As a result of a breast self-examination, Bonita's Stage I breast cancer was treated with **a removal of the tumor only, treatment with x-rays** and **circulation of cancer-destroying medicine throughout the body.**

6. Allen's prostate cancer was treated with the use of **radioactive beads directly in the tumor.**

7. Ellen was diagnosed with **cancer of white blood cells** and was treated with **cancer-destroying medicine throughout the body** and **bone marrow from a matching donor.**

Forty-five-year-old Clifford Walker, newly diagnosed with colon cancer, is part of a research project regarding familial patterns of cancer occurrence. During the course of the interview, Clifford tells the cancer registrar that his father and brother both died of colon cancer before their fiftieth birthdays. He hopes that the information he is providing can be used to help future colon cancer patients.

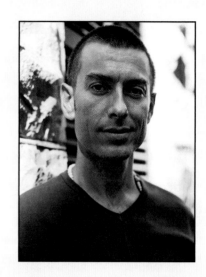

The cancer registrar stages Clifford's cancer by looking at the pathology report. From the size and level of invasion of the tumor recorded on the pathology report, she chooses T4. Because there were no lymph nodes positive for cancer, she chooses N0; because there were no metastases, she chooses M0. Using the rubric provided, she finds that a T4 N0 M0 is the equivalent of a stage II colon cancer. She notes that the pathologist has determined that the cancer is a grade 2, moderately to poorly differentiated.

The information Magda has collected on the familial pattern study will be used to devise better screening for cancers with suspected genetic components. The registry information she collects is continually merged with national data to determine the most efficient treatment protocols.

---

WALKER, CLIFFORD K - 578412 Opened by GOLDBERG, ALBERT MD

Task   Edit   View   Time Scale   Options   Help

As Of 08:40

**WALKER, CLIFFORD K**

Age: 45 years
DOB: 07/31/1965

Sex: Male
MRN: 578412

Loc: WHC-SMMC
FIN: 3506004

Reference Text Browser | Form Browser | Medication Profile

Orders | Last 48 Hours | ED | Lab | Radiology | Assessments | Surgery | **Clinical Notes** | Pt. Info | Pt. Schedule | Task List | I & O | MAR

Flowsheet: Clinical Notes      Level: Discharge Summary        ⦿ Table   ◯ Group   ◯ List

Navigator

✓ Discharge Summary

Diagnosis: Sigmoid colon cancer by colonoscopy
Procedure: Sigmoid colectomy and appendectomy
History: This 45-year-old male with a significant family history of colon cancer came to my office after a colonoscopy demonstrated a carcinoma at 18 cm. He comes now after having an outpatient bowel preparation.
Hospital Course: The patient was admitted, and a sigmoid colectomy was performed. At that time, an appendectomy was also done. His postoperative course was unremarkable. His diet was slowly advanced, and by day 4, he was able to be discharged to home.

His pathology report demonstrated a carcinoma through the wall with a microperforation. He had 12 nodes examined, all negative for carcinoma. His appendix was also positive for subacute appendicitis. He was scheduled for follow-up in my office in 10 days.

PROD | MAHAFC | 14 Dec 2010 | 08:40

## ⟳ Discharge Summary

*Using the Discharge Summary on p. 618, answer the following questions.*

1. What was the patient's diagnosis?

   _____

2. How was his cancer diagnosed?

   _____

3. What procedures were done?

   _____

4. How do we know that there was no cancer in the lymph nodes?

   _____

# Illustration Credits

Beare PG, Myers: *Adult health nursing,* ed 3, St Louis, 1998, Mosby (Fig. 11-19D).

Bird D, Robinson D: *Torres and Ehrlich modern dental assisting,* ed 8, Philadelphia, 2005, Saunders (Fig. 5-9).

Black JM, Hawks JH, Keene A: *Medical-surgical nursing: clinical management for positive outcomes,* ed 8, Philadelphia, 2009, Saunders (Figs. 5-11, 6-22, 8-16, 9-12, 11-15A, 12-17B, 12-20B, 14-11, 14-17, 14-26, 15-14).

Bolognia JL: *Dermatology,* ed 2, St Louis, 2008, Mosby (Figs. 5-8, 9-11).

Bonewit-West K: *Clinical procedures for medical assistants,* ed 7, Philadelphia, 2008, Saunders (Figs. 6-11, 6-12, 9-20).

Bontrager KL: *Textbook of radiographic positioning and related anatomy,* ed 7, St Louis, 2009, Mosby (Fig. 6-15).

Bork K, Brauninger W: *Skin disease in clinical practice,* ed 2, Philadelphia, 1999, Saunders (Fig. 4-15).

Brody HJ: *Chemical peeling,* ed 2, St Louis, 1997, Mosby (Fig. 4-36).

Callen JP, Greer KE, Saller AS, et al: *Color atlas of dermatology,* ed 3, Philadelphia, 2003, Saunders (Figs. 4-5, 4-12, 4-14, 4-18 to 4-20, 4-21).

The Centers for Disease Control: Figs. 4-28

Christian PE: *Nuclear Medicine and PET/CT: technology and techniques,* ed 7, 2012 (Fig. 16-8)

Christensen BL: *Foundations and adult health nursing,* ed 6, St Louis, 2010, Mosby (Fig. 11-19D)

Cotran RS, et al: *Robbins' pathologic basis of disease,* ed 6, 1999 (Fig. 10-17B)

De la Maza, et al: *Color atlas of diagnostic microbiology,* St Lous, 1997, Mosby (Fig. 7-15)

Damjanov I: *Anderson's pathology,* ed 10, St Louis, 2000, Mosby (Figs. 3-22, 4-25, 5-26, 6-10, 7-12, 8-12, 9-15, 10-19, 14-15, 15-9).

Damjanov I: *Pathology: a color atlas,* St Louis, 2000, Mosby (Figs. 5-12, 5-14A, 5-16, 5-17B, 10-15, 10-16BC, 11-6, 11-10, 12-11).

Early PJ, Sodee DB: *Nuclear medicine: principles and practice,* ed 2, St Louis, 1994, Mosby (Fig. 11-16).

Eisen D, Lynch DP: *The mouth: diagnosis and treatment,* St Louis, 1998, Mosby (Fig. 5-10).

Eisenberg RL, Johnson N: *Comprehensive radiographic pathology,* ed 4, St Louis, 2007, Mosby (Fig. 11-15B).

Elkin MK, Perry AG, Potter PA: *Nursing intervention and clinical skills,* ed 4, St Louis, 2008, Mosby (Figs. 4-16, 6-14).

Epstein E: *Common skin disorders,* ed 5, Philadelphia, 2001, Saunders (Fig. 4-7).

Feldman M, et al: *Sleisenger and Fordtran's gastrointestinal and lvier disease,* ed 8, Philadelphia, 2006, Saunders (Fig. 1-1).

Fletcher CD: Diagnostic histopathology of tumors, ed 3, London, 2008, Churchill Livingstone (Figs. 8-10B, 10-18).

Fortinash KM: *Psychiatric mental health nursing,* ed 4, St Louis, 2008, Mosby (Fig. 13-3).

Frank ED, Long BW, Smith BJ: *Merrill's atlas of radiographic positions and radiologic procedures,* ed 12, St Louis, 2012, Mosby (Figs. 2-3, 2-4, 3-12, 3-15B, 3-24, 5-22, 5-23, 5-24, 6-8, 6-13, 8-10A, 8-13, 9-17, 10-20, 10-22, 10-26, 12-21, 10-23A, 10-26, 15-11, 16-10).

Frazier MS, Drzymkowski JW: *Essentials of human diseases and conditions,* ed 4, Philadelphia, 2008, Saunders (Figs. 4-13, 5-18, 6-16B).

Fuller JK: *Surgical technology,* ed 4, Philadelphia, 2006, Saunders (Figs. 1-9, 3-23B, 5-28B, 5-29, 14-18)

Goldberg JG, Falcone T: Atlas of endoscopic techniques in gynecology, Philadelphia, 2000, Saunders (Fig. 8-19).

Habif TP: *Clinical dermatology,* ed 5, St Louis, 3010, Mosby (Figs 4-10, 4-23, 4-34, 9-19).

Hagen-Ansert SL: *Textbook of diagnostic sonography,* ed 7, St Louis, 2012, Mosby (Figs. 8-9, 8-14B, 8-15, 10-23B).

Herlihy B, Maebius NK: *The human body in health and illness,* ed 4, Philadelphia, 2011, Saunders (Figs. 9-6, 9-9, 12-24, 14-1, 14-9).

Hill MJ: *Skin disorders,* St Louis, 1994, Mosby (Figs. 4-11, 4-13).

Ignatavicius DD, Workman ML: *Medical-surgical nursing: critical thinking for collaborative care,* ed 6, Philadelphia, 2011, Saunders (Figs. 4-32, 6-7, 6-21AB, 11-21, 14-16, 14-20, 14-21, 15-5, 15-12).

Kowalczyk N: *Radiographic pathology for technologists,* ed 5, St Louis, 2009, Mosby (Figs. 3-26A, 3-31A, 16-7).

Kumar P, Clark ML: *Kumar and Clarks's clinical medicine,* ed 7, Philadelphia, 2009, Saunders (Figs. 6-9, 7-11, 9-10, 12-17).

Kumar V, Abbas AK, Fausto N: *Basic pathology,* ed 7, Philadelphia, 2003, Saunders (Fig. 12-19).

Kumar V, et al: *Robbins basic pathology,* ed 8, Philadelphia, 2007, Saunders (Fig. 11-13).

LaTrenta G: Atlas of aesthetic face and neck surgery, Philadelphia, 2004, Saunders (Fig. 4-35).

Lewis SM: *Medical-surgical nursing: assessment and management of clinical problems,* ed 8, St Louis, 2011, Mosby (Figs. 3-13, 3-23A, 6-5, 6-14, 10-9BC, 10-17, 12-26).

Lowdermilk DL, Perry SE, Bobak IM: *Maternity and women's health care,* ed 10, St Louis, 2012, Mosby (Figs. 8-11, 8-25).

Mahan LK, Escott-Stump S: *Krause's food and nutrition therapy,* ed 12, Philadelphia, 2008, Saunders (Fig. 5-17A).

Marks JG jr, Miller JJ: *Lookingbill & Marks' principles of dermatology,* ed 4, London, 2006, Saunders (Fig. 4-9).

McCance KL, Huether SE: *Pathophysiology: the biologic basis for disease in adults and children,* ed 6, St Louis, 2010, Mosby (Figs. 4-26, 4-30).

*Mosby's medical nursing and allied health dictionary,* ed 8, St Louis, 2009, Mosby (Figs. 7-9, 7-10, 15-4).

Murray SS: *Foundations of maternal newborn & women's health nursing,* ed 5, Philadelphia, 2010, Saunders (Figs. 1-11, 8-22, unn 8-7).

O'Neill WC: *Atlas of renal ultrasonography,* Philadelphia, 2001, Saunders (Fig. 6-6A).

Pagana KD, Pagana TJ: *Mosby's manual of diagnostic and lab tests,* ed 4, St Louis, 2010, Mosby (Fig. 12-22).

*PHTLS basic and advanced prehospital trauma life support,* ed 7, St Louis, 2011, Mosby (Fig. 14-10).

Potter PA, Perry AG: *Fundamentals of nursing,* ed 7, St Louis, 2011, Mosby (Figs. 5-26B, 11-19A-C).

Salvo SG: *Mosby's pathology for massage therapists,* ed 2, St Louis, 2009, Mosby (Fig. 5-17).

Seidel HM, et al: *Mosby's guide to physical examination,* ed 7, St Louis, 2011, Mosby (Figs. 3-11, 4-8, 4-29, 7-6, 7-7, 12-2A, 14-3, 14-4, 14-6 to 14-8).

Sorrentino SA: *Textbook for long-term care nursing assistants,* ed 6, St Louis, 2011, Mosby (Fig. 11-18).

Sorrentino SA: *Assisting with patient care,* ed 2, St Louis, 2004, Mosby (Fig. 14-4).

Stone DR, Gorbach SL: *Atlas of infectious diseases,* Philadelphia, 2000, Saunders (Fig. 14-23).

Stuart GW, Laraia MT: *Principles and practice of psychiatric nursing,* ed 9, St Louis, 2009, Mosby (Figs. 13-1, 13-2, 13-3).

Thibodeau GA, Patton KT: *Anatomy and physiology,* ed 7, St Louis, 2010, Mosby (Figs. 9-13, 10-17B).

Thibodeau GA, Patton KT: *The human body in health and disease,* ed 5, St Louis, 2010, Mosby (Figs. 12-5, 12-16, 12-23, 15-3, 15-7).

Wilson SF, Giddens JF: *Health assessment for nursing practice,* ed 4, St Louis, 2012, Mosby (Figs. 3-15A, 3-25, 4-6.

Young AP, Proctor DB: *Kinn's the medical assistant,* ed 11, Philadelphia, 2011, Saunders (Figs. 3-16, 10-24, 11-17).

Ziessman HA: *Nuclear medicine, the requisites,* ed 3, St Louis, 2011, Mosby (Fig. 15-10).

Zitelli BJ, Davis HW: *Atlas of pediatric physical diagnosis,* ed 5, St Louis, 2007, Mosby (Figs. 3-9 to 3-11, 5-6, 5-13, 5-19, 7-3, 11-4, 11-5, 12-9, 14-5, 14-24, 14-25, 14-28, 15-6, 15-20).

# References

**Chapter 1**

Beers MH, Berkow R, Burs M, editors: *Merck manual diagnosis and therapy*, Whitehouse Station, NJ, 1999, Merck & Co.

Haubrich WS, editor: *Medical meanings: a glossary of word origins*, Philadelphia, 1997, American College of Physicians.

Plato: The republic, New York, 1955, Viking Press (Translated by D Lee).

**Chapter 2**

Shakespeare W: Hamlet. In Montgomery W, Jowet J, Wells S, et al, editors: *Oxford Shakespeare: the complete works of William Shakespeare*, New York, 1999, Oxford University Press.

**Chapter 3**

Anderson GP: *Healing wisdom: wit, insight, and inspiration for anyone facing illness*, New York, 1994, EP Dutton.

Bureau of Labor Statistics: *Occupational outlook handbook*, Washington, DC, 2002-2003, U.S. Department of Labor.

Davis NM: *Medical abbreviations: 14,000 conveniences at the expense of communication and safety*, ed 9, Huntingdon Valley, PA, 1999, Neil M. Davis Associates.

Haubrich WS, editor: *Medical meanings: a glossary of word origins*, Philadelphia, 1997, American College of Physicians.

**Chapter 4**

Edison TA: Life. In Bartlett J, Kaplan J, editors: *Bartlett's familiar quotations: a collection of passages, phrases, and proverbs traced to their sources in ancient and modern literature*, ed 16, New York, 1992, Little, Brown.

Micozzi MS: *Fundamentals of complementary and alternative medicine*, ed 2, New York, 2001, Churchill -Livingstone.

Novey DW: Clinician's complete reference to complementary and alternative medicine, St Louis, 2000, Mosby.

**Chapter 5**

Byrne R: *The 2,548 best things anybody ever said*, New York, 2003, Simon & Schuster.

Franklin B: Letter to Jean-Baptiste Leroy (November 13, 1789). In Bartlett J, Kaplan J, editors: *Bartlett's familiar quotations: a collection of passages, phrases, and proverbs traced to their sources in ancient and modern literature*, ed 16, New York, 1992, Little, Brown.

Rybacki J, Long J: The essential guide to prescription drugs 2001: everything you need to know for safe drug use, New York, 2000, Harper Collins.

**Chapter 6**

Beers MH, Berkow R, Burs M, editors: *Merck manual of diagnosis and therapy*, 1999, Merck & Co.

Dinesen I (Karen Blixen): The dreamers. In *Seven gothic tales*, New York, 1934, Random House.

Smith H: Lectures on the kidney, Lawrence, 1943, University of Kansas. Available online: ACP-ASIM Medicine in Quotations, http://www.acponline.org/cgi-bin/medquotes.pl.

**Chapter 7**

Bureau of Labor Statistics: *Occupational outlook handbook*, Washington, DC, 2002-2003, U.S. Department of Labor.

Freeman L, Lawlin GF: *Mosby's complementary and alternative medicine: a research-based approach*, St Louis, 2001, Mosby.

Richardson B: Congressional record, 43905-43906, May 24, 1994.

**Chapter 8**

Fischbach F: A manual of laboratory and diagnostic tests, ed 6, Philadelphia, 2000, Lippincott Williams & Wilkins.

**Chapter 9**

Prescott L: Novel anti-IgE monoclonal antibody promising against allergic diseases, *Inpharma* 1232:7-8, 2000.

Quote from http://www.quoteablequotes.net.

**Chapter 11**

American College of Physicians—American Society of Internal Medicine: A pulmonologist's valentine, *N Engl J Med* 304:739, 1981. Available online: ACP-ASIM Medicine in Quotations, http://www.acponline.org/cgi-bin/medquotes.pl.

**Chapter 12**

Quereshi B: Review of Jones L, Sidell M: The challenge of promoting health: exploration and action, *J R Soc Med* 90:705, 1997. Available online: ACP-ASIM Medicine in Quotations, http://www.acponline.org/cgi-bin/medquotes.pl.

**Chapter 13**

Dubos RJ: The three faces of medicine, *Bull Am Coll Phys* 2:162-166, 1961.

**Chapter 14**

Quote from http://www.quoteablequotes.net.

**Chapter 16**

Mayo CH, Hendricks WA: Carcinomas of the right segment of the colon, *Ann Surg* 83:357-363, 1926.

# Appendix A

## Word Parts and Definitions

| Word Part | Meaning | Word Part | Meaning |
|-----------|---------|-----------|---------|
| -a | noun ending | ana- | up, apart, away |
| a- | no, not, without | andr/o | male |
| ab- | away from | angi/o | vessel |
| abdomin/o | abdomen | ankyl/o | stiffening |
| -ablation | removal | ante- | forward, in front of, before |
| -abrasion | scraping of | anter/o | front |
| -ac | pertaining to | anthrop/o | man |
| acid/o | acid | anti- | against |
| acous/o | hearing | antr/o | antrum, cavity |
| acro- | heights, extremes, extremities | aort/o | aorta (largest artery) |
| acromi/o | acromion | -apheresis | removal |
| acu- | sharp | aphth/o | ulceration |
| -acusis | hearing | apic/o | pointed extremity, apex |
| -ad | toward | apo- | separate, away from |
| ad- | toward | append/o | vermiform appendix, that which is added |
| aden/o | gland | | |
| adenoid/o | adenoid (pharyngeal tonsil) | appendic/o | vermiform appendix, that which is added |
| adip/o | fat | | |
| adnex/o | accessory | -ar | pertaining to |
| adren/o | adrenal gland | -arche | beginning |
| aer/o | air | arteri/o | artery |
| af- | toward | arteriol/o | arteriole (small artery) |
| agglutin/o | clumping | arthr/o | articulation (joint) |
| agora- | marketplace | articul/o | articulation (joint) |
| -al | pertaining to | -ary | pertaining to |
| albin/o | white | -ase | enzyme |
| albumin/o | protein | astr/o | star |
| -algia | pain | ather/o | fatty plaque |
| aliment/o | nutrition | -atic | pertaining to |
| allo- | other, different | -ation | process of |
| alveol/o | alveolus | atri/o | atrium |
| ambly/o | dull, dim | audi/o | hearing |
| ambul/o | walking | aur/o | ear |
| amni/o | amnion | auricul/o | ear |
| -amnios | amnion, inner fetal sac | auto- | self |
| amphi- | both | axill/o | axilla (armpit) |
| amyl/o | starch | az/o | nitrogen |
| -an | pertaining to | azot/o | nitrogen |
| an- | no, not, without | bacteri/o | bacteria |
| an/o | anus | balan/o | glans penis |

*Continued*

## Word Parts and Definitions—cont'd

| Word Part | Meaning | Word Part | Meaning |
|-----------|---------|-----------|---------|
| bar/o | pressure, weight | cellul/o | cell |
| bartholin/o | Bartholin gland | -centesis | surgical puncture |
| bas/o | base, bottom | cephal/o | head |
| bi- | two | cerebell/o | cerebellum |
| bi/o | life, living | cerebr/o | cerebrum |
| bil/i | bile | cerumin/o | cerumen (earwax) |
| bin- | two | cervic/o | neck, cervix |
| -blast | embryonic, immature | -chalasia | condition of relaxation, slackening |
| blast/o | embryonic, immature | -chalasis | relaxation, slackening |
| blephar/o | eyelid | cheil/o | lips |
| bol/o | to throw, throwing | chem/o | drug, chemical |
| brachi/o | arm | -chezia | condition of stools |
| brachy- | short | chol/e | bile, gall |
| brady- | slow | cholangi/o | bile vessel |
| bronch/o | bronchus | cholecyst/o | gallbladder |
| bronchi/o | bronchus | choledoch/o | common bile duct |
| bronchiol/o | bronchiole | cholesterol/o | cholesterol |
| bucc/o | cheek | chondr/o | cartilage |
| bunion/o | bunion | chord/o | cord, spinal cord |
| burs/o | bursa | chori/o | chorion (outer fetal sac) |
| calc/o, calc/i | calcium | chorion/o | chorion (outer fetal sac) |
| calcane/o | calcaneus (heelbone) | choroid/o | choroid, vascular membrane |
| calcul/o | stone, calculus | chrom/o | color |
| cali/o | calyx, calix | chromat/o | color |
| calic/o | calyx, calix | chym/o | juice |
| calyc/o | calyx, calix | circum- | around |
| cancer/o | cancer, malignancy | cirrh/o | orange-yellow |
| canth/o | canthus (corner of eye) | -cision | process of cutting |
| capit/o | head | -clasis | intentional breaking |
| capn/o | carbon dioxide | -clast | breaking down |
| carcin/o | cancer | claustr/o | closing |
| -carcinoma | cancer of epithelial origin | clavicul/o | clavicle (collarbone) |
| cardi/o | heart | cleid/o | clavicle (collarbone) |
| -cardia | condition of the heart | clitorid/o | clitoris |
| carp/o | carpus (wrist) | -coagulation | process of clotting |
| cartilag/o | cartilage | coccyg/o | coccyx (tailbone) |
| cata- | down | cochle/o | cochlea |
| caud/o | tail | col/o | colon (large intestine) |
| cauter/i | burning | coll/o | neck |
| cec/o | cecum (first part of large intestine) | colon/o | colon (large intestine) |
| -cele | herniation, protrusion | colp/o | vagina |
| celi/o | abdomen | commissur/o | connection |

## Word Parts and Definitions—cont'd

| Word Part | Meaning |
| --- | --- |
| con- | together |
| con/o | cone |
| condyl/o | condyle, knob |
| coni/o | dust |
| conjunctiv/o | conjunctiva |
| contra- | opposite, against |
| cor/o | pupil |
| cord/o | cord, spinal cord |
| cordi/o | heart |
| core/o | pupil |
| corne/o | cornea |
| coron/o | crown, heart |
| corpor/o | body |
| cortic/o | cortex (outer portion) |
| cost/o | costa (rib) |
| cox/o | coxa (hip) |
| crani/o | cranium (skull) |
| crin/o | to secrete, secreting |
| -crine | to secrete, secreting |
| -crit | to separate, separating |
| crur/o | leg |
| cry/o | extreme cold |
| crypt- | hidden |
| cubit/o | elbow, forearm |
| culd/o | cul-de-sac (rectouterine pouch) |
| -cusis | hearing |
| cut/o | skin |
| cutane/o | skin |
| cyan/o | blue |
| cycl/o | ciliary body, recurring, round |
| -cyesis | pregnancy, gestation |
| cyst/o | bladder, sac |
| cyt/o | cell |
| -cyte | cell |
| -cytosis | abnormal increase in cells |
| dacry/o | tear |
| dacryoaden/o | lacrimal gland |
| dacryocyst/o | lacrimal sac |
| dactyl/o | digitus (finger or toe) |
| de- | down, lack of |
| dendr/o | dendrite, tree |
| dent/i | teeth |
| derm/o | skin |

| Word Part | Meaning |
| --- | --- |
| dermat/o | skin |
| -desis | binding |
| dextr/o | right |
| di- | two, both |
| dia- | through, complete |
| diaphragm/o | diaphragm |
| diaphragmat/o | diaphragm |
| digit/o | finger or toe |
| dipl/o | double |
| dips/o | thirst |
| -dipsia | condition of thirst |
| dis- | bad, abnormal, apart |
| dist/o | far |
| diverticul/o | diverticulum, pouch |
| dors/o | back |
| -drome | to run, running |
| duct/o | to carry, carrying |
| duoden/o | duodenum |
| dur/o | dura mater, hard |
| -dynia | pain |
| dys- | bad, difficult, painful, abnormal |
| -e | noun ending |
| e- | outward, out |
| -eal | pertaining to |
| ec- | out, outward |
| echo- | sound, reverberation |
| -ectasia | condition of expansion, dilation |
| -ectasis | expansion, dilation |
| ecto- | outward, outer |
| -ectomy | removal, excision |
| -edema | swelling |
| ef- | away from |
| electr/o | electricity |
| -emesis | vomiting, vomit |
| -emia | blood condition |
| -emic | pertaining to blood condition |
| en- | in |
| encephal/o | brain |
| end- | within |
| endo- | within |
| endocardi/o | inner lining of the heart |
| endometri/o | endometrium |
| enter/o | small intestines, intestines |

*Continued*

## Word Parts and Definitions—cont'd

| Word Part | Meaning | Word Part | Meaning |
|---|---|---|---|
| eosin/o | rosy-colored | fornic/o | arched structure, fornix |
| epi- | above, upon | foss/o | hollow, depression |
| epicardi/o | epicardium | front/o | front, forehead |
| epicondyl/o | epicondyle | fund/o | fundus (base, bottom) |
| epididym/o | epididymis | fung/i | fungus |
| epiglott/o | epiglottis | -fusion | process of pouring |
| episi/o | vulva (external female genitalia) | galact/o | milk |
| epitheli/o | epithelium | gastr/o | stomach |
| erg/o | work | -gen | producing, produced by |
| erythr/o | red | gen/o | origin, originate |
| erythrocyt/o | red blood cell | -genesis | production, origin |
| eschar/o | scab | -genic | pertaining to produced by |
| -esis | state of | -genous | pertaining to originating from |
| eso- | inward | ger/o | old age |
| esophag/o | esophagus | geus/o | taste |
| esthesi/o | feeling, sensation | gingiv/o | gums |
| ethmoid/o | ethmoid bone | glauc/o | gray, bluish green |
| eu- | healthy, normal | -glia | glia cell, glue |
| ex- | out | -globin | protein substance |
| exanthemat/o | rash | -globulin | protein substance |
| -exia | condition | glomerul/o | glomerulus |
| exo- | outside | gloss/o | tongue |
| extra- | outside | gluc/o | sugar, glucose |
| faci/o | face | glute/o | gluteus (buttocks) |
| fallopi/o | fallopian tube | glyc/o | sugar, glucose |
| fasci/o | fascia | glycos/o | sugar, glucose |
| fec/a | feces, stool | gnath/o | jaw, entire |
| femor/o | femur (thigh bone) | gnos/o | knowledge |
| fer/o | to bear, carry | gon/o | seed |
| -ferous | pertaining to carrying | gonad/o | gonad, sex organ |
| ferr/o | iron | goni/o | angle |
| fet/o | fetus | -gram | record, recording |
| fibr/o | fiber | granul/o | little grain |
| fibrin/o | fibrous substance | -graph | instrument to record |
| fibul/o | fibula (lower lateral leg bone) | graph/o | to write, writing |
| -fida | to split, splitting | -graphy | process of recording |
| flex/o | to bend, bending | gravid/o | pregnancy, gestation |
| fluor/o | to flow, flowing | -gravida | pregnancy, gestation |
| -flux | to flow, flowing | gynec/o | female, woman |
| follicul/o | follicle, small sac | halit/o | breath |
| foramin/o | hole, foramen | hal/o | to breathe, breathing |

## Word Parts and Definitions—cont'd

| Word Part | Meaning |
|---|---|
| hedon/o | pleasure |
| hem/o | blood |
| hemangi/o | blood vessel |
| hemat/o | blood |
| hemi- | half |
| hemorrhoid/o | hemorrhoid |
| hepat/o | liver |
| herni/o | hernia |
| heter/o | different |
| hiat/o | an opening |
| hidr/o | sweat |
| hidraden/o | sudoriferous gland (sweat gland) |
| hil/o | hilum |
| hist/o | tissue |
| home/o | same |
| homo- | same |
| humer/o | humerus (upper arm bone) |
| humor/o | liquid |
| hydr/o | water, fluid |
| hymen/o | hymen |
| hyper- | excessive, above |
| hypo- | deficient, below, under |
| hypophys/o | hypophysis, pituitary |
| hyster/o | uterus |
| -i | noun ending |
| -ia | condition, state of |
| -iac | pertaining to |
| -iasis | condition, presence of |
| iatr/o | treatment |
| -iatric | pertaining to treatment |
| -iatrician | one who specializes in treatment |
| -iatrist | one who specializes in treatment |
| -iatry | process of treatment |
| -ic | pertaining to |
| ichthy/o | fishlike |
| -ician | one who studies |
| -icle | small, tiny |
| -id | pertaining to |
| idi/o | unique, unknown |
| -ile | pertaining to |
| ile/o | ileum (third part small intestines) |

| Word Part | Meaning |
|---|---|
| ili/o | ilium (superior, widest pelvic bone) |
| immun/o | safety, protection |
| -in | substance |
| in- | in, not |
| -ine | pertaining to |
| infer/o | downward |
| infra- | down |
| inguin/o | groin |
| insulin/o | insulin |
| inter- | between |
| interstit/o | space between |
| intestin/o | intestine |
| intra- | within |
| -ion | process of |
| -ior | pertaining to |
| ipsi- | same |
| ir/o | iris |
| irid/o | iris |
| -is | structure, thing, noun ending |
| is/o | equal |
| isch/o | hold back, suppress |
| ischi/o | ischium (lower part of pelvic bone) |
| -ism | condition, state of |
| -ist | one who specializes |
| -itis | inflammation |
| -itic | pertaining to |
| -ium | structure, membrane |
| -ive | pertaining to |
| -ization | process of |
| jejun/o | second part of small intestine jejunum |
| kal/i | potassium |
| kary/o | nucleus |
| kathis/o | sitting |
| kerat/o | hard, horny, cornea |
| ket/o | ketone |
| keton/o | ketone |
| -kine | movement |
| kinesi/o | movement |

*Continued*

## Word Parts and Definitions—cont'd

| Word Part | Meaning |
|---|---|
| -kinin | movement substance |
| klept/o | to steal, stealing |
| kyph/o | roundback |
| labi/o | lips, labia |
| labyrinth/o | labyrinth (inner ear) |
| lacrim/o | tear |
| lact/o | milk |
| -lalia | condition of babbling |
| lamin/o | lamina, thin plate |
| lapar/o | abdomen |
| -lapse | falling, dropping, prolapse |
| laryng/o | larynx (voice box) |
| later/o | side |
| lei/o | smooth |
| leiomy/o | smooth muscle |
| -lepsy | seizure |
| leuk/o | white |
| leukocyt/o | white blood cell |
| levo- | left |
| lex/o | word, speech |
| ligament/o | ligament |
| ligat/o | to tie, tying |
| lingu/o | tongue |
| lip/o | fat |
| lipid/o | lipid, fat |
| -listhesis | slipping |
| lith/o | stone, calculus |
| -lithotomy | removal of a stone |
| lob/o | lobe, section |
| lobul/o | small lobe |
| log/o | study |
| -logist | one who specializes in the study of |
| -logy | study of |
| long/o | long |
| lord/o | swayback |
| lumb/o | lower back |
| lumin/o | lumen (space within vessel) |
| lymph/o | lymph |
| lymphaden/o | lymph gland (lymph node) |
| lymphangi/o | lymph vessel |
| lymphat/o | lymph |

| Word Part | Meaning |
|---|---|
| lys/o | break down, dissolve |
| -lysis | breaking down, dissolving, loosening, freeing from adhesions |
| -lytic | pertaining to breaking down |
| macro- | large |
| macul/o | macula, macule, macula lutea, spot |
| mal- | bad, poor |
| -malacia | condition of softening |
| malle/o | malleus, hammer |
| malleol/o | distal process lower leg, little malleolus |
| mamm/o | breast |
| man/o | scanty pressure |
| mandibul/o | lower jaw |
| -mania | condition of madness |
| man/u | hand |
| mast/o | breast |
| mastoid/o | mastoid process |
| maxill/o | maxilla (upper jaw bone) |
| meat/o | meatus (opening) |
| medi/o | middle |
| mediastin/o | mediastinum (space between lungs) |
| medull/o | medulla, inner portion |
| -megaly | enlargement |
| melan/o | black, dark |
| men/o | menstruation, menses |
| mening/o | meninges |
| meningi/o | meninges |
| menisc/o | meniscus, crescent |
| menstru/o | menstruation |
| ment/o | mind, chin |
| meso- | middle |
| meta- | beyond, change |
| metacarp/o | metacarpal (hand bone) |
| metatars/o | metatarsal (foot bone) |
| -meter | instrument to measure |
| metr/o | uterus |
| metri/o | uterus |
| -metry | process of measurement |
| micro- | small |

## Word Parts and Definitions—cont'd

| Word Part | Meaning | Word Part | Meaning |
|-----------|---------|-----------|---------|
| mid- | middle | odont/o | teeth |
| -mission | to send, sending | -oid | resembling, like |
| mitochondri/o | mitochondria | olecran/o | elbow |
| mono- | one | olig/o | scanty, few |
| morph/o | shape, form | -oma | tumor, mass |
| muc/o | mucus | omphal/o | umbilicus (navel) |
| multi- | many | onc/o | tumor |
| muscul/o | muscle | -on | structure |
| mut/a | change | -one | hormone, substance that forms |
| my/o | muscle, to shut | onych/o | nail |
| myc/o | fungus | oophor/o | ovary (female gonad) |
| myel/o | bone marrow, spinal cord | ophthalm/o | eye |
| myocardi/o | myocardium (heart muscle) | -opia | vision condition |
| myos/o | muscle | -opsia | vision condition |
| myring/o | eardrum | -opsy | process of viewing |
| myx/o | mucus | opt/o | vision |
| narc/o | sleep, stupor | optic/o | vision |
| nas/o | nose | or/o | mouth, oral cavity |
| nat/o | birth, born | orbit/o | orbit |
| natr/o | sodium | orch/o | testis, testicle (male gonad) |
| necr/o | death, dead | orchi/o | testis, testicle (male gonad) |
| neo- | new | orchid/o | testis, testicle (male gonad) |
| nephr/o | kidney | orex/o | appetite |
| neur/o | nerve | organ/o | organ, viscus |
| neutr/o | neutral | orth/o | straight, upright |
| nev/o | nevus, birthmark | -ose | pertaining to, full of |
| nid/o | nest | -osis | abnormal condition |
| noct/i | night | osm/o | sense of smell |
| nod/o | node, knot | oss/i | bone |
| -noia | condition of mind | osse/o | bone |
| non- | not | ossicul/o | ossicle (tiny bone) |
| nuch/o | neck | oste/o | bone |
| nucle/o | nucleus | ot/o | ear |
| nulli- | none | -ous | pertaining to |
| nyctal/o | night | ov/o | ovum (egg) |
| nymph/o | woman, female | ovari/o | ovary (female gonad) |
| o/o | ovum, egg, female sex cell | ovul/o | ovum (female sex cell) |
| occipit/o | occiput, back of head | ox/i, ox/o | oxygen |
| occlus/o | to close, closing, a blockage | oxy- | rapid |
| -occlusion | condition of closure | palat/o | palate, roof of mouth, palatine bone |
| -occult | secret, hidden | | |
| ocul/o | eye | palm/o | palm |

*Continued*

## Word Parts and Definitions—cont'd

| Word Part | Meaning |
|---|---|
| palpebr/o | eyelid |
| pan- | all |
| pancreat/o | pancreas |
| papill/o | papilla, nipple, optic disk |
| papul/o | papule, pimple |
| par- | beside, near |
| -para | delivery, parturition |
| para- | near, beside, abnormal |
| parathyroid/o | parathyroid |
| parenchym/o | parenchyma |
| -paresis | slight paralysis |
| pariet/o | wall, partition |
| part/o | parturition (delivery) |
| -partum | parturition (delivery) |
| patell/o, patell/a | patella (kneecap) |
| path/o | disease |
| -pathy | disease process |
| -pause | stop, cease |
| pector/o | chest |
| ped/o | foot, child |
| pedicul/o | lice |
| pelv/i, pelv/o | pelvis |
| pen/i | penis |
| -penia | deficiency condition |
| -pepsia | digestion condition |
| per- | through |
| peri- | surrounding, around |
| pericardi/o | sac surrounding the heart |
| perine/o | perineum |
| peritone/o periton/o | peritoneum |
| perone/o | lower, lateral leg bone, fibula |
| -pexy | fixation, suspension |
| phac/o | lens |
| phag/o | to eat, swallow |
| phak/o | lens |
| phalang/o | phalanx (finger/toe bones) |
| phall/o | penis |
| pharyng/o | pharynx (throat) |
| phas/o | speech |
| phe/o | dark |

| Word Part | Meaning |
|---|---|
| -pheresis | removal |
| -phil | attraction |
| phil/o | attraction |
| -philia | condition of attraction; increase |
| phleb/o | vein |
| -phobia | condition of fear, extreme sensitivity |
| phon/o | sound, voice |
| phor/o | to carry, to bear |
| phot/o | light |
| phren/o | diaphragm, mind |
| -phylaxis | protection |
| physi/o | growth; nature |
| -physis | growth; nature |
| phyt/o | growth; nature |
| pil/o | hair |
| pituitar/o | pituitary |
| placent/o | placenta |
| -plakia | condition of patches |
| plant/o | sole of foot |
| plas/o | formation |
| -plasia | condition of formation, development |
| -plasm | formation |
| plasm/o | plasma |
| plast/o | formation |
| -plastin | forming substance |
| -plasty | surgical repair |
| -plegia | paralysis |
| pleur/o | pleura, membrane surrounding lungs |
| plethysm/o | volume |
| plic/o | fold, plica |
| -pnea | breathing |
| pne/o | to breathe, breathing |
| pneum/o | lung, air |
| pneumon/o | lung |
| -poiesis | formation, production |
| -poietin | forming substance |
| pol/o | pole |
| poly- | many, much, excessive, frequent |
| polyp/o | polyp |

## Word Parts and Definitions—cont'd

| Word Part | Meaning | Word Part | Meaning |
|---|---|---|---|
| poplite/o | back of knee | rhabd/o | striated |
| por/o | passage | rhabdomy/o | striated (skeletal) muscle |
| post- | behind, after | rheumat/o | watery flow |
| poster/o | back | rhin/o | nose |
| potass/o | potassium | rhiz/o | spinal nerve root, nerve root |
| prax/o | purposeful movement | rhythm/o | rhythm |
| pre- | before, in front of | rhytid/o | wrinkle |
| preputi/o | prepuce (foreskin) | rib/o | ribose |
| presby- | old age | rot/o | wheel |
| press/o | pressure | -rrhagia, -rrhage | bursting forth |
| primi- | first | | |
| pro- | forward, in front of, in favor of | -rrhaphy | suture, repair |
| proct/o | rectum and anus | -rrhea | discharge, flow |
| prolactin/o | prolactin | -rrheic | pertaining to discharge |
| prostat/o | prostate | -rrhexis | rupture |
| prosth/o, prosthes/o | addition | rug/o | rugae, ridge |
| | | sacr/o | sacrum |
| proxim/o | near | sagitt/o | arrow, separating the sides |
| psych/o | mind | salping/o | tube, fallopian or eustachian |
| -ptosis | drooping, prolapse, falling | -salpinx | fallopian, tube |
| -ptysis | spitting | sarc/o | flesh |
| pub/o | pubis, anterior pelvic bone | -sarcoma | connective tissue cancer |
| pulmon/o | lung | scapul/o | scapula (shoulder blade) |
| pupill/o | pupil | schiz/o | split |
| puerper/o | childbirth, puerperium | scler/o | sclera, hard |
| purpur/o | purple | -sclerosis | abnormal condition of hardening |
| pustul/o | pustule | scoli/o | curvature |
| py/o | pus | -scope | instrument to view |
| pyel/o | renal pelvis | -scopic | pertaining to viewing |
| pylor/o | pylorus | -scopy | process of viewing |
| pyr/o | fever, fire | scot/o | dark |
| pyret/o | fever, fire | scrot/o | scrotum (sac holding testes) |
| quadri- | four | sebac/o | sebum, oil |
| rachi/o | spinal column, backbone | seb/o | sebum, oil |
| radi/o | radius (lower lateral arm bone) | semin/i | semen |
| radi/o | rays | seps/o | infection |
| radicul/o | nerve root, spinal nerve root | -sepsis | infection |
| re- | back, backward, again | sept/o | septum, wall, partition |
| rect/o | rectum, straight | septic/o | infection |
| ren/o | kidney | ser/o | serum |
| reticul/o | network | sial/o | saliva |
| retin/o | retina | sialaden/o | salivary gland |
| retro- | backward | sider/o | iron |

*Continued*

## Word Parts and Definitions—cont'd

| Word Part | Meaning |
|---|---|
| -siderin | iron substance |
| sigmoid/o | sigmoid colon |
| sin/o | sinus, cavity |
| sinistr/o | left |
| sinus/o | sinus, cavity |
| -sis | state of, condition |
| skelet/o | skeleton |
| somat/o | body |
| somn/o | sleep |
| son/o | sound |
| -spadias | a rent or tear |
| -spasm | spasm, sudden, involuntary contraction |
| sperm/o | spermatozoon (male sex cell) |
| spermat/o | spermatozoon (male sex cell) |
| sphenoid/o | sphenoid |
| spin/o | spine |
| spir/o | to breathe, breathing |
| splen/o | spleen |
| spondyl/o | vertebra, backbone, spine |
| squam/o | scaly |
| -stalsis | contraction |
| staped/o | stapes (third ossicle in ear) |
| -stasis | controlling, stopping |
| steat/o | fat |
| -stenosis | abnormal condition of narrowing |
| ster/o | steroid |
| stere/o | 3-dimensional |
| stern/o | sternum (breastbone) |
| steth/o | chest |
| sthen/o | strength |
| -sthenia | condition of strength |
| stom/o | an opening, a mouth |
| stomat/o | mouth, oral cavity |
| -stomy | new opening |
| strom/o | stroma (supportive tissue) |
| sub- | under, below |
| sudor/i | sweat |
| sulc/o | sulcus, groove |
| super/o | upward |
| supra- | upward, above |
| sur/o | calf |

| Word Part | Meaning |
|---|---|
| sympath/o | to feel with |
| syn- | together, joined |
| syndesm/o | ligament (structure connecting bone) |
| synovi/o | synovium |
| tachy- | fast, rapid |
| tars/o | tarsal bone (ankle bone) |
| tax/o | order, coordination |
| tel/e | end, far, complete |
| tele/o | end, far, complete |
| tempor/o | temporal bone |
| ten/o | tendon (structure connecting muscles to bones) |
| tend/o | tendon (structure connecting muscles to bones) |
| tendin/o | tendon (structure connecting muscles to bones) |
| tens/o | stretching |
| -tension | process of stretching, pressure |
| terat/o | deformity |
| test/o | testis, testicle (male gonad) |
| testicul/o | testis, testicle (male gonad) |
| tetra- | four |
| thalam/o | thalamus |
| thalass/o | sea |
| thel/e | nipple |
| -therapy | treatment |
| therm/o | heat, temperature |
| thorac/o | thorax (chest) |
| -thorax | chest (pleural cavity) |
| thromb/o | clotting, clot |
| -thrombin | clotting substance |
| thrombocyt/o | clotting cell |
| thym/o | thymus gland, mind |
| -thymia | condition/state of mind |
| thyr/o | thyroid gland, shield |
| thyroid/o | thyroid gland |
| tibi/o | tibia (shinbone) |
| -tic | pertaining to |
| -tion | process of |
| toc/o | labor, delivery |
| -tocia | condition of labor, delivery |

## Word Parts and Definitions—cont'd

| Word Part | Meaning |
| --- | --- |
| tom/o | section, cutting |
| -tome | instrument to cut |
| -tomy | incision, cutting |
| ton/o | tension, tone |
| tonsill/o | tonsil |
| top/o | place, location |
| tox/o | poison |
| toxic/o | poison |
| trabecul/o | little beam |
| trache/o | trachea (windpipe) |
| tract/o | to pull, pulling |
| trans- | through, across |
| -tresia | condition of an opening |
| tri- | three |
| trich/o | hair |
| trigon/o | trigone |
| -tripsy | process of crushing |
| -tripter | machine to crush |
| -trite | instrument to crush |
| trochanter/o | trochanter |
| trop/o | to turn, turning |
| troph/o | development, nourishment |
| -trophy | process of nourishment, development |
| tub/o | tube, pipe |
| tubercul/o | tubercle, a swelling |
| tympan/o | eardrum, drum |
| -ule | small |
| uln/o | ulna (lower medial arm bone) |
| ultra- | beyond |
| -um | structure, thing, membrane |
| umbilic/o | umbilicus (navel) |
| ungu/o | nail |
| uni- | one |
| ur/o | urine, urinary system |
| ureter/o | ureter |
| urethr/o | urethra |
| -uria | urinary condition |
| urin/o | urine, urinary system |

| Word Part | Meaning |
| --- | --- |
| -us | structure, thing, noun ending |
| uter/o | uterus |
| uve/o | uvea |
| uvul/o | uvula |
| vag/o | vagus nerve |
| vagin/o | vagina |
| valv/o | valve |
| valvul/o | valve |
| varic/o | varices |
| vas/o | vessel, ductus deferens, vas deferens |
| vascul/o | vessel |
| ven/o | vein |
| ventr/o | belly side |
| ventricul/o | ventricle |
| venul/o | venule, small vein |
| -verse | to turn |
| vers/o | to turn |
| -version | process of turning |
| vertebr/o | vertebra, spine |
| vesic/o | bladder |
| vesicul/o | small sac, seminal vesicle, blister |
| vestibul/o | vestibule (small space at entrance to canal) |
| vill/o | villus |
| vir/o | virus |
| viscer/o | viscera, organ |
| vitre/o | vitreous humor, glassy |
| vol/o | volume |
| vomer/o | vomer |
| vulgar/o | common |
| vulv/o | vulva (external female genitalia) |
| xen/o | foreign |
| xer/o | dry |
| xiph/i | xiphoid process, sword |
| -y | process of; condition |
| zo/o | animal |
| zygom/o | zygoma (cheekbone) |
| zygomat/o | zygoma (cheekbone) |

# Appendix B

## Definitions and Word Parts

| Meaning | Word Part |
|---|---|
| 3-dimensional | stere/o |
| abdomen | abdomin/o, celi/o, lapar/o |
| abnormal | para-, dys- |
| abnormal condition | -osis |
| abnormal condition of hardening | -sclerosis |
| abnormal condition of narrowing | -stenosis |
| abnormal increase in cells | -cytosis |
| above, upon | epi- |
| accessory | adnex/o |
| acid | acid/o |
| acromion | -acromion |
| addition | prosth/o, prosthes/o |
| adenoid (pharyngeal tonsil) | adenoid/o |
| adrenal gland | adren/o |
| again | re- |
| against | anti- |
| air | aer/o, pneum/o |
| all | pan- |
| alveolus | alveol/o |
| amnion | amni/o |
| amnion (inner fetal sac) | -amnios |
| angle | goni/o |
| animal | zo/o |
| ankle bone (tarsal bone) | tars/o |
| antrum, cavity | antr/o |
| anus | an/o |
| aorta (largest artery) | aort/o |
| appendix, vermiform | append/o, appendic/o |
| appetite | orex/o |
| arm | brachi/o |
| armpit (axilla) | axill/o |
| around | circum- |
| arrow, separating the sides | sagitt/o |
| arteriole (small artery) | arteriol/o |
| artery | arteri/o |
| atrium | atri/o |

| Meaning | Word Part |
|---|---|
| attraction | phil/o, -phil |
| away from | ab-, ef-, apo- |
| back | dors/o, poster/o |
| backbone | rachi/o |
| back of knee | poplite/o |
| back, again | re- |
| backward | retro-, re- |
| bacteria | bacteri/o |
| bad, abnormal, apart | dis- |
| bad, difficult, painful, abnormal | dys- |
| bad, poor | mal- |
| Bartholin gland | bartholin/o |
| base, bottom | bas/o |
| bear, carry | fer/o, phor/o, duct/o |
| before, in front of | pre- |
| beginning | -arche |
| behind, after | post- |
| belly side | ventr/o |
| below | hypo- |
| bend, bending | flex/o |
| beside, near | par- |
| between | inter- |
| beyond | ultra- |
| beyond, change | meta- |
| bile, gall | bil/i, chol/e |
| bile vessel | cholangi/o |
| binding | -desis |
| birth, born | nat/o |
| black, dark | melan/o |
| bladder | vesic/o |
| bladder, sac | cyst/o |
| blister | vesicul/o |
| blood | hem/o, hemat/o |
| blood condition | -emia |
| blood vessel | hemangi/o |
| blue | cyan/o |
| blueish green | glauc/o |
| body | corpor/o, somat/o, som/o |

## Definitions and Word Parts—cont'd

| Meaning | Word Part |
|---|---|
| bone | oss/i, osse/o, oste/o |
| bone marrow, spinal cord | myel/o |
| both | amphi- |
| brain | encephal/o |
| break down, dissolve | lys/o |
| break down, freeing from adhesions, dissolving, loosening | -lysis |
| breaking down | -clast |
| breast | mamm/o, mast/o |
| breastbone (sternum) | stern/o |
| breath | halit/o |
| breathe, breathing | pne/o |
| breathing, to breathe | -pnea, spir/o, hal/o |
| bronchiole | bronchiol/o |
| bronchus | bronch/o, bronchi/o |
| bunion | bunion/o |
| burning | cauter/i |
| bursa | burs/o |
| bursting forth | -rrhagia, -rrhage |
| buttocks | glute/o |
| calcium | calc/o, calc/i |
| calf | sur/o |
| calyx, calix | cali/o, calic/o, calyc/o |
| cancer | carcin/o |
| cancer of epithelial origin | -carcinoma |
| cancer, malignancy | cancer/o |
| canthus (corner of eye) | canth/o |
| carbon dioxide | capn/o |
| carry, carrying | duct/o |
| carry, to bear | phor/o |
| cartilage | cartilag/o, chondr/o |
| cecum (first part of large intestine) | cec/o |
| cell | cellul/o, cyt/o, cyte |
| cerebellum | cerebell/o |
| cerebrum | cerebr/o |
| cervix | cervic/o |
| change | mut/a |
| cheek | bucc/o |
| cheekbone (zygoma) | zygom/o, zygomat/o |
| chest (thorax) | pector/o, steth/o, thorac/o |

| Meaning | Word Part |
|---|---|
| chest (pleural cavity) | -thorax |
| child, foot | ped/o |
| childbirth, puerperium | puerper/o |
| chin | ment/o |
| cholesterol | cholesterol/o |
| choroid | choroid/o |
| chorion (outer fetal sac) | chori/o, chorion/o |
| ciliary body | cycl/o |
| clitoris | clitorid/o |
| close, closing, a blockage | occlus/o |
| closing | claustr/o |
| clotting cell | thrombocyt/o |
| clotting substance | -thrombin |
| clotting, clot | thromb/o |
| clumping | agglutin/o |
| cochlea | cochle/o |
| collarbone (clavicle) | cleid/o, clavicul/o |
| color | chrom/o, chromat/o |
| common | vulgar/o |
| common bile duct | choledoch/o |
| condition of an opening | -tresia |
| condition of attraction; increase | -philia |
| condition of babbling | -lalia |
| condition of closure | -occlusion |
| condition of expansion, dilation | -ectasia |
| condition of fear, extreme sensivity | -phobia |
| condition of formation, development | -plasia |
| condition of labor, delivery | -tocia |
| condition of madness | -mania |
| condition of patches | -plakia |
| condition of relaxation, slackening | -chalasia |
| condition of softening | -malacia |
| condition of stools | -chezia |
| condition of strength | -sthenia |
| condition of the heart | -cardia |
| condition of thirst | -dipsia |
| condition, presence of | -iasis |

*Continued*

## Definitions and Word Parts—cont'd

| Meaning | Word Part | Meaning | Word Part |
|---|---|---|---|
| condition, state of | -exia, -ia, -ism, -y | duodenum | duoden/o |
| condition/state of mind | -thymia, -noia | dust | coni/o |
| condyle, knob | condyl/o | ear | aur/o, auricul/o, ot/o |
| cone | con/o | earwax, cerumen | cerumin/o |
| conjunctiva | conjunctiv/o | eardrum, drum | myring/o, tympan/o |
| connection | commissur/o | eat, swallow | phag/o |
| connective tissue cancer | -sarcoma | elbow | olecran/o |
| contraction | -stalsis | elbow (forearm) | cubit/o |
| controlling, stopping | -stasis | electricity | electr/o |
| cord, spinal cord | chord/o | embryonic, immature | -blast, blast/o |
| cornea | corne/o, kerat/o | end, far, complete | tel/e, tele/o |
| cortex (outer portion) | cortic/o | endocardium (inner lining of the heart) | endocardi/o |
| crown | coron/o | endometrium | endometri/o |
| curvature | scoli/o | enlargement | -megaly |
| dark | phe/o, scot/o | enzyme | -ase |
| death, dead | necr/o | epicardium | epicardi/o |
| deficiency condition | -penia | epicondyle | epicondyl/o |
| deficient, below, under | hypo- | epididymis | epididym/o |
| deformity | terat/o | epiglottis | epiglott/o |
| delivery, parturition | -para | epithelium | epitheli/o |
| dendrite, tree | dendr/o | equal | is/o |
| development | troph/o | esophagus | esophag/o |
| diaphragm | diaphragm/o, diaphragmat/o | ethmoid bone | ethmoid/o |
| diaphragm, mind | phren/o | excessive, above | hyper- |
| different | heter/o | expansion, dilation | -ectasis |
| digestion condition | -pepsia | extreme cold | cry/o |
| discharge, flow | -rrhea | eye | ocul/o, ophthalm/o |
| disease | path/o | eyelid | blephar/o, palpebr/o |
| disease process | -pathy | face | faci/o |
| distal process lower leg, little malleolus | malleol/o | falling, drooping, prolapse | -lapse, -ptosis |
| diverticulum, pouch | diverticul/o | fallopian tube | fallopi/o, salping/o, -salpinx |
| double | dipl/o | far | tel/e, tele/o |
| down | cata-, infra- | fascia | fasci/o |
| down, lack of | de- | fast, rapid | tachy- |
| downward | infer/o | fat | adip/o, lip/o, steat/o |
| drooping, prolapse | -ptosis | fatty plaque | ather/o |
| drug, chemical | chem/o | feces, stool | fec/a |
| dry | xer/o | feel with | sympath/o |
| dull, dim | ambly/o | feeling, sensation | esthesi/o |

## Definitions and Word Parts—cont'd

| Meaning | Word Part | Meaning | Word Part |
|---------|-----------|---------|-----------|
| female, woman | gynec/o, nymph/o | half | hemi- |
| femur (thighbone) | femor/o | hand | man/u |
| fetus | fet/o | hard (dura mater) | dur/o |
| fever, fire | pyr/o, pyret/o | hard, horny, cornea | kerat/o |
| fiber | fibr/o | head | capit/o, cephal/o |
| fibrous substance | fibrin/o | healthy, normal | eu- |
| fibula | fibul/o, perone/o | hearing | acous/o, audi/o, -acusis |
| finger or toe (digitus) | dactyl/o, digit/o | heart | cardi/o, cordi/o, coron/o |
| finger/toe bones (phalanx) | phalang/o | | |
| first | primi- | heat, temperature | therm/o |
| fishlike | ichthy/o | heelbone (calcaneus) | calcane/o |
| fixation, suspension | -pexy | heights, extremes, extremities | acro- |
| flesh | sarc/o | | |
| flow, flowing | fluor/o | hemorrhoid | hemorrhoid/o |
| fold, plica | plic/o | hernia | herni/o |
| follicle, small sac | follicul/o | herniation, protrusion | -cele |
| foot, child | ped/o | hidden | crypt- |
| foreign | xen/o | hilum | hil/o |
| foreskin (prepuce) | preputi/o | hip (coxa) | cox/o |
| formation, production | plas/o, plast/o, -poiesis, -plasm | hold back, suppress | isch/o |
| | | hole, foramen | foramin/o |
| forming substance | -plastin, -poietin | hollow, depression | foss/o |
| fornix | fornic/o | hormone, substance that forms | -one |
| forward, in front of | ante-, pro- | | |
| four | quadri-, tetra- | humerus (upper arm bone) | humer/o |
| frequent | poly- | | |
| front, forehead | anter/o, front/o | hymen | hymen/o |
| fungus | myc/o, fung/i | ileum | ile/o |
| fundus (base, bottom) | fund/o | ilium (superior, widest pelvic bone) | ili/o |
| gallbladder | cholecyst/o | | |
| gland | aden/o | in | en-, in- |
| glans penis | balan/o | in favor of | pro- |
| glomerulus | glomerul/o | incision, cutting | -tomy |
| glue, glia cell | -glia | infection | seps/o, -sepsis, septic/o |
| gonad, sex organ | gonad/o | | |
| groin | inguin/o | inflammation | -itis |
| growth; nature | physi/o, -physis, phyt/o | inner ear (labyrinth) | labyrinth/o |
| | | instrument to crush | -trite |
| gums | gingiv/o | instrument to cut | -tome |
| hair | pil/o, trich/o | instrument to measure | -meter |

*Continued*

## Definitions and Word Parts—cont'd

| Meaning | Word Part | Meaning | Word Part |
|---|---|---|---|
| instrument to record | -graph | lower jaw | mandibul/o |
| instrument to view | -scope | lumen (space within vessel) | lumin/o |
| insulin | insulin/o | lung | pneumon/o, pulmon/o, pneum/o |
| intentional breaking | -clasis | | |
| intestine | intestin/o, enter/o | lymph | lymph/o, lymphat/o |
| inward | eso- | lymph gland (lymph node) | lymphaden/o |
| iris | ir/o, irid/o | | |
| iron | ferr/o, sider/o | lymph vessel | lymphangi/o |
| iron substance | -siderin | machine to crush | -tripter |
| ischium | ischi/o | male | andr/o |
| jaw, entire | gnath/o | male sex cell, spermatozoon | spermat/o |
| jejunum | jejun/o | | |
| joint (articulation) | arthr/o, articul/o | malleus, hammer | malle/o |
| juice | chym/o | man | anthrop/o |
| ketone | ket/o, keton/o | many | multi- |
| kidney | nephr/o, ren/o | many, much, excessive | poly- |
| kneecap (patella) | patell/o, patell/a | marketplace | agora- |
| knowledge | gnos/o | mass | -oma |
| labor, delivery | toc/o | mastoid process | mastoid/o |
| lacrimal gland | dacryoaden/o | meatus (opening) | meat/o |
| lacrimal sac | dacrocyst/o | mediastinum | mediastin/o |
| lamina, thin plate | lamin/o | medulla | medull/o |
| large | macro- | meninges | mening/o, meningi/o |
| large intestine (colon) | col/o, colon/o | meniscus | menisc/o |
| left | levo-, sinistr/o | menstruation, menses | menstru/o, men/o |
| leg | crur/o | metacarpal (hand bone) | metacarp/o |
| lens | phac/o, phak/o | metatarsal (foot bone) | metatars/o |
| lice | pedicul/i | middle | medi/o, meso-, mid- |
| life, living | bi/o | milk | galact/o, lact/o |
| ligament | ligament/o, syndesm/o | mind | ment/o, phren/o, psych/o |
| light | phot/o | | |
| lipid, fat | lipid/o | mitochrondria | mitochondri/o |
| lips | cheil/o | mouth, oral cavity | or/o, stomat/o |
| lips (labia) | labi/o | movement | -kine, kinesi/o |
| liquid | humor/o | movement substance | -kinin |
| little beam | trabecul/o | mucus | muc/o, myx/o |
| little grain | granul/o | muscle | muscul/o, my/o, myos/o |
| liver | hepat/o | | |
| lobe, section | lob/o | myocardium (heart muscle) | myocardi/o, cardiomy/o |
| long | long/o | | |
| lower back | lumb/o | nail | onych/o, ungu/o |

## Definitions and Word Parts—cont'd

| Meaning | Word Part | Meaning | Word Part |
|---|---|---|---|
| near | proxim/o | organ, viscera | organ/o, viscer/o |
| near, beside, abnormal | para-, par- | origin, originate | gen/o |
| neck | nuch/o, coll/o | ossicle | ossicul/o |
| neck, cervix | cervic/o | other, different | allo- |
| nerve | neur/o | out, outward | ec-, ex- |
| nerve root | radicul/o, rhiz/o | outside | exo-, extra- |
| nest | nid/o | outward | e-, ecto- |
| network | reticul/o | ovary | oophor/o, ovari/o |
| neutral | neutr/o | ovum, egg | o/o, ovul/o, ov/o |
| nevus, birthmark | nev/o | oxygen | ox/i, ox/o |
| new | neo- | pain | -algia, -dynia |
| new opening | -stomy | palate, roof of mouth, palatine bone | palat/o |
| night | noct/i, nyctal/o | | |
| nipple | thel/e | palm | palm/o |
| nipple | papill/o | pancreas | pancreat/o |
| nitrogen | az/o, azot/o | papilla | papill/o |
| no, not, without | a-, an-, in-, non- | papule | papul/o |
| node, knot | nod/o | paralysis | -plegia |
| none | nulli- | paralysis, slight | -paresis |
| nose | nas/o, rhin/o | parathyroid | parathyroid/o |
| nourishment | troph/o | parenchyma | parenchym/o |
| noun ending | -a, -e, -i, -is, -um, -on, -ium, -us | parturition, delivery | part/o, -partum |
| | | passage | por/o |
| nucleus | kary/o, nucle/o | pelvis | pelv/i, pelv/o |
| nutrition | aliment/o | penis | pen/i, phall/o |
| occiput, back of head | occipit/o | perineum | perine/o |
| old age | ger/o, presby- | peritoneum | peritone/o, periton/o |
| one | mono-, uni- | peroneum | perone/o |
| one who specializes | -ist | pertaining to | -ac, -al, -an, -ar, -ary, -atic, -eal, -iac, -ac, -ic, -id, -ile, -ine, -ior, -itic, -ive, -ous, -tic |
| one who specializes in the study of | -logist | | |
| one who specializes in treatment | -iatrician, -iatrist | pertaining to blood condition | -emic |
| optic disk | papill/o | pertaining to breaking down | -lytic |
| one who studies | -ician | | |
| opening | hiat/o | pertaining to carrying | -ferous |
| opening, a mouth | stom/o | pertaining to discharge | -rrheic |
| opposite, against | contra- | pertaining to originating from | -genous |
| optic disk | papill/o | | |
| orange-yellow | cirrh/o | pertaining to produced by | -genic |
| order, coordination | tax/o | | |

*Continued*

## Definitions and Word Parts—cont'd

| Meaning | Word Part |
|---|---|
| pertaining to treatment | -iatric |
| pertaining to viewing | -scopic |
| pertaining to, full of | -ose |
| pimple | papul/o |
| pituitary, hypophysis | hypophys/o, pituitar/o |
| place, location | top/o |
| placenta | placent/o |
| plasma | plasm/a |
| pleasure | hedon/o |
| pleura (membrane surrounding lungs) | pleur/o |
| pointed extremity, apex | apic/o |
| poison | tox/o, toxic/o |
| pole | pol/o |
| polyp | polyp/o |
| potassium | kal/i, potass/o |
| pouch, diverticulum | diverticul/o |
| pregnancy, gestation | -cyesis, gravid/o, gravida |
| pressure | press/o |
| pressure, weight | bar/o |
| process of viewing | -opsy |
| process of | -ation, -ion, -ization, -tion, -y |
| process of clotting | -coagulation |
| process of crushing | -tripsy |
| process of cutting | -cision |
| process of measurement | -metry |
| process of nourishment, development | -trophy |
| process of pouring | -fusion |
| process of recording | -graphy |
| process of stretching, pressure | -tension |
| process of treatment | -iatry |
| process of turning | -version |
| process of viewing | -scopy |
| producing, produced by | -gen |
| production | -genesis |
| prolactin | prolact/o |
| prolapse | -ptosis |
| prostate | prostat/o |

| Meaning | Word Part |
|---|---|
| protection | -phylaxis |
| protein | albumin/o |
| protein substance | -globin, -globulin |
| pubis, anterior pelvic bone | pub/o |
| pull, pulling | tract/o |
| pupil | cor/o, core/o, pupill/o |
| purple | purpur/o |
| purposeful movement | prax/o |
| pus | py/o |
| pustule | pustul/o |
| pylorus | pylor/o |
| radius | radi/o |
| rapid, fast | oxy-, tachy- |
| rash | exanthemat/o |
| rays | radi/o |
| record, recording | -gram |
| rectouterine pouch (cul-de-sac) | culd/o |
| rectum and anus | proct/o |
| rectum, straight | rect/o |
| recurring, round | cycl/o |
| red | erythr/o |
| red blood cell | erythrocyt/o |
| relaxation, slackening | -chalasis |
| removal of a stone | -lithotomy |
| removal, excision | -ablation, -apheresis, -pheresis, -ectomy |
| renal pelvis | pyel/o |
| rent or tear | -spadias |
| repair | -rrhaphy |
| resembling, like | -oid |
| retina | retin/o |
| rhythm | rhythm/o |
| rib (costa) | cost/o |
| ribose | rib/o |
| right | dextr/o |
| rosy-colored | eosin/o |
| roundback | kyph/o |
| rugae, ridge | rug/o |
| run, running | -drome |
| rupture | -rrhexis |
| sac surrounding the heart | pericardi/o |

## Definitions and Word Parts—cont'd

| Meaning | Word Part |
|---|---|
| sacrum | sacr/o |
| safety, protection | immun/o |
| saliva | sial/o |
| salivary gland | sialaden/o |
| same | home/o, homo-, ipsi- |
| scab | eschar/o |
| scaly | squam/o |
| scanty, few | olig/o |
| scanty, pressure | man/o |
| sclera, hard | scler/o |
| scraping of | -abrasion |
| scrotum | scrot/o |
| sea | thalass/o |
| sebum, oil | seb/o, sebac/o |
| secret, hidden | -occult |
| secrete, secreting | crin/o, -crine |
| section, cutting | tom/o |
| seed | gon/o |
| seizure | -lepsy |
| self | auto- |
| semen | semin/i |
| send, sending | -mission |
| sense of smell | osm/o |
| separate, separating | -crit |
| separate, away | apo- |
| septum | sept/o |
| serum | ser/o |
| shape, form | morph/o |
| sharp | acu- |
| shinbone (tibia) | tibi/o |
| short | brachy- |
| shoulder blade (scapula) | scapul/o |
| side | later/o |
| sigmoid colon | sigmoid/o |
| sinus, cavity | sin/o, sinus/o |
| sitting | kathis/o |
| skeleton | skelet/o |
| skin | cut/o, cutane/o, derm/o, dermat/o |
| skull (cranium) | crani/o |

| Meaning | Word Part |
|---|---|
| sleep, stupor | narc/o, somn/o |
| slight paralysis | -paresis |
| slipping | -listhesis |
| slow | brady- |
| small | micro-, -ule |
| small intestines, intestines | enter/o |
| small lobe | lobul/o |
| small sac, seminal vesicle | vesicul/o |
| smooth | lei/o |
| smooth muscle | leiomy/o |
| sodium | natr/o |
| softening | -malacia |
| sole of foot | plant/o |
| sound | echo-, son/o |
| sound, voice | phon/o |
| space between | interstit/o |
| spasm | -spasm |
| speech | phas/o |
| spermatozoon | sperm/o |
| sphenoid | sphenoid/o |
| spinal column | rachi/o |
| spinal cord | cord/o, myel/o |
| spinal nerve root | rhiz/o, radicul/o |
| spine | spin/o, vertebr/o |
| spitting | -ptysis |
| spleen | splen/o |
| split | schiz/o, -fida |
| split, splitting | -fida |
| spot, macula lutea, macule | macul/o |
| stapes | staped/o |
| star | astr/o |
| starch | amyl/o |
| state of | -esis, -sis |
| state of relaxation | -chalasis |
| steal, stealing | klept/o |
| steroid | ster/o |
| stiffening | ankyl/o |
| stomach | gastr/o |
| stone (calculus) | calcul/o, lith/o |
| stop, cease | -pause |

*Continued*

## Definitions and Word Parts—cont'd

| Meaning | Word Part |
|---|---|
| straight, upright | orth/o |
| strength | sthen/o |
| stretching | tens/o |
| striated | rhabd/o |
| striated (skeletal) muscle | rhabdomy/o |
| stroma (supportive tissue) | strom/o |
| structure, membrane, thing | -um, -ium |
| structure, thing, noun ending | -us, -on, -is |
| study | log/o |
| study of | -logy |
| substance | -in |
| sugar, glucose | glycos/o, gluc/o, glyc/o |
| sulcus, groove | sulc/o |
| surgical puncture | -centesis |
| surgical repair | -plasty |
| surrounding, around | peri- |
| suture | -rrhaphy |
| swallow, eat | phag/o |
| swayback | lord/o |
| sweat | hidr/o, sudor/i |
| sweat gland (suderiferous gland) | hidraden/o |
| swelling | -edema, tubercul/o |
| synovium | synovi/o |
| tail | caud/o |
| tailbone (coccyx) | coccyg/o |
| taste | geus/o |
| tear | dacry/o, lacrim/o |
| teeth | dent/i, odont/o |
| temporal bone | tempor/o |
| tendon | ten/o, tend/o, tendin/o |
| tension, tone | ton/o |
| testis, testicle | orch/o, orchi/o, orchid/o, test/o, testicul/o |
| thalamus | thalam/o |
| thirst | dips/o |
| three | tri- |

| Meaning | Word Part |
|---|---|
| throat (pharynx) | pharyng/o |
| through | per- |
| through, across | trans- |
| through, complete | dia- |
| thymus gland, mind | thym/o |
| thyroid gland | thyroid/o |
| thyroid gland, shield | thyr/o |
| tissue | hist/o |
| throw, throwing | bol/o |
| tie, tying | ligat/o |
| to flow, flowing | fluor/o |
| together | con- |
| together, joined | syn- |
| tongue | gloss/o, lingu/o |
| tonsil | tonsill/o |
| to shut | my/o |
| toward | ad-, -ad, af- |
| treatment | iatr/o, -therapy |
| tree | dendr/o |
| trochanter | trochanter/o |
| trigone | trigon/o |
| tube, fallopian | -salpinx |
| tube, fallopian or eustachian | salping/o |
| tube, pipe | tub/o |
| tumor | onc/o |
| tumor, mass | -oma |
| tubercle | tubercul/o |
| turn, turning | trop/o, vers/o, -verse |
| twisting | tors/o |
| two | bi-, bin- |
| two (both) | di- |
| ulceration | aphth/o |
| ulna | uln/o |
| umbilicus (navel) | omphal/o, umbilic/o |
| under, below | sub-, hypo- |
| unique, unknown | idi/o |
| up, apart, away | ana- |
| upper jaw bone (maxilla) | maxill/o |
| upward | super/o, supra- |
| ureter | ureter/o |

## Definitions and Word Parts—cont'd

| Meaning | Word Part | Meaning | Word Part |
|---|---|---|---|
| urethra | urethr/o | vision condition | -opia, -opsia |
| urinary condition | -uria | vitreous humor, glassy | vitre/o |
| urine, urinary system | ur/o, urin/o | voice box (larynx) | laryng/o |
| uterus | hyster/o, metr/o, metri/o, uter/o | volume | plethysm/o, vol/o |
| | | vomer | vomer/o |
| uvea | uve/o | vomiting | -emesis |
| uvula | uvul/o | vulva | episi/o, vulv/o |
| vagina | colp/o, vagin/o | walking | ambul/o |
| vagus nerve | vag/o | wall, partition, septum | pariet/o, sept/o |
| valve | valv/o, valvul/o | water, fluid | hydr/o |
| varices | varic/o | watery flow | rheumat/o |
| vas deferens | vas/o | wheel | rot/o |
| vein | phleb/o, ven/o | white | albin/o, leuk/o |
| ventricle | ventricul/o | white blood cell | leukocyt/o |
| venule (small vein) | venul/o | windpipe (trachea) | trache/o |
| vertebra, spine | spondyl/o, vertebr/o | within | end, endo-, intra- |
| vessel | angi/o, vascul/o, vas/o | woman, female | nymph/o |
| vessel, ductus deferens, vas deferens | vas/o | word, speech | lex/o |
| | | work | erg/o |
| villus | vill/o | wrinkle | rhytid/o |
| vestibule | vestibul/o | wrist (carpus) | carp/o |
| virus | vir/o | write, writing | graph/o |
| vision | opt/o, optic/o | xiphoid process | xiph/i |

# Appendix C

## Abbreviations

| Abbreviation | Meaning |
|---|---|
| # | fracture |
| 3DCRT | three-dimensional computed radiography tomography |
| A | action |
| A1c | average glucose level |
| A+P | auscultation and percussion |
| A, B, AB, O | blood types |
| ABG | arterial blood gases |
| ABR | auditory brain response |
| Acc | accommodation |
| ACS | anterior ciliary sclerotomy; American College of Surgeons |
| ACTH | adrenocorticotropic hormone |
| AD | Alzheimer disease |
| ADH | antidiuretic hormone |
| ADHD | attention-deficit/hyperactivity disorder |
| ADL | activities of daily living |
| AEB | atrial ectopic beats |
| AF | atrial fibrillation |
| AFP | alpha-fetoprotein test |
| AHIMA | American Health Information Management Association |
| AI | artificial insemination |
| AIDS | acquired immunodeficiency syndrome |
| AK | astigmatic keratotomy |
| ALS | amyotrophic lateral sclerosis |
| ALL | acute lymphocytic leukemia |
| AMI | acute myocardial infarction |
| AML | acute myelogenous leukemia |
| ANA | antinuclear antibody |
| ANS | autonomic nervous system |
| AP | anteroposterior |
| APA | American Psychiatric Association |
| ARF | acute renal failure; acute respiratory failure |
| ARMD, AMD | age-related macular degeneration |
| AS | aortic stenosis |
| ASD | atrial septal defect |

| Abbreviation | Meaning |
|---|---|
| ASHD | arteriosclerotic heart disease |
| ASL | American sign language |
| Astigm, As, Ast | astigmatism |
| AV | atrioventricular |
| B2M | beta-2 microglobulin |
| BaS | barium swallow |
| basos | basophils |
| BBB | blood-brain barrier; bundle branch block |
| BCC | basal cell carcinoma |
| BD | bipolar disorder |
| BE | barium enema |
| BM | bowel movement |
| BMP | basic metabolic panel |
| BMT | bone marrow transplant |
| BP | blood pressure |
| BPH | benign prostatic hyperplasia/ hypertrophy |
| BPM | beats per minute |
| BSE | breast self-examination |
| BTA | bladder tumor antigen |
| BUN | blood urea nitrogen |
| bx | biopsy |
| C1-C7 | first cervical through seventh cervical vertebrae |
| C1-C8 | cervical nerves |
| CA | cancer |
| CA125 | tumor marker primarily for ovarian cancer |
| CA15-3 | tumor marker used to monitor breast cancer |
| CA19-9 | tumor marker for pancreatic, stomach, and bile duct cancer |
| CA27-29 | tumor marker used to check for recurrence of breast cancer |
| CABG | coronary artery bypass graft |
| CAD | coronary artery disease |
| CAM | complementary and alternative medicine |
| CAPD | continuous ambulatory peritoneal dialysis |

## Abbreviations—cont'd

| Abbreviation | Meaning |
|---|---|
| CAT | computed axial tomography |
| Cath | (cardiac) catheterization |
| CBC | complete blood cell (count) |
| CCB | calcium channel blocker(s) |
| CCF | congestive cardiac failure |
| CCPD | continuous cycling peritoneal dialysis |
| CEA | carcinoembryonic antigen |
| CF | cystic fibrosis |
| CHF | congestive heart failure |
| CIN | cervical intraepithelial neoplasia |
| CK | creatine kinase |
| CIS | carcinoma in situ |
| CLL | chronic lymphocytic leukemia |
| CML | chronic myelogenous leukemia |
| CMP | comprehensive metabolic panel |
| CNS | central nervous system |
| $CO_2$ | carbon dioxide |
| COPD | chronic obstructive pulmonary disease |
| CP | cerebral palsy |
| CPAP | continuous positive airway pressure |
| CPK | creatine phosphokinase |
| CPR | cardiopulmonary resuscitation |
| CPT | Current Procedural Terminology |
| CKD | chronic kidney disease |
| CS | cesarean section |
| CSF | cerebrospinal fluid |
| CST | contraction stress test |
| CT scan | computed tomography scan |
| CTA | clear to auscultation |
| CTR | certified tumor registrar |
| CTS | carpal tunnel syndrome |
| CV | cardiovascular |
| CVA | cerebrovascular accident |
| CVS | chorionic villus sampling |
| CWP | coal workers' pneumoconiosis |
| Cx | cervix |
| CXR | chest x-ray |
| D&C | dilation and curettage |
| D1-D12 | first dorsal through twelfth dorsal vertebrae |

| Abbreviation | Meaning |
|---|---|
| DAP | Draw-a-Person Test |
| Decub | pressure ulcer |
| DEXA, DXA | dual-energy x-ray absorptiometry |
| DI | diabetes insipidus |
| Diff | differential WBC count |
| DJD | degenerative joint disease |
| DLE | disseminated lupus erythematosus |
| DM | diabetes mellitus |
| DOE | dyspnea on exertion |
| DRE | digital rectal exam |
| DSA | digital subtraction angiography |
| DSM | Diagnostic and Statistical Manual of Mental Disorders |
| DT | delirium tremens |
| DTR | deep tendon reflex |
| DUB | dysfunctional uterine bleeding |
| DVT | deep vein thrombosis |
| EBV | Epstein-Barr virus |
| ECC | extracorporeal circulation |
| ECCE | extracapsular cataract extraction |
| ECG, EKG | electrocardiogram |
| ECHO | echocardiography |
| ECP | emergency contraceptive pills |
| ECT | electroconvulsive therapy |
| ED | emergency department |
| EDD | estimated delivery date |
| EEG | electroencephalogram |
| EF | external fixation |
| EGD | esophagogastroduodenoscopy |
| EM, em | emmetropia |
| EMG | electromyography |
| EOC | epithelial ovarian cancer |
| EOM | extraocular movements |
| eosins | eosinophils |
| EP | evoked potential |
| ERCP | endoscopic retrograde cholangiopancreatography |
| ERT | estrogen replacement therapy |
| ESR | erythrocyte sedimentation rate |
| ESRD | end-stage renal disease |
| EST | exercise stress test |

*Continued*

## Abbreviations—cont'd

| Abbreviation | Meaning |
|---|---|
| ESWL | extracorporeal shock wave lithotripsy |
| EVLT | endovenous laser ablation |
| FB | foreign body |
| FBS | fasting blood sugar |
| FHR | fetal heart rate |
| FOBT | fecal occult blood test |
| FPG | fasting plasma glucose |
| FSH | follicle-stimulating hormone |
| FTA-ABS | fluorescent treponemal antibody absorption test |
| G | grade, pregnancy |
| GAD | generalized anxiety disorder |
| GAF | global assessment of functioning |
| GARS | gait assessment rating scale |
| GB | gallbladder |
| Gc | gonococcus |
| GCT | germ cell tumor |
| GERD | gastroesophageal reflux disease |
| GFR | glomerular filtration rate |
| GH | growth hormone |
| GI | gastrointestinal |
| GIFT | gamete intrafallopian transfer |
| GN | glomerulonephritis |
| GPA | gravida, para, abortion |
| H | hypodermic |
| HAV | hepatitis A virus |
| Hb | hemoglobin |
| HBV | hepatitis B virus |
| hCG | human chorionic gonadotropin |
| Hct | hematocrit; packed-cell volume |
| HD | hemodialysis |
| HDL | high-density lipoproteins |
| HDN | hemolytic disease of the newborn |
| HF | heart failure |
| Hgb | hemoglobin |
| hGH | human growth hormone |
| HHN | hand-held nebulizer |
| HIV | human immunodeficiency virus |
| HIVD | herniated intervertebral disk |
| HPV | human papilloma virus |

| Abbreviation | Meaning |
|---|---|
| HRT | hormone replacement therapy |
| HSG | hysterosalpingography |
| HSV-1 | herpes simplex virus-1 |
| HSV-2 | herpes simplex virus-2; herpes genitalis |
| htn | hypertension |
| I&D | incision and drainage |
| IBS | irritable bowel syndrome |
| ICCE | intracapsular cataract extraction |
| ICD | implantable cardiac defibrillator; International Classification of Diseases |
| ICP | intracranial pressure |
| ICSH | interstitial cell-stimulating hormone |
| ICSI | intracytoplasmic sperm injection |
| ID | intradermal |
| IDC | infiltrating ductal carcinoma |
| IDDM | insulin-dependent diabetes mellitus |
| IF | internal fixation |
| Ig | immunoglobulin |
| IMRT | intensity-modulated radiation therapy |
| IOL | intraocular lens |
| IOP | intraocular pressure |
| IQ | intelligence quotient |
| IUD | intrauterine device |
| IVF | in vitro fertilization |
| IVU | intravenous urogram |
| KS | Kaposi sarcoma |
| KUB | kidney, ureter, bladder |
| L1-L5 | first lumbar through fifth lumbar vertebrae; lumbar nerves |
| LA | left atrium |
| Lap | laparoscopy |
| LASIK | laser-assisted in situ keratomileusis |
| lat | lateral |
| LCA | left circumflex artery; left coronary artery |
| LD | lactic dehydrogenase (formerly LDH) |
| LDH | lactate dehydrogenase |

## Abbreviations—cont'd

| Abbreviation | Meaning | Abbreviation | Meaning |
|---|---|---|---|
| LDL | low-density lipoproteins | NIDDM | non–insulin-dependent diabetes mellitus (type 2 diabetes) |
| LEEP | loop electrocautery excision procedure | NK | natural killer cell |
| LES | lower esophageal sphincter | NPDR | nonproliferative diabetic retinopathy |
| LH | luteinizing hormone | NSCLC | non–small cell lung cancer |
| LLL | left lower lobe | NSE | neuron-specific enolase (used to detect neuroblastoma, small cell cancer) |
| LLQ | lower left quadrant | | |
| LMP | last menstrual period | | |
| LN | luteinizing hormone | NSR | normal sinus rhythm |
| LP | lumbar puncture | NST | nonstress test |
| LRQ | lower right quadrant | NTG | nitroglycerin |
| LUL | left upper lobe | O | origin |
| LUQ | left upper quadrant | $O_2$ | oxygen |
| LV | left ventricle | OA | osteoarthritis |
| LVAD | left ventricular assist device | OAE | otoacoustic emissions |
| lymphs | lymphocytes | OB | obstetrics |
| MCH | mean corpuscular hemoglobin | OCD | obsessive-compulsive disorder |
| MCHC | mean corpuscular hemoglobin concentration | OCP | oral contraceptive pill |
| | | ODD | oppositional defiant disorder |
| MD | muscular dystrophy; medical doctor | OGTT | oral glucose tolerance test |
| MDI | metered dose inhaler | OM | otitis media |
| MDRTB | multidrug-resistant tuberculosis | Ophth | ophthalmology |
| mets | metastases | OSA | obstructive sleep apnea |
| MI | myocardial infarction | OT | oxytocin |
| MIDCAB | minimally invasive direct coronary artery bypass | Oto | otology |
| | | PA | posteroanterior; pulmonary artery |
| MMPI | Minnesota Multiphasic Personality Inventory | PAC | premature atrial contractions |
| | | PACAB | port-access coronary artery bypass |
| MR | mental retardation; mitral regurgitation | Pap | Papanicolaou test |
| MRI | magnetic resonance imaging | PCOS | polycystic ovary syndrome |
| MS | multiple sclerosis; mitral stenosis; musculoskeletal | PCV | packed-cell volume; hematocrit |
| | | PD | Parkinson disease; panic disorder |
| MSH | melanocyte-stimulating hormone | PDA | patent ductus arteriosus |
| MSLT | multiple sleep latency test | PDD | pervasive developmental disorders |
| MUGA | multigated (radionuclide) angiogram | | |
| | | PDR | proliferative diabetic retinopathy |
| MV | mitral valve | PEG | percutaneous endoscopic gastrostomy |
| MVP | mitral valve prolapse | | |
| MY | myopia | PET scan | positron emission tomography scan |
| neuts | neutrophils | | |
| NGU | nongonococcal urethritis | PGH | pituitary growth hormone |

Continued

## Abbreviations—cont'd

| Abbreviation | Meaning |
|---|---|
| pH | acidity/alkalinity |
| PICC | peripherally inserted central catheter |
| PID | pelvic inflammatory disease |
| PIP | proximal interphalangeal joint |
| PK | penetrating keratoplasty (corneal transplant) |
| PKU | phenylketonuria |
| Plats | platelets; thrombocytes |
| PMDD | premenstrual dysphoric disorder |
| PMNs, polys | polymorphonucleocytes |
| PMS | premenstrual syndrome |
| PNS | peripheral nervous system |
| pos | posterior |
| PPB | positive-pressure breathing |
| PPD | purified protein derivative |
| PRK | photorefractive keratectomy |
| PRL | prolactin |
| PSA | prostate-specific antigen |
| PSG | polysomnography |
| PT | prothrombin time |
| PTC/PTCA | percutaneous transhepatic cholangiography |
| PTCA | percutaneous transluminal coronary angioplasty |
| PTH | parathyroid hormone |
| PTSD | posttraumatic stress disorder |
| PTT | partial thromboplastin time |
| PUD | peptic ulcer disease |
| PUVA | psoralen plus ultraviolet A |
| PV | pulmonary vein |
| PVC | premature ventricular contraction |
| PVD | peripheral vascular disease |
| RA | rheumatoid arthritis; right atrium |
| RAD | reactive airway disease |
| RAIU | radioactive iodine uptake |
| RBC | red blood cell (count) |
| RCA | right coronary artery |
| RF | rheumatoid factor |
| RFCA | radiofrequency catheter ablation |
| Rh | rhesus |
| RIA | radioimmunoassay |

| Abbreviation | Meaning |
|---|---|
| RLL | right lower lobe |
| RLQ | right lower quadrant |
| RML | right middle lobe |
| ROM | range of motion |
| RSV | respiratory syncytial virus |
| RUL | right upper lobe |
| RUQ | right upper quadrant |
| RV | right ventricle |
| Rx | therapy |
| S1-S5 | first sacral through fifth sacral vertebrae; sacral nerves |
| SA | sinoatrial |
| SAD | seasonal affective disorder |
| SARS | severe acute respiratory syndrome |
| SCLC | small cell lung cancer |
| SCC | squamous cell carcinoma |
| SG | specific gravity; skin graft |
| SIADH | syndrome of inappropriate antidiuretic hormone |
| SIRS | systemic inflammatory response syndrome |
| SLS | systemic lupus erythmatosus |
| SNS | somatic nervous system |
| SOB | shortness of breath |
| SPECT | single-photon emission computed tomography |
| SSRI | selective serotonin reuptake inhibitor |
| SSS | sick sinus syndrome |
| STH | somatotropic hormone |
| STSG | split-thickness skin graft |
| sup | superior |
| SVT | superficial vein thrombosis |
| sx | symptoms |
| T1-T12 | first thoracic through twelfth thoracic vertebrae; thoracic nerves |
| $T_3$ | triiodothyronine |
| $T_4$ | thyroxine |
| TAH-BSO | total abdominal hysterectomy with a bilateral salpingo-oophorectomy |

## Abbreviations—cont'd

| Abbreviation | Meaning |
|---|---|
| TA-90 | tumor marker for spread of malignant melanoma |
| TAT | Thematic Apperception Test |
| TB | tuberculosis |
| TDN | transdermal nitroglycerin |
| TDNTG | transdermal nitroglycerin |
| TEA | thromboendarterectomy |
| TEE | transesophageal echocardiogram |
| TENS | transcutaneous electrical nerve stimulation |
| TFTs | thyroid function tests |
| THR | total hip replacement |
| TIA | transient ischemic attack |
| TKR | total knee replacement |
| TM | tympanic membrane |
| TMR | transmyocardial revascularization |
| TNM | tumor-node-metastasis |
| TS | tricuspid stenosis |
| TSE | testicular self-examination |
| TSH | thyroid-stimulating hormone |
| TTS | transdermal therapeutic system |
| TUR | transurethral resection |
| TURP | transurethral resection of the prostate |
| TV | tricuspid valve |
| UA | urinalysis |

| Abbreviation | Meaning |
|---|---|
| UAE | uterine artery embolization |
| ULQ | upper left quadrant |
| UNHS | Universal Newborn Hearing Screening test |
| URI | upper respiratory infection |
| URQ | upper right quadrant |
| US | ultrasound; sonography |
| UTI | urinary tract infection |
| VA | visual acuity |
| VAD | ventricular assist device |
| VBAC | vaginal birth after cesarean section |
| VCUG | voiding cystourethrography |
| VD | venereal disease |
| VDRL | Venereal Disease Research Laboratory (test for syphilis) |
| VEB | ventricular ectopic beats |
| VF | visual field |
| VMA | urine vanillylmandelic acid |
| VP | vasopressin (also known as ADH) |
| VSD | ventricular septal defect |
| WAIS | Wechsler Adult Intelligence Scale |
| WBC | white blood cell (count) |
| ZIFT | zygote intrafallopian transfer |

# ISMP's **List of _Error-Prone Abbreviations_, _Symbols_, and _Dose Designations_**

| Abbreviations | Intended meaning | Misinterpretation | Correction |
|---|---|---|---|
| µg | Microgram | Mistaken as "mg" | Use "mcg" |
| AD, AS, AU | Right ear, left ear, each ear | Mistaken as OD, OS, OU (right eye, left eye, each eye) | Use "right ear," "left ear," or "each ear" |
| OD, OS, OU | Right eye, left eye, each eye | Mistaken as AD, AS, AU (right ear, left ear, each, ear) | Use "right eye," "left eye," or "each eye" |
| BT | Bedtime | Mistaken as "BID" (twice daily) | Use "bedtime" |
| cc | Cubic centimeters | Mistaken as "u" (units) | Use "mL" |
| D/C | Discharge or discontinue | Premature discontinuation of medications if D/C (intended to mean "discharge") has been misinterpreted as "discontinued" when followed by a list of discharge medications | Use "discharge" and "discontinue" |
| IJ | Injection | Mistaken as "IV" or "intrajugular" | Use "injection" |
| IN | Intranasal | Mistaken as "IM" or "IV" | Use "intranasal" or "NAS" |
| HS | Half-strength | Mistaken as bedtime | Use "half-strength" or "bedtime" |
| hs | At bedtime, hours of sleep | Mistaken as half-strength | |
| IU** | International unit | Mistaken as IV (intravenous) or 10 (ten) | Use "units" |
| o.d. or OD | Once daily | Mistaken as "right eye" (OD-oculus dexter), leading to oral liquid medications administered in the eye | Use "daily" |
| OJ | Orange juice | Mistaken as OD or OS (right or left eye); drugs meant to be diluted in orange juice may be given in the eye | Use "orange juice" |
| Per os | By mouth, orally | The "os" can be mistaken as "left eye" (OS-oculus sinister) | Use "PO," "by mouth," or "orally" |
| q.d. or QOD** | Every day | Mistaken as q.i.d., especially if the period after the "q" or the tail of the "q" is misunderstood as an "i" | Use "daily" |
| qhs | Nightly at bedtime | Mistaken as "qhr" or every hour | Use "nightly" |
| qn | Nightly or at bedtime | Mistaken as "qh" (every hour) | Use "nightly" or "at bedtime" |
| q.o.d. or QD** | Every other day | Mistaken as "q.d." (daily) or "q.i.d." (four times daily) if the "o" is poorly written | Use "every other day" |
| q1d | Daily | Mistaken as q.i.d. (four times daily) | Use "daily" |
| q6PM, etc. | Every evening at 6 PM | Mistaken as every 6 hours | Use "daily at 6 PM" or "6 PM daily" |
| SC, SQ, sub q | Subcutaneous | SC mistaken as SL (sublingual); SQ mistaken as "5 every;" the "q" in "sub q" has been mistaken as "every" (e.g., a heparin dose ordered "sub q 2 hours before surgery" misunderstood as every 2 hours before surgery) | Use "subcut" or " subcutaneously" |
| ss | Sliding scale (insulin) or ½ (apothecary) | Mistaken as "55" | Spell out "sliding scale;" use "one-half" or "½" |
| SSRI | Sliding scale regular insulin | Mistaken as selective-serotonin reuptake inhibitor | Spell out "sliding scale (insulin)" |
| SSI | Sliding scale insulin | Mistaken as Strong Solution of Iodine (Lugol's) | |
| i/d | Once daily | Mistaken as "tid" | Use "1 daily" |
| TIW or tiw | 3 times a week | Mistaken as "3 times a day" or "twice in a week" | Use "3 times weekly" |
| U or u** | Unit | Mistaken as the number 0 or 4, causing a 10-fold overdose or greater (e.g., 4U seen as "40" or 4u seen as "44"); mistaken as "cc" so dose given in volume instead of units (e.g., 4u seen as 4cc) | Use "unit" |
| UD | As directed ("ut dictum") | Mistaken as unit dose (e.g., diltiazem 125mg IV infusion "UD" misinterpreted as meaning to give the entire infusion as a unit [bolus] dose) | Use "as directed" |

| Dose designations and other information | Intended meaning | Misinterpretation | Correction |
|---|---|---|---|
| **Trailing zero after decimal point** (e.g., 1.0 mg)** | 1 mg | Mistaken as 10 mg if the decimal point is not seen | Do not use trailing zeros for doses expressed in whole numbers |
| **"Naked" decimal point** (e.g., .5 mg)** | 0.5 mg | Mistaken as 5 mg if the decimal point is not seen | Use zero before a decimal point when the dose is less than a whole unit |
| **Abbreviations such as mg. or mL. with a period following the abbreviation** | mg<br><br>mL | The period is unnecessary and could be mistaken as the number 1 if written poorly | Use mg, mL, etc. without a terminal period |

## ISMP's List of *Error-Prone Abbreviations, Symbols,* and *Dose Designations* (continued)

| Dose designations and other information | Intended meaning | Misinterpretation | Correction |
|---|---|---|---|
| **Drug name and dose run together (especially problematic for drug names that end in "l" such as Inderal40 mg; Tegretol300 mg)** | Inderal 40 mg<br><br>Tegretol 300 mg | Mistaken as Inderal 140 mg<br><br>Mistaken as Tegretol 1300 mg | Place adequate space between the drug name, dose, and unit of measure |
| **Numerical dose and unit of measure run together (e.g., 10mg, 100mL)** | 10 mg<br><br>100 mL | The "m" is sometimes mistaken as a zero or two zeros, risking a 10- to 100-fold overdose | Place adequate space between the dose and unit of measure |
| **Large doses without properly placed commas (e.g., 100000 units; 1000000 units)** | 100,000 units<br><br>1,000,000 units | 100000 has been mistaken as 10,000 or 1,000,000; 1000000 has been mistaken as 100,000 | Use commas for dosing units at or above 1,000, or use words such as 100 "thousand" or 1 "million" to improve readability |

| Drug name abbreviations | Intended meaning | Misinterpretation | Correction |
|---|---|---|---|

To avoid confusion, do not abbreviate drug names when communicating medical information. Examples of drug name abbreviations involved in medication errors include:

| | | | |
|---|---|---|---|
| **ARA A** | vidarabine | Mistaken as cytarabine (ARA C) | Use complete drug name |
| **AZT** | zidovudine (Retrovir) | Mistaken as azathioprine or aztreonam | Use complete drug name |
| **CPZ** | Compazine (prochlorperazine) | Mistaken as chlorpromazine | Use complete drug name |
| **DPT** | Demerol-Phenergan-Thorazine | Mistaken as diphtheria-pertussis-tetanus (vaccine) | Use complete drug name |
| **DTO** | Diluted tincture of opium, or deodorized tincture of opium (Paregoric) | Mistaken as tincture of opium | Use complete drug name |
| **HCl** | hydrochloric acid or hydrochloride | Mistaken as potassium chloride (The "H" is misinterpreted as "K") | Use complete drug name unless expressed as a salt of a drug |
| **HCT** | hydrocortisone | Mistaken as hydrochlorothiazide | Use complete drug name |
| **HCTZ** | hydrochlorothiazide | Mistaken as hydrocortisone (seen as HCT250 mg) | Use complete drug name |
| **MgSO4\*\*** | magnesium sulfate | Mistaken as morphine sulfate | Use complete drug name |
| **MS, MSO4\*\*** | morphine sulfate | Mistaken as magnesium sulfate | Use complete drug name |
| **MTX** | methotrexate | Mistaken as mitoxantrone | Use complete drug name |
| **PCA** | procainamide | Mistaken as patient controlled analgesia | Use complete drug name |
| **PTU** | propylthiouracil | Mistaken as mercaptopurine | Use complete drug name |
| **T3** | Tylenol with codeine No. 3 | Mistaken as liothyronine | Use complete drug name |
| **TAC** | triamcinolone | Mistaken as tetracaine, Adrenalin, cocaine | Use complete drug name |
| **TNK** | TNKase | Mistaken as "TPA" | Use complete drug name |
| **ZnSO4** | zinc sulfate | Mistaken as morphine sulfate | Use complete drug name |

| Stemmed drug names | Intended meaning | Misinterpretation | Correction |
|---|---|---|---|
| **"Nitro" drip** | nitroglycerin infusion | Mistaken as sodium nitroprusside infusion | Use complete drug name |
| **"Norflox"** | norfloxacin | Mistaken as Norflex | Use complete drug name |
| **"IV Vanc"** | intravenous vancomycin | Mistaken as Invanz | Use complete drug name |

| Symbols | Intended meaning | Misinterpretation | Correction |
|---|---|---|---|
| ℨ | Dram | Symbol for dram mistaken as "3" | Use the metric system |
| ℳ | Minim | Symbol for minim mistaken as "mL" | |
| **x3d** | For three days | Mistaken as "3 doses" | Use "for three days" |
| **> and <** | Greater than and less than | Mistaken as opposite of intended; mistakenly use incorrect symbol; "< 10" mistaken as "40" | Use "greater than" or "less than" |
| **/ (slash mark)** | Separates two doses or indicates "per" | Mistaken as the number 1 (e.g., "25 units/10 units" misread as "25 units and 110 units") | Use "per" rather than a slash mark to separate doses |
| **@** | At | Mistaken as "2" | Use "at" |
| **&** | And | Mistaken as "2" | Use "and" |
| **+** | Plus or and | Mistaken as "4" | Use "and" |
| **°** | Hour | Mistaken as a zero (e.g., q2° seen as q 20) | Use "hr," "h," or "hour" |

\*\* These abbreviations are included on The Joint Commission's "minimum list" of dangerous abbreviations, acronyms, and symbols that must be included on an organization's "Do Not Use" list, effective January 1, 2004. Visit www.jointcommission.org for more information about this Joint Commission requirement.

© ISMP 2011. Permission is granted to reproduce material with proper attribution for internal use within healthcare organizations. Other reproduction is prohibited without written permission from ISMP. Report actual and potential medication errors to the ISMP National Medication Errors Reporting Program (ISMP MERP) via the Web at www.ismp.org or by calling 1-800-FAIL-SAF(E).

## English-to-Spanish Translation Guide: Key Medical Questions

The following is a guide to help you complete the history and examination of Spanish-speaking patients. Initial questions presented are general ones used at the beginning of the examination. Questions for pain assessment follow. The remainder of the translations are arranged in order of the body systems. Each system's section contains basic vocabulary, questions used for history taking, and instructions that would facilitate examination. The intent of this guide is to offer an array of questions and phrases from which the examiner can choose as appropriate for assessment.

### Hints for Pronunciation of Spanish Words

1. *h* is silent.
2. *j* is pronounced as *h*.
3. *ll* is pronounced as a *y* sound.
4. *r* is pronounced with a trilled sound, and *rr* is trilled even more.
5. *v* is pronounced with a *b* sound.
6. A *y* by itself is pronounced with a long *e* sound.
7. Accent marks over the vowel indicate the syllable that is to be stressed.

### Introductory

| | |
|---|---|
| I am _____. | Soy _____. |
| What is your name? | ¿Cómo se llama usted? |
| I would like to examine you now. | Quisiera examinarlo(a) ahora. |

### General

| | |
|---|---|
| How do you feel? | ¿Cómo se siente? |
|   Good |   Bien |
|   Bad |   Mal |
| Do you feel better today? | ¿Se siente mejor hoy? |
| Where do you work? | ¿Dónde trabaja? (Cuál es su profesión o trabajo?) (¿Qué hace usted?) |
| Are you allergic to anything? | ¿Tiene usted alérgias? |
|   Medications, foods, insect bites? |   ¿Medicinas, alimentos, picaduras de insectos? |
| Do you take any medications? | ¿Toma usted alguna medicina? |
| Do you have any drug allergies? | ¿Es usted alérgico(a) a algún médicamento? |
| Do you have a history of | ¿Padece usted: |
|   Heart disease? |   de alguna enfermedad del corazón? |
|   Diabetes? |   del diabetes? |
|   Epilepsy? |   la epilépsia? |
|   Bronchitis? |   de bronquitis? |
|   Emphysema? |   de enfisema? |
|   Asthma? |   de asma? |

From Seidel HM: *Mosby's guide to physical examination,* ed 5, St Louis, 2003, Mosby.

## Pain

| | |
|---|---|
| Have you any pain? | ¿Tiene dolor? |
| Where is the pain? | ¿Dónde está el dolor? |
| Do you have any pain here? | ¿Tiene usted dolor aquí? |
| How severe is the pain? | ¿Qué tan fuerte es el dolor? |
| Mild, moderate, sharp, or severe? | ¿Ligero, moderado, agudo, o severo? |
| What were you doing when the pain started? | ¿Qué hacía usted cuando le comenzóel dolor? |
| Have you ever had this pain before? | ¿Ha tenido este dolor antes? |
| | (¿Ha sido siempre así?) |
| Do you have a pain in your side? | ¿Tiene usted dolor en el costado? |
| Is it worse now? | ¿Está peor ahora? |
| Does it still pain you? | ¿Le duele todavía? |
| Did you feel much pain at the time? | ¿Sintió mucho dolor entonces? |
| Show me where. | Muéstreme dónde. |
| Does it hurt when I press here? | ¿Le duele cuando aprieto aquí? |

## Head

*Vocabulary*

| | |
|---|---|
| Head | La cabeza |
| Face | La cara |

*History*

| | |
|---|---|
| How does your head feel? | ¿Cómo siente la cabeza? |
| Have you any pain in the head? | ¿Le duele la cabeza? |
| Do you have headaches? | ¿Tiene usted dolores de cabeza? |
| Do you have migraines? | ¿Tiene usted migrañas? |
| What causes the headaches? | ¿Qué le causa los dolores de cabeza? |

*Examination*

| | |
|---|---|
| Lift up your head. | Levante la cabeza. |

## Eyes

*Vocabulary*

| | |
|---|---|
| Eye | El ojo |

*History*

| | |
|---|---|
| Have you had pain in your eyes? | ¿Ha tenido dolor en los ojos? |
| Do you wear glasses? | ¿Usa usted anteojos/gafas/lentes/espejuelos? |
| Do you wear contact lenses? | ¿Usa usted lentes de contacto? |
| Can you see clearly? | ¿Puede ver claramente? |
| Better at a distance? | ¿Mejor a cierta distancia? |
| Do you sometimes see things double? | ¿Ve las cosas doble algunas veces? |
| Do you see things through a mist? | ¿Ve las cosas nubladas? |
| Were you exposed to anything that could have injured your eye? | ¿Fue expuesto(a) a cualquier cosa que pudiera haberle dañado el ojo? |
| Do your eyes water much? | ¿Le lagrimean mucho los ojos? |

*Examination*

| | |
|---|---|
| Look up. | Mire para arriba. |
| Look down. | Mire para abajo. |

| | |
|---|---|
| Look toward your nose. | Mírese la nariz. |
| Look at me. | Míreme. |
| Tell me what number it is. | Digame qué número es éste. |
| Tell me what letter it is. | Digame qué letra es ésta. |

### Ears/Nose/Throat

*Vocabulary*

| | |
|---|---|
| Ears | Los oídos |
| Eardrum | El tímpano |
| Laryngitis | La laringitis |
| Lip | El labio |
| Mouth | La boca |
| Nose | La naríz |
| Tongue | La lengua |

*History*

| | |
|---|---|
| Do you have any hearing problems? | ¿Tiene usted problemas al oir? |
| Do you use a hearing aid? | ¿Usa usted un audífono? |
| Do you have ringing in the ears? | ¿Le zumban los oídos? |
| Do you have allergies? | ¿Tiene alérgias? |
| Do you use dentures? | ¿Usa usted dentadura postiza? |
| Do you have any loose teeth, removable bridges, or any prosthesis? | ¿Tiene dientes flojos, dientes postizos, o cualiquier prótesis? |
| Do you have a cold? | ¿Tiene usted un resfriado/resfrío? |
| Do you have a sore throat frequently? | ¿Le duele la garganta con frecuencia? |
| Have you ever had a strep throat? | ¿Ha tenido alguna vez infección de la garganta? |

*Examination*

| | |
|---|---|
| Open your mouth. | Abra la boca. |
| I want to take a throat culture. This will not hurt. | Quiero hacer un cultivo de la garganta. Esto no le va a doler. |

### Cardiovascular

*Vocabulary*

| | |
|---|---|
| Heart | El corazón |
| Heart attack | El ataque al corazón |
| Heart disease | La enfermedad del corazón |
| Heart murmur | El soplo del corazón |
| High blood pressure | Alta presión |

*History*

| | |
|---|---|
| Have you ever had any chest pain? Where? | ¿Ha tenido alguna vez dolor de pecho? ¿Dónde? |
| Do you notice any irregularity of heartbeat or any palpitations? | ¿Nota cualquier latido o palpitación irregular? |
| Do you get short of breath? When? | ¿Tiene usted problemas con la respiración? ¿Cuándo? |
| Do you take medicine for your heart? How often? | ¿Toma medicina para el corazón? ¿Con qué frecuencia? |

| | |
|---|---|
| Do you know if you have high blood pressure? | ¿Sabe usted si tiene la presión alta? |
| Is there a history of hypertension in your family? | ¿En su familia se encuentran varias personas con alta presión? |
| Are any of your limbs swollen? | ¿Están hinchados algunos de sus miembros? |
|    Hands, feet, legs? |    ¿Manos, pies, piernas? |
| How long have they been swollen like this? | ¿Desde cuándo están hinchados así? |
| | (¿Qué tanto tiempo tiene usted con esta hinchazón?) |

*Examination*

| | |
|---|---|
| Let me feel your pulse. | Déjeme tomarle el pulso. |
| I am going to take your blood pressure now. | Le voy a tomar la presión ahora. |

## Respiratory

*Vocabulary*

| | |
|---|---|
| Chest | El pecho |
| Lungs | Los pulmones |

*History*

| | |
|---|---|
| Do you smoke? | ¿Fuma usted? |
|    How many packs a day? |    ¿Cuántos paquetes al día? |
| Have you any difficulty in breathing? | ¿Tiene dificultad al respirar? |
| How long have you been coughing? | ¿Desde cuándo tiene tos? |
| Do you cough up phlegm? | ¿Al toser, escupe usted flema(s)? |
| What is the color of your expectorations? | ¿Cuándo usted escupe, qué color es? |
| Do you cough up blood? | ¿Al toser, arroja usted sangre? |
| Do you wheeze? | ¿Le silba a usted el pecho? |

*Examination*

| | |
|---|---|
| Take a deep breath. | Respìre profundo. |
| Breathe normally. | Respìre normalmente. |
| Cough. | Tosa. |
| Cough again. | Tosa otra vez. |

## Gastrointestinal

*Vocabulary*

| | |
|---|---|
| Abdomen | El abdomen |
| Intestines/bowels | Los intestinos/las entrañas |
| Liver | El hígado |
| Nausea | Náusea |
| Gastric ulcer | La úlcera gástrica |
| Stomach | El estómago, la panza, la barriga |
| Stomachache | El dolor de estómago |

*History*

| | |
|---|---|
| What foods disagree with you? | ¿Qué alimentos le caen mal? |
| Do you get heartburn? | ¿Suele tener ardor en el pecho? |
| Do you have indigestion often? | ¿Tiene indigestion con frecuencia? |
| Are you going to vomit? | ¿Va a vomitar (arrojar)? |
| Do you have blood in your vomit? | ¿Tiene usted vómitos con sangre? |

| | |
|---|---|
| Do you have abdominal pain? | ¿Tiene dolor en el abdomen? |
| How are your stools? | ¿Cómo son sus defecaciones? |
| Are they regular? | ¿Son regulares? |
| Have you noticed their color? | ¿Se ha fijado en el color? |
| Are you constipated? | ¿Está estreñido? |
| Do you have diarrhea? | ¿Tiene diarrea? |

### Genitourinary

*Vocabulary*

| | |
|---|---|
| Genitals | Los genitales |
| Kidney | El riñón |
| Penis | El pene, el miembro |
| Urine | La orina |

*History*

| | |
|---|---|
| Have you any difficulty passing water? | ¿Tiene dificultad en orinar? |
| Do you pass water involuntarily? | ¿Orina sin querer? |
| Do you have a urethral discharge? | ¿Tiene desecho de la uretra? |
| Do you have burning with urination? | ¿Tiene ardor al orinar? |

### Musculoskeletal

*Vocabulary*

| | |
|---|---|
| Ankle | El tobillo |
| Arm | El brazo |
| Back | La espalda |
| Bones | Los huesos |
| Elbow | El codo |
| Finger | El dedo |
| Foot | El pie |
| Fracture | La fractura |
| Hand | La mano |
| Hip | La cadera |
| Knee | La rodilla |
| Leg | La pierna |
| Muscles | Los músculos |
| Rib | La costilla |
| Shoulder | El hombro |
| Thigh | El muslo |

*History*

| | |
|---|---|
| Did you fall, and how did you fall? | ¿Se cayó, y cómo se cayó? |
| How did this happen? | ¿Cómo sucedió esto? |
|   How long ago? |   ¿Hace cuanto tiempo? |

*Examination*

| | |
|---|---|
| Raise your arm. | Levante el brazo. |
|   Raise it more. |   Más alto. |
|   Now the other. |   Ahora el otro. |
| Stand up and walk. | Parese y camine. |

| | |
|---|---|
| Straighten your leg. | Enderece la pierna. |
| Bend your knee. | Doble la rodilla. |
| Push | Empuje |
| Pull | Jale |
| Up | Arriba |
| Down | Abajo |
| In/out | Adentro/afuera |
| Rest | Descanse |
| Kneel | Arrodíllese |

## Neurologic

### Vocabulary

| | |
|---|---|
| Brain | El cerebro |
| Dizziness | El vertigo, el mareo |
| Epilepsy | La epilépsia |
| Fainting spell | El desmayo |

### History

| | |
|---|---|
| Have you ever had a head injury? | ¿Ha tenido alguna vez daño en la cabeza? |
| Do you have convulsions? | ¿Tiene convulsiones? |
| Do you have tingling sensations? | ¿Tiene hormigueos? |
| Do you have numbness in your hands, arms, or feet? | ¿Siente entumecidos las manos, los brazos, o los pies? |
| Have you ever lost consciousness? | ¿Perdió alguna vez el sentido? (inconsiente) |
|   For how long? |   ¿Por cuánto tiempo? |
| How often does this happen? | ¿Con qué frecuencia ocurre esto? |

### Examination

| | |
|---|---|
| Squeeze my hand. | Apriete mi mano. |
| Can you not do it better than that? | ¿No puede hacerlo más fuerte? |
| Turn on your left/right side. | Voltéese al lado izquierdo/al lado derecho. |
| Roll over and sit up over the edge of the bed. | Voltéese y siéntese sobre el borde de la cama. |
| Stand up slowly. Put your weight only on your right/left foot. | Párese despacio. Ponga peso solo en la pierna derecha/izquierda. |
| Take a step to the side. | Dé un paso al lado. |
| Turn to your left/right. | Doble a la izquierda/derecha. |
| Is this hot or cold? | ¿Está frío o caliente esto? |
| Am I sticking you with the point or the head of the pin? | ¿Le estoy pinchando con el punto o la cabeza del alfiler? |

## Endocrine/Reproductive

### Vocabulary

| | |
|---|---|
| Uterus | El útero, la matríz |
| Vagina | La vagina |

### History

| | |
|---|---|
| Have you had any problems with your thyroid? | ¿Ha tenido alguna vez problemas con tiroides? |
| Have you noticed any significant weight gain or loss? | ¿Ha notado pérdida o aumento de peso? |
| What is your usual weight? | ¿Cuál es su peso usual? |
| How is your appetite? | ¿Qué tal su apetito? |

*Women*

| How old were you when your periods started? | ¿Cuántos años tenía cuando tuvo la primera regla? |
| How many days between periods? | ¿Cuántos dias entre las reglas? |
| When was your last menstrual period? | ¿Cuándo fue su última regla? |
| Have you ever been pregnant? | ¿Ha estado embarazada? |
| How many children do you have? | ¿Cuántos hijos tiene? |
| When was your last Pap smear? | ¿Cuándo fue su última prueba de Papanicolau? |
| Would you like information on birth control methods? | ¿Quiere usted información sobre los métodos del control de la natalidad? |
| Do you have a vaginal discharge? | ¿Tiene desecho vaginal? |

# Answers to Exercises and Review Questions

## Chapter 1

### Exercise 1
| 1. C | 2. D | 3. E |
| 4. B | 5. F | 6. A |

### Exercise 2
| 1. C | 2. D | 3. A |
| 4. E | 5. B | |

### Exercise 3
| 1. B | 2. D | 3. E |
| 4. A | 5. C | |

### Exercise 4
1. ophthalm/o (eye) + -logy (study of)
   **Def: study of the eye**
2. ot/o (ear) + -plasty (surgical repair)
   **Def: surgical repair of the ear**
3. gastr/o (stomach) + -algia (pain)
   **Def: pain in the stomach**
4. arthr/o (joint) + -scope (instrument to view)
   **Def: instrument to view a joint**
5. rhin/o (nose) + -tomy (incision)
   **Def: incision of the nose**

### Exercise 5
| 1. E | 2. G | 3. J |
| 4. I | 5. H | 6. A |
| 7. C | 8. D | 9. F |
| 10. B | | |

11. cardi/o (heart) + -megaly (enlargement)
    **Def: enlargement of the heart**
12. oste/o (bone) + -malacia (softening)
    **Def: softening of the bone**
13. valvul/o (valve) + -itis (inflammation)
    **Def: inflammation of a valve**

14. cephal/o (head) + -ic (pertaining to)
    **Def: pertaining to the head**
15. gastr/o (stomach) + -ptosis (prolapse)
    **Def: prolapse of the stomach**

### Exercise 6
| 1. E | 2. I | 3. H |
| 4. F | 5. J | 6. C |
| 7. D | 8. A | 9. G |
| 10. B | | |

11. oste/o (bone) + -logist (one who specializes in the study of)
    **Def: one who specializes in the study of bones**
12. spir/o (breathing) + -meter (instrument to measure)
    **Def: instrument to measure breathing**
13. hyster/o (uterus) + -scopy (process of viewing)
    **Def: process of viewing the uterus**
14. cyst/o (bladder, sac) + -scope (instrument to view)
    **Def: instrument to view the bladder**
15. splen/o (spleen) + -ectomy (removal)
    **Def: removal of the spleen**

### Exercise 7
| 1. C | 2. H | 3. F |
| 4. I | 5. B | 6. D |
| 7. E | 8. J | 9. A |
| 10. G | | |

11. sub- (under) + hepat/o (liver) + -ic (pertaining to)
    **Def: pertaining to under the liver**
12. peri- (around) + cardi/o (heart) + -um (structure)
    **Def: structure around the heart**

13. dys- (difficult) + pne/o (breathing) + -ic (pertaining to)
    **Def: pertaining to difficult breathing**
14. per- (through) + cutane/o (skin) + -ous (pertaining to)
    **Def: pertaining to through the skin**
15. hypo- (deficient) + glyc/o (sugar) + -emia (blood condition)
    **Def: blood condition of deficient sugar**

### Exercise 8
1. esophagi
2. larynges
3. fornices
4. pleurae
5. diagnoses
6. myocardia
7. cardiomyopathies
8. hepatides

### Exercise 9
| z | x |
| f | ph |
| n | pn |
| u | eu |
| t | pt |
| s | ps |

## Chapter 1 Review

### Word Part Definitions
1. inter-
2. per-
3. par-
4. intra-
5. anti-
6. a-
7. peri-
8. para-
9. pre-
10. poly-
11. sub-
12. dys-
13. –dynia
14. –rrhea
15. –stenosis

16. –oma
17. –tripter
18. –itis
19. –rrhage
20. –scopy
21. –logy
22. –tomy
23. –plasty
24. –ectomy
25. –graphy
26. –meter
27. –rrhaphy
28. –stomy
29. –osis
30. –pathy
31. –ar
32. –ia

## Wordshop

1. condition (-ia) without (an-) eye (ophthalm/o)
   **Term: anophthalmia**
2. pertaining to (-id) near (para-) ear (ot/o)
   **Term: parotid**
3. pertaining to (-ic) under (sub-) liver (hepat/o)
   **Term: subhepatic**
4. inflammation (-itis) stomach (gastr/o) small intestines (enter/o)
   **Term: gastroenteritis**
5. instrument to view (-scope) ear (ot/o)
   **Term: otoscope**
6. structure (-um) surrounding (peri-) heart (cardi/o)
   **Term: pericardium**
7. new opening (-stomy) colon (col/o)
   **Term: colostomy**
8. process of recording (-graphy) artery (arteri/o)
   **Term: arteriography**
9. process of viewing (-scopy) within (endo-)
   **Term: endoscopy**
10. removal (-ectomy) uterus (hyster/o)
    **Term: hysterectomy**
11. study of (-logy) many (poly-) sleep (somn/o)
    **Term: polysomnology**
12. pertaining to (-al) before (pre-) birth (nat/o)
    **Term: prenatal**

13. pain (-algia) head (cephal/o)
    **Term: cephalalgia**
14. pertaining to (-ic) above (epi-) stomach (gastr/o)
    **Term: epigastric**
15. enlargement (-megaly) spleen (splen/o)
    **Term: splenomegaly**

## Chapter 2

### Exercise 1
1. D    2. E    3. A
4. C    5. B

### Exercise 2
1. C   2. A   3. D   4. B

### Exercise 3
1. D   2. F   3. A   4. B
5. H   6. C   7. E   8. G

### Exercise 4
1. pertaining to within the lumen
2. pertaining to the hilum
3. pertaining to around the apex
4. pertaining to the antrum
5. pertaining to the nucleus
6. pertaining to the cytoplasm
7. pertaining to outside the body
8. pertaining to the vestibule
9. pertaining to the fundus
10. lumen
11. hilum
12. apex
13. body, corporis
14. sinuses

### Exercise 5
1. F    2. H    3. C, I
4. A    5. G    6. E
7. J    8. B    9. L
10. D   11. K

### Exercise 6
1. J    2. G    3. A    4. I
5. D    6. E    7. H    8. B
9. C   10. F

### Exercise 7
1. the study of cells
2. one who specializes in the study of disease
3. process of viewing dead (tissue)

4. one who specializes in the study of tissue
5. process of viewing living (tissue)

### Exercise 8
1. G
2. M    3. J    4. K    5. R
6. A    7. P    8. D    9. T
10. B   11. F   12. I   13. Q
14. C   15. S   16. N   17. E
18. O   19. H   20. L

### Exercise 9
See Fig. 2-2.

### Exercise 10
1. I    2. P    3. N    4. L
5. M   6. J    7. R    8. B
9. K   10. F   11. D   12. O
13. G   14. A   15. Q   16. E
17. C   18. H

### Exercise 11
1. C    2. A    3. F    4. K
5. I    6. J    7. L    8. E
9. D   10. H   11. G   12. B

### Exercise 12
1. esophagus
2. esophagus and stomach
3. the beginning and middle portions of the esophagus were normal
4. distal esophagus

### Exercise 13
1. D   2. C   3. B   4. A
5. E

### Exercise 14
1. epigastric
2. lumbar
3. hypogastric
4. iliac or inguinal
5. hypochondriac

### Exercise 15
See Fig. 2-6.

### Exercise 16
1. transverse
2. midsagittal
3. frontal or coronal

### Exercise 17
1. closer to the toes
2. inner surface

3. during
4. front to back

## Chapter 2 Review

### Word Part Definitions

1. epi-
2. meta-
3. uni-
4. endo-
5. bi-
6. af-
7. ipsi-
8. contra-
9. ef-
10. viscer/o
11. infer/o
12. anter/o
13. dist/o
14. medi/o
15. axill/o
16. super/o
17. proxim/o
18. sinistr/o
19. brachi/o
20. caud/o
21. lapar/o
22. later/o
23. dextr/o
24. poster/o
25. hist/o
26. corpor/o
27. cephal/o
28. crani/o
29. cyt/o
30. inguin/o
31. cervic/o
32. thorac/o

### Wordshop

1. pertaining to (-al) middle (mid-) sagittal plane (sagitt/o)
   **Term: midsagittal**
2. pertaining to (-al) two (bi-) side (later/o)
   **Term: bilateral**
3. toward (-ad) right (dextr/o)
   **Term: dextrad**
4. pertaining to (-ior) back (poster/o) front (anter/o)
   **Term: posteroanterior**
5. pertaining to (-ic) chest (thorac/o)
   **Term: thoracic**
6. pertaining to (-ic) abdomen (abdomin/o) pelvis (pelv/o)
   **Term: abdominopelvic**

7. pertaining to (-ar) low back (lumb/o)
   **Term: lumbar**
8. pertaining to (-al) opposite (contra-) side (later/o)
   **Term: contralateral**
9. formation (-plasm) cell (cyt/o)
   **Term: cytoplasm**
10. pertaining to (-ior) upward (super/o)
    **Term: superior**
11. pertaining to (-ic) above (supra-) chest (thorac/o)
    **Term: suprathoracic**
12. study of (-logy) tissues (hist/o)
    **Term: histology**
13. pertaining to (-ic) under (hypo-) stomach (gastr/o)
    **Term: hypogastric**
14. pertaining to (-al) same (ipsi-) side (later/o)
    **Term: ipsilateral**
15. pertaining to (-al) within (intra-) skull (crani/o)
    **Term: intracranial**

### Term Sorting

**Organization of the body:** apex, cytoplasm, hilum, lumen, nucleus, organ, sinus, system, vestibule, viscera

**Positional and Directional Terms:** afferent, anterior, distal, efferent, lateral, posterior, prone superior, supine, ventral

**Body Cavities and Planes:** coronal, cranial, midsagittal, pleural, sagittal, spinal, thoracic, transverse

**Abdominal Regions and Quadrants:** epigastric, hypochondriac, hypogastric, iliac inguinal, lumbar, umbilical

### Translations

1. plantar, palmar
2. antecubital
3. bilateral
4. buccal
5. biopsy
6. lumen
7. thoracic
8. distal
9. mediastinum

10. contralateral
11. supine
12. inguinal or iliac
13. thoracic, coxal
14. epigastric

### Radiology Report

1. distal end, the end closest to the wrist
2. backward
3. joint
4. pertaining to the back
5. posteroanterior, back to front

## Chapter 3

### Exercise 1

1. E, J    2. C, D    3. I
4. G, L    5. H, K    6. A
7. F       8. B

9. articul/o (joint) + -ar (pertaining to)
   **Def: pertaining to a joint**
10. tendin/o (tendon) + -ous (pertaining to)
    **Def: pertaining to a tendon**
11. muscul/o (muscle) + -ar (pertaining to)
    **Def: pertaining to a muscle**
12. syndesm/o (ligament) + -al (pertaining to)
    **Def: pertaining to a ligament**
13. chondr/o (cartilage) + -al (pertaining to)
    **Def: pertaining to the cartilage**
14. osse/o (bone) + -ous (pertaining to)
    **Def: pertaining to a bone**

### Exercise 2

1. E    2. J    3. F    4. L
5. H    6. N    7. B    8. O
9. G    10. C   11. K   12. M
13. A   14. D   15. I

16. build, break down
17. diaphysis, epiphyses
18. periosteum, endosteum
19. depressions, processes
20. antrum

**Exercise 3**
See Fig. 3-2.

**Exercise 4**

1. I    2. K    3. F    4. G
5. N    6. J    7. M    8. B
9. E    10. D    11. A    12. O
13. C    14. H    15. L    16. P

17. sub- (under, below) + mandibul/o (mandible) + -ar (pertaining to)
**Def: pertaining to under the mandible**
18. cost/o (rib) + chondr/o (cartilage) + -al (pertaining to)
**Def: pertaining to ribs and cartilage**
19. lumb/o (lower back) + sacr/o (sacrum) + -al (pertaining to)
**Def: pertaining to lower back and sacrum**
20. thorac/o (chest) + -ic (pertaining to)
**Def: pertaining to the chest**
21. sub- (under, below) + stern/o (breastbone) + -al (pertaining to)
**Def: pertaining to under the breastbone**

**Exercise 5**
See Fig. 3-3, A.

**Exercise 6**
See Fig. 3-4, A.

**Exercise 7**
See Fig. 3-4, C.

**Exercise 8**
See Fig. 3-4, B.

**Exercise 9**

1. F    2. I    3. G    4. H
5. A    6. J    7. C    8. D
9. E    10. B    11. P    12. N
13. K    14. O    15. Q    16. R
17. T    18. L    19. U    20. S
21. M    22. V

23. inter- (between) + phalang/o (finger or toe bones) + -eal (pertaining to)
**Def: pertaining to between the finger or toe bones**
24. humer/o (upper arm bone) + uln/o (lower medial arm bone) + -ar (pertaining to)
**Def: pertaining to the upper arm bone and the lower medial arm bone**
25. infra- (below) + patell/o (kneecap) + -ar (pertaining to)
**Def: pertaining to below the kneecap**
26. femor/o (thigh bone) + -al (pertaining to)
**Def: pertaining to the thigh bone**
27. supra- (above) + clavicul/o (collarbone) + -ar (pertaining to)
**Def: pertaining to above the collarbone**

**Exercise 10**
See Fig. 3-5.

**Exercise 11**
See Fig. 3-6.

**Exercise 12**

1. E    2. G    3. B    4. D
5. H    6. F    7. I    8. A
9. J    10. C    11. K

12. pertaining to (-ar) within (intra-) muscle (muscul/o)
**Term: intramuscular**
13. pertaining to (-al) buttocks (glute/o)
**Term: gluteal**
14. pertaining to (-al) synovium (synovi/o)
**Term: synovial**

**Exercise 13**
See table on pp. 82 and 83.

**Exercise 14**

1. N    2. L    3. F    4. A
5. M    6. K    7. J    8. C
9. H    10. I    11. D    12. G
13. B    14. E

**Exercise 15**

1. A DIP is the joint between the two phalanges farthest from the point of attachment. A PIP is the joint between the two phalanges nearest to the point of attachment.
2. bend
3. first finger, right hand
4. hand

**Exercise 16**

1. B    2. A    3. C    4. D

5. process of (-y) fingers, toes (dactyl/o) joined (syn-)
**Term: syndactyly**
6. without (a-) cartilage (chondr/o) condition of formation (-plasia)
**Term: achondroplasia**
7. process of (-y) many (poly-) fingers, toes (dactyl/o)
**Term: polydactyly**

**Exercise 17**

1. A    2. C    3. F    4. L
5. G    6. D    7. J    8. I
9. H    10. B    11. E    12. K

13. pain (-dynia) bone (oste/o)
**Term: osteodynia**
14. inflammation (-itis) bursa (burs/o)
**Term: bursitis**
15. inflammation (-itis) tendon (tendin/o)
**Term: tendinitis**
16. abnormal condition (-osis) bone (oste/o) passage (por/o)
**Term: osteoporosis**
17. softening (-malacia) bone (oste/o)
**Term: osteomalacia**

**Exercise 18**

1. H    2. G    3. F    4. B
5. J    6. L    7. C    8. D
9. K    10. E    11. A    12. I

13. slipping (-listhesis) vertebra (spondyl/o)
**Term: spondylolisthesis**

14. abnormal condition (-osis) vertebra (spondyl/o)
    **Term: spondylosis**
15. abnormal condition (-osis) curvature (scoli/o)
    **Term: scoliosis**
16. pertaining to (-ar) inflammation (-itis) fascia (fasci/o) sole (plant/o)
    **Term: plantar fasciitis**
17. destruction (-lysis) striated muscle (rhabdomy/o)
    **Term: rhabdomyolysis**
18. inflammation (-itis) many (poly-) muscle (myos/o)
    **Term: polymyositis**

*Exercise 19*
1. A     2. D     3. F     4. G
5. I     6. E     7. B     8. H
9. C

*Exercise 20*
1. subluxation, dislocation
2. sprain
3. strain
4. compartment syndrome

*Exercise 21*
1. C     2. A     3. D     4. B

5. tumor (-oma) skeletal muscle (rhabdomy/o)
   **Term: rhabdomyoma**
6. tumor (-oma) bone (oste/o)
   **Term: osteoma**
7. tumor (-oma) smooth muscle (leiomy/o)
   **Term: leiomyoma**
8. tumor (-oma) cartilage (chondr/o)
   **Term: chondroma**
9. abnormal condition (-osis) bone (oste/o) out (ex-)
   **Term: exostosis**

*Exercise 22*
1. humerus, upper arm bone
2. closest to her shoulder
3. comminuted
4. fibromyalgia
5. cannot move toward the midline

*Exercise 23*
1. F     2. E     3. B     4. G
5. A     6. D     7. H     8. C

9. process of viewing (-scopy) joint (arthr/o)
   **Term: arthroscopy**
10. process of recording (-graphy) joint (arthr/o)
    **Term: arthrography**
11. process of recording (-graphy) electrical (electro-) muscle (my/o)
    **Term: electromyography**
12. process of recording (-graphy) spinal cord (myel/o)
    **Term: myelography**

*Exercise 24*
1. H     2. C     3. G     4. A
5. B     6. J     7. F     8. I
9. E     10. D

11. surgical repair (-plasty) joint (arthr/o)
    **Term: arthroplasty**
12. intentional breaking (-clasis) bone (oste/o)
    **Term: osteoclasis**
13. excision (-ectomy) bunion (bunion/o)
    **Term: bunionectomy**
14. surgical repair (-plasty) tendon (ten/o) muscle (my/o)
    **Term: tenomyoplasty**
15. removal (-ectomy) meniscus (menisc/o)
    **Term: meniscectomy**
16. surgical repair (-plasty) ligament (syndesm/o)
    **Term: syndesmoplasty**

*Exercise 25*
1. bisphosphonates
2. disease-modifying antirheumatic drugs
3. inflammation and pain
4. muscle relaxants

*Exercise 26*
1. fracture of the fifth lumbar vertebra
2. osteoarthritis, nonsteroidal antiinflammatory drugs
3. range of motion
4. carpal tunnel syndrome

## Chapter 3 Review

*Word Part Definitions*
1. –desis
2. –plasia
3. –centesis
4. syn-
5. –malacia
6. –listhesis
7. peri-
8. –clasis
9. –physis
10. –osis
11. cleid/o
12. oste/o
13. gnath/o
14. rhabdomy/o
15. humer/o
16. carp/o
17. zygomat/o
18. femor/o
19. cervic/o
20. spondyl/o
21. chondr/o
22. myel/o
23. dactyl/o
24. phalang/o
25. cost/o
26. my/o
27. olecran/o
28. coccyg/o
29. patell/a
30. arthr/o
31. mandibul/o
32. scapul/o

*Wordshop*
1. structure (-um) surrounding (peri-) bone (oste/o)
   **Term: periosteum**
2. inflammation (-itis) many (poly-) muscle (myos/o)
   **Term: polymyositis**
3. inflammation (-itis) surrounding (peri-) joint (arthr/o)
   **Term: periarthritis**
4. softening (-malacia) cartilage (chondr/o)
   **Term: chondromalacia**
5. condition (-y) many (poly-) fingers or toes (dactyl/o)
   **Term: polydactyly**
6. destruction (-lysis) skeletal muscle (rhabdomy/o)
   **Term: rhabdomyolysis**

7. abnormal condition (-osis) bone (oste/o) growth (phyt/o)
**Term: osteophytosis**
8. binding (-desis) joint (arthr/o)
**Term: arthrodesis**
9. suture (-rrhaphy) muscle (my/o)
**Term: myorrhaphy**
10. condition (-y) joined, together (syn-) fingers or toes (dactyl/o)
**Term: syndactyly**
11. tumor (-oma) cartilage (chondr/o)
**Term: chondroma**
12. binding (-desis) joined, together (syn-) vertebrae (spondyl/o)
**Term: spondylosyndesis**
13. surgical repair (-plasty) ligament (syndesm/o)
**Term: syndesmoplasty**
14. formation (-plasia) no, without (a-) cartilage (chondr/o)
**Term: achondroplasia**
15. surgical repair (-plasty) tendon (ten/o) muscle (my/o)
**Term: tenomyoplasty**

*Term Sorting*
**Anatomy and Physiology:** articulation, cartilage, costa, diaphysis, digitus, humerus, ligament, radius, sternum, ulna
**Pathology:** arthrosis, bunion bursitis, CTS, osteomyelitis, osteoporosis, osteosarcoma, spondylolisthesis, syndactyly, tendinitis
**Diagnostic Procedures:** arthrography, arthroscopy, DEXA, EMG, goniometry, MRI, myelogram, Phalen test, ROM, serum calcium
**Therapeutic Interventions:** arthrocentesis, arthrodesis, laminectomy, meniscectomy, myorrhaphy, osteoclasis, osteoplasty, prosthesis, tenomyoplasty, TKR

*Translations*
1. chondromalacia, Baker cyst
2. amputation, prosthesis
3. myorrhaphy

4. arthrocentesis, hemarthrosis
5. reduction, clavicle
6. Phalen test, carpal tunnel syndrome
7. osteophytosis, interphalangeal joints
8. kyphosis, osteoporosis
9. osteomyelitis, radius
10. plantar fasciitis, tendinitis
11. electromyography (EMG), muscular dystrophy
12. greenstick, humerus
13. polydactyly, syndactyly
14. bunionectomy, bunion

*Operative Report*
1. osteoarthritis
2. the front of the knee
3. kneecap
4. near the patella
5. incision of a joint
6. turned out, away from the midline
7. an instrument to cut bone
8. increasing the angle of the joint beyond normal range

# Chapter 4

*Exercise 1*
| 1. B | 2. H | 3. F | 4. A |
| 5. D | 6. E | 7. G | 8. I |
| 9. C | 10. J | | |

11. a- (without) + vascul/o (vessel) + -ar (pertaining to)
**Def: pertaining to without vessels**
12. sub- (under, below) + ungu/o (nail) + -al (pertaining to)
**Def: pertaining to under the nail**
13. hypo- (below) + derm/o (skin) + -ic (pertaining to)
**Def: pertaining to below the skin**

*Exercise 2*
See Fig. 4-1.

*Exercise 3*
1. the nail bed is the tissue under the nail and the nail plate is the actual nail

2. palm
3. an instrument for compression of blood vessels to control blood flow to and from the fingertip
4. the nail root

*Exercise 4*
| 1. E | 2. F | 3. C | 4. A |
| 5. B | 6. D | 7. C | 8. D |
| 9. A | 10. E | 11. B | 12. D |
| 13. E | 14. C | 15. A | 16. B |

*Exercise 5*
1. eczema
2. atopic dermatitis
3. contact dermatitis
4. seborrheic dermatitis
5. impetigo
6. furuncle
7. pilonidal cyst
8. folliculitis
9. cellulitis

*Exercise 6*
| 1. D | 2. C | 3. F | 4. B |
| 5. H | 6. A | 7. G | 8. E |

9. pediculosis
10. herpes simplex virus (HSV)
11. scabies
12. dermatomycosis

*Exercise 7*
1. psoriasis
2. hypertrichosis
3. alopecia
4. keratinous cyst
5. acne vulgaris
6. clavus
7. pressure sore, decubitus ulcer
8. milia
9. xeroderma

*Exercise 8*
1. abnormal condition (-osis) excessive (hyper-) sweat (hidr/o)
**Term: hyperhidrosis**
2. abnormal (dys-) color (chrom/o) condition (-ia)
**Term: dyschromia**
3. inflammation (-itis) sweat (hidr/o) gland (aden/o)
**Term: hidradenitis**

4. abnormal condition (-osis) no (an-) sweat (hidr/o)
   **Term: anhidrosis**
5. vitiligo
6. albinism
7. miliaria

### Exercise 9
1. C     2. D     3. B     4. E
5. A

6. softening (-malacia) nail (onych/o)
   **Term: onychomalacia**
7. abnormal condition (-osis) fungus (myc/o) nail (onych/o)
   **Term: onychomycosis**
8. abnormal condition (-osis) hidden (crypt/o) nail (onych/o)
   **Term: onychocryptosis**
9. separation (-lysis) nail (onych/o)
   **Term: onycholysis**

### Exercise 10
1. C     2. A     3. D     4. B

### Exercise 11
1. D     2. A     3. B     4. C
5. E

6. dermat/o (skin) + fibr/o (fiber) + -oma (mass, tumor)
   **Def: mass of fibrous skin**
7. angi/o (vessel) + -oma (mass, tumor)
   **Def: mass of vessels**
8. seb/o (sebum) + -rrheic (pertaining to discharge) kerat/o (hard, horny) + -osis (abnormal condition)
   **Def: abnormal horny condition pertaining to discharge of sebum**

### Exercise 12
1. C     2. D     3. A     4. B

### Exercise 13
1. excisional
2. needle aspiration
3. incisional

4. exfoliation
5. punch
6. F
7. C
8. E
9. B
10. G
11. A
12. D

### Exercise 14
1. pruritic means pertaining to itching
2. no previous history of dermatitis
3. elevated and contained fluid
4. rash

### Exercise 15
1. A. skin graft from self
   B. skin graft from another human
   C. skin graft from another species
2. full-thickness graft
3. dermatome
4. laser therapy
5. débridement
6. cauterization
7. cryosurgery
8. curettage
9. incision and drainage
10. shaving
11. occlusive therapy
12. Mohs surgery
13. removal (-ectomy) wrinkle (rhytid/o)
    **Term: rhytidectomy**
14. removal (-ectomy) fat (lip/o)
    **Term: lipectomy**
15. surgical repair (-plasty) eyelid (blephar/o)
    **Term: blepharoplasty**
16. scraping of (-abrasion) skin (derm/o)
    **Term: dermabrasion**
17. surgical repair (-plasty) skin (dermat/o)
    **Term: dermatoplasty**

### Exercise 16
1. intradermal
2. topical
3. hypodermic

4. transdermal therapeutic system
5. anesthetic agent
6. keratolytics
7. antifungals
8. antibacterial
9. scabicide
10. aspirin, prednisone, fluocinonide (Lidex), triamcinolone (Kenalog), hydrocortisone (Cortizone)

11. D     12. C     13. A     14. B
15. E     16. G     17. F

### Exercise 17
1. ID          2. UV
3. SG          4. Decub
5. FB          6. I&D
7. Bx          8. PPD
9. TTS         10. TB

## Chapter 4 Review

### Word Part Definitions
1. hyper-
2. –osis
3. trans-
4. intra-
5. –cide
6. sub-
7. crypt-
8. –itis
9. par-
10. –lytic
11. hidr/o
12. melan/o
13. onych/o
14. chrom/o
15. rhytid/o
16. follicul/o
17. vascul/o
18. papul/o
19. macul/o
20. hemat/o
21. xen/o
22. exanthemat/o
23. kerat/o
24. hidraden/o
25. cutane/o
26. pedicul/o
27. seb/o
28. eschar/o
29. squam/o
30. pil/o
31. adip/o
32. myc/o

## Wordshop

1. abnormal condition (-osis) excessive (hyper-) hair (trich/o)
   **Term: hypertrichosis**
2. condition (-y) no (a-) development (troph/o)
   **Term: atrophy**
3. removal (-ectomy) wrinkle (rhytid/o)
   **Term: rhytidectomy**
4. pertaining to discharge (-rrheic) oil (seb/o)
   **Term: seborrheic**
5. condition (-ia) near (par-) nail (onych/o)
   **Term: paronychia**
6. abnormal condition (-osis) no (an-) sweat (hidr/o)
   **Term: anhidrosis**
7. surgical repair (-plasty) eyelid (blephar/o)
   **Term: blepharoplasty**
8. softening (-malacia) nail (onych/o)
   **Term: onychomalacia**
9. inflammation (-itis) follicle (follicul/o)
   **Term: folliculitis**
10. condition (-ia) abnormal (dys-) color (chrom/o)
    **Term: dyschromia**
11. pertaining to (-ous) under (sub-) skin (cutane/o)
    **Term: subcutaneous**
12. abnormal condition (-osis) fungus (myc/o) skin (dermat/o)
    **Term: dermatomycosis**
13. tumor (-oma) fiber (fibr/o) skin (dermat/o)
    **Term: dermatofibroma**
14. destruction/loosening (-lysis) nail (onych/o)
    **Term: onycholysis**
15. abnormal condition (-osis) hidden (crypt-) nail (onych/o)
    **Term: onychocryptosis**

## Term Sorting

**Anatomy and Physiology:** epidermis, eponychium, follicle, lunula, melanocyte, papilla, perspiration, sebaceous gland, sebum, strata

**Pathology:** alopecia, dermatomycosis, ecchymosis, eczema, hyperhidrosis, onychomycosis, plaque, tinea pedis, verruca, vesicle

**Diagnostic Procedures:** bacterial analysis, excisional bx, Mantoux test, punch biopsy, Tzanck test, Wood's light

**Therapeutic Interventions:** allograft, blepharoplasty, cauterization, curettage, débridement, dermabrasion, dermatoplasty, escharotomy, rhytidectomy, xenograft

## Translations

1. tinea pedis
2. pruritis, scabies
3. hyperhidrosis
4. onychocryptosis, paronychia
5. keloid
6. impetigo, papules, vesicles
7. pediculosis, pediculicide
8. acne vulgaris, retinoid
9. emollient, xeroderma
10. verruca (wart), cryosurgery
11. escharotomy, allograft
12. rhytidectomy (face-lift), blepharoplasty
13. decubitus ulcer

## ED Record

1. B. partial thickness
2. mottled (indicates redness), pain, and blisters are signs of 2nd degree burns
3. circumscribed, ½ cm elevated lesion containing fluid

## Chapter 5

### Exercise 1

| | | |
|---|---|---|
| 1. M | 2. H | 3. F |
| 4. E, I | 5. D, K | 6. C, G |
| 7. B | 8. N | 9. J |
| 10. L | 11. A | |

12. peri- (surrounding, around) + or/o (mouth) + -al (pertaining to)
    **Def: pertaining to around the mouth**
13. gingiv/o (gums) + -al (pertaining to)
    **Def: pertaining to the gums**
14. peri- (around) + odont/o (teeth) + -al (pertaining to)
    **Def: pertaining to around the teeth**
15. sub- (under, below) + mandibul/o (mandible) + -ar (pertaining to)
    **Def: pertaining to under the mandible**
16. nas/o (nose) + pharyng/o (pharynx) + -eal (pertaining to)
    **Def: pertaining to the nose and pharynx**

### Exercise 2
See Fig. 5-2.

### Exercise 3

| | | | |
|---|---|---|---|
| 1. H | 2. I | 3. M | 4. G |
| 5. N | 6. L | 7. O | 8. J |
| 9. F | 10. B | 11. P | 12. E |
| 13. D | 14. K | 15. A | 16. C |

17. peri- (around, surrounding) + rect/o (rectum) + -al (pertaining to)
    **Def: pertaining to around the rectum**
18. intra- (within) + lumin/o (lumen) + -al (pertaining to)
    **Def: pertaining to within the lumen**
19. epi- (above) + gastr/o (stomach) + -ic (pertaining to)
    **Def: pertaining to above the stomach**

### Exercise 4
See Figs. 5-3 and 5-4.

### Exercise 5

| | | | |
|---|---|---|---|
| 1. G | 2. D | 3. A | 4. C |
| 5. B | 6. E | 7. F | |

8. pancreat/o (pancreas) + -ic (pertaining to)
   **Def: pertaining to the pancreas**
9. bil/i (bile) + -ary (pertaining to)
   **Def: pertaining to bile**
10. sub- (under, below) + hepat/o (liver) + -ic (pertaining to)
    **Def: pertaining to below the liver**

## Exercise 6
See Fig. 5-5.

## Exercise 7
1. upper GI tract—pharynx, esophagus, stomach, duodenum
2. close to
3. fundus
4. gastroesophageal sphincter, cardiac sphincter

## Exercise 8
1. G    2. H    3. D    4. F
5. A    6. I    7. B    8. C
9. E    10. D    11. B    12. E
13. C    14. A

15. condition of stools (-chezia) blood (hemat/o)
    **Term: hematochezia**
16. vomiting (-emesis) blood (hemat/o)
    **Term: hematemesis**
17. abnormal (dys-) condition of digestion (-pepsia)
    **Term: dyspepsia**

## Exercise 9
1. esophageal atresia
2. cleft palate
3. Hirschsprung disease
4. congenital megacolon
5. pyloric stenosis

## Exercise 10
1. A    2. F    3. D    4. E
5. G    6. C    7. B

8. inflammation (-itis) gums (gingiv/o)
   **Term: gingivitis**
9. discharge (-rrhea) pus (py/o)
   **Term: pyorrhea**
10. condition of patches (-plakia) white (leuk/o)
    **Term: leukoplakia**

## Exercise 11
1. F          2. D, E
3. C          4. A, H, I
5. B          6. G

## Exercise 12
1. G    2. I    3. L    4. B
5. O    6. M    7. C    8. F
9. J    10. E    11. D    12. K
13. P    14. H    15. N    16. A

17. inflammation (-itis) appendix (appendic/o)
    **Term: appendicitis**
18. abnormal condition (-osis) diverticulum (diverticul/o)
    **Term: diverticulosis**
19. inflammation (-itis) rectum and anus (proct/o)
    **Term: proctitis**

## Exercise 13
1. cirrhosis
2. cholelithiasis
3. cholangitis
4. choledocholithiasis
5. pancreatitis
6. hepatitis
7. cholecystitis
8. jaundice

## Exercise 14
1. A    2. B    3. F    4. C
5. D    6. E

## Exercise 15
1. polyp
2. hepatocellular carcinoma, hepatoma
3. adenocarcinoma
4. odontogenic tumor

## Exercise 16
1. sonography
2. barium swallow
3. computed tomography scan (CT scan)
4. barium enema
5. manometry
6. stool culture
7. guaiac, hemoccult
8. biopsy
9. total bilirubin
10. gamma-glutamyl transferase (GGT)
11. transhepatic cholangiography

12. cholecyst/o (gallbladder) + -graphy (process of recording)
    **Def: process of recording the gallbladder**
13. proct/o (rectum and anus) + -scopy (process of viewing)
    **Def: process of viewing the rectum and anus**
14. cholangi/o (bile vessels) + -graphy (process of recording)
    **Def: process of recording the bile vessels**
15. colon/o (colon) + -scopy (process of viewing)
    **Def: process of viewing the colon**

## Exercise 17
1. colonoscopy
2. colonoscope
3. diverticula
4. pertaining to surrounding the rectum

## Exercise 18
1. B    2. E    3. A    4. F
5. H    6. N    7. J    8. M
9. G    10. L    11. D    12. I
13. K    14. C    15. O

16. pylor/o (pylorus) + my/o (muscle) + -tomy (incision)
    **Def: incision of the pylorus**
17. col/o (colon) + -stomy (new opening)
    **Def: new opening into the colon**
18. herni/o (hernia) + -rrhaphy (suture)
    **Def: suture of a hernia**
19. gastr/o (stomach) + -ectomy (removal)
    **Def: removal of the stomach**
20. polyp/o (polyp) + -ectomy (removal)
    **Def: removal of a polyp**

## Exercise 19
1. E    2. C    3. D    4. F
5. A    6. B

## Exercise 20
1. bowel movement
2. gallbladder

3. nausea and vomiting
4. gastroesophageal reflux disease
5. irritable bowel syndrome

## Chapter 5 Review

### Word Part Definitions
1. –rrhea
1. –scopy
3. –tresia
4. –stomy
5. –rrhaphy
6. –emesis
7. –chezia
8. –phagia
9. –stalsis
10. –pepsia
11. lingu/o
12. gingiv/o
13. inguin/o
14. phren/o
15. esophag/o
16. sial/o
17. cholangi/o
18. choledoch/o
19. stomat/o
20. py/o
21. gastr/o
22. proct/o
23. labi/o
24. hepat/o
25. bucc/o
26. odont/o
27. an/o
28. cholecyst/o
29. pharyng/o
30. lumin/o
31. col/o
32. enter/o

### Wordshop
1. pertaining to (-eal) stomach (gastr/o) esophagus (esophag/o)
   **Term: gastroesophageal**
2. condition of an opening (-tresia) no (a-)
   **Term: atresia**
3. pertaining to (-al) surrounding (peri-) teeth (odont/o)
   **Term: periodontal**
4. pertaining to (-ic) nose (nas/o) stomach (gastr/o)
   **Term: nasogastric**

5. new opening (-stomy) colon (col/o)
   **Term: colostomy**
6. inflammation (-itis) gall-bladder (cholecyst/o)
   **Term: cholecystitis**
7. new opening (-stomy) esophagus (esophag/o) stomach (gastr/o)
   **Term: esophagogastrostomy**
8. removal (-ectomy) gallbladder (cholecyst/o)
   **Term: cholecystectomy**
9. discharge (-rrhea) pus (py/o)
   **Term: pyorrhea**
10. condition of swallowing (-phagia) difficult, painful (dys-)
    **Term: dysphagia**
11. condition of digestion (-pepsia) difficult, bad (dys-)
    **Term: dyspepsia**
12. condition (-iasis) stone (lith/o) bile (chol/e)
    **Term: cholelithiasis**
13. condition (-iasis) stone (lith/o) common bile duct (choledoch/o)
    **Term: choledocholithiasis**
14. incision (-tomy) abdomen (lapar/o)
    **Term: laparotomy**
15. surgical repair (-plasty) mouth (stomat/o)
    **Term: stomatoplasty**

### Term Sorting
**Anatomy and Physiology:** cholecystokinin, deglutition, esophagus, jejunum, LES, lipid, mastication, oropharynx, peristalsis, rugae
**Pathology:** achalasia, cheilitis, cystoadenoma, dyspepsia, halitosis, hematemesis, hematochezia, jaundice, leukoplakia, pyrosis
**Diagnostic Procedures:** barium enema, BaS, cholecystography, CT scan, ERCP, GGT, manometry, PTCA, stool guaiac, total bilirubin

**Therapeutic Interventions:** anastomosis, cholecystectomy, colostomy, gastric gavage, herniorrhaphy, laparotomy, ligation, paracentesis, PEG, stomatoplasty

### Translations
1. colonoscopy, polypectomy
2. hepatitis, jaundice
3. inguinal hernia, herniorrhaphy
4. achalasia, manometry
5. stool guaiac or hemoccult test
6. ligation, cholecystectomy
7. colostomy, Crohn disease
8. laxative, constipation
9. flatus, diarrhea
10. appendicitis, peritonitis
11. gingivitis, malocclusion
12. cleft palate, Hirschsprung disease
13. regurgitation, esophageal atresia
14. hematochezia, hemorrhoids

### Operative Report
1. diagnosis of cholelithiasis
2. cholecystitis
3. laparoscopic cholecystectomy
4. back
5. to tie it off

## Chapter 6

### Exercise 1
1. C    2. F    3. D    4. A
5. E    6. G    7. B    8. L
9. J    10. H    11. M    12. I
13. K
14. trans- (through) + urethr/o (urethra) + -al (pertaining to)
    **Def: pertaining to through the urethra**
15. para- (near) + nephr/o (kidney) + -ic (pertaining to)
    **Def: pertaining to near the kidney**
16. retro- (backward) + peritone/o (peritoneum) + -al (pertaining to)
    **Def: pertaining to the back of the peritoneum**

17. supra- (above) + ren/o (kidney) + -al (pertaining to)
**Def: pertaining to above the kidney**
18. peri- (surrounding) + vesic/o (bladder) + -al (pertaining to)
**Def: pertaining to surrounding the bladder**

**Exercise 2**
See Figs. 6-1, 6-2, and 6-3.

**Exercise 3**
1. retention
2. edema
3. abscess
4. azotemia or uremia
5. enuresis
6. diuresis
7. urgency
8. incontinence
9. urinary condition (-uria) pus (py/o)
**Term: pyuria**
10. excessive (poly-) thirst (-dipsia)
**Term: polydipsia**
11. urinary condition (-uria) painful (dys-)
**Term: dysuria**
12. glycos/o (sugar) + -uria (urinary condition)
**Def: condition of sugar in the urine**
13. hemat/o (blood) + -uria (urinary condition)
**Def: condition of blood in the urine**
14. an- (without) + -uria (urinary condition)
**Def: condition of no urine**

**Exercise 4**
1. C    2. F    3. D    4. E
5. G    6. A    7. B

8. presence of (-iasis) stones (lith/o) kidney (nephr/o)
**Term: nephrolithiasis**
9. presence of (-iasis) stones (lith/o) ureter (ureter/o)
**Term: ureterolithiasis**
10. presence of (-iasis) stones (lith/o) bladder (cyst/o)
**Term: cystolithiasis**

11. presence of (-iasis) stones (lith/o) urethra (urethr/o)
**Term: urethrolithiasis**

**Exercise 5**
1. L    2. I     3. D    4. G
5. J    6. C     7. H    8. A
9. F    10. B    11. K   12. E

13. hydr/o (water) + nephr/o (kidney) + -osis (abnormal condition)
**Def: abnormal condition of water in the kidney**
14. cyst/o (urinary bladder) + -cele (herniation)
**Def: herniation of the urinary bladder**
15. nephr/o (kidney) + lith/o (stones) + -iasis (presence of)
**Def: presence of stones in the kidney**
16. ren/o (kidney) + -al (pertaining to) + sclerosis (a hardening)
**Def: pertaining to hardening of the kidney**

**Exercise 6**
1. E    2. C    3. F    4. B
5. A    6. D

**Exercise 7**
1. inability to hold urine (incontinence)
2. herniation of the bladder (cystocele)
3. barium enema and CT scan

**Exercise 8**
1. F    2. G    3. E    4. H
5. D    6. C    7. B    8. A

9. machine that crushes (-tripter) stone (lith/o)
**Term: lithotripter**
10. instrument to view (-scope) kidney (nephr/o)
**Term: nephroscope**
11. instrument to measure (-meter) urine (urin/o)
**Term: urinometer**

**Exercise 9**
1. tube that remains in the body to drain urine
2. post-
3. urinalysis and culture

**Exercise 10**
1. C    2. E    3. B    4. F
5. D    6. A

7. destruction of adhesions (-lysis) urethra (urethr/o)
**Term: urethrolysis**
8. process of crushing (-tripsy) stone (lith/o)
**Term: lithotripsy**
9. incision (-tomy) bladder (vesic/o)
**Term: vesicotomy**

**Exercise 11**
1. D    2. E    3. A    4. F
5. C    6. B

**Exercise 12**
1. diabetes mellitus
2. chronic kidney disease, hemodialysis
3. urinalysis, specific gravity, diabetes insipidus
4. urinary tract infection
5. voiding cystourethrography

## Chapter 6 Review

**Word Part Definitions**
1. –lithotomy
2. –cele
3. –lysis
4. –tripter
5. –dipsia
6. –scopy
7. –pexy
8. –ptosis
9. –uria
10. –esis
11. glycos/o
12. cyst/o or vesic/o
13. ureter/o
14. kal/i
15. noct/i
16. trigon/o
17. natr/o
18. ur/o
19. lith/o

20. meat/o
21. nephr/o or ren/o
22. olig/o
23. glomerul/o
24. ren/o or nephr/o
25. calic/o
26. pyel/o
27. urethr/o
28. vesic/o or cyst/o
29. albumin/o
30. azot/o
31. cortic/o

*Wordshop*
1. pertaining to (-al) surrounding (peri-) bladder (vesic/o)
   **Term: perivesical**
2. process of recording (-graphy) section (tom/o) kidney (nephr/o)
   **Term: nephrotomography**
3. instrument to visually examine (-scope) kidney (nephr/o)
   **Term: nephroscope**
4. herniation (-cele) ureter (ureter/o)
   **Term: ureterocele**
5. urinary condition (-uria) difficult or painful (dys-)
   **Term: dysuria**
6. urinary condition (-uria) blood (hemat/o)
   **Term: hematuria**
7. inflammation (-itis) glomerulus (glomerul/o) kidney (nephr/o)
   **Term: glomerulonephritis**
8. condition of (-iasis) stone (lith/o) urinary system (ur/o)
   **Term: urolithiasis**
9. urinary condition (-uria) no, not, without (an-)
   **Term: anuria**
10. process of crushing (-tripsy) stone (lith/o)
    **Term: lithotripsy**
11. blood condition (-emia) urea nitrogen (azot/o)
    **Term: azotemia**
12. freeing from adhesions (-lysis) urethra (urethr/o)
    **Term: urethrolysis**

13. urinary condition (-uria) excessive (poly-)
    **Term: polyuria**
14. inflammation (-itis) renal pelvis (pyel/o) kidney (nephr/o)
    **Term: pyelonephritis**
15. condition of thirst (-dipsia) excessive (poly-)
    **Term: polydipsia**

*Term Sorting*
**Anatomy and Physiology:** cortex, glomeruli, hilum, medulla, micturition, renal medulla, trigone, urea, urethra, urinary meatus
**Pathology:** albuminuria, DM, enuresis, nephroptosis, nephritis, pyuria, renal adenoma, renal colic, urethral stenosis, UTI
**Diagnostic Procedures:** BUN, cystoscopy, cystourethroscopy, GFR, IVU, KUB, nephrotomography, urinalysis, urinometer, VCUG
**Therapeutic Interventions:** CAPD, hemodialysis, lithotripsy, meatotomy, nephrolithotomy, nephropexy, nephrostomy, renal dialysis, urethrolysis, vesicotomy

*Translations*
1. edema, hypertension
2. BUN, creatinine clearance test
3. renal colic, urolithiasis
4. nephrolithiasis, lithotripsy
5. urinary tract infection (UTI), enuresis
6. cystoscope, cystocele
7. oligouria, azotemia
8. nephroptosis, nephropexy
9. nephrotomography, renal oncocytoma
10. polyuria, polydipsia
11. diabetes mellitus, diabetes insipidus
12. pyelonephritis
13. renal hypertension, renal failure
14. renal dialysis, renal transplant

*Operative Report*
1. a stone in the left ureter
2. normal caliber distal ureter
3. acute

4. yes; hydronephrosis is a backup of fluid in the kidney caused by obstruction of the flow of urine
5. CT scan, cystoscopy, abdominal x-ray, renal ultrasound, ureteroscopy, retrograde pyelogram
6. atraumatically

## Chapter 7

*Exercise 1*
1. D
2. K   3. A   4. G   5. B
6. I   7. J   8. L   9. H
10. F   11. E   12. C   13.

uni- (one) + testicul/o (testicle) + -ar (pertaining to)
**Def: pertaining to one testicle**
14. preputi/o (prepuce) + -al (pertaining to)
**Def: pertaining to the prepuce**
15. vesicul/o (seminal vesicle) + -ar (pertaining to)
**Def: pertaining to the seminal vesicle**
16. peri- (around) + prostat/o (prostate) + -ic (pertaining to)
**Def: pertaining to around the prostate**
17. intra- (within) + scrot/o (scrotum) + -al (pertaining to)
**Def: pertaining to within the scrotum**

*Exercise 2*
See Fig. 7-1.

*Exercise 3*
1. G   2. A   3. E   4. F
5. H   6. D   7. C   8. B

9. inflammation (-itis) glans penis (balan/o)
   **Term: balanitis**
10. condition (-ia) no (a-) living (zo/o) sperm (sperm/o)
    **Term: azoospermia**

11. inflammation (-itis) prostate (prostat/o)
**Term: prostatitis**
12. excessive (hyper-) formation (-plasia) pertaining to (-ic) prostate (prostat/o)
**Term: prostatic hyperplasia**
13. orch/o (testis) + -itis (inflammation)
**Def: inflammation of the testis**
14. olig/o (scanty) + sperm/o (sperm) + -ia (pertaining to)
**Def: pertaining to scanty sperm**
15. vesicul/o seminal vesicle + -itis = inflammation
**Def: inflammation of the seminal vesicle**

### Exercise 4
1. condylomata
2. syphilis
3. nongonococcal urethritis
4. gonorrhea
5. chancres
6. asymptomatic
7. human papillomavirus
8. herpes simplex virus-2

### Exercise 5
1. C
2. E  3. D  4. B  5. A
6.

tumor (-oma) semen (semin/i)
**Term: seminoma**
7. cancerous tumor of epithelial tissue (-carcinoma) gland (aden/o)
**Term: adenocarcinoma**

### Exercise 6
1. E    2. F    3. G    4. D
5. C    6. A    7. B

8. plethys/o (volume) + -graphy (process of recording)
**Def: process of recording volume**

9. epididym/o (epididymis) + vesicul/o (vesicle) + -graphy (process of recording)
**Def: process of recoding the epididymis and seminal vesicle**

### Exercise 7
1. F    2. B    3. C    4. A
5. G    6. D    7. E

8. vas/o (vas deferens) + vas/o (vas deferens) + -stomy (new opening)
**Def: new opening between the vas deferens**
9. trans- (through) + urethr/o (urethra) + -al (pertaining to)
**Def: pertaining to through the urethra**
10. prostat/o (prostate) + -ectomy (resection)
**Def: resection of the prostate**

### Exercise 8
1. through the rectum
2. increased chance of BPH
3. contribute to seminal fluid

### Exercise 9
1. D    2. A    3. B    4. E
5. C

### Exercise 10
1. BPH
2. STI or VD
3. syphilis
4. digital rectal examination, diagnose BPH
5. HPV
6. genitourinary

## Chapter 7 Review

### Word Part Definitions
1. hypo-
2. hyper-
3. –oma
4. trans-
5. –itis
6. circum-
7. –graphy
8. –cele
9. a-
10. crypt-
11. –ectomy
12. –genesis
13. –cision
14. –spadias
15. –plasia
16. andr/o
17. semin/i
18. balan/o
19. sperm/o
20. epididym/o
21. orchid/o
22. preputi/o
23. vesicul/o
24. pen/i or phall/o
25. scrot/o
26. vas/o
27. olig/o
28. prostat/o
29. plethysm/o
30. hydr/o
31. zo/o
32. phall/o or pen/i

### Wordshop
1. condition of (-ia) scanty (olig/o) sperm (sperm/o)
**Term: oligospermia**
2. inflammation (-itis) seminal vesicle (vesicul/o)
**Term: vesiculitis**
3. fixation (-pexy) testicle (orchi/o)
**Term: orchiopexy**
4. surgical repair (-plasty) glans penis (balan/o)
**Term: balanoplasty**
5. removal (-ectomy) prostate (prostat/o)
**Term: prostatectomy**
6. inflammation (-itis) glans penis (balan/o)
**Term: balanitis**
7. study of (-logy) male (andr/o)
**Term: andrology**
8. production (-genesis) sperm (spermat/o)
**Term: spermatogenesis**
9. condition of (-ia) no (a-) animals (zo/o) sperm (sperm/o)
**Term: azoospermia**
10. process of cutting (-cision) around (circum-)
**Term: circumcision**

11. condition of (-ism) hidden (crypt-) testicle (orchid/o)
**Term: cryptorchidism**
12. inflammation (-itis) epididymis (epididym/o)
**Term: epididymitis**
13. removal (-ectomy) epididymis (epididym/o)
**Term: epididymectomy**
14. condition of (-ism) no (an-) testicle (orch/o)
**Term: anorchism**
15. removal (-ectomy) testicle (orchid/o)
**Term: orchidectomy**

*Term Sorting*
**Anatomy and Physiology:** corpora cavernosa, ductus deferens, epididymis, gametes, genitalia, glans penis, prepuce, semen, spermatogenesis, tunica vaginalis
**Pathology:** anorchism, balanitis, BPH, ED, epididymitis, gonorrhea, hydrocele, oligospermia, phimosis, seminoma
**Diagnostic Procedures:** FTA-ABS, DRE, epididymovesiculography, PSA, Gram stain, plethysmography, sonography, sperm analysis, TSE, VDRL
**Therapeutic Interventions:** ablation, castration, circumcision, orchidectomy, orchiopexy, prostatectomy, sterilization, TUIP, TURP, vasectomy

*Translations*
1. sperm analysis, oligospermia (or azoospermia)
2. benign prostatic hyperplasia/hypertrophy (BPH), transurethral incision of the prostate (TUIP)
3. epididymitis
4. circumcision, phimosis
5. chancre, syphilis
6. Gram stain, gonorrhea
7. vasectomy, vasovasostomy
8. orchidectomy, cryptorchidism
9. erectile dysfunction (ED), plethysmography

10. condylomata, herpes genitalis (herpes simplex virus, HSV-2)
11. seminoma
12. urologist, varicocele
13. gynecomastia
14. azoospermia (or oligospermia), sterilization

*Operative Report*
1. abnormal enlargement of the prostate gland surrounding the urethra, leading to difficulty with urination.
2. A. painful urination
   B. inability to hold urine
   C. sensation of the need to urinate immediately
   D. urinating more often than normally
   E. condition of blood in the urine
3. two
4. transurethral resection of the prostate – removal of the prostate through the urethra
5. surrounding the prostate

## Chapter 8

*Exercise 1*

| | | | |
|---|---|---|---|
| 1. E | 2. F | 3. A | 4. A |
| 5. B | 6. G | 7. C | 8. D |
| 9. F | 10. A | 11. B | 12. H |

13. supra- (above) + cervic/o (cervix) + -al (pertaining to)
**Def: pertaining to above the cervix**
14. intra- (within) + uter/o (uterus) + -ine (pertaining to)
**Def: pertaining to within the uterus**
15. pre- (before) + menstru/o (menstruation) + -al (pertaining to)
**Def: pertaining to before menstruation**
16. trans- (across, through) + vagin/o (vagina) + -al (pertaining to)
**Def: pertaining to through the vagina**

*Exercise 2*
See Fig. 8-1.

*Exercise 3*

| | | |
|---|---|---|
| 1. B, J | 2. D, F | 3. G |
| 4. A, I | 5. L | 6. E, K |
| 7. H | 8. C | 9. M |

10. inter- (between) + labi/o (labia) + -al (pertaining to)
**Def: pertaining to between the labia**
11. intra- (within) + mamm/o (breast) + -ary (pertaining to)
**Def: pertaining to within the breast**

*Exercise 4*

| | |
|---|---|
| 1. C, I, K | 2. B, E |
| 3. A, H | 4. M |
| 5. D | 6. F, J |
| 7. L | 8. G |

9. ante- (before) + nat/o (birth) + -al (pertaining to)
**Def: pertaining to before birth**
10. peri- (surrounding) + umbilic/o (umbilicus) + -al (pertaining to)
**Def: pertaining to surrounding the umbilicus**

*Exercise 5*
See Fig. 8-4.

*Exercise 6*
1. pyosalpinx
2. adhesions
3. salpingitis
4. hydrosalpinx
5. polycystic ovary syndrome
6. oophar/o (ovary) + -itis (inflammation)
**Def: inflammation of the ovary**
7. an- (without) + ovul/o (ovum) + -ation (process of)
**Def: process of without (release of) an ovum**
8. hemat/o (blood) + -salpinx (fallopian tubes)
**Def: blood in the fallopian tubes**

*Exercise 7*
1. leukorrhea
2. retroflexion of the uterus

3. endometriosis
4. endometri/o (endometrium) + -itis (inflammation)
   **Def: inflammation of the endometrium**
5. hyster/o (uterus) + -ptosis (drooping)
   **Def: drooping of the uterus**
6. cervic/o (cervix) + -itis (inflammation)
   **Def: inflammation of the cervix**

### Exercise 8
1. vaginal prolapse
2. vulvitis
3. vulvodynia
4. thelitis
5. mastitis
6. vulvovaginitis
7. galact/o (milk) + -rrhea (flow, discharge)
   **Def: abnormal discharge of milk**
8. mast/o (breast) + -ptosis (drooping)
   **Def: drooping of the breast**
9. vagin/o (vagina) + -itis (inflammation)
   **Def: inflammation of the vagina**

### Exercise 9
1. menorrhagia
2. metrorrhagia
3. premenstrual syndrome
4. menometrorrhagia
5. premenstrual dysphoric disorder
6. dysfunctional uterine bleeding
7. dys- (painful) + men/o (menses) + -rrhea (discharge)
   **Def: painful menstrual discharge**
8. a- (without) + men/o (menses) + -rrhea (discharge)
   **Def: without menstrual discharge**

9. poly- (many) + men/o (menses) + -rrhea (discharge)
   **Def: many (frequent) menstrual discharge**
10. olig/o (scanty) + men/o (menses) + -rrhea (discharge)
    **Def: scanty menstrual discharge**

### Exercise 10
1. meconium
2. nuchal cord
3. abruptio placentae
4. cephalopelvic disproportion
5. ectopic pregnancy
6. abortion
7. preeclampsia
8. placenta previa
9. eclampsia
10. erythroblastosis fetalis
11. condition (-ia) without (a-) milk (galact/o)
    **Term: agalactia**
12. excessive (poly-) amnion (-amnios) fluid (hydr/o)
    **Term: polyhydramnios**
13. scanty (olig/o) amnion (-amnios) fluid (hydr/o)
    **Term: oligohydramnios**

### Exercise 11
| | | | |
|---|---|---|---|
| 1. E | 2. F | 3. D | 4. C |
| 5. B | 6. G | 7. A | 8. A |
| 9. C | 10. G | 11. F | 12. E |
| 13. D | 14. B | | |

### Exercise 12
1. 1 pregnancy, 1 delivery
2. pelvic inflammatory disease
3. dysmenorrhea
4. blood test

### Exercise 13
1. hysterosalpingography
2. pelvimetry
3. cervicography
4. hysteroscopy
5. sonohysterography
6. laparoscopy
7. hormone levels
8. Pap smear
9. culd/o (cul-de-sac) + -centesis (removal of fluid)
   **Def: removal of fluid from the cul-de-sac**

10. mamm/o (breast) + -graphy (process of recording)
    **Def: process of recording the breast**
11. culd/o (cul-de-sac) + -scopy (visual examination)
    **Def: process of viewing the cul-de-sac**
12. colp/o (vagina) + -scopy (visual examination)
    **Def: process of viewing the vagina**

### Exercise 14
1. human chorionic gonadotropin
2. Apgar score
3. contraction stress test
4. nonstress test
5. alphafetoprotein
6. congenital hypothyroidism
7. chorionic villus sampling
8. removal of fluid for diagnostic purposes (-centesis) amnion (amni/o)
   **Term: amniocentesis**

### Exercise 15
1. hysteropexy
2. salpingolysis
3. bilateral oophorectomy
4. TAH-BSO
5. lumpectomy
6. pelvic exenteration
7. uterine artery embolization
8. dilation and curettage
9. colpoplasty
10. mastopexy
11. clitorid/o (clitoris) + -ectomy (removal)
    **Def: removal of the clitoris**
12. culd/o (cul-de-sac) + -plasty (surgical repair)
    **Def: surgical repair of the cul-de-sac**
13. hymen/o (hymen) + -tomy (incision)
    **Def: incision of the hymen**
14. removal (-ectomy) ovary (oophor/o) cyst (cyst/o)
    **Term: oophorocystectomy**
15. surgical repair (-plasty) nipple (thel/e)
    **Term: theleplasty**

## Exercise 16
1. tubal ligation
2. VBAC
3. eutocia
4. cephalic version
5. C-section
6. sterilization
7. cerclage

8. A    9. C    10. B    11. D
12. E

13. episi/o (vulva) + -tomy (incision)
   **Def: incision of the vulva**
14. oxy- (rapid) + -tocia (labor)
   **Def: rapid labor**
15. salping/o (fallopian tube) + salping/o (fallopian tube) + -stomy (new opening)
   **Def: new opening between the fallopian tubes**

## Exercise 17
1. sterilization = surgical procedure that renders a person incapable of producing children multiparity = multiple (two or more) deliveries
2. multiparous = many (two or more) deliveries multigravida = many (two or more) pregnancies
3. laparoscopic
4. tie off
5. infraumbilical (below the navel)

## Exercise 18
1. OCP
2. barrier methods
3. condoms
4. IUDs
5. abortifacient
6. rhythm method
7. abstinence
8. spermicides
9. ECP

## Exercise 19
1. increase
2. hormone replacement therapy
3. soy beans
4. induce
5. tocolytics

## Exercise 20
1. H    2. D    3. F    4. B
5. G    6. E    7. C    8. A

## Chapter 8 Review

### Word Part Definitions
1. neo-
2. primi-
3. –gravida
4. –para
5. –salpinx
6. multi-
7. nulli-
8. –ptosis
9. –rrhea
10. –tocia
11. cervic/o
12. gravid/o
13. lact/o
14. mast/o or mamm/o
15. nat/o
16. papill/o or thel/e
17. mast/o or mamm/o
18. amni/o
19. thel/e or papill/o
20. gynec/o
21. o/o
22. olig/o
23. hyster/o or metr/o
24. men/o
25. part/o
26. chori/o
27. colp/o
28. hyster/o or metr/o
29. culd/o
30. salping/o
31. oophor/o
32. episi/o

### Wordshop
1. no (a-) menstruation (men/o) flow (-rrhea)
   **Term: amenorrhea**
2. process of recording (-graphy) uterus (hyster/o) fallopian tube (salping/o)
   **Term: hysterosalpingography**
3. frequent (poly-) menstruation (men/o) flow (-rrhea)
   **Term: polymenorrhea**
4. no (nulli-) pregnancy (-gravida)
   **Term: nulligravida**
5. after (post-) delivery (-partum)
   **Term: postpartum**
6. many (multi-) deliveries (-para)
   **Term: multipara**
7. painful (dys-) menstruation (men/o) flow (-rrhea)
   **Term: dysmenorrhea**
8. removal (-ectomy) uterus (hyster/o)
   **Term: hysterectomy**
9. freeing from adhesions (-lysis) fallopian tube (salping/o)
   **Term: salpingolysis**
10. fixation (-pexy) breast (mast/o)
   **Term: mastopexy**
11. pus (py/o) fallopian tube (-salpinx)
   **Term: pyosalpinx**
12. condition (-ia) without (a-) milk (galact/o)
   **Term: agalactia**
13. incision (-tomy) perineum (episi/o)
   **Term: episiotomy**
14. condition of labor, delivery (-tocia) healthy, normal (eu-)
   **Term: eutocia**
15. surgical repair (-plasty) nipple (thel/e)
   **Term: theleplasty**

### Term Sorting
**Anatomy and Physiology:** areola, cervix, endometrium, fimbriae, gestation, hCG, menopause, parturition, progesterone, puerperium
**Pathology:** anovulation, eclampsia, hematosalpinx, hysteroptosis, leiomyoma, menorrhagia, oophoritis, polyhydramnios, pyosalpinx, vulvodynia
**Diagnostic Procedures:** AFP, amniocentesis, Apgar, colposcopy, CST, culdocentesis, CVS, Pap smear, pelvimetry, PKU

**Therapeutic Interventions:**
cerclage, cervicectomy, colpopexy, D&C, LEEP, mastopexy, oophorectomy, salpingolysis, theleplasty, tubal ligation

## Translations

1. gynecologist, dysmenorrhea
2. obstetrician, amniocentesis
3. neonate, nuchal cord
4. leukorrhea, cervicitis
5. fallopian adhesions, salpingolysis
6. ectopic pregnancy, tubal ligation
7. primigravida, nonstress test (NST)
8. mastectomy, infiltrating ductal carcinoma (IDC)
9. Pap smear, colposcopy
10. mastitis, thelitis (or acromastitis)
11. hysterosalpingography, salpingitis
12. hysterectomy, leiomyosarcoma
13. oxytocia, episiotomy
14. cephalopelvic disproportion, cesarian section

## Operative Report

1. premature
2. first feces of the newborn
3. umbilical cord wrapped around the neck of the neonate
4. physical health of the infant at 1 and 5 minutes after birth
5. the health of the fetus

## Chapter 9

### Exercise 1

| | | | |
|---|---|---|---|
| 1. I | 2. J | 3. E | 4. A |
| 5. M | 6. K | 7. L | 8. F |
| 9. D | 10. C | 11. H | 12. G |
| 13. B | 14. N | 15. J | 16. A |
| 17. E | 18. H | 19. I | 20. B |
| 21. G | 22. D | 23. C | 24. F |

25. poly- (many) + nucle/o (nucleus) + -ar (pertaining to)
    **Def: pertaining to many nuclei**

26. a- (without) + granul/o (little grain) + cyt/o (cell) + -ic (pertaining to)
    **Def: pertaining to cells without little grains**
27. lymphat/o (lymph) + -ic (pertaining to)
    **Def: pertaining to the lymph**
28. a- (without) + nucle/o (nucleus) + -ar (pertaining to)
    **Def: pertaining to without a nucleus**
29. poly- (many) + morph/o (shape) + -ic (pertaining to)
    **Def: pertaining to many shapes**

### Exercise 2

1. A, B, AB, O
2. antigens
3. A, AB
4. universal donor, universal recipient
5. Rh

### Exercise 3

| | | | |
|---|---|---|---|
| 1. D | 2. A | 3. H | 4. J |
| 5. E | 6. C | 7. G | 8. F |
| 9. B | 10. I | | |

11. pertaining to (-ary) armpit (axill/o)
    **Term: axillary**
12. pertaining to (-al) groin (inguin/o)
    **Term: inguinal**
13. pertaining to (-al) neck (cervic/o)
    **Term: cervical**

### Exercise 4
See Fig. 9-7.

### Exercise 5

1. Nonspecific immunity is a general defense against pathogens. Specific immunity involves recognition of a given pathogen and a reaction against it.
2. mechanical—skin, mucus/physical—sneezing, coughing, vomiting, diarrhea/chemical—saliva, tears, perspiration

3. phagocytosis, inflammation, fever, protective proteins
4. active artificial
5. passive natural
6. passive artificial
7. active natural

| | | | |
|---|---|---|---|
| 8. B | 9. F | 10. D | 11. E |
| 12. C | 13. A | 14. G | 15. H |
| 16. I | 17. J | | |

### Exercise 6

1. sickle-cell anemia
2. autoimmune acquired hemolytic anemia
3. thalassemia
4. aplastic anemia
5. pancytopenia
6. pernicious anemia
7. acute posthemorrhagic anemia
8. hypo- (deficient) + vol/o (volume) + -emia (blood condition)
   **Def: blood condition of deficient volume**
9. hem/o (blood) + -lytic (pertaining to destruction)
   **Def: pertaining to the destruction of blood**
10. sider/o (iron) + -penia (deficiency)
    **Def: deficiency of iron**

### Exercise 7

| | | | |
|---|---|---|---|
| 1. G | 2. B | 3. E | 4. D |
| 5. C | 6. F | 7. A | |

8. deficiency (-penia) lymph cells (lymphocyt/o)
   **Term: lymphocytopenia**
9. abnormal increase (-cytosis) white blood cells (leuk/o)
   **Term: leukocytosis**
10. inflammation (-itis) lymph vessels (lymphangi/o)
    **Term: lymphangitis**
11. condition (-ism) excessive (hyper-) spleen (splen/o)
    **Term: hypersplenism**
12. lymphaden/o (lymph gland) + -pathy (disease)
    **Def: disease of the lymph gland**

13. lymphangi/o (lymph vessel) + -itis (inflammation)
   **Def: inflammation of the lymph vessels**
14. thromb/o (clot) + cyt/o (cell) + -penia (deficiency)
   **Def: deficiency of clotting cells**
15. lymph/o (lymph) + -cytosis (abnormal increase of cells)
   **Def: increase in lymph cells**

### Exercise 8
1. D    2. B    3. A    4. F
5. C    6. E

### Exercise 9
1. G    2. I    3. B    4. D
5. F    6. H    7. A    8. E
9. C

### Exercise 10
1. K    2. H    3. G    4. A
5. I    6. B    7. L    8. M
9. D   10. A   11. D   12. C
13. E   14. J   15. F

16. process of recording (-graphy) lymph vessels (lymphangi/o)
   **Term: lymphangiography**
17. process of recording (-graphy) artery (arteri/o) pertaining to (-ic) spleen (splen/o)
   **Term: splenic arteriography**
18. process of recording (-graphy) lymph gland (lymphaden/o)
   **Term: lymphadenography**

### Exercise 11
1. potassium level = 3.7 mEq/L
2. sodium level = 142 mEq/L
3. 15 mg/dL

### Exercise 12
1. E    2. D    3. C    4. A
5. F    6. B

7. splen/o (spleen) + -ectomy (removal)
   **Term: splenectomy**

8. adenoid/o (adenoid) + -ectomy (removal)
   **Term: adenoidectomy**
9. platelet + -pheresis (removal)
   **Term: plateletpheresis**
10. lymphaden/o (lymph gland) + -ectomy (removal)
   **Term: lymphadenectomy**

### Exercise 13
1. mildly pyrexic
2. pharyngeal inflammation
3. cervic/o (neck) + -al (pertaining to) + lymphaden/o (lymph gland) + -pathy (disease)
   **Def: lymph gland disease pertaining to the neck**
4. splenomegaly
5. lymphocytosis
6. He produced antibodies to the EB antigen.

### Exercise 14
1. J    2. C    3. E    4. I
5. B    6. A    7. H    8. G
9. F   10. D

### Exercise 15
1. Epstein-Barr virus
2. hematocrit, hemoglobin
3. acquired immunodeficiency syndrome, human immunodeficiency virus
4. comprehensive metabolic panel
5. bone marrow transplant

## Chapter 9 Review

### Word Part Definitions
1. –cyte
2. –gen
3. –cytosis
4. –globin
5. –poiesis
6. –edema
7. –philia
8. –penia
9. –siderin
10. –emia
11. hemat/o
12. eosin/o
13. inguin/o
14. nucle/o

15. lymphangi/o
16. myel/o
17. splen/o
18. pyr/o
19. erythr/o
20. thromb/o
21. lymphaden/o
22. cyt/o
23. neutr/o
24. axill/o
25. leuk/o
26. ser/o
27. granul/o
28. plasm/o
29. thym/o
30. lymph/o
31. morph/o
32. tonsill/o

### Wordshop
1. deficiency (-penia) all (pan-) cell (cyt/o)
   **Term: pancytopenia**
2. abnormal increase of cells (-cytosis) white (leuk/o)
   **Term: leukocytosis**
3. inflammation (-itis) lymph gland (lymphaden/o)
   **Term: lymphadenitis**
4. deficiency (-penia) clotting cells (thrombocyt/o)
   **Term: thrombocytopenia**
5. process of recording (-graphy) lymph gland (lymphaden/o)
   **Term: lymphadenography**
6. abnormal increase of cells (-cytosis) red (erythr/o)
   **Term: erythrocytosis**
7. removal (-ectomy) adenoids (adenoid/o)
   **Term: adenoidectomy**
8. swelling (-edema) lymph (lymph/o)
   **Term: lymphedema**
9. stopping/controlling (-stasis) blood (hem/o)
   **Term: hemostasis**
10. breakdown (-lysis) blood (hem/o)
   **Term: hemolysis**
11. substance (-in) iron (sider/o) blood (hem/o)
   **Term: hemosiderin**

12. deficiency (-penia) iron (sider/o)
    **Term: sideropenia**
13. process of recording (-graphy) lymph vessel (lymphangi/o)
    **Term: lymphangiography**
14. conditon of (-ism) excessive (hyper-) spleen (splen/o)
    **Term: hypersplenism**
15. removal (-ectomy) spleen (splen/o)
    **Term: splenectomy**

### Term Sorting

**Anatomy and Physiology:** agglutination, antibody, coagulation, eosinophil, hematopoiesis, hemoglobin, hemostasis, plasma, thrombocyte, thymus
**Pathology:** anaphylaxis, dyscrasia, edema, hypovolemia, leukocytosis, lymphangitis, mononucleosis, septicemia, sideropenia, thalassemia
**Diagnostic Procedures:** BMP, CBC, CMP, diff count, ELISA, Hct, lymphangiography, MCHC, monospot, Schilling test
**Therapeutic Interventions:** adenoidectomy, antiretrovirals, apheresis, blood transfusion, BMT, hematinic, hemostatic, plateletpheresis, splenectomy, vaccine

### Translations

1. splenomegaly, splenectomy
2. pancytopenia, aplastic anemia
3. leukocytosis, blood cultures
4. anaphalaxis
5. bone marrow transplant, acute myelogenous leukemia (AML)
6. sickle cell crisis, hypersplenism
7. plateletpheresis, thrombocytopenia
8. posthemorrhagic anemia, blood transfusion
9. lymphadenopathy, mononucleosis
10. hemophilia, partial thromboplastin time (PTT)
11. pernicious anemia, Schilling test

12. purpura, septicemia
13. leukopenia, neutropenia
14. polycythemia vera

### Clinical Notes

1. principal diagnosis: Sickle-Cell crisis
2. Motrin and Darvon
3. appendix

## Chapter 10

### Exercise 1

| | | |
|---|---|---|
| 1. D, F | 2. E | 3. G |
| 4. L | 5. H | 6. B |
| 7. K | 8. J | 9. A, C, I |

10. endo- (within) + vascul/o (vessel) + -ar (pertaining to)
    **Def: pertaining to within the vessel**
11. intra- (within) + ven/o (vein) + -ous (pertaining to)
    **Def: pertaining to within the vein**
12. peri- (around) + cardi/o (heart) + -al (pertaining to)
    **Def: pertaining to around the heart**

### Exercise 2

| | | | |
|---|---|---|---|
| 1. K | 2. I | 3. A | 4. B |
| 5. D | 6. C | 7. L | 8. E |
| 9. H | 10. F | 11. G | 12. J |

13. pertaining to (-ar) between (inter-) ventricle (ventricul/o)
    **Term: interventricular**
14. pertaining to (-al) surrounding (peri-) apex (apic/o)
    **Term: periapical**
15. pertaining to (-al) before (pre-) heart (cordi/o)
    **Term: precordial**
16. pertaining to (-al) through (trans-) heart muscle (myocardi/o)
    **Term: transmyocardial**

### Exercise 3
See Fig. 10-5B.

### Exercise 4
1. pulmonary arteries
2. tricuspid

3. mitral
4. competent
5. ejection fraction

### Exercise 5
1. during
2. neck, brain
3. within
4. narrowing

### Exercise 6

| | | | |
|---|---|---|---|
| 1. G | 2. A | 3. M | 4. F |
| 5. H | 6. D | 7. K | 8. L |
| 9. J | 10. B | 11. N | 12. E |
| 13. I | 14. C | | |

15. brady- (slow) + -cardia (heart condition)
    **Def: slow heart condition**
16. tachy- (rapid) + -cardia (heart condition)
    **Def: rapid heart condition**
17. cardi/o (heart) + -megaly (enlargement)
    **Def: enlargement of the heart**

### Exercise 7

| | | | |
|---|---|---|---|
| 1. C | 2. D | 3. B | 4. A |

### Exercise 8

| | | | |
|---|---|---|---|
| 1. C | 2. D | 3. B | 4. A |
| 5. E | | | |

### Exercise 9
1. dysrhythmia
2. fibrillation
3. flutter
4. atrioventricular block
5. sick sinus syndrome
6. ventricular ectopic beats
7. ventricular tachycardia

### Exercise 10
1. myocardial infarction
2. heart failure
3. cardiac tamponade
4. angina pectoris
5. coronary artery disease
6. inflammation (-itis) pericardium (pericardi/o)
   **Term: pericarditis**

7. inflammation (-itis) endocardium (endocardi/o)
   **Term: endocarditis**
8. disease (-pathy) heart muscle (cardiomy/o)
   **Term: cardiomyopathy**

*Exercise 11*
1. aneurysm
2. claudication
3. primary, essential
4. secondary
5. hemorrhoids
6. esophageal varices
7. peripheral artery disease
8. Raynaud disease
9. varicose veins
10. vascul/o (vessel) + -itis (inflammation)
    **Def: inflammation of the vessels**
11. hypo- (below, deficient) + tens/o (stretching) + -ion (process of)
    **Def: deficient pressure**
12. hyper- (excessive) + -tension (pressure)
    **Def: excessive pressure**
13. thromb/o (clot) + phleb/o (vein) + -itis (inflammation)
    **Def: inflammation of a clot in a vein**

*Exercise 12*
1. hemangioma
2. cardiac myxosarcoma
3. atrial myxoma
4. hemangiosarcoma

*Exercise 13*
1. heart vessels
2. normal heartbeat
3. arrhythmia
4. the upper chambers of the heart
5. enlarged
6. electrocardiogram

*Exercise 14*
1. MUGA scan
2. lipid profile
3. cardiac enzymes test
4. digital subtraction angiography
5. myocardial perfusion imaging

6. radiography
7. exercise stress test
8. cardiac catheterization
9. PET scan
10. incision (-tomy) vein (phleb/o)
    **Term: phlebotomy**
11. process of recording (-graphy) heart (cardi/o) vessel (angi/o)
    **Term: angiocardiography**
12. process of recording (-graphy) vein (phleb/o)
    **Term: phlebography**
13. process of recording (-graphy) electricity (electr/o) heart (cardi/o)
    **Term: electrocardiography**
14. process of recording (-graphy) heart (cardi/o) sound (echo-)
    **Term: echocardiography**

*Exercise 15*
1. PACAB
2. CABG
3. CPR
4. PICC
5. commissurotomy
6. PTCA
7. MIDCAB
8. RFCA
9. LVAD
10. EVLT
11. AICD
12. phleb/o (vein) + -ectomy (removal)
    **Def: removal of a vein**
13. pericardi/o (pericardium) + -centesis (surgical puncture)
    **Def: surgical puncture of the pericardium**
14. hemorrhoid/o (hemorrhoid) + -ectomy (removal)
    **Def: removal of a hemorrhoid**
15. scler/o (hard) + -therapy (treatment)
    **Def: treatment (by) hardening (veins)**
16. valvul/o (valve) + -plasty (surgical repair)
    **Def: surgical repair of a valve**

17. ather/o (fatty plaque) + -ectomy (removal)
    **Def: removal of plaque**

*Exercise 16*
1. C
2. A, C, D
3. A, E
4. A, D, E
5. A, D, E
6. A, E
7. B
8. F
9. G

*Exercise 17*
1. H  2. J  3. D  4. F
5. A  6. B  7. I  8. C
9. E  10. G

**Chapter 10 Review**

*Word Part Definitions*
1. –cardia
2. tetra-
3. –pathy
4. brady-
5. –sclerosis
6. echo-
7. tachy-
8. –graphy
9. –um
10. –megaly
11. arteri/o
12. cardi/o or coron/o
13. pulmon/o
14. vascul/o or angi/o
15. lumin/o
16. endocardi/o
17. angi/o or vascul/o
18. pariet/o
19. myocardi/o
20. phleb/o
21. hemangi/o
22. aort/o
23. corpor/o
24. coron/o or cardi/o
25. ather/o
26. epicardi/o
27. thromb/o
28. atri/o
29. sept/o
30. isch/o
31. cyan/o
32. pericardi/o

*Wordshop*
1. inflammation (-itis) surrounding (peri-) heart (cardi/o)
   **Term: pericarditis**

2. inflammation (-itis) clot (thromb/o) vein (phleb/o)
**Term: thrombophlebitis**
3. condition of (-ia) rapid (tachy-) heart (cardi/o)
**Term: tachycardia**
4. process of recording (-graphy) sound (echo-) heart (cardi/o)
**Term: echocardiography**
5. process of recording (-graphy) vessel (angi/o)
**Term: angiography**
6. surgical repair (-plasty) vessel (angi/o)
**Term: angioplasty**
7. condition of (-ia) abnormal (dys-) rhythm (rhythm/o)
**Term: dysrhythmia**
8. abnormal condition of hardening (sclerosis) artery (arteri/o)
**Term: arteriosclerosis**
9. pain (-dynia) heart (cardi/o)
**Term: cardiodynia**
10. removal (-ectomy) fatty plaque (ather/o)
**Term: atherectomy**
11. pertaining to (-ary) heart (cardi/o) lung (pulmon/o)
**Term: cardiopulmonary**
12. removal (-ectomy) vein (phleb/o)
**Term: phlebectomy**
13. pertaining to (-eal) outside (extra-) body (corpor/o)
**Term: extracorporeal**
14. pertaining to(-al) through (trans-) heart muscle (myocardi/o)
**Term: transmyocardial**
15. process of recording (-graphy) vein (phleb/o)
**Term: phlebography**

*Term Sorting*
**Anatomy and Physiology:**
aorta, atrium, bundle of His, capillary, diastole, endocardium, Purkinje fibers, septum, systole, ventricle
**Pathology:** aneurysm, arrhythmia, bradycardia, bruit, CAD, claudication, endocarditis, hemangiosarcoma, HTN, SOB

**Diagnostic Procedures:**
angiocardiography, auscultation, BP, ECG, EST, fluoroscopy, lipid profile, phlebography, phlebotomy, MUGA scan
**Therapeutic Interventions:**
CABG, commissurotomy, ECC, EVLT, LVAD, MIDCAB, pericardiocentesis, PTCA, thromboendarterectomy, valvuloplasty

*Translations*
1. patent ductus arteriosus (PDA), murmur
2. tetralogy of Fallot, echocardiography
3. pulmonary edema, heart failure (HF)
4. coronary artery disease (CAD), cardiodynia or angina
5. phlebography, thrombophlebitis
6. diaphoresis, tachycardia
7. cardiac enzymes test, electrocardiography
8. endovenous laser ablation (EVLT), varicose veins
9. angina pectoris, nitrate or antianginals
10. pericardiocentesis, cardiac tamponade
11. cardiac pacemaker, sick sinus syndrome (SSS)
12. percutaneous transluminal coronary angioplasty (PTCA), transmyocardial revascularization (TMR)
13. tricuspid stenosis, valvuloplasty
14. cardiomyopathy, left ventricular assist device (LVAD)

*Discharge Summary*
1. A. difficult or painful breathing
   B. profuse secretion of sweat
   C. high blood pressure
2. substernal (under the breastbone)
3. no cyanosis
4. echocardiography
5. coronary artery bypass graft
6. lungs

**Chapter 11**

*Exercise 1*

| | | |
|---|---|---|
| 1. T | 2. N | 3. S |
| 4. V | 5. E, O | 6. Q |
| 7. H | 8. C | 9. Z |
| 10. AA | 11. F | 12. G |
| 13. R | 14. D, L | 15. U |
| 16. B | 17. X | 18. DD |
| 19. J, P | 20. BB | 21. Y |
| 22. K | 23. CC | 24. W |
| 25. I | 26. M | 27. A |

28. inter- (between) + cost/o (rib) + -al (pertaining to)
**Def: pertaining to between the ribs**
29. in- (in) + spir/o (breathe) + -atory (pertaining to)
**Def: pertaining to breathing in**
30. para- (near) + nas/o (nose) + -al (pertaining to)
**Def: pertaining to near the nose**
31. endo- (within) + trache/o (trachea) + -al (pertaining to)
**Def: pertaining to within the trachea**

*Exercise 2*
See Figs. 11-1 and 11-2.

*Exercise 3*
1. difficulty breathing unless in an upright position
2. a nosebleed
3. hiccup or hiccough
4. tachypnea
5. make sounds
6. apnea
7. cyanosis
8. crackles
9. pleurodynia
10. wheezing
11. clubbing
12. discharge (-rrhea) nose (rhin/o)
**Term: rhinorrhea**
13. pain (-dynia) chest (thorac/o)
**Term: thoracodynia**
14. spitting (-ptysis) blood (hem/o)
**Term: hemoptysis**

15. good, normal (eu-) breathing (-pnea)
    **Term: eupnea**
16. excessive (hyper-) breathing (-pnea)
    **Term: hyperpnea**

## Exercise 4
1. coryza
2. URI
3. deviated septum
4. vocal polyps
5. pleurisy
6. croup
7. atelectasis
8. emphysema
9. asthma
10. pulmonary abscess
11. pneumoconiosis
12. cystic fibrosis
13. flail chest
14. pertussis
15. pneumon/o (lungs) + -ia (condition)
    **Def: condition of the lungs**
16. pneum/o (air) + -thorax (pleural cavity, chest)
    **Def: air in the pleural cavity**
17. py/o (pus) + -thorax (pleural cavity, chest)
    **Def: pus in the pleural cavity**
18. blood (hem/o) pleural cavity, chest (-thorax)
    **Term: hemothorax**
19. inflammation (-itis) bronchi (bronchi/o)
    **Term: bronchitis**
20. bronchi (bronch/o) spasm (-spasm)
    **Term: bronchospasm**

## Exercise 5
1. benign
2. chondroadenoma
3. non–small cell lung cancer
4. oat cell carcinoma

## Exercise 6
1. clear to auscultation
2. no wheezes
3. no crackles (rales)

4. chest x-ray
5. atelectasis

## Exercise 7
1. Mantoux skin test
2. ABG
3. sweat test
4. lung ventilation scan
5. pulmonary angiography
6. process of viewing (-scopy) bronchi (bronch/o)
   **Term: bronchoscopy**
7. process of viewing (-scopy) voice box (laryng/o)
   **Term: laryngoscopy**
8. process of measurement (-metry) breathing (spir/o)
   **Term: spirometry**

## Exercise 8
1. lungs
2. breathing in
3. bronchoscopy
4. lungs
5. URI

## Exercise 9
1. E    2. H    3. I    4. G
5. F    6. D    7. A    8. B
9. C

10. excision (-ectomy) voice box (laryng/o)
    **Term: laryngectomy**
11. surgical repair (-plasty) nose (rhin/o)
    **Term: rhinoplasty**
12. new opening (-stomy) windpipe (trache/o)
    **Term: tracheostomy**

## Exercise 10
1. C    2. E    3. D    4. A
5. B

6. nebulizer
7. inhaler
8. ventilator

## Exercise 11
1. chest x-ray, right middle lobe
2. purified protein derivative, tuberculosis
3. upper respiratory infection
4. chronic obstructive pulmonary disease, dyspnea on exertion

5. coal workers' pneumoconiosis
6. respiratory syncytial virus

## Chapter 11 Review

### Word Part Definitions
1. eu-
2. hyper-
3. hypo-
4. a-
5. –pnea
6. –ptysis
7. –rrhea
8. dys-
9. –metry
10. –ectasis
11. capn/o
12. pneum/o or pulmon/o
13. steth/o, pector/o or thorac/o
14. spir/o
15. orth/o
16. pleur/o
17. rhin/o or nas/o
18. sept/o
19. thorac/o, steth/o or pector/o
20. py/o
21. pharyng/o
22. muc/o
23. ox/i
24. phren/o
25. pulmon/o or pneum/o
26. pector/o, thorac/o or steth/o
27. cost/o
28. sin/o
29. tonsill/o
30. salping/o
31. laryng/o
32. rhin/o or nas/o

### Wordshop
1. difficult (dys-) breathing (-pnea)
   **Term: dyspnea**
2. rapid (tachy-) breathing (-pnea)
   **Term: tachypnea**
3. abnormal condition (-osis) dust (coni/o) lung (pneum/o)
   **Term: pneumoconiosis**
4. discharge (-rrhea) nose (rhin/o)
   **Term: rhinorrhea**

5. process (-ation) breathing (spir/o) out (ex-)
   **Term: expiration**
6. pus (py/o) chest (-thorax)
   **Term: pyothorax**
7. inflammation (-itis) pleurae (pleur/o)
   **Term: pleuritis**
8. surgical repair (-plasty) nose (rhin/o)
   **Term: rhinoplasty**
9. blood (hem/o) chest (-thorax)
   **Term: hemothorax**
10. narrowing (-stenosis) windpipe (trache/o)
    **Term: tracheostenosis**
11. incision (-tomy) windpipe (trache/o)
    **Term: tracheotomy**
12. pertaining to (-al) between (inter-) ribs (cost/o)
    **Term: intercostal**
13. pertaining to (-al) within (endo-) windpipe (trache/o)
    **Term: endotracheal**
14. abnormal condition (-osis) fungus (myc/o) nose (rhin/o)
    **Term: rhinomycosis**
15. process of viewing (-scopy) chest (thorac/o)
    **Term: thoracoscopy**

**Term Sorting**

**Anatomy and Physiology:** alveolus, diaphragm, epiglottis, eustachian tube, inhalation, mediastinum, olfaction, oropharynx, pleura, trachea

**Pathology:** aphonia, apnea, bronchiectasis, emphysema, epistaxis, hemoptysis, pleurisy, rhinomycosis, rhonchi, SARS

**Diagnostic Procedures:** ABG, bronchoscopy, CT, CXR, mediastinoscopy, PFT, pulse oximetry, spirometry, QFT, throat culture

**Therapeutic Interventions:** bronchodilator, bronchoplasty, CPAP, laryngectomy, septoplasty, sinusotomy, thoracocentesis, tonsillectomy, tracheostomy, tracheotomy

*Translations*
1. dyspnea, wheezing
2. dysphonia, laryngitis
3. stridor, croup
4. thoracodynia, pleural effusion
5. chest x-ray, pneumonia
6. pharyngitis, throat culture
7. pulse oximetry, spirometry
8. deviated septum, septoplasty
9. thoracocentesis, hemothorax
10. bronchiectasis, COPD
11. laryngeal, tracheostomy
12. Mantoux skin test, tuberculosis
13. anthracosis, pneumoconiosis
14. sweat test, cystic fibrosis

*ED Record*
1. slight profuse sweating, slight blueness of the nail bed
2. clip attached to ear lobe or finger
3. wheezes (whistling sounds) and rhonchi (rumbling sound heard when airways are blocked)
4. to measure breathing capacity
5. hand-held nebulizer

## Chapter 12

*Exercise 1*
1. central nervous system (CNS), peripheral nervous system (PNS)
2. transmit, to
3. efferent, from
4. somatic, autonomic

*Exercise 2*
1. stimulus → dendrite → cell body → axon → synapse

2. D    3. B    4. E    5. A
6. C

7. peri- (around) + neur/o (nerve) + -al (pertaining to)
   **Def: pertaining to around the nerve**

8. olig/o (few) + dendr/o (dendrite) + -itic (pertaining to)
   **Def: pertaining to few dendrites**
9. micro- (tiny) + gli/o (glue) + -al (pertaining to)
   **Def: pertaining to tiny glue (cells)**

*Exercise 3*
1. H    2. J    3. F    4. A
5. C    6. I    7. D    8. B
9. G    10. E    11. H    12. B
13. A    14. D    15. C    16. F
17. I    18. E    19. G    20. J

21. intra- (within) + ventricul/o (ventricle) + -ar (pertaining to)
    **Def: pertaining to within the ventricule**
22. epi- (above) + dur/o (dura mater) + -al (pertaining to)
    **Def: pertaining to above the dura mater**
23. para- (near) + sin/o (sinus) + -al (pertaining to)
    **Def: pertaining to near the sinus**
24. infra- (below) + cerebell/o (cerebellum) + -ar (pertaining to)
    **Def: pertaining to below the cerebellum**

*Exercise 4*
See Figs. 12-2 and 12-3.

*Exercise 5*

1. D    2. A    3. C    4. G
5. F    6. E    7. B    8. H
9. I

10. condition (-ia) without (an-) sense of smell (osm/o)
    **Term: anosmia**
11. condition (-ia) without (a-) taste (geus/o)
    **Term: ageusia**
12. condition of without knowing
    **Term: agnosia**
13. condition (-ia) difficult (dys-) sleep (somn/o)
    **Term: dyssomnia**

14. condition (-ia) difficult (dys-) eat (phag/o)
    **Term: dysphagia**
15. condition (-ia) without (a-) speech (phas/o)
    **Term: aphasia**

### Exercise 6
1. Huntington chorea
2. Tay-Sachs disease
3. cerebral palsy
4. coma
5. concussion
6. cerebral contusion
7. herniated intervertebral disk
8. mass (-oma) blood (hemat/o)
   **Term: hematoma**
9. spine (spin/o) split (-fida) two (bi-)
   **Term: spina bifida**
10. water (hydr/o) head (-cephalus)
    **Term: hydrocephalus**

### Exercise 7
1. Bell palsy
2. Tourette syndrome
3. Parkinson disease
4. amyotrophic lateral sclerosis
5. Alzheimer disease
6. Guillain-Barré syndrome
7. epilepsy
8. multiple sclerosis
9. narcolepsy

### Exercise 8
1. shingles
2. migraine
3. sciatica
4. hemiplegia
5. transient ischemic attack
6. paraparesis
7. cerebrovascular accident

8. C    9. E    10. A    11. F
12. D    13. B    14. G

15. radicul/o (nerve root) + -itis (inflammation)
    **Def: inflammation of a nerve root**
16. encephal/o (brain) + -itis (inflammation)
    **Def: inflammation of the brain**

17. hemi- (half) + -paresis (slight paralysis)
    **Def: slight paralysis of half of the body**
18. quadri- (four) + -plegia (paralysis)
    **Def: paralysis of four (limbs)**
19. inflammation (-itis) meninges (mening/o)
    **Term: meningitis**
20. inflammation (-itis) nerve (neur/o)
    **Term: neuritis**
21. inflammation (-itis) many (poly-) nerve (neur/o)
    **Term: polyneuritis**

### Exercise 9
1. E    2. D    3. B    4. F
5. A    6. C

### Exercise 10
1. grand mal
2. an attack resembling an epileptic seizure but having purely psychological causes
3. bending and straightening
4. pharynx is clear
5. II-XII, or 2-12

### Exercise 11
1. gait assessment rating scale (GARS)
2. cerebrospinal fluid analysis
3. lumbar puncture, or spinal tap
4. Babinski sign
5. multiple sleep latency test (MSLT)
6. cerebral angiography
7. single-photon emission computed tomography (SPECT)
8. positron emission tomography (PET)
9. electr/o (electricity) + encephal/o (brain) + -graphy (process of recording)
   **Def: process of recording electrical activity of the brain**
10. echo- (sound) + encephal/o (brain) + -graphy (process of recording)

**Def: process of recording the brain with sound**
11. neur/o (nerve) + endo- (within) + -scopy (visual examination)
    **Def: visual examination within the nerves**
12. process of recording (-graphy) spinal cord (myel/o)
    **Term: myelography**
13. process of recording (-graphy) brain (encephal/o) sound (echo-)
    **Term: echoencephalography**
14. process of recording (-graphy) many (poly-) sleep (somn/o)
    **Term: polysomnography**

### Exercise 12
1. cerebrovascular accident
2. no paresthesia
3. no ataxia
4. unable to express her words
5. major stroke

### Exercise 13
1. A    2. B    3. I    4. E
5. C    6. J    7. F    8. G
9. H    10. D    11. K

12. cord/o (spinal cord) + -tomy (incision)
    **Def: incision of the spinal cord**
13. neur/o (nerve) + -lysis (destruction)
    **Def: destruction of a nerve**
14. ventricul/o (ventricle) + peritone/o (peritoneum) + -al (pertaining to)
    **Def: to drain fluid from a ventricle to the peritoneum through a shunt**
15. suture (-rrhaphy) nerve (neur/o)
    **Term: neurorrhaphy**
16. incision (-tomy) vagus nerve (vag/o)
    **Term: vagotomy**
17. removal (-ectomy) skull (crani/o)
    **Term: craniectomy**

## Exercise 14
| 1. H | 2. G | 3. E | 4. C |
|------|------|------|------|
| 5. B | 6. D | 7. F | 8. A |

## Exercise 15
1. lumbar puncture, cerebrospinal fluid
2. second cervical vertebra
3. magnetic resonance imaging, multiple sclerosis
4. polysomnography
5. activities of daily living, cerebrovascular accident

## Chapter 12 Review

### Word Part Definitions
1. quadri-
2. –paresis
3. hemi-
4. poly-
5. mono-
6. –lepsy
7. –oma
8. para-
9. –esthesia
10. –plegia
11. cortic/o
12. phag/o
13. geus/o
14. rhiz/o or radicul/o
15. cerebell/o
16. esthesi/o
17. blast/o
18. myel/o or cord/o
19. dur/o
20. phas/o
21. ventricul/o
22. encephal/o
23. cord/o or myel/o
24. dendr/o
25. narc/o or somn/o
26. neur/o
27. cerebr/o
28. gnos/o
29. radicul/o or rhiz/o
30. somn/o or narc/o
31. osm/o
32. mening/o

### Wordshop
1. inflammation (-itis) many (poly-) nerve (neur/o)
   **Term: polyneuritis**
2. inflammation (-itis) brain (encephal/o)
   **Term: encephalitis**
3. paralysis (-plegia) four (quadri-)
   **Term: quadriplegia**
4. process of recording (-graphy) brain (encephal/o) sound (echo-)
   **Term: echoencephalography**
5. incision (-tomy) nerve (neur/o)
   **Term: neurotomy**
6. condition (-ia) no, not, without (a-) recognition (gnos/o)
   **Term: agnosia**
7. condition (-ia) no, not, without (an-) sense of smell (osm/o)
   **Term:anosmia**
8. nerve (neur/o) pain (-algia)
   **Term: neuralgia**
9. abnormal (para-) condition of sensation (-esthesia)
   **Term: paresthesia**
10. process of recording (-graphy) many (poly-) sleep (somn/o)
    **Term: polysomnography**
11. resection (-tomy) spinal nerve root (rhiz/o)
    **Term: rhizotomy**
12. destruction (-lysis) nerve (neur/o)
    **Term: neurolysis**
13. condition (-ia) of no, not, without (a-) sense of taste (geus/o)
    **Term: ageusia**
14. condition (-ia) difficult (dys-) sleep (somn/o)
    **Term: dyssomnia**
15. slight paralysis (-paresis) four (quadri-)
    **Term: quadriparesis**

### Term Sorting
**Anatomy and Physiology:** axon, cauda equina, cerebellum, CNS, CSF, meninges, neuron, neurotransmitter, synapse, ventricle
**Pathology:** agraphia, ALS, amnesia, fasciculation, HIVD, hydrocephalus, sciatica, spina bifida, syncope, TIA
**Diagnostic Procedures:** ADL, Babinski reflex, echoencephalography, evoked potential, GARS, LP, MRI, neuroendoscopy, polysomnography, SPECT
**Therapeutic Interventions:** cordotomy, craniectomy, hypnotic, nerve block, neurolysis, neuroplasty, neurorrhaphy, rhizotomy, TENS, vagotomy

### Translations
1. CVA, contralateral
2. hemiparesis, aphasia
3. hematoma, amnesia
4. vertigo, syncope
5. spina bifida, meningocele
6. hydrocephalus, ventriculoperitoneal shunt
7. tremors, hypokinesia
8. narcolepsy, MSLT
9. lumbar puncture (spinal tap), meningitis
10. polysomnography, hypersomnia
11. rhizotomy, trigeminal neuralgia
12. migraine, aura
13. neuralgia, paresthesia
14. sciatica, HIVD

### Discharge Summary
1. dizziness, sensation of movement when there is none, fainting
2. magnetic resonance angiography (imaging the carotid arteries with contrast agent)
3. within and outside the skull
4. incoordination

## Chapter 13

### Exercise 1
| 1. G | 2. J | 3. K | 4. H |
|------|------|------|------|
| 5. B | 6. C | 7. I | 8. E |
| 9. A | 10. F | 11. D | |

12. mood
13. labile
14. projection
15. abnormal condition (-osis) of mind (psych/o)
    **Term: psychosis**
16. condition of (-ism) sleep (somn/o) walking (ambul/o)
    **Term: somnambulism**
17. condition of (-ia) well (eu-) mind (thym/o)
    **Term: euthymia**

18. condition of (-ia) no (an-) pleasure (hedon/o)
    **Term: anhedonia**

### Exercise 2
1. severe mental retardation
2. Asperger syndrome
3. Tourette syndrome
4. conduct disorder
5. mild mental retardation
6. moderate mental retardation
7. attention-deficit/hyperactivity disorder
8. autistic disorder
9. oppositional defiant disorder
10. Rett disorder

### Exercise 3
1. alcohol
2. inhalants
3. controlling substance use
4. schizophrenia
5. dream
6. hallucination, delusions
7. persistent delusional
8. disorganized

### Exercise 4
1. social phobia
2. claustrophobia
3. generalized anxiety disorder
4. obsessive-compulsive disorder
5. posttraumatic stress disorder
6. dissociative identity disorder
7. hypochrondriacal disorder
8. bipolar disorder
9. depressive disorder
10. hypomania
11. cyclothymia
12. dysthymia
13. somnambulism
14. satyriasis
15. premature ejaculation
16. panic disorder
17. anorexia nervosa
18. pyromania
19. paranoid personality disorder
20. sadomasochism

21. acrophobia
22. ped/o (child) + phil/o (attraction) + -ia (condition)
    **Def: condition of attraction to a child**
23. para- (abnormal) + somn/o (sleep) + -ia (condition)
    **Def: condition of abnormal sleep**
24. klept/o (steal) + -mania (condition of madness)
    **Def: condition of stealing madness**
25. agora- (marketplace) + -phobia (fear)
    **Def: condition of fear of the marketplace (open spaces)**
26. trich/o (hair) + till/o (pulling) + –mania (condition of madness)
    **Def: condition of pulling hair madness**

### Exercise 5
1. D    2. B    3. F    4. C
5. G    6. A    7. E

### Exercise 6
1. euthymic
2. affect was appropriate to verbal content and showed broad range
3. no evidence of delusions
4. posttraumatic stress disorder

### Exercise 7
1. behavioral
2. light therapy
3. ECT
4. psychoanalysis
5. cognitive therapy
6. hypnosis
7. narcosynthesis
8. pharmacotherapy

### Exercise 8
1. G    2. C    3. E    4. H
5. D    6. B    7. A    8. F

### Exercise 9
1. chronic struggle to fall asleep or stay asleep

2. psychologist
3. hypnotics
4. anxiety

### Exercise 10
1. seasonal affective disorder
2. generalized anxiety disorders
3. mental retardation, intelligence quotient, Wechsler Adult Intelligence Scale
4. attention-deficit/hyperactivity disorder
5. posttraumatic stress disorder

## Chapter 13 Review

### Word Parts
1. –lalia
2. –mania
3. an-
4. –phobia
5. –thymia
6. agora-
7. eu-
8. –logist
9. bi-
10. –ia
11. acro-
12. –iatrist
13. dys-
14. hedon/o
15. cycl/o
16. orex/o
17. phren/o, psych/o or thym/o
18. somat/o
19. anthrop/o
20. nymph/o
21. kathis/o
22. pol/o
23. psych/o, phren/o or thym/o
24. klept/o
25. ped/o
26. iatr/o
27. somn/o
28. thym/o, psych/o or phren/o
29. phil/o
30. pyr/o
31. claustr/o
32. phor/o

## Wordshop

1. condition of (-ia) no (an-) pleasure (hedon/o)
**Term: anhedonia**
2. study of (-logy) mind (psych/o)
**Term: psychology**
3. condition of fear (-phobia) man (anthrop/o)
**Term: anthropophobia**
4. abnormal condition (-osis) mind (psych/o)
**Term: psychosis**
5. condition of madness, compulsion (-mania) fire (pyr/o)
**Term: pyromania**
6. condition of fear (-phobia) closing (claustr/o)
**Term: claustrophobia**
7. state of mind (-thymia) good/normal (eu-)
**Term: euthymia**
8. condition of fear (-phobia) heights (acro-)
**Term: acrophobia**
9. condition of (-ia) split (schiz/o) mind (phren/o)
**Term: schizophrenia**
10. condition of (-ism) sleep (somn/o) walking (ambul/o)
**Term: somnambulism**
11. condition of madness/ compulsion (-mania) hair (trich/o) pulling (till/o)
**Term: trichotillomania**
12. abnormal (para-) condition (-ia) sleep (somn/o)
**Term: parasomnia**
13. condition of fear (-phobia) marketplace (agora-)
**Term: agoraphobia**
14. condition of babbling (-lalia) reverberation (echo-)
**Term: echolalia**
15. condition of (-ia) no (an-) appetite (orex/o)
**Term: anorexia**

## Term Sorting

**Pathology:** acrophobia, ADHD, akathisia, anhedonia, anxiety, catatonia, confabulation, cyclothymia, delusion, DTs, GAD, hallucination, hypomania OCD, PD, psychosis, PTSD, pyromania, schizophrenia, somnambulism,
**Diagnostic Procedures:** Bender Gestalt, DAP, DSM-IV-TR, GAF, MMPI, Rorschach, TAT, WAIS
**Therapeutic Interventions:** antidepressants, anxiolytics, ECT, detoxification, hypnosis, psychoanalysis, sedatives, stimulants

## Translations

1. blunt affect, dysthymia
2. anorexia nervosa, agoraphobia
3. parasomnia, somnambulism
4. SAD, libido, anhedonia
5. dysphoria, euphoria, bipolar disorder
6. anxiety, PTSD
7. psychologist, acrophobia, claustrophobia
8. psychiatrist, OCD
9. psychosis, hallucinations
10. ADHD
11. oppositional defiant disorder, pyromania
12. trichotillomania
13. pharmacotherapy

## SOAP Note

1. depression
2. no
3. gastroesophageal reflux disease
4. antidepressants
5. cognitive therapy

## Chapter 14

### Exercise 1

| | | |
|---|---|---|
| 1. B | 2. E, G | 3. A, I |
| 4. C | 5. H | 6. D, F |
| 7. K | 8. J | |

9. pertaining to (-ar) two (bin-) eyes (ocul/o)
**Term: binocular**
10. pertaining to (-al) above (supra-) the orbit (orbit/o)
**Term: supraorbital**
11. pertaining to (-ar) outside (extra-) the eye (ocul/o)
**Term: extraocular**

### Exercise 2

See Fig. 14-1.

### Exercise 3

| | | |
|---|---|---|
| 1. J | 2. L | 3. I, M |
| 4. B | 5. B | 6. K |
| 7. H | 8. E | 9. F |
| 10. D | 11. G | 12. A |
| 13. C | | |

14. extra- (outside) + ocul/o (eye) + -ar (pertaining to)
**Def: pertaining to outside the eye**
15. pre- (in front of) + retin/o (retina) + -al (pertaining to)
**Def: pertaining to in front of the retina**
16. intra- (within) + scler/o (sclera) + -al (pertaining to)
**Def: pertaining to within the sclera**

### Exercise 4

See Fig. 14-2A.

### Exercise 5

| | | | |
|---|---|---|---|
| 1. D | 2. I | 3. F | 4. B |
| 5. L | 6. E | 7. G | 8. J |
| 9. K | 10. H | 11. C | 12. A |

13. xer/o (dry) + ophthalm/o (eye) + -ia (condition)
**Def: condition of dry eye**
14. eso- (inward) + trop/o (turning) + -ia (condition)
**Def: condition of turning inward**
15. blephar/o (eyelid) + -chalasis (relaxation, slackening)
**Def: relaxation or slackening of the eyelid**
16. dacryocyst/o (lacrimal sac) + -itis (inflammation)
**Def: inflammation of the tear sac**
17. inflammation (-itis) eyelid (blephar/o)
**Term: blepharitis**
18. inflammation (-itis) lacrimal gland (dacryoaden/o)
**Term: dacryoadenitis**

19. drooping (-ptosis) eyelid (blephar/o)
    **Term: blepharoptosis**
20. process of (-ion) turning (trop/o) in (en-)
    **Term: entropion**

## Exercise 6
1. J    2. I    3. F    4. G
5. K    6. B    7. L    8. A
9. E    10. D    11. H    12. C
13. M

14. nyctal/o (night blindness) + -opia (vision condition)
    **Def: night blindness vision condition**
15. a- (without) + chromat/o (color) + -opsia (vision condition)
    **Def: without color vision condition**
16. a- (lack of) + phak/o (lens) + -ia (condition)
    **Def: condition of no lens**
17. hemi- (half) + an- (without) + -opsia (vision)
    **Def: without half vision condition**
18. opt/o (vision) + -ic (pertaining to) neur/o (nerve) + -itis (inflammation)
    **Def: inflammation of the nerve pertaining to vision**
19. inflammation (-itis) cornea (kerat/o)
    **Term: keratitis**
20. vision condition (-opia) old age (presby-)
    **Term: presbyopia**
21. inflammation (-itis) uvea (uve/o)
    **Term: uveitis**
22. disease (-pathy) retina (retin/o)
    **Term: retinopathy**

## Exercise 7
1. retinoblastoma
2. intraocular melanoma
3. choroidal hemangioma

## Exercise 8
1. E    2. H    3. F    4. B
5. I    6. G    7. C    8. D
9. A    10. J    11. K

## Exercise 9
1. H    2. G    3. L    4. A
5. J    6. K    7. I    8. F
9. D    10. M    11. E    12. B
13. C

14. trabecul/o (little beam) + -tomy (incision)
    **Def: incision of the little beam (orbital network of the eye)**
15. dacryocyst/o (lacrimal sac) + rhin/o (nose) + -stomy (new opening)
    **Def: new opening between the lacrimal sac and the nose**
16. vitr/o (vitreous humor) + -ectomy (removal)
    **Def: removal of vitreous humor**

## Exercise 10
1. C    2. E    3. B    4. A
5. D

## Exercise 11
1. cataracts
2. preoperatively (before the surgery)
3. destroyed by breaking into small pieces
4. posterior lens implant
5. topical anesthetic

## Exercise 12
1. myopia
2. laser in situ keratomileusis, photorefractive keratectomy
3. visual acuity
4. age-related macular degeneration
5. ophthalmology
6. intraocular pressure
7. visual field

## Exercise 13
1. E, I    2. B    3. C
4. A    5. H    6. F
7. G, J    8. D

9. pre- (before) + auricul/o (ear) + -ar (pertaining to)
    **Def: pertaining to before (in front of) the ear**

10. supra- (above) + tympan/o (eardrum) + -ic (pertaining to)
    **Def: pertaining to above the eardrum**
11. circum- (around) + aur/o (ear) + -al (pertaining to)
    **Def: pertaining to around the ear**

## Exercise 14
See Fig. 14-22.

## Exercise 15
1. A    2. H    3. K    4. G
5. F    6. I    7. B    8. D
9. C    10. E    11. J    12. L

13. ear (ot/o) pain (-algia)
    **Term: otalgia**
14. condition (-ia) small (micro-) ears (ot/o)
    **Term: microtia**
15. abnormal condition (-osis) of hardening (-sclerosis) ear (ot/o)
    **Term: otosclerosis**

## Exercise 16
1. acoustic neuroma
2. ceruminoma

## Exercise 17
1. no lymphadenopathy
2. no wheezing
3. tympanic membrane
4. oropharynx
5. otitis media

## Exercise 18
1. E    2. D    3. F    4. A
5. B    6. C

7. ot/o (ear) + -scopy (visual exam)
    **Def: visual exam of the ear**
8. tympan/o (eardrum) + -metry (process of measurement)
    **Def: process of measurement of the eardrum**
9. audi/o (hearing) + -metric (pertaining to measurement)
    **Def: pertaining to measurement of hearing**

## Exercise 19
1. E     2. B     3. C     4. A
5. D

## Exercise 20
1. C     2. D     3. A     4. B

## Exercise 21
1. E     2. C     3. A     4. D
5. B

## Chapter 14 Review

### Word Part Definitions
1. –plasty
2. extra-
3. –itis
4. exo-
5. –cusis
6. an-
7. presby-
8. –opsia
9. macro-
10. micro-
11. lacrim/o
12. kerat/o
13. cerumin/o
14. tympan/o or myring/o
15. dacryocyst/o
16. ot/o or auricul/o
17. opt/o
18. audi/o or acous/o
19. blephar/o or palpebr/o
20. labyrinth/o
21. myring/o or tympan/o
22. ophthalm/o or ocul/o
23. core/o
24. ocul/o or ophthalm/o
25. acous/o or audi/o
26. papill/o
27. palpebr/o or blephar/o
28. irid/o
29. auricul/o or ot/o
30. phac/o
31. salping/o
32. dacryoaden/o

### Wordshop
1. condition (-ia) small (micro-) ear (ot/o)
   **Term: microtia**
2. condition (-ia) no (a-) lens (phak/o)
   **Term: aphakia**
3. discharge (-rrhea) ear (ot/o)
   **Term: otorrhea**
4. old age (presby-) hearing (-cusis)
   **Term: presbycusis**
5. incision (-tomy) eardrum (tympan/o)
   **Term: tympanotomy**
6. abnormal (para-) hearing (-cusis)
   **Term: paracusis**
7. abnormal condition of hardening (-sclerosis) ear (ot/o)
   **Term: otosclerosis**
8. inflammation (-itis) inner ear (labyrinth/o)
   **Term: labyrinthitis**
9. vision condition (-opsia) no (a-) color (chromat/o)
   **Term: achromatopsia**
10. process of measurement (-metry) hearing (audi/o)
    **Term: audiometry**
11. inflammation (-itis) tear gland (dacryoaden/o)
    **Term: dacryoadenitis**
12. drooping (-ptosis) eyelid (blephar/o)
    **Term: blepharoptosis**
13. pertaining to (-al) nose (nas/o) tear (lacrim/o)
    **Term: nasolacrimal**
14. condition of aversion to (-phobia) light (phot/o)
    **Term: photophobia**
15. process of measurement (-metry) pressure (ton/o)
    **Term: tonometry**

### Term Sorting
**Anatomy and Physiology:** accommodation, cerumen, cochlea, fovea, labyrinth, lacrimation, pinna, refraction, sclera, stapes
**Pathology:** anacusis, chalazion, exophthalmia, nyctalopia, otalgia, otorrhea, otosclerosis, scotoma, strabismus, tinnitus
**Diagnostic Procedures:** Amsler grid, audiometer, diopters, gonioscopy, ophthalmoscopy, otoscopy, slit lamp, tonometry, tympanometry, VA
**Therapeutic Interventions:** coreoplasty, IOLs, iridotomy, miotics, otoplasty, phacoemulsification, scleral buckling, stapedectomy, tympanostomy, tympanotomy

### Translations
1. photophobia, epiphora
2. otoscope, otitis media
3. anisocoria, hyphema
4. achromatopsia, myopia
5. audiologist, presbycusis
6. glaucoma, tonometry
7. blepharoplasty, blepharoptosis
8. scleral buckling, retinal detachment
9. tinnitus, vertigo
10. dacryocystorhinostomy, lacrimal
11. Schirmer tear test, xerophthalmia
12. nyctalopia, retinitis pigmentosa
13. otoplasty, macrotia
14. anacusis, otosclerosis

### Medical Letter
1. Diplopia means double vision; cephalgia means headache
2. nearsightedness with malcurvature of the lens
3. Goldmann applanation tonometry
4. pertaining to around the border of the sclera and the cornea

## Chapter 15

### Exercise 1
1. hypophysis
2. hypothalamus
3. adenohypophysis
4. metabolism, calcium
5. kidneys
6. medulla, cortex
7. glucagon, insulin
8. ketones
9. mediastinum, immune
10. pineal, melatonin, sleep

11. Q     12. K     13. R     14. X
15. Y     16. V     17. D     18. W
19. T     20. A     21. U     22. M
23. I     24. G     25. P     26. O
27. J     28. F     29. N     30. B
31. E     32. S     33. C     34. L
35. H

36. peri- (surrounding) + thyroid/o (thyroid) + -al (pertaining to)
**Def: pertaining to surrounding the thyroid gland**

37. hypo- (deficient) + glyc/o (sugar) + -emic (pertaining to blood condition)
**Def: pertaining to deficient blood sugar condition**

38. retro- (behind) + pancreat/o (pancreas) + -ic (pertaining to)
**Def: pertaining to behind the pancreas**

39. inter- (between) + lob/o (lobe) + -ar (pertaining to)
**Def: pertaining to between lobes**

### Exercise 2
See Fig. 15-1.

### Exercise 3
1. D   2. E   3. J   4. F
5. H   6. G   7. A   8. C
9. B   10. I

11. hypo- (deficient) + glyc/o (sugar) + -emia (blood condition)
**Def: condition of deficient sugar in the blood**

12. par- (abnormal) + esthesi/o (feeling) + -ia (condition)
**Def: condition of abnormal feeling**

13. hyper- (excessive) + calc/o (calcium) + -emia (blood condition)
**Def: condition of excessive calcium in the blood**

14. hypo- (deficient) + natr/o (sodium) + -emia (blood condition)
**Term: hyponatremia**

15. hyper- (excessive) + kal/i (potassium) + -emia (blood condition)
**Term: hyperkalemia**

16. -uria (urine condition) + glucos/o (sugar)
**Term: glycosuria**

### Exercise 4
1. hormones
2. thyroid
3. cortex
4. pituitary
5. Hypoparathyroidism
6. cretinism, myxedema
7. SIADH
8. type 1 diabetes, type 2 diabetes
9. hyper- (excessive) + insulin (insulin/o) + -ism (condition)
**Def: condition of excessive insulin**
10. hypo- (deficient) + thyroid/o (thyroid gland) + -ism (condition)
**Def: condition of deficient thyroid gland (hormones)**
11. acr/o (extremities) + -megaly (enlargement)
**Def: enlargement of the extremities**

### Exercise 5
1. B   2. F   3. D   4. C
5. E   6. A

### Exercise 6
1. type 2
2. diabetic retinopathy
3. peripheral vascular disease, foot ulcer
4. normal (without fever)

### Exercise 7
1. sonography
2. magnetic resonance imaging
3. A1c
4. total calcium
5. urine glucose
6. glucometer

### Exercise 8
1. excision (-ectomy) pancreas (pancreat/o)
**Term: pancreatectomy**
2. excision (-ectomy) adrenal gland (adrenal/o)
**Term: adrenalectomy**
3. excision (-ectomy) pituitary gland (hypophys/o)
**Term: hypophysectomy**
4. excision (-ectomy) parathyroid gland (parathyroid/o)
**Term: parathyroidectomy**
5. excision (-ectomy) thyroid gland (thyroid/o)
**Term: thyroidectomy**

### Exercise 9
1. C   2. A   3. D   4. B

### Exercise 10
1. type 2
2. dehydration
3. Glucophage
4. IV fluids

### Exercise 11
1. E   2. C   3. F   4. B
5. A   6. D   7. G

## Chapter 15 Review

### Word Parts
1. -graphy
2. pan-
3. endo-
4. hyper- or poly-
5. supra-
6. hypo-
7. -emia
8. exo-
9. -crine
10. acro-
11. poly- or hyper-
12. –ectomy
13. kal/i
14. pituitar/o or hypophys/o
15. chrom/o
16. natr/o
17. glyc/o or gluc/o
18. gonad/o
19. parathyroid/o
20. trop/o
21. aden/o
22. thym/o
23. gluc/o or glyc/o
24. phe/o
25. crin/o
26. thyr/o
27. thalam/o
28. adren/o
29. calc/o
30. pancreat/o
31. cyt/o
32. hypophys/o or pituitar/o

## Wordshop

1. blood condition (-emia) of excessive (hyper-) sodium (natr/o)
   **Term: hypernatremia**
2. enlargement (-megaly) of the extremities (acro-)
   **Term: acromegaly**
3. urine condition (-uria) of sugar (glucos/o)
   **Term: glucosuria**
4. condition (-ia) of an eye (ophthalm/o) outward (ex-)
   **Term: exophthalmia**
5. instrument to measure (-meter) sugar (gluc/o)
   **Term: glucometer**
6. excessive (poly-) urinary condition (-uria)
   **Term: polyuria**
7. urinary condition (-uria) of ketones (keton/o)
   **Term: ketonuria**
8. abnormal condition (-osis) of acidity (acid/o) due to ketones (ket/o)
   **Term: ketoacidosis**
9. condition (-ia) of excessive (poly-) eating (phag/o)
   **Term: polyphagia**
10. abnormal (par-) sensation condition (-esthesia)
    **Term: paresthesia**
11. removal (-ectomy) of the parathyroid gland (parathryroid/o)
    **Term: parathyroidectomy**
12. excessive (poly-) condition of thirst (-dipsia)
    **Term: polydipsia**
13. study of (-logy) glands that secrete (crin/o) within (endo-)
    **Term: endocrinology**
14. blood condition (-emia) of excessive (hyper-) sugar (glyc/o)
    **Term: hyperglycemia**
15. blood condition (-emia) of deficient (hypo-) potassium (kal/i)
    **Term: hypokalemia**

## Term Sorting

**Anatomy and Physiology:** ACTH, cortex, endocrine, epinephrine, GH, glucagon, hypophysis, oxytocin, pancreas, vasopressin

**Pathology:** anorexia, diabetes insipidus, GHD, gigantism, goiter, hirsutism, hyperinsulinism, polydipsia, SIADH, thymoma

**Diagnostic Procedures:** A1c, FPG, glucometer, MRI, OGTT, RAIU, RIA, sonography, TFT, urinalysis

**Therapeutic Interventions:** adrenalectomy, antidiabetics pancreatoduodenectomy hypophysectomy, orchiectomy, pancreatectomy, parathyroidectomy, prednisone, thymectomy, thyroidectomy

## Translations

1. polydipsia, polyuria
2. exophthalmia, hyperthyroidism
3. hypocalcemia, tetany, hypoparathyroidism
4. cretinism, myxedema
5. hirsutism, hyperglycemia, hypokalemia
6. hyperinsulinism, hypoglycemia
7. islet cell carcinoma, pancreatoduodenectomy (Whipple procedure)
8. type 1 diabetes, glucometer
9. thyroidectomy, goiter
10. hyponatremia, SIADH
11. gestational diabetes, type 2 diabetes
12. FPG, prediabetes
13. acromegaly, adenohypophysis
14. anorexia, paresthesia

## Office Visit Summary

1. excessive urination
2. polydipsia
3. A. fasting plasma glucose
   B. oral glucose tolerance test
   C. urinalysis
4. insulin

## Chapter 16

### Exercise 1

| | | | |
|---|---|---|---|
| 1. F | 2. H | 3. J | 4. G |
| 5. B | 6. E | 7. A | 8. I |
| 9. D | 10. C | | |

11. malignant
12. carcinoma
13. sarcoma
14. myeloma
15. well
16. grading
17. staging
18. primary

### Exercise 2

1. packs
2. history
3. tumor markers
4. biopsy
5. breast

### Exercise 3

1. benign growth that may occur in the intestines: considered precancerous lesions
2. colon carcinoma
3. colonoscopy, upper GI endoscopy (esophagogastro-duodenoscopy)
4. instrument used to visually examine the colon
5. procedure to visually examine the colon and surgical removal of five polyps

### Exercise 4

1. brachytherapy
2. mapping
3. sentinel
4. en bloc resection
5. margins
6. immunotherapy
7. CAM
8. 3DCRT

### Exercise 5

1. protocol
2. kill
3. replication
4. antineoplastic hormones
5. alkylating agents
6. antimetabolites
7. mitotic inhibitors

### Exercise 6

1. Cancer has spread beyond breast tissue.
2. neck and liver

3. surgery and chemotherapy
4. decreased level of sodium in the blood
5. She probably will live only a few months.

## Exercise 7
1. biopsy
2. grade 4
3. cancer, fecal occult blood test
4. certified tumor registrar, tumor, nodes, metastases
5. single-photon emission computed tomography, metastases

## Chapter 16 Review

### Word Parts
1. neo-
2. –plasia
3. –oma
4. apo-
5. dys-
6. –genesis
7. ana-
8. –blast
9. –carcinoma
10. ecto-
11. –stasis
12. –sarcoma
13. meta-
14. –plasm
15. hyper-
16. –ptosis
17. mut/a
18. blast/o
19. sarc/o
20. onc/o
21. path/o
22. nod/o
23. derm/o
24. carcin/o

### Wordshop
1. tumor (-oma) of a nerve (neur/o)
   **Term: neuroma**
2. tumor (-oma) of a blood vessel (hemangi/o)
   **Term: hemangioma**
3. malignant tumor (-sarcoma) of bone (oste/o)
   **Term: osteosarcoma**
4. tumor (-oma) of a gland (aden/o)
   **Term: adenoma**
5. tumor (-oma) of embryonic (blast/o) retina [retinal cells] (retin/o)
   **Term: retinoblastoma**
6. treatment (-therapy) using short distance (brachy-)
   **Term: brachytherapy**
7. condition of formation (-plasia) apart (ana-)
   **Term: anaplasia**
8. falling (-ptosis) away (apo-)
   **Term: apoptosis**
9. process of (-tion) change (mut/a)
   **Term: mutation**
10. tumor (-oma) of the meninges (mening/o)
    **Term: meningioma**
11. star (astr/o) cell (cyt/o) tumor (-oma)
    **Term: astrocytoma**
12. kidney (nephr/o) tumor (-oma)
    **Term: nephroma**
13. dark (phe/o) color (chrom/o) cell (cyt/o) tumor (-oma)
    **Term: pheochromocytoma**

### Term Sorting
**Benign neoplasms:** acoustic neuroma, BPH, dermatofibroma, fibroids, leiomyoma, meningioma, neuroma, osteoma, pheochromocytoma, thymoma
**Malignant neoplasms:** adenocarcinoma, Ewing sarcoma, hemangiosarcoma, hypernephroma, Kaposi sarcoma, leukemia, myxosarcoma, retinoblastoma, seminoma, Wilms tumor
**Diagnostic Procedures:** AFP, biopsy, BTA, CA125, CT scan, hCG, mammogram, PET, PSA, SPECT
**Therapeutic Interventions:** 3DCRT, BMT, brachytherapy, chemotherapy, gamma knife, immunotherapy, IMRT, lumpectomy, mastectomy, radiotherapy

### Translations
1. seminoma, multiple myeloma, adenocarcinoma
2. grade I, well differentiated
3. metastasis
4. Pap smear, severe dysplasia
5. lumpectomy, radiotherapy (radiation, radiation therapy), chemotherapy
6. brachytherapy
7. leukemia, chemotherapy, BMT

### Discharge Summary
1. sigmoid colon cancer
2. colonoscopy
3. sigmoid colectomy, appendectomy
4. all nodes were negative for carcinoma

Page references followed by "f" refer to
figures, by "t" refer to tables, and by "b"
refer to boxes.